I0197757

I tell you truly...

"He who drinks from my mouth will become like me.
As for me, I will become what he is, and what is hidden will be revealed to him."

"Thou shalt love thy neighbor as thyself."

"Is it not written in your law, I said, Ye are gods?"

"The Kingdom of God is within of you."

"I and [my] Father are one."

"The Kingdom of the Father is spread upon the earth
and men do not see it!"

"He who has ears to hear, let him hear!"

—Jesus

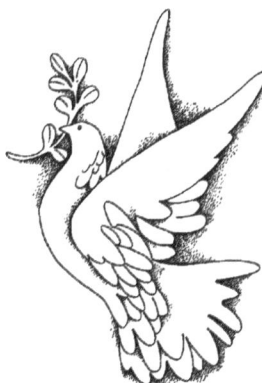

On the front cover: *The Glory of Divine Grace*

The cover design was produced from a painting by the author, Dr. Muata Ashby. It is composed of Jesus sitting in a cross-legged position within a fish Mandorla. Over his head is the golden sun, shining its rays within the fish. Gold is the color of God, the Supreme Being. Below Jesus is a crescent moon. On his chest is an Ankh cross, and outside the fish there is a dove with a sun disk over its head. The painting of Jesus is based on the descriptions of him from *Revelation 1* and *Ezekiel 8* in the Bible, and the writings of one Jewish Historian, *Josephus*. The sun over his head is the forerunner of the halo and a symbol of the dynamic power of the Spirit as it engenders life in all creation which is symbolized by the Mandorla-fish. The Mandorla or vertical oval, ◊, is related to the Madonna, Mary, the mother of Jesus. It is at once a symbol of her divinity as well as her feminine gender. The upright oval symbol is also known as the "almond." It has been regarded as a symbol of the goddess all over the world, and it has become one of the icons of Mary. It is also known as the *Vesica Piscis* or "Vessel of the Fish." The fish, ◁▷, is an ancient symbol of life. It is related to Christ. It relates to transcendence of the world as well as to material and spiritual abundance. The melding of the Mandorla with the fish in this painting denotes the Christ (fish) essence coming forth from the womb of creation (Mandorla-Mary) which has been begotten by the Holy Spirit (Dove). The color red symbolizes the blood of Mary at the birth of Jesus as well as the blood of Christ which was shed to atone for the sins of humanity. The deep blue-purple in which the picture is immersed is the formless ocean prior to creation, before the spirit of God stirred up the waters and caused them to take form as creation, the physical universe. Blue is the color which symbolizes Mary. The moon symbolizes the mind of God, on which the light of the Spirit (sun) shines and reflects. This is an allusion to the mystical teaching that the light of the Cosmic Mind of God reflects as the mind of all human beings and brings life and enlightenment to the their hearts through the teachings. The Ankh symbolizes the life giving essence of Christ, who unifies the opposites of Creation into one divinity. Its use in early Christianity affirms the Ancient Egyptian roots of Christianity. The dove symbolizes the Supreme Spirit, God, whose omnipresence enables Creation, Christ, the sun, the moon, human beings, etc., to exist by Divine Grace. Hence, the title of the painting, *The Glory of Divine Grace*.

On the back cover: At top two Ancient Egyptian-Christian Ankh crosses. At the bottom the Christian relief uses the Ancient Ankh.

Prints of the original painting used for the front cover are available from C. M. Books 8" X 10" $9.95, 11" X 17" $19.95

Cruzian Mystic Books
P.O.Box 570459
Miami, Florida, 33257
(305) 378-6253 Fax: (305) 378-6253

The author is available for group lectures and individual counseling. For further information contact the publisher.

Publisher's Cataloging-in-Publication
(Provided by Quality Books, Inc.)

Ashby, Muata.
Christian Yoga: the mystical journey from Jesus to Christ. Book I, Initiation into the history and philosophy of mystical Christianity / Muata Ahbaya Ashby. -- 1 st ed.
  p. cm.
  Includes bibliographical references and index.

  ISBN: 1-884564-05-4

    1. Christianity and yoga. 2. Christianity--Origin.
  3. Mysticism--Christianity. 4. Yoga. 1. Title. II.
  Title: Initiation into the history and philosophy of mystical Christianity

  BR128.Y63A74 1998   248.2'2
                             QBI98-950

OTHER BOOKS BY MUATA ASHBY

EGYPTIAN YOGA VOLUME I: THE PHILOSOPHY OF ENLIGHTENMENT

EGYPTIAN YOGA VOLUME II: THE SUPREME WISDOM OF ENLIGHTENMENT

INITIATION INTO EGYPTIAN YOGA

BLOOMING LOTUS OF DIVINE LOVE

MYSTICISM OF USHET REKHAT

EGYPTIAN PROVERBS

THEF NETERU: THE MOVEMENT OF THE GODS AND GODDESSES

THE CYCLES OF TIME

THE HIDDEN PROPERTIES OF MATTER

THE WISDOM OF ISIS: GOD IN THE UNIVERSE

THE MYSTICAL TEACHINGS OF
THE AUSARIAN RESURRECTION

THE WISDOM OF MAATI

THE SERPENT POWER

EGYPTIAN TANTRA YOGA

MEDITATION: THE ANCIENT EGYPTIAN PATH TO ENLIGHTENMENT

(For additional titles by Dr. Ashby see the back section of this book
and send for the free catalog.)

TABLE OF CONTENTS

Dedication...9

Foreword 10

The biblical authority for this work..15

  What is the Biblical Authority for this Book?   15
    Christian Yoga Volume II: 16

Introduction to The bible, the Christian Gospels from Ancient Egypt and The key terms for understanding spiritual philosophy 18

    How this Book Was Created...18
    Who Am I? 18
  What is the Bible?   19
    The Bible and its Translations 20
    ENGLISH TRANSLATIONS...22
    The Construction of the Bible Gospels...22
    A History of Modern Jewish Zionism 25
    The Nag Hammadi Library and its Relation to The Bible...27
    Yoga Philosophy and the World Religious Philosophies Defined.....................................35
      Hinduism and Mahayana Buddhism 36
    Selected Spiritual Philosophies Compared 37
  Religious Philosophies   37
  Religious Categories   38
      Theism 38
      Atheism...38
      Ethicism..38
      Ritualism...38
      Monism 38

Chapter I The Origins of creation, humanity, Religion and yoga philosophy 39

  The Origins of Humankind   39
  The Ancient Creation Myths   40
    The Forms of Creation...41
  the Common Ancestry of Humanity According to the Bible and the myth of race and racism   42
    Conclusion: One World, One Humanity, One Destiny...44
      DNA and The Spirit..45
  the Origins of Philosophy   46
    Ancient Mystical Philosophy..47
    The Purpose of Religion: Religion as a Yoga Philosophy 49

Chapter II The ancient Egyptian origins of Judaism 51

  Ancient Origins: Who Were the Ancient Egyptians?   51
    The History of Manetho..53
    The Company of Gods and Goddesses of Anu 54
    More on The Dynastic Period of Ancient Egypt...54
    The Ancient Egyptian Creation Myths and Their Relationship to Christianity and Gnosticism 55
    The Ausarian Resurrection, Its Historical and Mystical Implications 58
    The Christian Eucharist and the Eucharist of the Ancient Egyptian Mysteries 60
    Theban Theology and The Triad of Creation 62

Judaism and Ancient Egyptian Religion   65
   Ancient Egypt and the Exodus...70
   Ancient Egypt, Sumeria and Judaism 72
      ANCIENT EGYPTIAN RELIGION 73
Judaism in Ethiopia   75
   Rastafarianism and the Judeo-Christian Religion...................................76

Chapter iii: the ancient Egyptian origins of christianity 78

The Ancient Egyptian Origins of Christianity   78
The Ancient African Ancestry of Jesus   81
   The Descriptions of Jesus...87
   The Personality of Jesus and the Mystical Christ   88
   The Apostles Creed: 90
Christianity and the Ancient Egyptian Religion   94
The Evolution of the Cross   97
   The Christian Crosses and the Mystical Ankh Cross.............................100

Chapter iiii: how other spiritual traditions influenced christianity 103

Other Saviors of the Ancient World   103
The Ancient Egyptian and Indian Background of Christianity   103
   The Birth Stories of Heru, Jesus, Krishna, and Buddha 104
The Philosophy of Buddha (C. 600 B.C.E.)   107
   Jesus and Buddha...110

Chapter v: The origins and hidden meaning of the bible............................115

The Compilation of the Canonical Gospels   115
The Hints of a Secret Teaching in the Traditional Bible   116
The Ten Commandments and The Precepts of Maat   118
The Significance of The Precepts of Maat   121
    Maat Principles of Ethical Conduct 123
The Effect of Zoroastrianism on Western Religions   124
Islam and Christianity   127
   Islam in America: Malcolm X and The Nation of Islam 130
   The Origins of Esoteric (Mystical) Islam: Sufism (c. 700 A.C.E)............131
What is the Philosophy of Gnosticism?   132
Gnostic Christianity and Chinese Taoism   134

Chapter vi: The development of the Christian church................................137

Problems in the early Christian church   137
The Coptic Church   138
The impact of ancient Greek Philosophy on Christian philosophy   139
   Neo-Platonism 141
   Hellenism..141
   Alexander The Great...141
Druidism, Celtic Christianity and The Arthurian Legends   143
   Celtic Christianity..144
   The Arthurian Legends...144
   The Fall of Rome and the Breakup of the Church 146
   Protestantism - Martin Luther (c. 1517 A.C.E.) 147
    The Church of England, The King James Bible and the Struggle for Power between the Protestants and The
    Pope in Rome...148
   Racism in the Christian Church and The Heroism of the Quaker Movement 150
   The Methodist and African Methodist Episcopal Churches 153
   The Revival Movement 153

Modern Developments in the Christian Churches 155
Fundamentalism and the Second Birth 155
Born Again in the Bible and in the Christian Church 156
The Difficult Nature of True Christian Living...156
Overview of Christianity in Africa and The Missionary Movements.............................161
CONCLUSION..163
A History Of Modern Christian and Non-Christian Mysticism   163
New Age Spirituality   166

Chapter VII: Initiation into Christianity Yoga **167**
Christianity as a Spiritual Discipline 167
For Spiritual Transformation 167
A deeper look at yoga philosophy   167
Introduction 167
Vedanta and Yoga In India   167
Basic Yoga Philosophy   168
Yoga Stage 1: Listening to the Wisdom Teachings 168
Yoga Stage 2: Reflecting on the Teachings and Practicing them in Everyday Life 169
Yoga-Vedanta Philosophy Continued: Human Desire as the Cause of Pain and Suffering 170
Yoga Stage 3: Meditation on the Teachings 172
Introduction to Yoga In Christianity   172
The General Plan of Christian Yoga   174
The Initiatic Way of Education   174
The Aspirant   175
The Qualities of a Spiritual Aspirant 175
The Teacher   177

Chapter viii: The Female Aspect of Christianity **182**
God as Mother   182
Jesus and Mary Magdalene...183
Mary, the Mother of Jesus, and Aset, the Mother of Heru and the Black Madonna..............185
ASET (Isis): The Egyptian Goddess - Prototype of Mother Mary 188
The Black Madonna...189
The Female Savior of Humankind...191
Mary Magdalene, the Female Sage and Apostle of Christianity and Partner of Jesus.......191

Chapter ix: Christian yoga wisdom **195**
What is Knowledge?   195
What is the Mind from The Gnostic Philosophical Point Of View?   196
Who is God? The Ancient Egyptian Origins of Monotheism and The Concepts of God in The World Religions
and The Christian Gospels   198
Akhenaton, Moses and the Concept of One God in Ancient Egyptian Mythology 198
Hymns to Aten 201
The concepts of god in world religions and mystical philosophies   202
The Concept of God in Vedanta and Yoga Philosophies from India.................................202
The Concept of God in Confucianism 202
The Concept of God in Buddhism 202
The Concept of God in Shintoism 202
The Concept of God in Taoism..202
The Concept of God in Hinduism...202
The Concept of God in Sikhism 202
The Concept of God in Islam...202
The Concept of God and Creation According to the New Testament and the Gnostic Gospels.........202
The Concept of God and Creation According to Ancient Egyptian Religion and Mystical Philosophy 202

Male   Female 203
God as The All and The Absolute   205

Chapter x: The deeper meaning of symbols, rituals of Christianity **207**

The Power of Symbolism   207
Paganism and Idolatry in the Christian Church 208
The Origins of Angels 215
The Symbol of the Eyes and Trinity of God 215
Secret Codes in the Bible? 217
The Message of Rituals   217
Yoga, Christianity, Reincarnation and transpersonal psychology   219
The purpose of Mental Concepts in spiritual study   220
The Idea of Christhood   221
Self-knowledge and The Baptism of Truth   223
What is Consciousness?   228
Body Consciousness   230
Where can True Happiness be Found?   232

Chapter Xi: The pearls of mystical Christian wisdom **234**

The Wisdom of the Sermon on the Mount and the Ten Commandments 234
The Sermon on the Mount and Its Virtuous Qualities 235
The Ten Commandments and Their Origins in Ancient Egyptian Wisdom 236
The Ten Commandments and the Teachings of Maat: 236
The Teachings of the Bible and The Teachings of Sage Amenemope 237
The Teachings of the Bible and The Teachings of Sage Ptahotep 238
The Teachings of the Bible 238
The Teachings of Ptahotep 238
The Commandments of Jesus 239
Teachings of Ancient Egypt 239
Jesus on prayer 239
Teachings of Sage Ani on prayer 239
The Transitory and Illusory Nature of the World   240
Attachment: The source of Human Pain and Suffering   242
The Illusoriness of Family and Relationships   243
Health of the Mind and Body: Vegetarianism and Christianity, the diet of Christian initiates   247
Sin, Evil, the Devil   249
What is The Ego and Egoism?   251
The Greatest Secret: God is the Mystery, the Light Within   252
Purification by the Fire of Wisdom   256

Chapter XII: Introduction to Christian yoga meditation **259**

The next step in the journey from Jesus to Christ   259
How to Begin the Journey from Jesus to Christ   259
Materials needed for Christian Yoga Meditation 260
Time-line of Major World Religions and Mystical Philosophies and selected world events   263

Index **264**

Bibliography **279**

Copyrights **280**

Other Books From C M Books 281

Music Based on the Prt M Hru and other Kemetic Texts 288

DEDICATION

To the Christ in all,

☥

Which is the underlying reality behind the whole universe and the innermost reality of every individual.

Also,
To Swami Jyotirmayananda,
Who is the supreme exponent of Universal Religion, Yoga, and Vedanta Philosophy and illuminer of the highest philosophy in every mystical tradition.

Om Namo Bhagavate Jyotirmayananda ya!

To my spiritual partner and Managing Editor,
Karen Vijaya Clarke-Ashby,
whose editorial management,
devotion to and knowledge of the teachings of Yoga
and mystical spirituality made this work possible.

To
Carmen Ashby, my first teacher in this birth, who gave me the feeling of religious practice and the tenderness which only a mother can give. To my father, Reginald T. Ashby, my father, a man of caring, and a source of love for his children and associates, who, though not a church going person, taught me the meaning of love in the way that only a true father can teach.

To Archana (Ellen Fiur) for her editorial assistance, Hamsa Yogi (Lou Lochard) and Asar Oronde Reid for their artwork and others who have contributed to the production of this work.

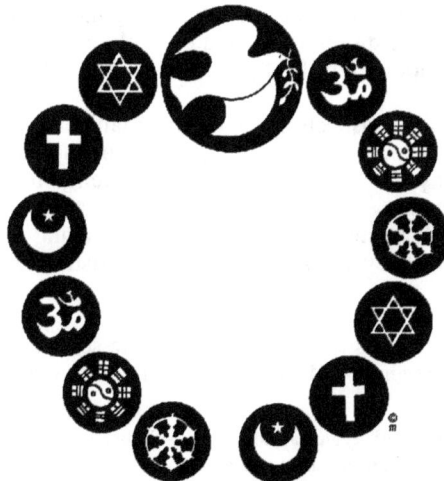

FOREWORD

Jesus practiced Yoga!

This was my realization after so many years away from the church. After seeking spiritual upliftment in books on ancient philosophies, mystical religions from Africa, "the South" and Eastern wisdom, I realized that when the New Testament is read from the perspective of Yoga Philosophy, it becomes clear that Jesus practiced the yoga disciplines which have been espoused since the beginning of civilization in Ancient Egypt and India. But how is this possible? This was one of the questions that gave impetus to my desire for the exploration of early Christianity and Ancient Egyptian religion. *Christian Yoga: The Mystical Journey From Jesus To Christ* is the fruit of that exploration.

Why the title *"Christian Yoga?"* For the last 1700 years Christianity has been thought of as a religion or system of worshiping a God through the teachings of a personality known as Jesus Christ. However, if we look deeper into the history and philosophy of Christianity, a new picture emerges. It is possible to discover that Christianity contains heretofore unknown secrets of spiritual life which can promote the spiritual evolution of all human beings. But what are these teachings embedded in the very heart of the Christian doctrines? The term *Yoga* is most often associated with India and Eastern forms of meditation and exercise postures. However, these disciplines are only a small part of Yoga. Yoga is a vast discipline and philosophy of spiritual life including mental and physical practices which promote spiritual evolution. These include exercise, meditation, ethical behavior, metaphysics, harnessing the subtle energy of the body, sublimation of desires and a host of other teachings which lead to spiritual transformation. Yoga is not a religion. It is the universal science of spiritual living which can be used by all religions to enhance their religious practices. In Christianity, these very same Yoga teachings were and are at the very heart of its early philosophy. In this volume we will trace origins of the practice of Yoga in Ancient Egypt and India, and then in Christianity, revealing that Christianity incorporates most of the Yogic disciplines which have been espoused by all of the worlds great Saints and Sages, including Jesus Christ, from time immemorial.

The study of the deeper implications of Christianity has been an undertaking which I have pondered for many years. Having grown up as a devout Catholic within the Roman Catholic religion and having attended Catholic schools in my youth, I share a common tradition and history along with millions of other baby-boomers who experienced the social, political and religious struggles of the sixties as well as the unprecedented opening up of society since that time. With the advent of worldwide communications and global economies, the world communities have become more aware of themselves in relation to cultural differences as well as similarities. At no time in the past has it been so easy to access information from differing cultures[1] and study it in context with the increasingly accurate picture of the historical past of humanity.

Yet, even with the major technological advances which we have had in recent years, today societies are still plagued by crime, racism, sexism, religious intolerance, economic inequality and disease. These conditions have only served to further intensify the debate on the question of the validity of religion and philosophy, and their explanation of the current state of society. Even with the burgeoning nature of modern society, many of those who grew up in the Catholic faith have become disappointed and even bitter about what they perceive as a dissatisfying and even contradictory doctrine which does not fulfill their needs as they move through life.

While many will agree that the ritualistic aspects of the Catholic faith are or were very endearing and emotionally comforting, especially in their youth, many feel that the teachings of the church are not in touch with their life. Many who have had occasion to study the history of the Catholic religion from a scholarly perspective become aghast at the discovery of the atrocities, crimes, death and destruction which has occurred in the name of Christianity or under the direction of Christian authorities. Others, having studied various philosophies from an impersonal and atheistic perspective, have even turned away from Christianity in favor of other religions or none at all.

As a youth, being taught by Catholic nuns and priests in Catholic school, I learned that God was someone who existed in fact, sitting on a throne somewhere in heaven, with definite features and cultural characteristics. From a

---

[1] Over the years, historians have recognized Western or occidental culture and philosophy, implying European history, and Eastern culture and philosophy, implying India, China, etc., and Mesopotamian culture and philosophy, implying the Middle East. This book will use the term "the South" to refer to African culture and philosophy (in particular Ancient Egypt) in the same manner as European culture is referred to as "the West" and Indian and Chinese cultures are referred to as "the East."

distance he watches us and hates when we commits sins and loves it when we are good. Jesus, his son, was sitting at the right hand side of God's throne from where he judged the good or bad deeds of human beings. I was taught that all those who are "good" get to go and live with Jesus and God forever, but others who are "sinful" go either to hell for eternity or to purgatory for an extended period of time. I was taught that at the end of time, Jesus would return and that all people would be resurrected bodily from their graves. Those who were "righteous" would go to heaven or "purgatory" while the "sinners" would go to hell forever. At Easter time, the many passion plays of Jesus' death scenes which were re-enacted evoked strong feelings in all those who witnessed them. I remember feeling shocked at the brutality and wanton violence of the scenes by the actors who played the roles of Roman soldiers and consequently, I carried an indelible impression in my mind of sorrow for this person, Jesus, who had somehow "died for me" so many years ago. Strange feelings emerged through those experiences, perhaps a combination of pity, sorrow, fear and confusion, along with an eerie sense of devotion to this person (Jesus) who had cared for me and all humanity enough to give up his life to "pay for my sins." I felt an almost reciprocal feeling, "you died for me, therefore the least I can do is follow you."

As I grew up, I became disillusioned by what I felt were contradictions between what was said and what was done by priests and parishioners. The actual accounts of the history of religion, such as they are, also conflicted with the message of the church. Although church ideas were sublime, the actions of church goers, employees and clergy contradicted the messages given by the church. In historical terms, the countless atrocities, murders and other injustices such as the Atlantic Slave Trade and the plundering of Africa and the Americas, which the church had condoned, further eroded my faith in the church. I developed a feeling of mistrust toward all religions and a confused notion about what religion was supposed to be. However, I never did lose faith in the existence of an all-encompassing "Supreme Being" or "Creator."

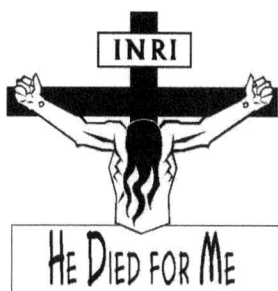

I had no basis of truth to engender discrimination at that young age. The excessive freedom allowed to young people in modern times and the tendency towards externalizing ourselves into television, movies, games, etc., provided a substitute or distraction, as it were, for what I needed: positive role models, introspection and inner growth. My search led me to meet others like myself in an effort to find the answers to some fundamental questions. This was the beginning of my journey into Christian mystical philosophy, Ancient Egyptian Mystical Philosophy and Indian Mystical Philosophy.

The questions, *Why do I exist? What is existence?*, and *Who am I?*, are a most important part of every human being's self-development. As such, the search for an explanation of the meaning of human existence took the form of disciplined modes of inquiry and thinking which were later called "religion" or "philosophy." The search for one's "reason" to exist and the "meaning of life" are central issues which relate to one's feeling of fulfillment in life. Philosophy, therefore, is an integral part of everyone's existence, whether they adhere to a particular philosophical or religious idea or not.

Through my own journey of self-discovery, I have realized the value of study, reflection and meditation on oneself. Reflection and meditation are arts seldom discussed in the general course of our Western educational system and thus, they are often misunderstood or altogether neglected. Learning how to think about things and then to transcend the thinking mind through meditation are arts in which ancient mystical philosophy and religion, in their original essence, specialized. Early Christianity, being founded on mystical philosophy, was no exception to this. In modern civilization, meditation is thought to be the practice of active pondering of a question or problem. In mystical traditions, meditation is a highly developed discipline for discovering the depths of the psyche which lie beyond the conscious level of the mind. When these practices are explored in depth and applied to one's life, it is possible to make philosophy an integral part of every activity, not just reserving it for some specific time, place or activity.

Through my studies of early Christianity, Ancient Egyptian religion, modern day world religions, mystery religions, Yoga philosophy and modern science, I was able to rediscover the feelings which were unique to my early experiences in the Catholic Church and have also been able to relate them to the highest mystical philosophies of other cultures. It is my hope that others such as myself as well as others in different religious traditions may discover the reasons for their own disappointments with religious doctrines and dogmas, and in this way, move beyond them. In order for the modern church to hold its members, it must be able to carry them beyond that which is simply ritualistic and compulsory. While many of the changes made by the Vatican Councils may seem to be enlightening, non-dogmatic and progressive, the present stance of the church with respect to fundamental issues of religious understanding differs greatly with the original teachings of the church prior to the emergence of orthodox Catholicism as the dominant form of Christianity. This is why the modern Christian Churches are suffering from so many people leaving in search of new religions.

Modern church ideas such as the reduced emphasis on private confession between the confessor and the priest in favor of individuals making their peace with God "directly" were seen as heretical not very long ago. Ironically, the ideas of self-absolution, self-baptism and self-salvation existed long before the advent of Christianity and was indeed a part of early Christianity. However, at various points in history, Christianity became a tool to control and assume power over others rather than a discipline for spiritual enlightenment. With very few exceptions, this calamity has occurred in almost all other major religious systems as well. Therefore, it is, as it always has been, the task of the individual to discover the hidden jewels which are latent in all traditions and to apply them to his/her life for the purpose of enlightening himself or herself and humanity. When we discover the true essence of spirituality within ourselves, we discover the means to overcome pain and sorrow as well. In this discovery, the passion of our own Christ within transcends both pleasure and pain and we achieve the promise of eternal peace, the Kingdom of Heaven.

In relating to Christianity as a mythology with psychological and mystical implications, I will draw heavily on several non-western spiritual texts because these explicitly express the deeper implications of the mythology inherent in religious and mystical thought. Among these are: *The Bhagavad Gita, The Dhamapada, The Pyramid Texts, The Egyptian Book of Coming Forth By Day and By Night, Thrice Greatest Hermes* and *The Yoga Vasistha*. *The Bhagavad Gita* or "The Song of the Lord," is the Hindu "Bible." It relates the story of Krishna and Arjuna. Krishna, as the incarnated Divine Self (God), instructs his student, Arjuna, as to the mysteries of creation and how to grow spiritually. *The Dhamapada* is the compilation of teachings of Buddha. *The Pyramid Texts, The Book of Coming Forth By Day and Night* and *Thrice Greatest Hermes* represent the religious teachings of Ancient Egypt in their earliest, intermediate, and later forms, respectively.

Unlike the others, *The Yoga Vasistha* is not very well known outside of India. *The Yoga Vasistha* is a work of nearly 30,000 stanzas, containing the essence of all the Indian scriptures. It is also known as *The Maha Ramayana* or simply as *The Vasistha*. It contains the teachings which were given to Lord Rama, an incarnation of God, by his Guru (spiritual preceptor) Sage Vasistha, which led him to remember his divine nature and attain Enlightenment. *The Vasistha* has been revered in the circles of Yoga Philosophy as *the high Vedanta* or the most advanced mystical philosophy because it holds the purest form of the Vedantic teachings which lead to spiritual Enlightenment. It is revered as the culmination of all teachings on the paths to Enlightenment. *The Vasistha* is a blessing to all who have had an opportunity to read and understand it, even more so for those who can study its teachings as they are translated by a living master. I have had the privilege to experience this blessing, thanks to my spiritual preceptor Swami Jyotirmayananda, a world renowned teacher of Indian Yoga philosophy.

Each of these texts, especially the Ancient Egyptian texts, exerted an influence on early Christian thought, and therefore, offer insight into the teachings of Christianity. In this work I will attempt to give an introductory view of Gnosticism, Yoga philosophy and Ancient Egyptian and Indian mysticism mythology, and mystical philosophy. The goal will be to study these traditions comparatively in order to gain insight into the meanings of the Christian texts, and also to explore the Ancient Egyptian and Indian origins of the philosophies espoused in the texts of early Christianity.

The purpose of this volume is not to prove or disprove the origins of Christian mythology, but to show the similarities to other mythologies, to determine the tenets of early Christianity and to trace those teachings into modern times. The goal will be to gain insight into the *"psycho-mythology"* or psychological implications of Christian mythology for the psycho-spiritual transformation of the individual, leading to the attainment of spiritual Enlightenment or Christhood. The attainment of Christhood is the goal of Christianity. The state of Christhood is known as the Kingdom of Heaven in Christianity. In other spiritual philosophies, it is known by other names such as Cosmic Consciousness, Nirvana, Enlightenment, Liberation, Self-Realization, Resurrection, etc.

Here, the term *psycho* must be understood as far more than simply that which refers to the mind. I will be using *psycho* to mean everything that constitutes human consciousness in all of its stages and states. *Mythology* refers to the codes, messages, ideas, directives, beliefs, etc., that affect the psyche through the conscious, subconscious and unconscious mind of an individual, specifically those effects which result in transpersonal or transcendental changes in the personality of the individual or those which constitute anti-transcendental movements.

This journey into mystical Christianity is in reality a *Transpersonal* view of Christian philosophy and mythology. What is presently considered to be a new field of psychological thought (Transpersonal Psychology) has appeared throughout recorded history in the writings of Ancient Egypt, the early Greek philosophers and other ancient mystery religions. Nowhere, however, has it received more extensive literary exposition than in the religious and philosophical schools of the East. The spiritual practice of India in particular, having enjoyed an unbroken tradition for over 2,500 years, is yet an undiscovered treasure of psychological understanding and experience. Carl Jung, the eminent western psychiatrist, remarked that the West is far behind the East in the understanding of the psyche. The advent of the "New Age" movement in modern society, coupled with the availability of foreign ideas due to modern technology and mass communications, has allowed a renaissance, as it were, to occur in Western thinking about human psychology and the understanding of consciousness itself. While ordinary psychology and psychiatry seek to help a person to discover and integrate the aspects of their human personality, transpersonal psychology seeks to assist a person in integrating the transcendental aspects of the personality as well. This includes the spirit, as well as the mind and body, and it also takes into account the problems of human life as well. Our journey will reveal the vast transpersonal wisdom of Christianity. Modern western science is confirming many ancient mystical ideas, thereby expanding the understanding about the universe outside of us as well as within.

In its complete form religion is composed of three aspects, mythology, ritual and mysticism. While many religions contain rituals, traditions, metaphors and myths, there are few professionals (scholars, clergy) trained in the understanding of their deeper aspects and their mystical and psychological implications. Thus, there is disappointment, frustration and disillusionment among many followers as well as leaders within many religions, particularly in the Western Hemisphere, because it is difficult to evolve spiritually without proper spiritual understanding. Proper spiritual understanding requires adept preceptorship or spiritual guidance. Many Christians, feeling out of touch with the church, have left it feeling guilt and a deep sense of loss. Through self-search and research, it is possible to discover mythological vistas within early Christianity which can rekindle the true spirit of Christianity in the human heart. The exoteric (outer, ritualistic) practices of Christianity with which we are mostly familiar is only the tip of an iceberg, so to speak; it is only a beginning movement towards a deeper discovery of the transcendental truths of existence. After journeying through this work, the reader will be able to understand Christianity as the great Sufi mystic *Mansur al-Hallaj* understood Islam. Prior to his crucifixion (like Jesus) he was reported to have said:

"The function of the orthodox community is to give the mystic his desire."

Perhaps the most important theme of this work is the exploration of *The Philosophy of Oneness*. Though it will be developed in more detail in Volume II of this project, it is appropriate to give a working definition of *The Philosophy of Oneness* as it applies to this study here. There are universal themes which are reflected in various societies and philosophies throughout the history of humankind. The strongest theme in all periods of history is *The Philosophy of Oneness*, specifically, that all things are one. In *The Philosophy of Oneness*, humanity, nature, and God are not understood as separate entities, but are regarded as being part of the singular essence of existence. If all things are one then the question arises, why does there appear to be such vast differentiation in nature and among human beings? These themes have been explored at various times and attempts have been made to explain them. The problem has been that the search for an explanation of these themes has led those who have tried to convey their impressions (Sages, Saints, visionaries, etc.) to an area not easily conveyed in language and not easily understood intellectually. From their efforts, various religions and philosophies have emerged, but the essence of the teaching has often diffused into the clouds of ritual and dogma as the founders of those religions and philosophies passed on. Thus, the following quotations are found in *The Gospel of Thomas*, a Gnostic Christian text, and three of the world's major religious philosophies. They refer to a transcendental essence which goes beyond the phenomenal world of human existence, which some people refer to as God, Goddess, Pure Consciousness, Higher Self, Jehovah, Allah, Pa Neter, Great Spirit, Brahman, Supreme Being, etc.

First from *The Gospel of Thomas*:

> Jesus said: "I shall give you what no eye has seen and what no ear has heard and what no hand has touched and what has never occurred to the human mind."

From the Ancient Egyptian Wisdom Texts:

> "We use Metu Neter symbols (hieroglyphs) to convey the essence of the meaning; thoughts and words get in the way of knowledge. This is why the Metu Neter (Divine Speech) conveys the image, picture of what is meant. The image may be separated from the words but not from essence. Only essence is the reality; words are a sign of degeneration. Concentrate on these with body and mind still. The Supreme Being creates all through the Word (speech) so our use of the speech must be as the divine form not human, Neter Metu (speech is divine)."[16]

From the *Kena Upanishad* we have the statement:

> "He truly knows Brahman (God, Absolute reality) who knows him as beyond knowledge; he who thinks that he knows, knows not. The ignorant think that Brahman is known, but the wise know him to be beyond knowledge."[47]

And from the Chinese *Tao Te Ching* we have:

"The Tao that can be told is not the eternal Tao.
The name that can be named is not the eternal name.
The nameless is the beginning of heaven and earth."[69]

In the words of Heinrich Zimmer, an eminent mythologist and student of psychology: *The best things can't be said and the second best are misunderstood.* The *"best things"* being referred to here are the things which are beyond thought, the transcendental realities. The *"second best"* are the objects of time and space reality which are considered as manifestations of the first. The problem comes in because we are using the second best to interpret the best and this leads us back to knowledge in the realm of time and space thinking, to the relative instead of the absolute. Further, verbal communication is less efficient than symbolic communication since it is also based on the description of objects in time and space.

Thus, the visionary authors of the world's spiritual texts sought to convey their ideas and impressions about a reality (God, Buddha, Brahman, Tao, etc.), which lies beyond ordinary human comprehension, through the use of symbolic imagery and mythology. Communication through symbol and myth has the ability to convey information at the subconscious level. Studies have shown that symbolic forms of communication may reach areas of the subconscious mind without the subject even being aware of it.[70] Therefore, as we begin our journey into *Christian Yoga: The Mystical Journey From Jesus To Christ*, we must keep in mind that there is a higher essence underlying everything in creation, to which we must to direct our attention. However, the writings can only point us in the correct direction. They are not in themselves the truth.

It is further stipulated that mental understanding is in reality a sophisticated system of symbolism. The modes of understanding symbolism and mythology may be classified into two categories, those that allude to concrete realities and those that point to a reality which is not readily grasped by the intellect. For example, a concrete symbol might be a no smoking sign with a picture of a cigarette enclosed by a circle and a back-slash (\ ) over it. Cigarettes are objects which can be touched. The circle singles them out and the \ signifies the message *"please do not light up here."* The symbols convey the message faster than if you had to read the words. However, the meaning must be first understood and then the symbols act to carry the message instantaneously. Similarly, a symbol such as a picture of a human figure dancing while holding a drum in one hand and a torch in the other can lead one to reflect on deeper realities which sustain our consciousness if the symbol is understood to be tied to teachings which are related to those deeper realities. In the same manner, religious symbols and myths affect the zone of the psyche which is beyond conscious thought but which may yet be partially understood with the use of conscious thought. This is the realm of experience that can be known and intuitionally experienced, but not thought about, because it is not possible to encapsulate it with thoughts. This is the realm of experience that we will explore in this journey through the evolution of mystical Christian thought and practice.

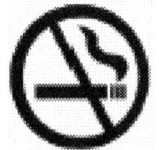

—Muata Abhaya Ashby 1995

THE BIBLICAL AUTHORITY FOR THIS WORK

WHAT IS THE BIBLICAL AUTHORITY FOR THIS BOOK?

The authority for the creation of this book comes from the Bible itself, and the Christian tradition. The Bible tradition is clear on the legitimacy and even the necessity of speaking about spiritual matters. This tradition is most prominently visible in the Biblical writings of the Apostle Paul, whose letters form the backbone of the New Testament. The only requirements are that the speaker should not have egoistic designs for personal gain or aggrandizement, and that he or she should not speak out of ignorance. Rather, they should have a sincere desire to impart the knowledge which will lead to peace, harmony and enlightenment. The ego in a human being is the source of all of their pain and sorrow. It is also the ego, in the form of pride, desire for wealth and pleasure, etc, that prevents a person from finding spirituality in their lives. Humility is the key ingredient in spirituality. Humility will allow a person's ego to become subservient to the Higher Self, the Holy Spirit. Only when a person is successful in putting down their ego is it then possible for the Spirit to guide them in their actions, words and thoughts. The following passages from the Christian Bible attest to this teaching.

Mark 13:11

11 But when they shall lead [you], and deliver you up, be not anxious beforehand what ye shall speak, neither do ye premeditate: but whatever shall be given you in that hour, that speak ye: for it is not ye that speak, but the Holy Spirit.

Acts 2:4

4 And they were all filled with the Holy Spirit, and began to speak in other languages, as the Spirit gave them utterance.

Acts 4:31

31 And when they had prayed, the place was shaken where they were assembled; and they were all filled with the Holy Spirit, and they spoke the word of God with boldness.

This speaking out on the nature of the teachings and their practice has been an integral part of Christianity since its inception. The words of Moses and the words of the Apostle Paul were instrumental in the creation of the Old and New Testaments, respectively, and they affirmed that it was God, the spirit, who inspired them. Sometimes this speaking out causes controversy or differences in the ranks of Christian followers (Body of Christ), but this is also an integral part of the Christian tradition. Jesus himself, the founder of Christianity affirmed this in his own statements.

Matthew 10

34 Think not that I am come to send peace on earth: I came not to send peace, but a sword.
35 For I am come to set a man at variance against his father, and the daughter against her mother, and the daughter in law against her mother in law.
36 And a man's foes [shall be] they of his own household.
37 He that loveth father or mother more than me is not worthy of me: and he that loveth son or daughter more than me is not worthy of me.
38 And he that taketh not his cross, and followeth me, is not worthy of me.
Matthew 12
30 He that is not with me is against me; and he that gathereth not with me scattereth abroad.

Jesus did not come to destroy the Jewish religion, but as an Enlightened Sage he understood that the religion needed to be revised. Judaism had become bogged down in rituals and corruption and Jesus' task was to bring forth the beauty and glory of what was always there, but which had, over time, been misunderstood or forgotten. This is why he tells us in Matthew 10 that he has come, not to smooth things out and soothe people's feelings, but to fulfill the teachings and to bring forth their true, higher meaning. Sometimes it is hard for people to change their long established ways, to reevaluate the comfortable concepts that they hold. When confronted with the fact that the things they have believed for a long time are flawed or incomplete, it is natural that they may become hostile, bitter or otherwise upset in the beginning. But this updating of the teachings is not a task which was to occur once and for all times. Did not Moses try to reform the religion that came before him? The ten commandments were a refinement on the covenant between God and Abraham. Jesus came to upset the status quo of his times because the religion of Moses needed revitalization. The following passage from Matthew, Chapter 19, tell us why Jesus brought an improvement over the laws given by Moses.

> 7 They say to him, Why did Moses then command to give a writing of divorcement, and to put
> her away?
> 8 He saith to them, Moses, because of the hardness of your hearts, permitted you to put away your
> wives: but from the beginning it was not so.

The law given in the time of Moses was for people of that time with the way of thinking of that time. The task of bringing forth the teachings of any spiritual tradition requires an ongoing ministry carried on by those who attain the exalted level of communing with the Spirit and who have attained a level of scholarly refinement. From this communion arises the living word, and this living word should carry as much weight as the scripture itself, since books cannot teach anything without a wise teacher to explain them. This is how Christianity was born. It was not a discarding of the old but an expansion in the understanding of it. Thus, a vast science, called Christology, has developed over the years. It is the study of everything that encompasses Christianity. One of its most important endeavores is "Exegesis" or the critical explanation or analysis, especially of a text. Another important area of study in religion is Eschatology. Eschatology is the branch of theology, or doctrines, dealing with death, resurrection, judgment, immortality, etc. These areas, along with genesis (origins), genealogy and history from antiquity to the present, will be primary concerns of this volume.

Whenever a body of water such as a stream stops flowing, it will stagnate and its contents will putrefy. If you live in a closed room and do not ever open your windows, the air will become musty and stale. That which does not grow stagnates, and eventually decays until a new vision is born which can revitalize and reaffirm its true meaning for the times. This stagnation of spiritual understanding and practice has been the problem in Christianity, and it has become progressively worst particularly in the last 300 years.

I believe *Christian Yoga* is a work of literature which can bring forth a new vision to Christianity. Its intent is not to push people to discard Christianity, but to understand its development and deeper philosophy, and in so doing, allow for a deeper vision to emerge which will not only reaffirm the Bible and other Christian texts, but also engender a deeper understanding and respect for other religions and spiritual traditions, in order to bring forth the greater fulfillment of the Christian plan for all humanity. This work has been divided into two volumes. This is Volume I. The first part of this volume will trace the origins of Christianity and Yoga to Ancient Egypt and Ethiopia. It will explore the background and origins of Christianity and other contemporary philosophies in the time of Jesus and preceding his birth. It will also seek to establish early Christian thought as a mystical system of human transformation akin to the Shetaut Neter or Ancient Egyptian Mysteries and Indian Yoga through comparisons to these systems of philosophy. This present book will define Yoga and Religion in detail, showing that the goals of Yoga and Religion are identical, varying only in certain nuances of the practices employed by the practitioners. It will show that Jesus indeed practiced Yoga just as countless Sages and Saints have since the dawn of history, and will outline the teachings of Christian Yoga. It will then trace the development of Christianity over the last 1,700 years and last, but certainly not least, it will present an introduction to Mystical Christian Wisdom and Philosophy.

Christian Yoga Volume II:

The forthcoming book *Christian Yoga Volume II* will outline the disciplines of Christian Yoga or the Mystical Christian Wisdom and Philosophy, in more detail. It will also explore the philosophy, disciplines and practice of Christianity as a Yogic spiritual discipline in more detail. Volume II will explore the climax of Christian Yoga as a mystical philosophy for psychological transformation leading to union with the Divine, i.e., *The Mystical Journey*

From Jesus To Christ. It will also explore the Christian paths of righteousness, devotion, mystical experience and the mystical path of meditation.

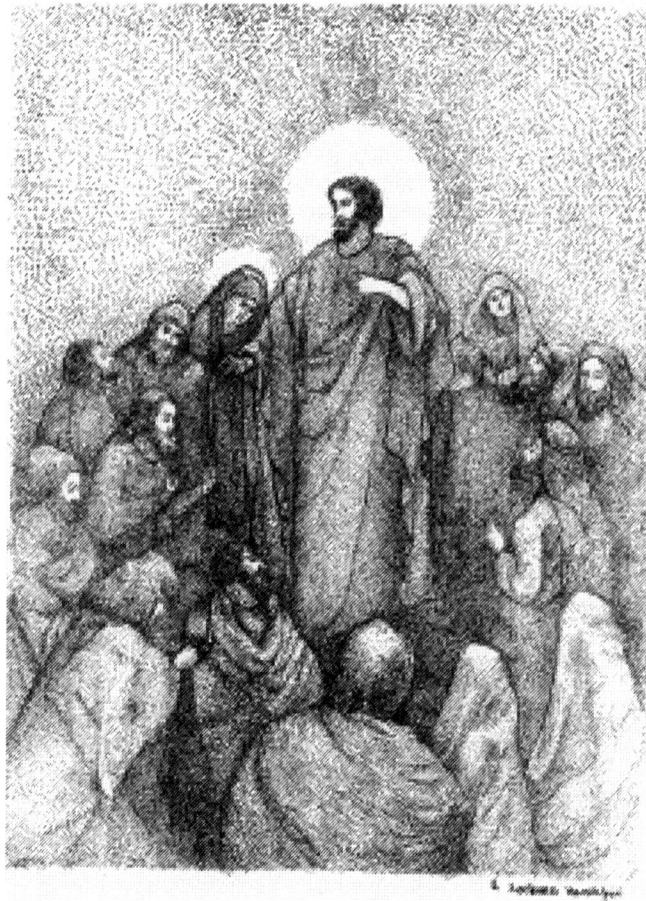

Above: Jesus and his disciples.
The disciples include Mary, his mother, and Mary Magdalene.
Drawing by Lou Lochard.

INTRODUCTION TO THE BIBLE, THE CHRISTIAN GOSPELS FROM ANCIENT EGYPT AND THE KEY TERMS FOR UNDERSTANDING SPIRITUAL PHILOSOPHY

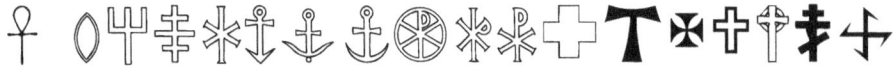

How this Book Was Created

This book is in reality two books in one. It was created with the idea of providing a history, reference source and instructional manual for understanding and practicing mystical Christianity. Thus, it was put together with the idea of providing two important aspects for all those who would like to learn about pre-Roman and post-Roman Catholic Christianity. The introduction provides important keys to understanding the entire work. Chapters 1 through 6 present the origins and history of Christianity and introduce the similarities between Christianity and Ancient Egyptian Religion. This part of the book also discusses the mystical Christianity, that is, Christianity in its original form, and Orthodox Christianity, Christianity after the folklore and traditions were added, as well as the reason why so many Christian denominations have developed. Chapters 7 through 11 present an introduction to Yoga philosophy and to the Yogic practices contained in early Christianity which still survive in Gnostic Gospels and also in the Bible. It has been necessary to include much information in the history portion of this book because it is extremely important to understand the social, political and human forces which affected the way in which Christianity is currently understood and promoted to the masses world over. Though it may at times seem tedious or irrelevant, the historical facts brought forth here are essential in clearing up certain questions which many people have about Christianity, that have also been causing strife and misunderstanding in the world for centuries. Some may want to believe it is not important, that it is all in the past, but what is today came out of what was yesterday.

> Galatians 6:7
> 7 Be not deceived; God is not mocked: for whatever a man soweth, that shall he also reap.

Therefore, in order to understand why things are the way they are, we need to understand the process and factors that contributed to their creation. Religion is no different. Having knowledge and removing these obstacles is essential for the proper understanding of the mystical Christian philosophy. Therefore, the reader should thoroughly read through the history section of this book before venturing into the later chapters.

Who Am I?

"Who am I? Where do I come from?, Where am I going? Why am I here?" These are perhaps the most important questions to every human being. Some people believe that there is a God who created humanity and the universe. These people are called *theists*. Others believe that there is no God and that Creation occurred by chance. These people are known as *atheists*. The theists rely on faith while the atheists say that nothing outside of what the senses can perceive is real, and anything that is perceived outside of the senses represents imagination or insanity. The *agnostic* believes that there can be no proof of the existence of God but does not deny the possibility that God exists. The *Gnostics* (Ancient Egyptians and Greeks who practiced Yoga as well as Christian and non-Christian Mystical Spirituality before and during the early Christian era), on the other hand, believe that there is a spiritual basis for all existence and that this essence can be discovered and experienced. The Bible is a compilation of various writings which tell the story of Christianity, thus, it is a theistic text.

WHAT IS THE BIBLE?

The Bible is a compilation of scriptures which form the basis of Judaism, Christianity and Islam. It is thought of as being the source of divine stories, revelations, prohibitions and prescriptions for Christian moral living which will lead a human being to find God and experience eternal life with God. Excluding the Apocrypha, the Hebrew Bible or Old Testament is accepted as sacred by both the Christians and the Jews. The Roman Catholic Church and the Eastern Orthodox Church accept parts of the Apocrypha as sacred, while Jews and Protestants do not. Only Christians accept the New Testament as sacred.

Thus the Bible, especially the Old Testament, is a very important book since so many followers of Judaism, Christianity and Islam base their faith on it. However, if this is true, why are there three separate religions, especially since they all claim to believe in the same God? In the Bible, the Old Testament speaks of prophets and of a savior who would come to save all believers. While the Jews and Christians generally believe in the same Old Testament, they differ in their belief in the New Testament. The early Christians were a sect of Jews. They believed that Jesus was the definitive prophet and savior who brought the ultimate teachings of spirituality. They thought that he instituted an advanced and expanded teaching which should be added to the Old Testament. The orthodox Jews, however, did not agree, so they continued to believe in the teachings instituted by Moses and continued to follow the teachings of the Old Testament.

> 2 Kings 13:5
> 5 And the LORD gave Israel[I] a saviour, so that they went out from under the hand of the Syrians: and the children of Israel dwelt in their tents, as in times past.

> Isaiah 19:20
> 20 And it shall be for a sign and for a witness to the LORD of hosts in the land of Egypt: for they shall cry to the LORD because of the oppressors, and he shall send them a saviour, and a great one, and he shall deliver them.

So Jews do not believe that the savior spoken of in the Old Testament has yet come, while the Christians have accepted Jesus as that savior. In the time of Jesus, most Jews were looking for a military leader like David or a miracle worker like Moses to save them, and not a spiritual philosopher like Jesus. Therefore, the Jews continue to wait for a savior and consequently, they have developed separate rituals and traditions related to their beliefs. In Judaism these separate customs and traditions are referred to as the Talmudic Tradition. As the Christians believe that Jesus was the prophesied savior, they have developed an independent tradition based on that system of belief. The Muslims believe in the Old Testament. They believe that Abraham existed and that his son, Ishmael, was the progenitor of their nation, as the Bible says. They also believe that Jesus existed and that he was a prophet who performed miracles, but that he only paved the way for one who would come after him. They believe that his mother, Mary, gave birth to him as a virgin, as the Bible says. However, they believe that a new prophet came to bring a more advanced teaching. His name was Muhammad. They believe that he brought the definitive and final teaching, and that the worship of God in the manner and custom which he brought forth is correct. As the Jews and Christians disagree, there is strife between the three groups, the irony being that they worship the same God.

Through their association with Egypt from the time of Abraham, Moses, Joseph, and the early years of Jesus, the early Jews and Christians adopted many of the Ancient Egyptian ideas and rituals into the developing Jewish and Christian faiths, respectively. According to the Bible, the Jews owe their existence to Ancient Egypt, having originated there through Abraham's marriage to an Egyptian woman and the assimilation of hundreds of Egyptians into his family which had previously been just he, his wife and children along with some close relatives. Abraham had a son with the Egyptian slave of his wife Sarah. In the biblical tradition, Abraham's son, Ishmael, is held as the progenitor of the Arabian peoples. The word "Ishmael" means "God will hear."

The Koran (Quran)[II] acknowledges that Abraham was the progenitor of the Arabs. It recognizes Ismail's (Ishmael) line as well as of Israel's line as originating from Abraham. It extols the virtues of Ismail and further states that Abraham with Ismail built the Kaba (Temple of Mecca) and purified it, thus establishing the religion of Islam.

[I] Definition: **Israel,** Biblical name, borne by the Hebrew patriarch Jacob, and by the 12 tribes descended from him.
[II] The sacred text of Islam, believed to contain the revelations made by Allah to Mohammed.

The Koran

> 2:125 Remember We made the House a place of assembly for men and a place of safety; and take ye the Station of Abraham as a place of prayer; and We covenanted with Abraham and Ismail, that they should sanctify My house for those who compass it round, or use it as a retreat, or bow, or Prostrate themselves (therein in prayer).
> 2:126 And remember Abraham said: "My Lord, make this a City of Peace, and feed its People with fruits, -- such of them as believe in Allah and the Last Day." He said: "(Yea), and such as reject Faith, -- for a while will I grant them their pleasure, but will soon drive them to the torment of Fire, -- An evil destination (indeed)!"
> 2:127 And remember Abraham and Ismail raised the foundations of the House (with this prayer): "Our Lord! Accept (this service) from us: For Thou art the All-Hearing, the All-Knowing."
> 2:128 "Our Lord! Make of us Muslims, bowing to Thy (Will), and of our progeny a people Muslim, bowing to Thy (Will); and show us our places for the celebration of (due) rites; and turn unto us (in Mercy); for Thou art the Oft-Returning, Most Merciful."

So how can we unravel the intricate web of philosophies, faiths, doctrines, customs and traditions in order to discover the true meaning of spirituality in religion which transcends differences which lead to wars and strife? First we must understand what religion is and what is its purpose. Then we need to trace its origins and development. This journey will give us insights into the original intent and meaning, and show us how the forces of politics, economics and history and have impacted and changed the doctrines and teachings of religion down to the present. Then we will be in a position to practice religion with an informed intellect and a heart which has been cleared of all diffidence.

The Bible and its Translations

Before we discuss the nature of the translations of the Bible, we need to understand what the Bible is in more depth. Many people see the Bible as an historical text, while others see it as a work of literature, and still others see it as mythology. The Bible is one of the primary sources containing information regarding the beliefs of the Christian faith. It is a compilation of selected portion of writings[1] by different authors who wrote over a period of 1000-2000 years (1,500 B.C.E.- 200 A.C.E.). It is composed of two main sections, the Old Testament and the New Testament, which are made up of smaller books. The original form of the Old Testament is in the ancient Hebrew language. Later, about 250 B.C.E., the Old Testament was translated into Greek. The original form of the New Testament is in the ancient Aramaic, Greek and Hebrew. These forms serve as the primary "original" texts of the Bible. However, since most of the people of the world do not understand ancient Aramaic, Hebrew or Greek, it became necessary to make translations of the Bible into forms that people of modern times could understand. The Bible translations pose important problems because the meanings of some of the ancient Hebrew words are not understood in part or at all by the church or religious scholars. Present day English speaking people would not be able to understand the original King James Version of the Bible which was written only 387 years ago, much less scriptures that were written over 1,700 years ago. However, the essence of a teaching can be discerned and brought forth by those who are initiated into the correct understanding and practice of religious philosophy in its three steps[II]. This is why updates to the translations are necessary.

However, the necessity for translations also opens the door to corruption and misunderstanding, as some translators may want to present a certain view of the scriptures to prove their own points or to mislead others, or they may simply not produce a correct translation because they do not understand the philosophy which the original Bible Sages were trying to impart. Many people do not see the Bible as a book of spiritual principles. Rather, they insist that it is to be believed word for word. If this is the case, and it certain words, customs or ideas cannot be understood by theologians and scholars, as discussed earlier, the Bible will become the object of many different interpretations and consequently, arguments as well. Some of these controversies will be presented later in this volume. For this reason, the religious beliefs of the translator which may or may not be in agreement with the original scriptural meaning, may influence the translation and therefore, the reader should exercise caution when choosing a translation to use for study.

[I] The Bible does not include the entire group of scriptures that were written in biblical times.

[II] Myth, Ritual and metaphysical (Mysticism).

Since languages change over time, it is necessary to update the translations on a regular basis. Another important factor is that there are new discoveries that arise from time to time which may alter the timelines of the Bible or elucidate a new meaning of the old text, which in turn may affect the meaning of the teachings. This has been a major task which this volume, *Christian Yoga*, has attempted to perform in reference to the Nag Hammadi scriptures (discussed below) and their relation to the traditional Christian canonical scriptures. If the church is honest with itself and with its followers, it will welcome the new discoveries and make the necessary adjustments to the doctrine since this will lead followers in a better way. However, the church, as a whole, has been reluctant to accept any new changes because the church hierarchy fear this would undermine their authority. This, among many other problems, has fueled the controversy over the correctness of the Pope in Rome, the head of the Catholic Church, and specifically, his right to exert authority over the Christian doctrine itself. The doctrine of "Infallibility" will be discussed in more detail throughout this volume.

The question and struggle is to determine how best to provide a translation without reinterpreting the text. Some translators provide a word-for-word translation which means that each word is translated individually, but this is often difficult to understand since the nuances of the culture, inflections and grammar of ancient times is pretty much alien to modern society. Some translators work individually, while others work in committees. It is thought that committees would do a better job since its individual members would be less susceptible to deviation from the original texts. Some translators work individually, but their work is checked by a committee. The chart below illustrates the most popular English translations of the Bible. However, there are several thousand Bibles produced for people in various languages. Unfortunately, some of the Bibles were produced by translators who were not checked by any committee. Others could not even read the original texts but gave their rendition anyway, and still others were simply paraphrased by people who thought they were conveying a meaning, but instead deviated from the original texts substantially. Some may want to promote a conservative agenda or a liberal agenda. Others may want to highlight a particular doctrine or political view over another, etc. So under these circumstances, it is not surprising that in the days of slavery, when Christian slave owners wanted to justify their ownership of slaves, some Bibles were produced espousing interpretations of scriptures and commentaries on those scriptures which promote racist ideals. These have not been included in the list. So, as we have seen, paraphrases can convey the meaning of certain texts more easily than the word for word translations, but can also more easily reflect the doctrinal viewpoints of the translators more easily. Therefore, it is important to know who has produced the book and if they have or had any ulterior motives or hidden agendas in their work. Many people feel that when they pick up a Bible, they are holding the "Word of God." This idea has been engrained in the minds of many people for so many years that most do not question the contents of the Bible they are reading, and even become hostile when their illusions are challenged. They brand anyone who deviates from the concepts they have accepted as blasphemers or worse. All the while they are filling themselves with ignorance which will hurt their own spiritual evolution and accordingly, humanity as a whole.

There have been four major discoveries in the last 100 years which directly affect the Bible and consequently, also the Christian doctrine. Since 1611, when the King James Version was written, evidence that allows for more accurate translations has been discovered:

1. The Codex Sinaiticus (Aleph). It was discovered in 1844 locked away in the monastery of St. Catherine. This monastery is located in the Sinai Peninsula. It is estimated that it was written in the 4th century. It contains most of the New Testament.

2. In 1895 the New Testament papyri was discovered in Egypt. It was fragmented but has proven to be valuable.

3. The Dead Sea Scrolls were discovered in 1947 near the Dead Sea. They provide nearly all of the Book of Isaiah as well as many other portions of the Old Testament. They are believed to date from 150 B.C.E. to 68 A.C.E.

4. The Nag Hammadi Library discovered in Egypt in 1945. These scriptures contain invaluable texts of the New Testament, non-canonized Gospels, which were not included in the Bible, as well as non-Christian Gnostic texts which completely revolutionize the Christian faith by introducing a strong mystical component. The powerful nature of these texts and their far reaching implications for the

understanding of the true doctrines of Christianity are the main reasons why these texts are rarely, if ever, acknowledged by Christian theologians, priests or ministers of the various Christian denominations.

The following is a list of English translations, who translated them and when the translation was done.

ENGLISH TRANSLATIONS	TRANSLATOR	DATE OF TRANSLATION
Bishops Bible	Church of England	1568
Rheims-Douay Bible	Roman Catholic	1582-1610
King James Bible	Church of England	1611+
Authorized (King James) Version	*	1769
Authorized (King James) Version	Webster Update	1833
Youngs Literal Translation	(Robert Young)	1863
English Revised Version	Church of England (KJV rev.)	1881-85
American Standard Version	American Revision Committee	1901
Weymouth Modern Speech NT	(R. F. Weymouth)	1903+
Twentieth Century	Inter-denominational	1904
Jewish Version of 1917 (OT)		1917
Moffat's New Translation	(James Moffatt)	1924, 1935
Smith-Goodspeed Version	(Edgar Goodspeed)	1931
Charles B. Williams NT	(Charles B. Williams)	1937
Ronald Knox's Catholic Version	Roman Catholic	1944-50
Revised Standard Version	(KJV revised later Catholic)	1946-52
Confraternity Version	(Rheims-Douay-Challoner rev.)	1948
New World Translation	Watchtower Society	1950-60
NT in Modern English	J. B. Philips	1958
Berkeley version	*	1959
New American Standard	Lockman Foundation (ASV rev.)	1971
Wuest's Expanded Trans. (NT)	Kenneth Wuest	1961
New English Bible	*	1970
NT in Plain English	Charles Kingsley Williams	1963
NT in Language of Today	William F. Beck (a Lutheran)	1964
Amplified Bible	*	1965
Today's English or Good News	American Bible Society	1966
Jerusalem Bible	Roman Catholic	1966
Living Bible	*	1972
New International Version	New York Bible Society	1978
	*(not available)	

This book (*Christian Yoga*) has made use of the Authorized (King James) Version, 1769 edition, with Webster Update of 1833 and the New Revised Standard Version 1990, which is an authorized version of the Revised Standard Version, published in 1952, which was a revision of the American Standard Version, published in 1901, which itself was a revision of the King James Version, published in 1611. It is a word-for-word translation which is good to begin your serious studies in understanding the Christian teachings. However, as you work through *Christian Yoga, The Mystical Journey From Jesus to Christ*, which will provide many of the Nag Hammadi scriptures and their mystical interpretation, it is recommended that you also read the New International Version. This version is a paraphrase which is very accurate and easy to understand. It is written with the world community, as well as the female gender, in mind. Thus, it is less patriarchal and biased in reference to sex, ethnicity and culture. It is also recommended that you obtain the Nag Hammadi Library itself. It is now published as a complete volume.

The Construction of the Bible Gospels

Since there is no evidence to support the events given in the Bible, except the Bible itself, it cannot be treated as a history text. From a literary point of view, most scholars, even Jewish Biblical scholars, feel that it is poor literature. Thus, the scriptures of the Bible may be more accurately regarded as mythology, that is, a collection of stories which carry a message of religion. The primary books of mythology in the Bible which relate the Christian story are the

Gospels. There are four Gospels in the Christian Bible. Three of these are referred to as *Synoptic Gospels,* because they relate a synopsis of the story of Jesus, and their wording in many cases is identical. The fourth gospel, The Gospel of John, gives a different account of the story and as such, has caused much controversy for theologians. The purpose of selecting the first three Gospels was probably to provide some consistency in the single scripture (Bible). However, the church cannot explain the inclusion of a gospel that contains a different version. Most likely the gospel was included as a compromise since the exclusion of so many other Gospels was surely a source of great friction between the sects of Christianity which struggled to compile a cannon of texts to be included in the Bible.

Some of the differences between the Gospel of John and the other three Gospels in the Bible are as follows. Some of the events appear at different times in the Gospel of John such as the cleansing of the temple which appears at the beginning, whereas in the other Gospels it appears after Jesus' triumphant entry into Jerusalem. John places the Last Supper before the feast of the Passover and the crucifixion before the first day of the Passover. John describes the ministry of Jesus as lasting for two years whereas the other three describe it as lasting only one year. The three Gospels are presented as paradoxical statements whereas John provides allegorical discourses for reflection and meditation on the Christian teachings. Another important characteristic of the Synoptic Gospels is that they emphasize a messianic[1] message and religious matters. Thus, the Synoptic Gospels are concerned with establishing Jesus as the savior and therefore, also faith in the church. The Gospel of John is more concerned with the teaching itself and is therefore more akin to the Gnostic form of spirituality.

Modern scholars generally agree that a person other than the authors of the Synoptic Gospels wrote The Gospel of John. They also believe that it was written later. The very idea that three similar Gospels should be chosen from the dozens available is motive to inquire about the reasoning behind the choices. At the time of the creation of the Bible there was much debate about which Gospels should be included in it. Like the books based on the letters of Paul, Gospels were designed to consolidate the philosophy of Christianity, to promote the faith in and practice of Christianity and to assist the various churches in understanding and delivering the Christian message. The New Testament contains thirteen letters which bear Paul's name as their author. Scholars believe that seven of them were written by Paul himself. These are: 1 Thessalonians, Galatians, 1 Corinthians, 2 Corinthians, Romans, Philippians, and Philemon. So the choice of Gospels and books to include in the Bible was based on their adherence to a particular view of the story of Jesus. Also, it was based on the desire of the early church to engender faith in the chosen Christian story and to foment the desire in people to adhere to the newly forming churches based on that story. This is when the traditional Jewish leaders began to separate themselves from the newly forming Christian worshipers consisting of Jews who were still attending the Jewish Synagogues but also following the Christian faith (the teachings of Jesus). As previously discussed, the traditional Jews, then and now, believe that the Messiah has not yet come to the earth and therefore, do not believe in Jesus or the Christian story.

Many writings that were called "Gnostic" or "Knowing" Gospels were "deleted" from the standard text by Roman Emperor Constantine and the church authorities under the control of the Roman Empire. In the *Essene Gospel of Peace,* translated by Edmond Bordeaux Szekeley in the early twentieth century from a copy which was locked away in the Vatican, Jesus states that his teachings are to help guide others to attain his level of consciousness, Cosmic Consciousness, to become as he was: Christ. The same teaching is found in the *Gospel of Thomas,* one of several early Gnostic Christian texts which were found in Egypt, and then edited and altered by the Nicean Council and the Roman Emperor Constantine. Thus, in the light of the Gnostic texts, the phrase *"being saved through Jesus"* refers more to a metaphorical reliance on Jesus rather than to a literal understanding. It means that an individual may effect his or her own salvation by studying and practicing the teachings of Jesus, and not that you need Jesus himself to act as mediator between you and God to attain salvation.

"Salvation is accomplished through the efforts of the individual. There is no mediator between a person and his/her salvation."

Ancient Egyptian Proverb

For 300 to 600 years after the Nicean council, the Roman emperors, and later on, the Christian leaders, set about to destroy any vestige of religious doctrines that did not comply with the doctrines of their new religion. The crusades, inquisitions and excommunications were later attempts to promote ignorance among the masses of people and subjugation to the church authorities in all matters.

Along with the four Gospels used by the present day Christian Church as the accounts of the life and teachings of Jesus, there were at least eight other Gospels written by other Christian sects during the first centuries of the Christian era. It is not possible to know the exact number, but some scholars estimate that prior to the Catholic Church's destruction of other faiths, it is possible that there may have been hundreds of other Gospels. At that time

---

[1] Hebrew *mashiah*, meaning "anointed," savior. Messianic: saving work or message.

there were dozens of Christian sects claiming to be the bearers of the true doctrine. There was a wide variation in some of their views. Some insisted on the doctrine of reincarnation. Before Christianity was accepted by the Roman Empire, some Christian sects held that it was wrong to martyr oneself by following the teachings openly, since the teachings represented an inner faith, while others held that they must defy the Roman authorities by pledging allegiance to Jesus instead of to Caesar (the emperor). Other Gospels from different sects spoke of God as being female. Many Christian sects incorporated elaborate rituals which included sexuality in their symbolism as well as in the performance of the mystery rites. Still others laid emphasis on the mystical Christian understanding that all people are potential Christs[1] if they follow the teachings of Jesus.[81]

And you, answered Jesus, *be true sons of God that you also may partake in his power and in the knowledge of all secrets.* (Essene *Gospel of Peace* Book 1, p 34)[72]

The same idea is found in the *Gospel of Thomas* (a) and *The Secret Book of James* (b):

(a) 112. Jesus says: "He who drinks from my mouth *will become like me.* As for me, I will become what he is, and what is hidden will be revealed to him."

(b) But if you are afflicted and persecuted by Satan, and do the Father's will, I say this:
The Father will love you, and *make you my equal...* (Chapter 3:4-5)

The Gospel According to Thomas is one of several Nag Hammadi papyruses which were discovered in Egypt in 1945.[82] Like the *Dead Sea Scrolls,* discovered in Qumran, they show a view of early Christianity which encompassed many sects whose spiritual beliefs were originally based on doctrines that differed from that of the Roman church. The specific form of Christianity adopted by the Roman emperor in c.325 A.C.E.[80] was clearly an altered version of earlier Gnostic (knowing) Christianity which developed out of the Ancient Egyptian Religion. The Ancient Egyptian gods and goddesses, Ra, Asar (Osiris), Aset (Isis) and Heru (Horus) were transformed into the Father, Son, Holy Ghost and Mary of modern day Christianity.[58]

Alexandria, the city in Egypt founded by *Alexander the Great* upon his conquest of Egypt, became the center of scholarship and learning in the entire ancient world from 300 B.C.E. to 250 A.C.E. It was here that the doctrines of the Religion of Asar (Osiris) and Hermeticism from Ancient Egypt (5,500 B.C.E-300 B.C.E), the Buddhist missionaries from India, the cult of Christos from the Near East and the teachings of Zarathustra (Zoroaster) melded into an amalgam of several Jewish and Christian sects. *Dionysius the Areopagite* played an important role in bridging the gap between the mystical religious teachings, Judaism and Christianity. Up to this time the symbols associated with Gnosticism, Hermeticism and Christianity were known to be metaphors to describe the ultimate reality of the universe and man's relationship to it. It was not until the time of the Christians from the Byzantine throne, the Jewish leaders who followed Yahweh (a name for God used by the ancient Hebrews), and then later, the Muslims who followed Allah (the supreme being in Islam), that the symbols and metaphors of religion began to be understood literally, as facts rather than as metaphors to explain the mystery behind every individual. The idea of "God" became circumscribed by a particular doctrine, which was the exclusive property belonging to certain "chosen people." Thus, they saw all other God-forms as idols or devils. All other religions were seen as heresies. Consequently, the followers of those forms were considered as pagans who must be subdued and converted or destroyed. This point is most strongly illustrated in the Bible itself in several passages. This point is of great importance because the concept of a proprietary God is central to Western religions.

The Bible - Genesis 12: 1-3
"The Lord... said to Abraham... "I will make you into a great nation and I will bless you; I will make your name great, and you will be a blessing. I will bless those who bless you, and whoever curses you I will curse; and all peoples on earth will be blessed through you."

The Bible Exodus 33 1-2
"The Lord said to Moses, Go, leave this place, you and the people whom you have brought out of the land of Egypt, and go to the land of which I swore to Abraham, Isaac, and Jacob, saying, "To your descendents I will give it. I will send an angel before you, and I will drive out the Canaanites, the Amorites, the Hittites, the Perizzites, the Hivites, and the Jesubites."

The Bible 2 Kings 5.15
"Now I know that there is no God in all earth except in Israel..."

The Bible - Genesis 1.28

---

[1] *Gospel of Thomas, Essene Gospel of Peace.*

"Be fruitful and multiply, and fill the earth and subdue it; and have dominion over the fish of the sea and over the birds in the air and over every living thing that moves upon the earth."

The preceding statement contains a mandate and a tacit authorization to subdue the earth and to control it. In the extreme, these statements could be interpreted as permission or consent to conquer any and all parts of the earth and its peoples, since their inhabitants are disqualified as being worthy to live or possess property, due to their pagan status, i.e., not believing in the true and only God, the god of Christianity. An atmosphere was created in Europe wherein other peoples could be thought of and classified as "non-human," deserving less consideration and respect.[70]

At the end of the Middle Ages, passages such as those in Exodus 33: 1-2 led to the idea that a particular piece of land was bequeathed to the Jews by God, and that the heathen peoples should be removed from the land and a Jewish state established there. This idea, which some people felt based on the passages above, was a contributing factor towards the belief that the crusades were biblically sanctioned. This doctrine was to have severe repercussions for the Native Americans who were almost completely annihilated and for the Africans who were captured and enslaved during the conquest of the New World. Thus, racism, with all its repercussions, is related to spiritual ignorance. It is estimated that over 50 million Native Americans and over 100 million Africans were killed as a result of the wars for conquest of the Americas (Native American Holocaust[I]) and the slave trade (African Holocaust) by the various European countries, respectively.[79] In modern times this feeling has led to the birth of Zionism[II] and the State of Israel,[84] located in Palestine, which has not only displaced the Palestinian people who have lived there for centuries, but has also destabilized the entire region and fostered many wars and animosity between the Jewish and Muslim peoples.

A History of Modern Jewish Zionism

Beginning with Abraham (c. 2,100 B.C.E?) and ending with the creation of a Jewish state in 1948 A.C.E., the events surrounding Palestine and the creation of the Jewish state of Israel shows the long struggle of the Jewish people to establish a permanent country for themselves and the conflict which ensued when the Jews were successful in taking control of the land which has been considered as the Holy Land for Jews, Christians, and Muslims. The creation of Israel had begun in ancient times, but it was not until the late 1800s that the movement took on strength due to the ability of the Jews to develop political clout and financial backing from their own sources and from the Western countries. The Balfour Declaration of 1917 was crucial to the plans of the Israeli leaders. In the aftermath of World War II when the Palestinians were weak militarily and the western countries were stronger, Britain took control of the area. This was the opportunity that the Jewish leaders were waiting for since 1896. These factors, coupled with the Western interest in Middle Eastern oil, enabled the Jewish leaders to promote the partitioning of Palestine and obtain the permission and financing to start a settlement in Palestine. The establishment of a Jewish State was not officially part of the original settlement idea as authorized by the previous declarations of the United Nations or the British mandate. Having succeeded in occupied the land, the Jews then set out to establish and expand a Jewish State by military force.

Many Christians support the cause of Zionism, some because they believe it is sanctioned by the Bible as a God given right of the Jews which is ordained under penalty of death and damnation for those who oppose it. They follow this teaching out of fear because the Old Testament in the Bible says that those who go against the chosen people (the Jews) will be destroyed by God himself. The passage below from the Bible is one of several which espouse this idea.

[I] The killing of many victims, often savagely: massacre, mass murder, etc.

[II] Definition: **Zionism** is a political movement advocating the reestablishment of a Jewish homeland in Palestine, the "promised land" of the Bible, with its capital Jerusalem, the "city of Zion." **Zi·on:** The historic land of Israel as a symbol of the Jewish people. **b.** The Jewish people; Israel. **2.** A place or religious community regarded as sacredly devoted to God. **3.** An idealized, harmonious community; utopia.

THE MYSTICAL JOURNEY FROM JESUS TO CHRIST

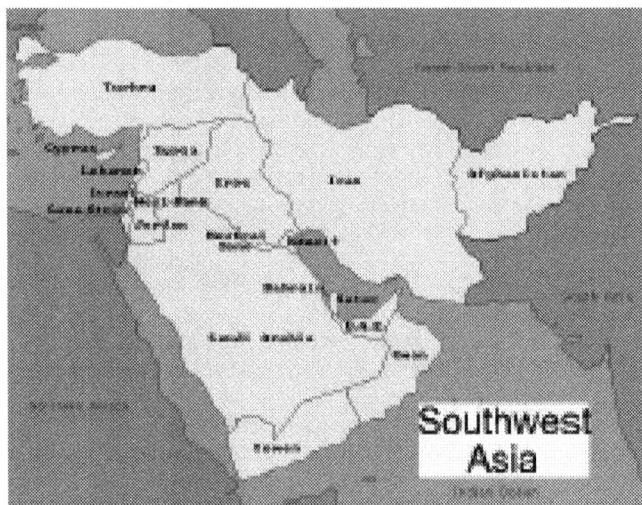

Left: Map of the countries involved in the modern struggle to control the Biblical Holy Land.

Southwest Asia

1 Chronicles 17

9 Also I will ordain a place for my people Israel, and will plant them, and they shall dwell in their place, and shall be moved no more; neither shall the children of wickedness waste them any more, as at the beginning,
10 And since the time that I commanded judges [to be] over my people Israel. Moreover I will subdue all thy enemies. Furthermore I tell thee that the LORD will build thee an house.

We need to have a deeper understanding of the history of those who started the religion of Judaism and those who have adhered to it, in order to have a deeper understanding of why the Zionist movement has received such impetus in the mythology, ritual and secular life of Jews. Christians, Jews and Muslims will have a better understanding of Judaism and will also better understand their own position on the Zionist movement. Only correct insight and understanding will allow one to act out of truth and righteousness instead of fear and ignorance. Thus, all peoples will be benefited accordingly.

Mattew 3
8 Bring forth therefore fruits in keeping with repentance.

If the Jews wanted to set up a new nation or state they should have entered into negotiations with the people living in the area (Palestinians and other Arabs). Then they could have come to a mutual agreement that might have been beneficial to both. Having taken the land by force and expulsed the people who have been living there for several generations, and having committed atrocities on them, all with the financial backing from Jews abroad and from western countries such as the United States, the Jews in the newly formed state of Israel have promoted a climate of mistrust, hatred and revenge. They have adopted the principle used by many western countries, that military might and financial power can be used to control, steal from or enslave others. In response, the Palestinians and other Arab nations have engaged in militant attacks and demonstrations against the Jews as well. Both sides have caused the deaths of children and other innocent civilians. Although the land was unjustly taken, what is needed now is justice, forgiveness and understanding. What is needed is a kind of justice that allows people an opportunity to live together and forgiveness for those who acted wrongly, out of spiritual ignorance. Also, those who have committed the wrongs, on both sides, need to forgive themselves. However, forgiveness involves making amends for one's wrongdoing. This is not necessarily to be understood as paying someone in the form of money to redress a wrong. A person can pay a fine and remain just as ignorant and harbor the same feelings which led to the past mistake until it occurs again in the future. Those who commit wrongs need to face up to them and correct their feelings, thoughts and actions so that the error will not occur again. Both the Jews and the Arabs need to reconcile their anger and forgive the attacks which both have perpetrated on each other. This is self-forgiveness and making amends. True repentance and amends for a wrongdoing means eradicating the ignorance which led to the error and, in the future, acting in ways that will promote harmony instead of strife and violence. True peace does not come from getting more guns in order to hold an opponent at bay. It comes from making an opponent into a friend. This can only occur when there is good feeling amongst people which comes from caring, sharing, trust, respect, honesty and acceptance. Ultimately, the Jews and Palestinians and other Arabs need to realize and affirm that they both have a right to exist and that both come from and are sustained by the same God. This is the only way to have true reconciliation and peace.

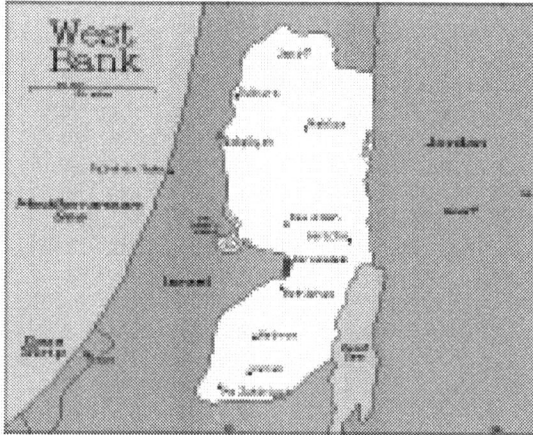

The disputed territory between the Arabs and the Jews. Also, the land which was disputed in the time of the Crusades.

Acceptance cannot come when one sees oneself as superior and others as inferior or when one sees oneself as all right and the other as all wrong. True friendship cannot come from injustice and a true coming together cannot occur if there is segregation of peoples. The idea of race and racism has become intermixed with ideas of religion in Jewish philosophy. In modern times the idea of racism, which developed out of the European kidnapping and enslaving of African peoples, also adversely affects the Jews. The Europeans who considered themselves as "white" saw them as Semitic or mixed 0.05"with non-white blood and discriminated against them. From a genetic standpoint, all peoples from the Middle East were of mixed African and Asian descent in biblical times. This was confirmed by Herodotus and other historians of ancient times as well as the writings of the Bible itself. Many people do not realize that there were no "white" or lighter skinned Jews until the latter part of the first millennium of our era (between the fifth and ninth centuries A.C.E.) when the Jews moved into Europe and began to mix with Europeans. It must be clearly understood that Judaism is supposed to be a religion and not an ethnic group or race. This idea is proven easily by the existence of the Falashas. The Falashas are a native Jewish sect of Ethiopia. Their origin is unknown, but believed to be ancient. The Falashas are dark skinned African peoples who follow the Jewish faith from a time even before the Jews moved into Europe. More importantly, however, let us not forget that in the remote past human beings originated in Africa and therefore, are African in ancestry, just as all humans are of "one blood" (Acts 17:26) and "one flesh" (1 Corinthians 15:39) in God. Therefore, this means that racial distinctions are a bogus and illusory expression of a person's level of spiritual ignorance, a feeling of separation from others which is fueled by frustration, misunderstanding, greed, anger, etc. All human beings deserve compassion, love and caring, regardless of their faith, skin color, etc. Anything less than this is inhuman and un-spiritual, and therefore, sinful. Sin brings on an effect wherein the sinner receives a punishment for the sinful behavior in the form of suffering and frustration either in this lifetime or a future one. Therefore, those who believe that might makes right or that they have gotten away with something which they know is wrong are overlooking the greater plan of cosmic order which administers absolute justice to all beings. So it is important to be fair, compassionate and forgiving, since those who you treat in this way will more easily be able to respond to you in kind. On the other hand, those whom you have treated badly will in all likelihood treat you with fear, hatred and mistrust in return.

Job 4:8
Even as I have seen, they that plow iniquity, and sow wickedness, reap the same.

Around the time of Jesus, Christianity brought in a new message to the Jews. The Kingdom of Heaven was not an exclusive place where only Jews would be able to enter. Rather, anyone would be able to enter if they did what was required, practice the Christian principles in their life just as Jesus did and taught. This message drew new converts from all lands. It was a principal reason why the Jewish political and religious leaders opposed Christianity. Even though Christianity has been associated with Western civilization and with an elitist church organization based in Rome in the last 1,300 years, it was originally conceptualized as a universal religion. The following passages from Matthew in the New Testament illustrate the universal appeal of Christianity to all peoples.

Matthew 7:21
21. Not every one that says to me, Lord, Lord, shall enter into the kingdom of heaven; but he that doeth the will of my Father who is in heaven.

Matthew 8:11
11 And I say to you, That many shall come from the east and the west, and shall sit down with Abraham, and Isaac, and Jacob, in the kingdom of heaven.

The Nag Hammadi Library and its Relation to The Bible

Having fascinated scholars ever since their discovery in 1945, the 52 Gnostic texts found at Nag Hammadi, Egypt constitute an extremely important discovery relating to the understanding of early Christianity. Nag Hammadi is a modern name for a town which is located in east central Egypt, and 48 km (about 30 mi.) south of Qina. These texts which date back to the time of the biblical Jesus have redefined the manner in which the social climate and history during the time of Jesus are being viewed. Up to the time of their discovery, it was known that many sects of Christian groups existed. These groups were considered to be outcasts and heretics by the Orthodox Roman Catholic groups. It was also known that the early councils of the Roman Catholic Bishops had altered, edited and even omitted from the Bible, many existing scriptures of the time claimed to be inspired by Jesus. By the time the Roman Catholic Church had compiled and canonized the scriptures which would make up the present day Christian Bible, these works had undergone many revisions and changes. The term *gnostic* is derived from the Greek word *gnostikos*, meaning "one who knows," which is based on a word for "knowledge," *gnosis*. In Gnostic Christianity, Jesus Christ is only the revealer of knowledge. Gnosis means knowledge gained from the source, referring to Christhood itself as the ultimate source, superceding even the scriptures (Bible, Gospels, etc.) themselves. Knowledge is of two types, information and experience. The gnostic form of knowledge relates to having experience of the Divine as opposed to just simply having information about the Divine from scriptures, wisdom teachings and other such texts. This is the difference between someone describing to you what ice cream tastes like (information) as opposed to your actually tasting it for yourself (gnosis, experience).

In 1769, the first Gnostic texts turned up in modern times when a Scottish tourist purchased a Coptic (Late Ancient Egyptian) manuscript near Thebes (Waset) in Upper Egypt. It contained a record of Jesus' teachings to his disciples, a group composed of both men and women. In 1773 a collector discovered another Coptic text which contained a conversation on the "mysteries" between Jesus and his disciples. In 1896, a German Egyptologist purchased manuscripts in Cairo, Egypt, which contained the *Gospel of Mary* (Magdalene) and the *Apocryphon* (secret book) *of John* (which was also found at Nag Hammadi in 1945).

By the time of the translation of the *Essene Gospel of Peace* in 1929, a Gnostic Christian text written by the Essenes, it became evident that many of those ancient Gnostic (knowing) texts survived. The Essenes were a group of Jewish ascetic communities which had cultural and religious ties to Ancient Egypt and the Near East. The Essenes, along with the *Therapeuts,* another Jewish sect of Egypt that did not follow the established Jewish authorities, claimed to follow the true teachings of their leader, whose title was "Teacher of Righteousness*.*"

The entire group of texts discovered at Nag Hammadi are referred to as the *Nag Hammadi Library.* Some of the texts are Christian in nature, while others have no mention of a person called Jesus. However, they all deal with the same theme as other Gnostic texts, that is, knowing the mystery of life within oneself. Among the texts discovered at Nag Hammadi are: *The Gospel of Thomas, The Gospel of Philip, The Gospel of Truth, The Gospel to the Egyptians, The Secret Book of James, The Apocalypse of Paul, The Letter of Peter to Philip,* and *The Apocalypse of Peter.*

The discoveries in Egypt in 1945 coupled with the discovery of the Dead Sea Scrolls in Qumran (Palestine) in 1947 have been the source of controversy as well as speculation into the true nature of Christianity and Judaism, respectively, as to their origins and teachings. Consequently, many scholarly studies have been undertaken to completely catalogue and translate the texts and to attempt to ascertain the meanings intended by them. While the discovery of the *Dead Sea Scrolls* received much publicity, the discovery of the *Nag Hammadi Library* was shrouded in secrecy by the authorities. It was not until several years after the discovery that they were fully translated and made available to the world. This extraordinary discovery was finally published and translated into English in 1977 as 'The Nag Hammadi Library.' As one begins to see their importance, it becomes clear why modern day officials of the church and government would be apprehensive about releasing information related to ancient literary works that might completely revolutionize the current understanding of the teachings which so many people have held for over fifteen hundred years. One in particular, *The Gospel of Thomas,* opens with: *"These are the secret words which the living Jesus spoke, and which the twin, Judas Thomas, wrote down."* It contains many of the sayings from the New Testament but in different contexts from the Bible gospel versions. The new perspective from the newly found texts is fueling the speculation and controversy over the teachings of Christianity as they have been given by the mainstream biblical tradition, the Roman Catholic Church as well as the other Christian churches that emerged after.

For example, some texts like *The Gospel of Thomas* seem to suggest that Jesus had a twin and that he gave secret teachings to his disciples. The Roman Catholic Bible itself establishes the idea that there is a secret or inner teaching through the following statement, but does not elaborate on it further. It simply suggests that there is a secret understanding but does not tell us what it is.

> Mark 4:11
> And he said to them, "To you it is given to know the mystery of the Kingdom of God: but to them that are outside, all [these] things are done in parables..."

THE HISTORY AND PHILOSOPHY OF MYSTICAL CHRISTIANITY

The Gospel of Philip states that the companion of Jesus was Mary Magdalene, that he kissed her on the mouth and that he loved her more than the other disciples. Other Gnostic texts strongly refute the Catholic view of bodily resurrection and the virgin birth, calling these notions ridiculous and misunderstood by the orthodox community. The following excerpt from the Gnostic *Gospel of Phillip* brings home this point.

> "Those who say that the Lord died first and then rose up are in error, for he rose up and then died. We are to receive the resurrection while we live."

Gnosticism developed during a period of time (600 B.C.E - 100 C.E) when the whole world was undergoing a renaissance (if not revolution) in the way in which religion, social justice, and the nature of existence were viewed throughout the entire ancient world from Egypt, Africa in the South to Rome in the West, and China and India in the East.

In the East, *Buddha* and *Mahavira* emerged in India with new views on a philosophy of self-knowledge based on the oneness of creation and humankind. During the same time, farther East in China, Confucius and Lao-Tsu emerged with basically the same philosophy. By contrast, in Persia, Zoroaster became a proponent of a dualistic philosophy of creation which saw good and evil in everything as well as rigid religious rules that must be followed in order to live according to "God's will." It is notable that in later times the Judeo-Christian-Islamic orthodox traditions developed a dualistic view of nature, God, and humanity, being influenced by Zoroastrianism and Aristotelian rationalism rather than the "Monistic" and "Panentheistic" traditions (Ancient Egyptian religion, Gnosticism, Eastern Philosophy) which originally gave birth to them and influenced their early development. Monism is the belief that all reality comes from and exists in one source. Panentheism is the belief that all existence is a manifestation of (one) God, but also that God is more than the phenomenal universe. A major reason for this fundamental change in the basic concepts of the philosophy lies in the development of the of Christianity, Islam and Judaism in Western civilization. As we move through our study of religion and yoga philosophy, we will discover the points in history where the original philosophies of Western civilization diverged from their common origins with Eastern religions and we will see how these diverging views branched off into seemingly new doctrines. With this insight we will be able to work back from the present in order to discover the ancient meaning of the teachings.

As the Ancient Egyptian society and government organizations deteriorated after more than 5,000 years of high civilization, the early Greek philosophers such as *Thales* and *Pythagoras* began their studies in the Egyptian temples.[44] Later on, when the Druids, Therapeuts and others left Egypt, this same philosophy which was originally espoused in Ancient Egypt became masked under the local folklore and customs of individual tribes and religious groups in Europe and the Middle East.[64]

The ultimate truth, God, is revered by all peoples but culture and folk differences color the expression of that reverence. This is what is called the *folk expression of religion based on culture and local traditions.* For example, the same ultimate reality, God, is expressed by Christians based on European culture and traditions. The same ultimate reality is expressed by Muslims based on Arab culture and traditions. The same ultimate and transcendental reality is worshipped by Jews based on Hebrew culture and traditions. If people who practice religion stay at the outer levels (culture, myths and traditions) they will always see differences between faiths. Mysticism allows any person in any religion to discover that the same Supreme Being is being worshipped by all under different names and forms. Therefore, the task of all true spiritual seekers is to go beyond the veil of the outer forms of religion, including the symbols, but more importantly, the doctrines, rituals and traditions (see model below).

Below: The Culture-Myth Model, showing how the folk expression of religion is based on culture and local traditions.

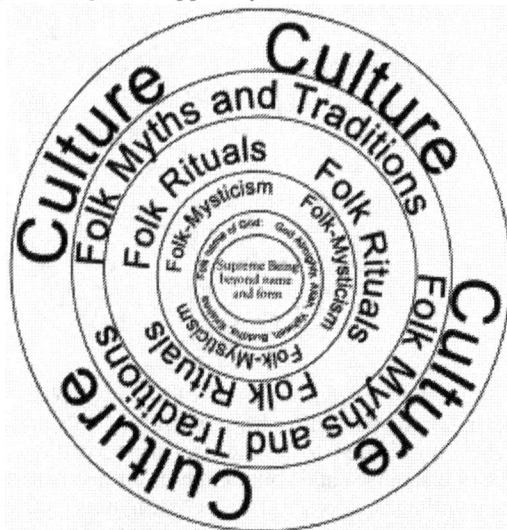

It is possible to focus on the apparent differences between cultures and religious philosophies. This has been the predominant form of philosophical discourse and study of Western scholarship. The seeming differences between religions have led to innumerable conflicts between the groups throughout history, all because of the outer expression of religion. However, throughout this work I will attempt to focus on the synchretic aspects of the philosophies and religions in question because it is in the similarities wherein harmony is to be found, harmony in the form of concurrence in ideas and meaning. In light of this idea of harmony it is possible to look at the folklore of cultural traditions throughout the world and see the same psycho-mythological message being espoused through the various cultural masks. They are all referring to the same Supreme Being. While giving commentary and adding notes which I feel will be helpful to the understanding of the texts which I will compare, I have endeavored to use the actual texts wherever possible so that you, the reader, may see for yourself and make your own judgment.

One text in particular, *The Gospel of Thomas*, seems to be most representative of the combined Gnostic Christian philosophy of Oneness. The other texts I will focus on are the *Bhagavad Gita* from India, and *Thrice Greatest Hermes* and the *Book of Coming Forth By Day and Night* from Ancient Egypt. These texts are either contemporary with the advent of Christianity or were already in existence prior to the development of Gnosticism and Christianity.

The *Bhagavad Gita,* or the *Song of God,* is part of the Indian epic book *Mahabharata*. It is possibly the most influential Hindu text. In the Gita, Krishna is the Supreme Being who teaches his beloved devotee, *Arjuna,* the subtleties of the various paths of Yoga and how they can lead an aspirant to discover his/her own self as one with the Supreme through wisdom of and devotion to God. It emphasizes devotion (*Bhakti Yoga* — Yoga of Divine Love) while giving a concise discourse on the wisdom teachings of the Vedas and Upanishads, along with a comprehensive summary of the main aspects of yoga philosophy.

Below: The Culture-Myth Models of four world spiritual systems, showing how the folk expression of each religion is based on culture and local traditions.

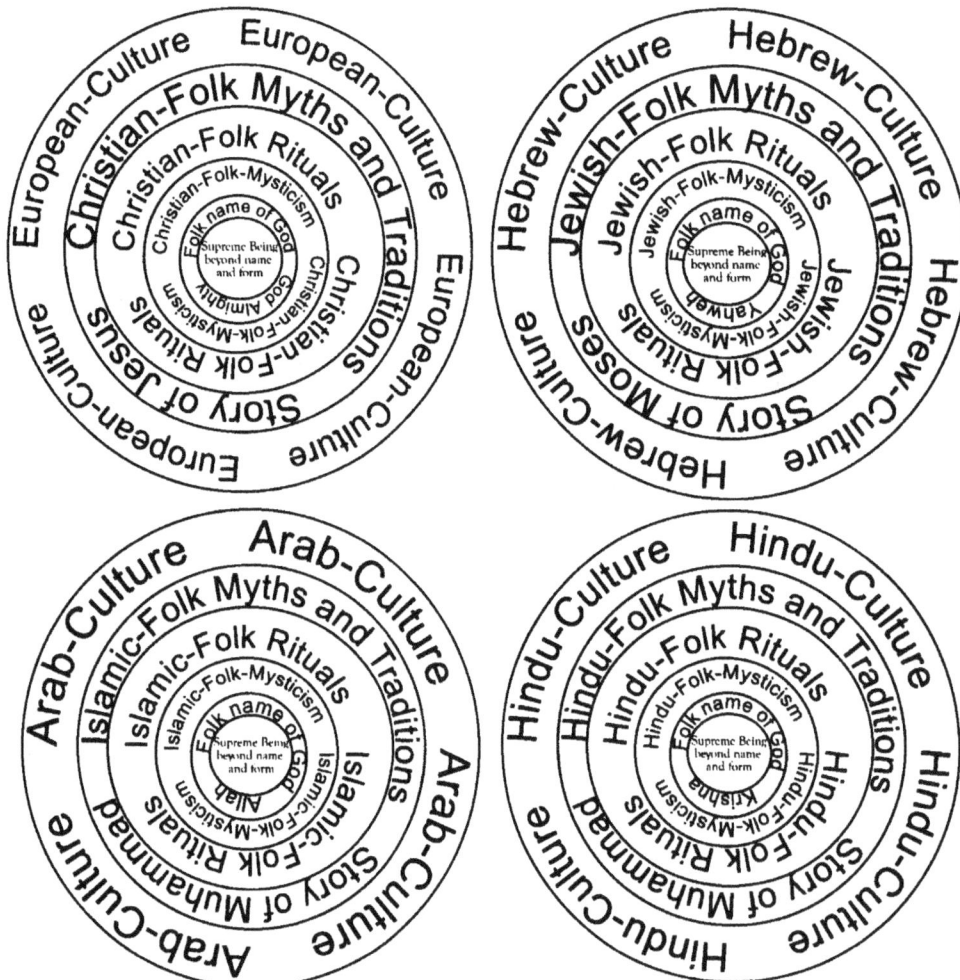

The Hindu sacred tradition is the basis of Indian society. This tradition is composed of sacred written texts and oral traditions passed on from generation to generation in an unbroken link. They are divided into *Sruti* and *Smrti*. *Sruti* is considered to be the primary revelation, and Smrti is everything else besides. Thus, Smriti includes the literary discourses and commentaries on the main scriptures by the numerous Indian Saints and Sages throughout the last two thousand years. The Vedas, hymns exalting and glorifying contain the liturgy for ritual sacrifices, and are generally held to be the most sacred texts. The great epic poems contain important sacred material.

Thrice Greatest Hermes is a compilation of Hermetic philosophy which descended from the Ancient Egyptian Mystery Religion (5,500 B.C.E.-100 B.C.E.). It was popular during the formative years of early Greek philosophy (900? B.C.E.-200 B.C.E.) and Christianity (100 BCE-450 A.C.E.). The many versions of the Ancient Egyptian *"Book of Coming Forth by Day and Night,"* beginning with the *Ancient Egyptian Pyramid Texts,* are the oldest known philosophical and spiritual texts in the world. Having existed since the time of the earliest Ancient Egyptian dynasties (5,500 BCE), the Pyramid Texts describe the journey of the human soul in the realm of the afterlife and what each man and woman must do and know while still on earth, to survive death and thereby *"come forth"* into the light of *"day"* (life, illumination, self-knowledge, eternal happiness, resurrection, enlightenment).

Keeping the preceding in mind, another important task of this study is to focus on the psychological significance of the mythology, symbols and rituals, rather than their historical or ethnic features.[1] This psycho-mythical point of view is supported by the Gnostic Christian texts. It is evident that many of the traditional Biblical texts originated from or were inspired by the Gnostic understanding, but were at some point edited or toned down, as it were, to a form which became ambiguous and which placed greater importance on historicity rather than on mystical significance of the scriptures. For example, the idea of self-salvation through the practice of the teachings which was held by pre-Roman Catholic Christians was transformed into the idea of salvation through the church by later Orthodox Catholic Church authorities.

Below are two corresponding verses, first as it is presented in the Gnostic Christian text, and then as it appears in the Bible (Orthodox Christianity). The statement which appears in the Bible not only falls short of providing a deeper meaning, but it also turns the meaning away from the individual interpretation for every Christian follower and transforms it into what might be called a church or group statement. Thus, from a psychological standpoint, we move to a sectarian understanding of the statement in the Orthodox Church version. So the Orthodox Church was the first denominational movement in Christianity since it sought to set itself apart from the other Christians. Therefore, it is not surprising that the sectarian orthodox movement in the development of Christianity opposed the Gnostic or psycho-mystical movement which had its roots in the Ancient Egyptian, Yogic, Hindu, Taoist and Buddhist teachings which are themselves essentially psychological teachings designed for individual practice and self-transformation leading to a mystical spiritual awakening.

Gnostic text from the *Gospel of Thomas* where Jesus is speaking to his disciples:

55. If they ask you, "Whence have you come from?" tell them "We have come from the Light, from the place whence the Light is produced of itself." If someone says to you: "What are you?" say, "We are the sons and we are the elect of the living Father."

Now let's compare the previous statement to the traditional Bible text:

John 8

14 Jesus answered and said to them, Though I testify concerning myself, [yet] my testimony is true: for I know from where I came, and where I go; but ye cannot tell from where I come, and where I go.

It is evident that the Gnostic statement which originally sought to impart specific knowledge as to the origin of the disciple has been transformed into an ambiguous statement which relates the reader to a worldly form of thinking based on a connection to the church rather than to a transcendental reference which is to be experienced in the heart of the individual. In the Bible, the emphasis is on the personal, rather than the transpersonal Jesus. Further, the Biblical statement takes the form of a riddle with respect to the origins and status of the disciples. The latter text also uses "I" rather than "you." Thus, the focus of attention is in the personality of Jesus as an entity outside and separate from ourselves rather than the inner or self-application of the teaching as a psychological metaphor.

Before proceeding with the main body of this work, it would be helpful to establish some working definitions for the disciplines which will be discussed in order to provide a common basis for understanding the journey we will undertake. These terms will be further defined and explored throughout the course of this work.

---

[1] The word "ethnic" may have originated from the Bible term "ethnos" meaning "of or pertaining to a group of people recognized as a class on the basis of certain distinctive characteristics, such as religion, language, ancestry, culture, or national origin."[124]

Philosophy

Philosophy has been defined as the speculative inquiry concerning the source and nature of human knowledge and a system of ideas based on such thinking. In this work, the idea of philosophy will be confined to the modes of thinking employed for the purpose of transforming the human mind, leading it to achieve transpersonal states of consciousness. In its original sense philosophy is a mental discipline for leading a person to enlightenment. In modern times this lofty notion of philosophy has come to be regarded as unscientific speculation or even as an opinion or belief of one person or group versus another. Specifically, we will look at Christianity as a philosophy of psychological transformation.

"Never forget, the words are not the reality, only reality is reality; picture symbols are the idea, words are confusion."[I]

"The Self {ultimate reality} is not known through study of scriptures, nor through subtlety of the intellect, nor through much learning; but by him who longs for it is it known."[II]

One caveat which any true philosophy must follow is the understanding that words in themselves cannot capture the ultimate essence of reality. Words can be a trap to the highly developed intellect. Therefore, we must always keep in mind that words and philosophical discourse can only point the way to the truth. In order to discover the truth we must go beyond all words, all thoughts, and all of our mental concepts and philosophies because the truth, as *Hermetic* and *Vedanta* philosophy would say, can only be experienced; it cannot be encapsulated in any way, shape or form.

The study of philosophy in its highest form is to assist the student in understanding his/her own mind in order to be able to transcend it, and thus, experience the "transcendental" reality which lies beyond words, thoughts, concepts and mental notions. Mental conceptions are based on our own worldly experiences. They help us to understand the world as the senses perceive it. However, clinging to these experiences as the only reality precludes our discovery of other forms of reality or existence which lies beyond the capacity of the senses. A dog's olfactory sense and the vision of a hawk are much superior to that of the human being. The world of a dog or hawk is much different because they have an expanded range of sensitivity in their senses. Human beings use instruments such as telescopes and microscopes to expand the capability of the senses, but these are also limited and cannot capture reality as it truly is. If the human senses cannot even perceive the atoms which scientists tell us comprise all material objects in creation, how can they be expected to perceive that which is even subtler than the atom, the Spirit of God?

> 1. In the beginning God created the heaven and the earth.
> 2 And the earth was without form, and void; and darkness [was] upon the face of the deep. And
> the Spirit of God moved upon the face of the waters.

However, the human has one advantage which is superior to all senses and scientific instruments, the intuitional mind when it is purified by the practice of Yoga philosophy and disciplines. Ancient mystical philosophical systems have as their main goal the destruction of the limited concepts and illusions of the mind. In essence, the philosophies related to understanding nature and a human being's place in it were the first disciplines which practiced what would today be called Transpersonal Psychology, that is, a system of psychology which assists us in going beyond the personal or ego-based aspects of the psyche in order to discover what lies beyond (trans) the personal (relating to the personality).

> 1. Let him who seeks go on seeking until he finds. When he finds he will become astonished {troubled}. When he becomes troubled, he will be awed and he will reign over the universe {all}.

> 98. He who seeks will find and whomever knocks will be let in.
>
> —Gospel of Thomas

Metaphysics

Metaphysics is the branch of philosophy that systematically investigates first causes of nature, the universe and ultimate reality. The term comes from the Greek "*meta physika*," meaning "after the things of nature." In Aristotle's

---

[I] Hermetic proverb.

[II] Mystery religions based on the Egyptian mysteries of Isis and Osiris and those of Buddha and Krishna (India).

works, he envisioned that the first philosophy came after the physics. Metaphysics has been divided into *ontology*, or the study of the essence of being or that which is or exists, and *cosmology*, the study of the structure and laws of the universe and the manner of its creation. From time immemorial, philosophers, such as those who wrote the Ancient Egyptian Creation myths, to Greek philosophers such as Plato and Aristotle, to more modern philosophers such as Whitehead and Kant, have written on metaphysics. Skeptics, however, have charged that speculation which cannot be verified by objective evidence is useless. However, these skeptics do not realize that what they consider as "objective reality" is not objective at all, since objectivity is based on the perceptions of the senses, and as just discussed, modern science itself has proven that the human senses cannot perceive the phenomenal universe as it really is. Further, the objective information that can be gathered by scientific instruments is only valid under certain conditions. This makes it relative and not absolute information. Thus, what people ordinarily consider to be real and abiding is not. Einstein's proof of relativity confirms this. There must be something real beyond the phenomenal world which sustains it. The search for that higher essence is the purpose of philosophy and metaphysics. Therefore, the value of metaphysical and mystical philosophy studies is evident.

Psychology

Psychology, as used by ordinary practitioners of society, has been defined as the study of the thought processes characteristic of an individual or group (mind, psyche, ethos, mentality). In this work we will focus on Christianity as a psychological discipline for understanding the human mind, its source, higher development and transformation. However, Mystical Psychology in reality does not relate only to the mind since a human being is composed of several complex aspects. The term personality, as it is used in Yoga, implies mind, body and spirit, as well as the conscious, subconscious and unconscious aspects of the mind. Therefore, the discipline of psychology must be expanded to include physical as well as spiritual dimensions. Once again, modern medical science has, within the last twenty years, acknowledged the understanding that health cannot be treated as a physical problem only, but as one which involves the mind, body and spirit. Likewise, spiritual teaching must be related as a discipline which involves not only the soul of an individual, but the mind and body as well – in other words, the entire human being.

Yoga

The literal meaning of the word Yoga is to *"yoke"* or to *"link"* back. The implication is to link back individual consciousness (human personality) to its original source, the original essence: Universal Consciousness. In a broad sense Yoga is any process which helps one to achieve liberation or freedom from bondage to the pain and spiritual ignorance of ordinary human existence. So whenever you engage in any activity with the goal of promoting the discovery of your true Self, be it studying the spiritual wisdom teachings, exercising, fasting, meditation, breath control, rituals, chanting, prayer, etc., you are practicing yoga. If the goal is to help you to discover your essential nature as one with God or the Supreme Being, Consciousness, then it is Yoga.

Yoga (Sanskrit for "union") is a term used for a number of disciplines, the goal of each being to lead the practitioner to attain union with Universal Consciousness. Present day Yoga philosophy is based on several Indian texts such as the *Upanishads, Bhagavad Gita* and the *Yoga-sutras* of Patañjali and several other Yoga treatises developed in India. The practice of Yoga generally involves meditation, moral restraints, and the awakening of energy centers (in the body) through specific postures (asanas) or physical exercises and breathing exercises. All Yoga disciplines are devoted to freeing the soul or individual self from worldly (mental) restraints. They have become popular in the West as a means of self-control and relaxation.

Yoga, in all of its forms as the disciplines for spiritual development, was practiced in Ancient Egypt earlier than anywhere else in history. From here the teachings of Ancient Egyptian Religion and Yoga influenced the development of Christianity and other religions which survive to this day. The disciplines of Yoga fall under five major categories. These are: *Yoga of Wisdom, Yoga of Devotional Love, Yoga of Meditation, Tantric Yoga* and *Yoga of Selfless Action.* Within these categories there are subsidiary forms which are part of the main disciplines. The important point to remember is that all aspects of yoga can and should be used in an integral fashion to effect an efficient and harmonized spiritual movement in the practitioner. Therefore, while there may be an area of special interest to a person, other elements are bound to become part of the yoga program as needed. For example, while a yogin (practitioner of Yoga) may place emphasis on the yoga of wisdom, they may also practice devotional yoga and meditation yoga along with the wisdom studies.

While it is true that yogic practices may be found in religion, strictly speaking, yoga is neither a religion or a philosophy. It should be thought of more as a way of life or discipline for promoting greater fullness and experience of life, physically, mentally and spiritually. Yoga was developed at the dawn of history by those who wanted more out of life. These special men and women wanted to discover the true origins of creation and of themselves.

Therefore, they set out to explore the vast reaches of consciousness within themselves. They are sometimes referred to as "Seers," "Sages," "Saints," etc. Awareness or consciousness can only be increased when the mind is in a state of peace and harmony. Thus, the disciplines of devotion to the higher Self, meditation, right action and study of the wisdom teachings (which are all part of Yoga) are the primary means to controlling the mind and allowing the individual to mature psychologically and spiritually.

Religion

All religions tend to be deistic at the elementary levels. Most often it manifests as an outgrowth of the cultural concepts of a people as they try to express the deeper feeling which they perceive, though not in its entirety. Thus, deism is based on limited spiritual knowledge. Deism, as a religious belief or form of theism, holds that God's action was restricted to an initial act of creation, after which he retired (separated) to contemplate the majesty of his work. Deists hold that the natural creation is regulated by laws put in place by God at the time of creation and inscribed with perfect moral principles. A deeper study of religion will reveal that in its original understanding, it seeks to reveal the deeper essential nature of creation, the human heart and their relation to God, which transcends the deistic model or doctrine. The term religion comes from the Latin *"Relegare"* which uses the word roots *"Re"* which means *"Back"* and *"Ligon"* which means *"to hold, to link, to bind."* Therefore, the essence of true religion is the same as yoga, that is, of linking back, specifically, linking the soul of its follower back to its original source: God. So, although religion in its purest form is a Yoga system, incorporating the yoga disciplines within its teachings, the original intent and meaning of the religious scriptures are often misunderstood, if not distorted. This occurs because religions have developed in different geographic areas. As a result, the lower levels of religion which are mixed with culture (historical accounts, stories and traditions) have developed independently, and thereby appear to be different from each other on the surface. This leads to confusion and animosity among people who are ignorant of the true process of religious movement. Religion consists of three levels: *myth, ritual and mystical experience*. If the first two levels are misunderstood or accepted literally, the spiritual movement will fail to proceed to the next higher level. In order for a religious experience to lead one to have a mystical experience, all three levels of religion must be completed. This process will be fully explained throughout the text of this volume.

Mysticism

Mysticism is a spiritual discipline for attaining union with the Divine through the practice of deep meditation or contemplation, and other spiritual disciplines such as austerity, detachment, renunciation, etc. In this aspect, Mysticism and Yoga are synonymous.

Dualism

Similar to Deism, Dualism is the belief that all things in nature are separate and real, and that they exist independently from any underlying essence or support. It is the belief in the pairs of opposites wherein everything has a polar counterpart. For example: male - female, here - there, hot - cold, etc. While these elements seem real and abiding to the human mind, mystical philosophers throughout history have been claiming that this is only an outer expression of the underlying essence from which they originate. In reality, the underlying essence of all things is non-dual and all-encompassing. It is the substratum of all that exists. Modern science has been confirming this view of matter. The latest experiments in quantum physics show that all matter is composed of energy. Most importantly for this study, dualism is a state of mind that occurs at an immature level of mental understanding of reality. It is akin to egoism and egoistic tendencies which tend to make a person see himself/herself as separate and distinct from the world and from other living beings. Through the study and practice of mystical spiritual teachings, dualism is replaced with non-dualism and salvation, spiritual enlightenment, then occurs. Therefore, salvation or resurrection is related to a non-dualistic view of existence and bondage and death are related to dualism and egoism.

A dualistic view of life can lead to agitation, suffering and even catastrophic events in human experience because the mind is trained to see either good or evil, acceptable or unacceptable, you or me, etc., and not the whole of creation composed of many parts. In the dualistic state of mind, the attitudes of separation and exclusivism are exaggerated. These render the mind agitated. Mental agitation prevents the mind from achieving greater insights into the depths of spiritual teachings. Thus, agitated people are usually frustrated and unable to discover inner peace and spiritual fulfillment.

When societal institutions such as the church rationalize and even sanction dualism, then egoistic sentiments hold sway over the heart of human beings. In this sense, dualism and egoism go hand in hand. When universal love and humility are replaced by egoism and arrogance, then it becomes possible to hurt others and to hurt nature. When we forget our common origin and destiny, we easily fall into the vast pit of egoism. We see ourselves as an individual in a world of individuals, fighting a battle of survival for wealth in order to gain pleasures of the senses, rather than

34

seeing ourselves as divine beings who are made in the same image, with the same frailties and potential. This degraded condition opens the doors to the deep-rooted fears and sense of inadequacy which translate into anger, resentment, hatred, greed and all negative tendencies in the human personality. The concept of dualism is the basis of the atrocities and injustices that have been committed in the history of the world. Under its control, human beings seek to control others and nature, and to satisfy their inner urges through violence because they cannot control themselves and express their deeper needs in constructive ways. In the Indian Vedantic tradition, duality or *dvaita* is seen as the greatest error of the human mind. For this reason all of the disciplines of Vedanta, Shetaut Neter, Yoga, Buddhism, Taoism and other forms of creation-centered spirituality are directed toward developing a correct understanding of human existence. When the underlying unity behind the duality is discovered, there can be no violence or ill will against others. This is the basis of non-violence. Harmony and spiritual enlightenment then arise spontaneously. Egoism now gives way to universal love and peace.

Spiritual Transformation

Transformation here is to be understood as not merely a change in specific behavior patterns or a change in feeling based on temporary circumstances, but as a complete re-orientation of the psychology of the individual. This re-orientation will lead to a permanent improvement in behavior and genuine metamorphosis of the innermost levels of the mind. Specifically, we will focus on Christianity as a system for psychological transformation wherein the individual ceases to be a limited individual, subject to the foibles and follies of human nature, and attains the state of transcendence of these failings.

Mythology

Most people hold the opinion that mythology is a lie, an illusion, fiction or fantasy. Mythology can be best understood as a language. However, it is a unique kind of language. An ordinary language is sometimes similar to another because it is a part of a family of languages. For example, Italian and Spanish words are similar. This similarity makes it possible for a person whose native language is Spanish to understand the meanings of some Italian words and somewhat follow along a conversation in Italian. Even so, mythology is much more intelligible than this. Mythology is more akin to music in its universality. If the key elements of this language of mythology are well understood, then it is possible to understand and relate any mythological system to another and thereby gain the understanding of the message being imparted.

Enlightenment

Enlightenment is the central topic of our study and the coveted goal of all practitioners of Yoga and Religion. Enlightenment is the term used to describe the highest level of spiritual awakening. It means attaining such a level of spiritual awareness that one discovers the underlying unity of the entire universe as well as the fact that the source of all creation is the same source from which the innermost Self within every human heart arises.

All forms of spiritual practice are directed toward the goal of assisting every individual to discover the true essence of the universe both externally, in physical creation, and internally, within the human heart, as the very root of human consciousness. Thus, many terms are used to describe the attainment of the goal of spiritual knowledge and the eradication of spiritual ignorance. Some of these terms are: *Enlightenment, Resurrection, Salvation, The Kingdom of Heaven, Christ Consciousness, Cosmic Consciousness, Moksha or Liberation, Buddha Consciousness, One With The Tao, Self-realization, Know Thyself, Horushood, Nirvana, Sema, Yoga,* etc.

Yoga Philosophy and the World Religious Philosophies Defined

Yoga philosophy and disciplines have developed independently as well as in conjunction with religious philosophies. It may be accurate to say that Yoga is a science unto itself which religions have used and incorporated into their religious philosophies and practices by relating the yogic principles to symbols such as deities, gods, goddesses, angels, saints, etc. The following is a brief description of yoga philosophy in comparison to the philosophies which developed along side it.

Yoga Philosophy[64]

Human consciousness and universal consciousness are in reality one and the same. The appearance of separation is a mental illusion. Yoga is the mystical and mindful (thoughtful, aware, observant) union of individual and universal consciousness by integrating the aspects of individual personality, thereby allowing the personality to be purified so that it may behold its true essence.

Monotheism[84]

Monotheism means the belief in the existence of a single God in the universe. Christianity, Judaism, and Islam are the major monotheistic religions. It must be noted here that the form of monotheism espoused by the major Western religions is that of an exclusive, personified deity who exists in fact and is separate from creation. In contrast, the monotheism of Ancient Egyptian, Hindu and Gnostic Christian traditions envisions a single Supreme Deity that is expressed as the Supreme Deity of all other traditions, as well as the phenomenal world. It is not exclusive, but universal.

Polytheism[84]

Polytheism means the belief in or worship of many gods. Such gods usually have specific attributes or functions.

Totemism[123]

Totemism is the belief in the idea that there is a relationship between kinship groups and specific animals and plants. Many scholars believe that religions which use these symbols are primitive because they are seen as worshipping those animals themselves. However, when the mythology behind the beliefs is examined more closely, the totems are understood as symbols of specific tutelary deities which relate the individuals to a group, but also to the greater workings of nature, and ultimately, to God.

Pantheism[84]

1- Absolute Pantheism: Everything there is, is God. God and Creation are one.
2- Modified Pantheism: God is the reality or principle behind nature.

Panentheism[66]

Term coined by KC F. Krause (1781-1832) to describe the doctrine that God is immanent in all things but also transcendent, so that every part of the universe has its existence in God, but He is more than the sum total of the parts.

Shetaut Neter: Ancient Egyptian Philosophy - Egyptian Yoga[64]

1-Monotheistic Polytheism - Ancient Egyptian religion encompasses a single and absolute Supreme Deity that expresses as the cosmic forces (gods and goddesses), human beings and nature.

Hinduism and Mahayana Buddhism

1-Monotheistic Polytheism.

Vedanta Philosophy[84]

1- Absolute Monism: Only God is reality. All else is imagination.
2- Modified Monism: God is to nature as soul is to body.

While on the surface it seems that there are many differences between the philosophies, upon closer reflection there is only one major division, that of belief or non-belief. Among the believers there are differences of opinion as to how to believe. This is the source of all the trouble between religions. This is because ordinary religion is deistic, based on traditions and customs which are themselves based on culture, as we saw earlier. Since culture varies from place to place and from one time in history to another, there will always be some variation in spiritual traditions. These differences will occur not only between cultures, but even within the same culture. An example of this is Christianity with its myriad of denominations.

Therefore, those who cling to the idea that religion has to be related to a particular culture and its specific practices or rituals will always have some difference with someone else's conception. There are three stages of religion, Myth, Ritual and Mystical. Culture belongs to the myth stage of religious practice, the most elementary level.

Myth ➙ Ritual ➙ Mysticism

An important theme, which will be developed throughout this volume, is the complete practice of religion. In its complete form, religion is composed of three aspects, *mythology, ritual* and *metaphysical* or the *mystical experience* (mysticism - mystical philosophy). At the first level a human being learns the stories and traditions of the religion. At the second level rituals are learned and practiced. At the third level a spiritual aspirant is led to actually go beyond myths and rituals and to attain the ultimate goal of religion. This is an important principle because many religions present different aspects of philosophy at different levels and an uninformed onlooker may label it as primitive or idolatrous, etc., without understanding what is going on. For example, Hinduism and Ancient Egyptian Religion present polytheism and duality at the first two levels of religious practice. However, at the third level, mysticism, the practitioner is made to understand that all of the gods and goddesses being worshipped do not exist in fact but are in reality aspects of the single, transcendental Supreme Self.

In the area of Yoga Philosophy and the category of Monism, there are little, if any, differences. This is because these disciplines belong to the third level of religion wherein mysticism reaches its height. The goal of all mysticism is to transcend the phenomenal world and all mental concepts. Ordinary religion is a part of the world and the mental concepts of people, and must too be ultimately transcended.

Selected Spiritual Philosophies Compared

The Sages of ancient times created philosophies through which it might be possible to explain the origins of creation, as we saw above. Then they set out to create disciplines which could lead a person to discover for themselves the spiritual truths of life and thereby realize the higher reality which lies beyond the phenomenal world. These disciplines are referred to as religions and spiritual philosophies (mysticism-yoga). Below is a basic listing of world religious and spiritual philosophies.

RELIGIOUS PHILOSOPHIES				
Shetaut Neter	**Vedanta**	**Samkhya**	**Buddhism**	**Yoga**
Non-dualist metaphysics. God manifests as nature and cosmic forces (neteru). Union with the Divine through wisdom, devotion and identification with the Divine.	Non-dualist metaphysics. God alone exists. Union with the Divine through wisdom, devotion and identification with the Divine.	Dualist Philosophy. Discipline of understanding what is real (God) from what is unreal (transient world of time and space).	Union with the Absolute through extinction of desire.	Mystical tradition: union of individual consciousness with the Absolute Consciousness (God) through cessation of mental activity by wisdom, devotion and identification with the Divine. Example ↓ Egyptian Yoga Indian Yoga Christian Yoga Buddhist Yoga Chinese (Taoist) Yoga

RELIGIOUS CATEGORIES				
Theism	*Atheism*	*Ethicism*	*Ritualism*	*Monism*
Belief in a God which will save you.	Salvation by doing what makes you happy. There is no God, only existence, which just happened on its own without any help.	Salvation by performing the right actions.	Salvation by performing the correct rituals.	Salvation by understanding that all is the Self (God).
↓	↓	↓	↓	↓
Example	Example	Example	Example	Example
Orthodox Christian Orthodox Islam Orthodox Judaism	Epicureans Charvacas Atheists Existentialists Stoics Humanists	Zoroastrianism Jainism Confucianism Aristotelianism	Brahmanism Priestcraft	Taoism Spinoza Cabalism Sufism Idealism Christian Science Gnosticism Gnostic Christian Vedanta Shetaut Neter Buddhism

CHAPTER 1 THE ORIGINS OF CREATION, HUMANITY, RELIGION AND YOGA PHILOSOPHY

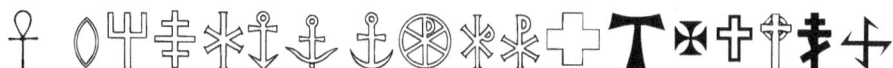

THE ORIGINS OF HUMANKIND

n order to begin our journey of discovery into mystical spirituality, we will need a reference point. Science offers a useful reference point to understand the origins of life classifying the evolution of human life on earth. However, as we will see, science does not provide all of the answers about history. Therefore, we will eventually need to move beyond the confining ideas of evolution and scientific thinking. The Stone Age is a period that is regarded as being early in the development of human cultures. The Stone Age refers to the period before the use of metals. The artifacts used by people as tools and weapons were made of stone. The dates given for the Stone Age differ greatly for different parts of the world due to varying rates of development among societies and also due to the limitations of science. In Europe, Asia, and Africa, it is thought to have begun about two million years ago and to have ended in most parts of Northeast Africa (Ancient Egypt), Southwest Asia (Middle East) and Southeast Asia, by about 6000 B.C.E. It is also thought to have lingered in Europe, the rest of Asia, and other parts of Africa until 4,000 B.C.E. or later. However, the remarkable new evidence surrounding the Ancient Egyptian Sphinx shows that Ancient Egypt has a much older history than was previously thought and therefore, did not experience the ages of time as did the rest of the world. The Stone Age has been divided into three periods: Paleolithic, Mesolithic, and Neolithic.

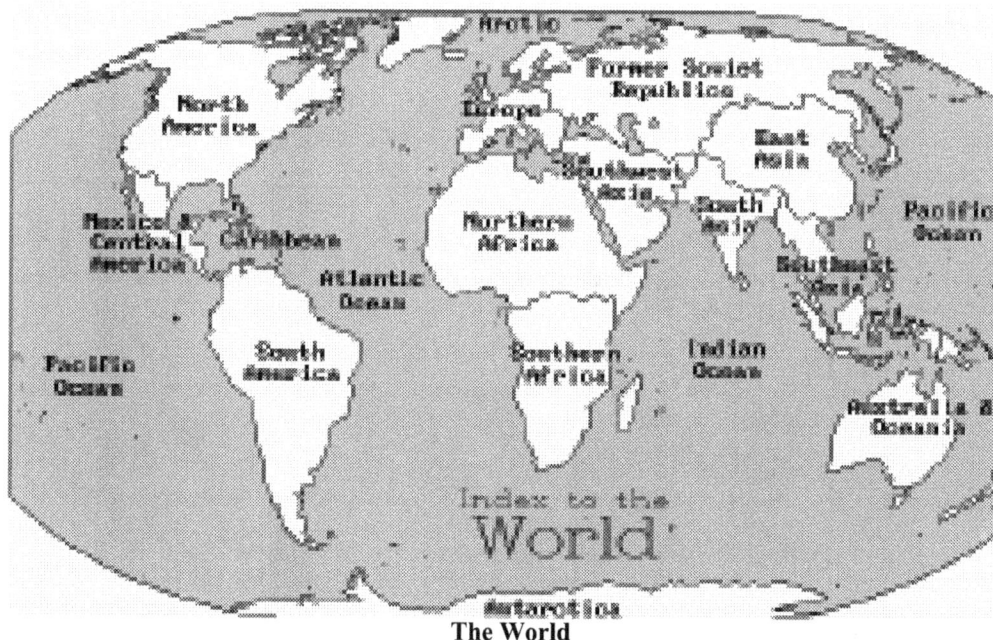

The World

The Paleolithic Age lasted from two million years ago to the end of the last ice age, which was about 13,000 B.C.E. Agricultural villages began to develop by the year 8,000 B.C.E. By the year 6,000 B.C.E. pottery began to appear in the regions of the ancient Middle East, and the use of copper began for the first time in some regions. The Mesolithic or Middle Stone Age followed the Paleolithic Age. It is thought to have begun about 10,000 B.C.E. in Europe. In the Neolithic Age or New Stone Age which followed the Mesolithic Age, human beings first lived in settled villages, bred and domesticated animals, cultivated grain crops, and practiced pottery, flint-mining, and weaving.

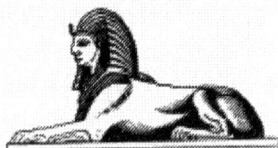

The Ancient Egyptian *Horemakhet* (Sphinx)

The theories about the origins of humanity are not firm because much of the evidence of the evolutionary development of human beings has been swept away by the active nature of the planet. Volcanoes, storms, floods, etc., eventually wipe away all remnants of everything that happens on the surface of the earth as they recycle matter to bring forth life sustaining conditions again. For example, the city of Rome was buried in several feet of dust, ash and other natural particles, which eventually claim the surface of the earth through the action of wind and other natural phenomena of weather. Further, new scientific evidence compels scientists to revise their estimates to account for the new findings. One important example in this area relates to the Ancient Egyptian Sphinx, in the area today known as Giza, in Egypt. The Great Sphinx was once known as *Horemakhet* or "Heru in the Horizon." It was later known by the Greeks as Harmachis. New discoveries show the Ancient Egyptian Sphinx to be much older than previously thought. The importance of this discovery is that it places advanced civilization first in northeast Africa (Ancient Egypt), at the time when Europe, Mesopotamia[I] and the rest of Asia were just coming out of the Paleolithic Age. Thus, when Ancient Egypt had already created the Sphinx, the Temple complexes and the Great Pyramids, the rest of the world was just beginning to learn how to practice farming and to use sleds, boats and other elementary instruments which were just being invented there. The new findings related to the Sphinx, which are supported by many ancient writings, are leading us to realize the true depths of human origins and the starting point for civilization. This means that we must begin to open up to expand our present concepts of reality, history and religion beyond the limitations of antiquated beliefs in order to discover the secrets of existence. Mystical philosophy and religion are the disciplines that will show us the true origin and destiny of humankind. This is the ultimate purpose of Christian Yoga.

THE ANCIENT CREATION MYTHS

The creation stories of Ancient Egypt, the Bible, Cabalism (Jewish Mysticism) and the Hindu-Vedantic tradition are remarkably similar in the notion of the existence of a primeval formlessness which subsequently gave rise to different forms resulting in the differentiation and objectification of matter.

Ancient Egyptian Shabaka Inscription:

"Ptah conceived in his heart (reasoning consciousness) all that would exist and at his utterance (the word - will, power to make manifest), created Nun, the primeval waters (unformed matter-energy).

Then, not having a place to sit Ptah causes Nun to emerge from the primeval waters as the Primeval Hill so that he may have a place to sit. Atom (Atum) then emerges and sits upon Ptah. Then came out of the waters four pairs of Gods, the Ogdoad (eight Gods)...

In the Ancient Egyptian creation story involving the Ausarian Mysteries, The Supreme Being (Nebertcher, Neberdjer) assumes the role of Asar and creates the universe in the form of Khepra (Khepera) and Tem:

"Neb-er-tcher saith, I am the creator of what hath come into being, and I myself came into being under the form of the god Khepra (Khepera), and I came into being in primeval time. I had union with my hand, and I embraced my shadow in a love embrace; I poured seed into my own mouth, and I sent forth from myself issue in the form of the gods Shu (air) and Tefnut (moisture)."

"I came into being in the form of Khepera, and I was the creator of what came into being, I formed myself out of the primeval matter, and I formed myself in the primeval matter. My name is Ausares (Asar).

I was alone, for the gods were not yet born, and I had emitted from myself neither Shu nor Tefnut. I brought into my own mouth, *hekau* (utterance – the word), and I forthwith came into being under the form of things which were created under the form of Khepera."

[I] Mesopotamia (from a Greek term meaning "between rivers") lies between the Tigris and Euphrates rivers, a region that is part of modern Iraq[75]

Genesis 1 (Bible)
> 1. In the beginning God created the heaven and the earth.
> 2 And the earth was without form, and void; and darkness [was] upon the face of the deep. And the Spirit of God moved upon the face of the waters.

From the Sepher (Sefir) Yezirah (Cabalism):
> These are the ten spheres of existence, which came out of nothing. From the spirit of the Living God emanated air, from the air water, from the water, fire or ether, from the ether, the height and the depth, the East and the West, the North and the South.

From the Zohar (Cabalism):
> Before God manifested Himself, when all things were still hidden in him... He began by forming an imperceptible point; this was His own thought. With this thought He then began to construct a mysterious and holy form...the Universe.

From the Laws of Manu (Indian):
> Manu is a Sage-Creator God of Indian Hindu-Vedic tradition who recounts the process of Creation wherein the *Self Existent Spirit* (God) felt desire. Wishing to create all things from his own body, God created the primeval waters (Nara) and threw a seed into it. From the seed came the golden cosmic egg. The Self-Existent Spirit (Narayana) developed in the egg into Brahma (Purusha, God) and after a year of meditation, divided into two parts (male and female).

The Forms of Creation

When we think of our body, we don't differentiate between the lips and the face, or the fingers and the arm, etc. In a mysterious way we consider all of the parts as a whole and call this "me" or "my body." In the same way, in the state of Enlightenment, Christhood (Horushood, Buddhahood, etc.), the entire universe is understood as "me." This is the state wherein the Kingdom of Heaven is experienced. A psychological understanding of consciousness in terms of Christian Gnostic philosophy would render Jesus as the ego within us and Christ as the underlying source of consciousness, which supports and transcends the ego. Thus, Jesus' journey was to go from being Jesus, an ordinary human being, to Christ, a human being who is aware of the grander reality beyond the body and is one with God. The attainment of his Christhood occurred as a result of his movement towards enlightenment through his practices of Yoga. This is what is supposed to be the goal of every Christian, to become Christlike while alive by following the teachings of Jesus Christ (Christian Yoga). The consciousness of every human being is essentially pure, deep down (Christlike), until the mind associates with the ego. Then the Christ Consciousness becomes submerged. When this occurs, multiplicity and duality appear to exist, but as the following Cabalistic passage explains, the multiplicity of creation is merely the forms which energy takes on as it moves and interacts in different polarities or the pairs of opposites. This same concept of vibrations being the underlying cause of the phenomenal world existed prior to Cabalism within the Shabaka Inscription (above) and the Ancient Egyptian metaphysical text, *Kybalion* (below). This teaching is equivalent to the concept of *Ying and Yang* of Taoism which holds that Creation is composed of two opposite but complementary forces which balance each other and form a transcendental harmony.

From the Kabbalah (Cabala):
> Polarity is the principle that runs through the whole of creation, and is in fact, the basis of manifestation. Polarity really means the flowing of force from a sphere of high pressure to a sphere of low pressure, high and low being always relative terms. Every sphere of energy needs to receive the stimulus of an influx of energy at higher pressure, and to have an output into a sphere of lower pressure. The source of all energy is the Great Unmanifest (God), and it makes its own way down the levels, changing its form from one to the other, till it is finally "earthed" in matter.
>
> The pure impulse of dynamic creation is formless; and being formless, the creation it gives rise to can assume any and every form.

The following passage comes from *Lao-Tzu*, the classical Taoist writer who popularized Taoism in China at the same time that *Buddha* and *Mahavira* developed Buddhism and Jainism in India, respectively. He further illustrates the idea of undifferentiated versus differentiated consciousness.

There was something undifferentiated and yet complete, which existed before heaven and earth.
Soundless and formless, it depends on nothing and does not change.
It operates everywhere and is free from danger.
It may be considered the mother of the universe.

The same idea of *"formlessness"* or *"undifferentiated"* matter occurs in the *Rig* (Rik) *Veda*, the Upanishads and the Bhagavad Gita from India as well. The only difference between the following texts is that the Gita applies all of the attributes of the manifest and unmanifest nature of divinity and incorporates them in the anthropomorphic personality of Krishna.

From the Rig Veda:
There was neither non-existence nor existence then; there was neither the realm of space nor the sky beyond.
There was no distinguishing sign of night nor of day...
Desire came upon that one in the beginning; that was the first seed of mind.

From the Upanishads:
 There are, assuredly, two forms of the Eternal: the formed and the formless, the mortal and the immortal, the
    stationary and the moving, the actual and the yon (that one or those yonder).

Gita: Chapter 9:17
 I am the Father of the universe; I am the Mother, the sustainer, as well as the Grandfather. I am the goal of
 Vedic knowledge, I am the sacred Om, and I am verily the Vedas in the form of Rik, Yaju and Sama.

The following passages from the Kybalion, an Ancient Egyptian metaphysical text, contain the same idea of energy in different levels of manifestation and show how this knowledge may be applied to control one's mind:

"To change your mood or mental state, change your vibration."
"Mastery of self consists not in abnormal dreams, visions and fantastic imaginings or living, but in using the higher forces against the lower thus escaping the pains of the lower by vibrating on the higher."
"Mind, as matter, may be transmuted from state to state, degree to degree, condition to condition, pole to pole; and vibration to vibration. Transmutation is a Mental Art."
"To destroy an undesirable rate of mental vibration, concentrate on the opposite vibration to the one to be suppressed."
"The wise ones serve the higher planes and rule the lower, in this way one operates the laws instead being a slave to them."
"Those who may come to understand the law of vibrations will hold the scepter of power in their hand."
"Nothing rests, everything moves; everything vibrates."
"Gender is in everything; everything has its Masculine and Feminine Principles; Gender manifests on all planes."
"Everything is dual; everything has poles; everything has its pair of opposites; like and unlike are the same; opposites are identical in nature, but different in degree; extremes meet; all truths are but half- truths; all paradoxes may be reconciled."
"Everything flows out and in; everything has its tides; all things rise and fall; the pendulum-swing manifests in everything; the measure of the swing to the right is the measure to the left; rhythm compensates."
"Every cause has its Effect; every Effect has its Cause; everything happens according to Law; Chance is a name for Law unrecognized; there are many planes of causation, but nothing escapes the Law."

THE COMMON ANCESTRY OF HUMANITY ACCORDING TO THE BIBLE AND THE MYTH OF RACE AND RACISM

The Bible explains the most important question of humanity, where the world came from. This knowledge provides a reference point to understand how everything came into existence. The next question is more profound. When you look around you see a world of multiplicity and seemingly endless variety, how did this come about and why is it so? This question and its misunderstanding has been the greatest cause of strife among people throughout history, because people also see themselves as they see nature, as separate and different elements in competition for survival. However, an in depth study of the Bible reveals the answers to the most divisive issue of modern times, the question of race, the origin of humanity and the relationship between all human beings.

Acts 17

26 And hath made of one blood all nations of men to dwell on all the face of the earth, and hath determined the times before appointed, and the bounds of their habitation...

There are some very important Bible texts found in the books of Acts and Corinthians, which illuminate and clarify the question of race. In Acts 17: 26 we are told that God made only one blood out of which all nations emerged (Nations: i.e. Africans, Europeans, Asiatics, Native Americans, etc.). This means that all human beings share one common physiology, that there is no difference between human beings from different parts of the world. According to Strong's Concordance of ancient Hebrew, blood also has a deeper meaning than just the medium which carries oxygen throughout the body. It is the seat of life itself, the essence of life which sustains a human being.

1 Corinthians 15

39 All flesh [is] not the same flesh: but [there is] one [kind of] flesh of men, another flesh of beasts, another of fishes, [and] another of fowls.

1 Corinthians 15

44 It is sown a natural body; it is raised a spiritual body. There is a natural body, and there is a spiritual body.

In 1 Corinthians 15, we learn that all living beings are classified according to their physiology. The word used in the Bible is "flesh." It relates to the outer appearance of a living being as well as the group it belongs to exclusively. The word flesh in the Bible may be likened to the modern term "species." According to the American Heritage Dictionary, species means *1. a. A fundamental category of taxonomic classification consisting of organisms capable of interbreeding. 1. b. an organism belonging to such a category. 2. A kind, variety, or type.* We are to understand that while every species is unique within its own group, there is no such thing as different species within the human populations of the world. All human beings belong to the same flesh, i.e. species. Also, there is no such thing as racial difference within the human population. All human beings can interbreed and produce offspring. All human beings can bleed and feel the same pain. All human beings desire the same thing, happiness. The body of every human being is constructed in basically the same way. Even distinctions based on gender are not reliable for distinguishing human beings. The spirit is beyond the body. This is the lesson from 1 Corinthians 15: 44. So gender is only a superficial difference, as is skin color. Therefore, all human beings are members of one single group, regardless of their physical appearance. It is interesting that all dogs are referred to as dogs regardless of the breed,[1] but some human beings are classified as "different" than others. The fallacy of racial distinctions is self-evident for the discerning and honest student of life and the scriptures of the Bible. This is exactly the same teachings presented in the Ancient Egyptian Hymns of Amun and the Ausarian Resurrection Myth.

"Thou makest the color of the skin of one race to be different from that of another, but however many may be the varieties of mankind, it is thou that makes them all to live."
-Ancient Egyptian Proverb from *The Hymns of Amun*

"Souls, Heru, son, are of the self-same nature, since they came from the same place where the Creator modeled them; nor male nor female are they. Sex is a thing of bodies, not of Souls."
-Ancient Egyptian Proverb from *The Ausarian Resurrection*

Romans 12

3 For, through the grace given to me, I say, to every man that is among you, not to think [of himself] more highly than he ought to think; but to think soberly, according as God hath dealt to every man the measure of faith. {Soberly: Gr. to sobriety}

---

[1] **breed** *n.* **1.** A group of organisms having common ancestors and certain distinguishable characteristics, especially a group within a species developed by artificial selection and maintained by controlled propagation.

4 For as we have many members in one body, and all members have not the same office:
5 So we, [being] many, are one body in Christ, and every one members one of another.

The message of Romans 12: 3-5 is that human beings should not engage in self-important and egoistic acts or thoughts. In light of the other teachings, this would be ridiculous. Egoism is like a spark which can ignite the greatest fires of human conflict if it is not checked before it gets out of control. Ignorance as to the true origins of humanity is the source of strife between nations. Therefore, the study of the teachings along with the insights of modern science pave the way to harmony in society and spiritual enlightenment for every human being. The differences in abilities such as artistic capacity or intellectual capacity cannot be ascribed to groups of people since there are intelligent individuals as well as less intelligent individuals in all ethnic groups. The gifts given to each human being by God are for the purpose of allowing every individual to fulfill their own special mission in life, and to fulfill the needs of the society into which they are born. One individual may need to work as an engineer while another as a storekeeper. Through these tasks they both assist society, and neither should look down on the other. Imagine all the garbage that would pile up in the streets and in your home if there were no garbage persons. It would not serve society well to have everyone be a doctor or an engineer. At the time of death all people go to the grave, the crematorium, etc. Therefore, the higher reality is that a human being needs to affirm the higher essence of life instead of concentrating on the transient and unpredictable occurrences of life. So all human beings, while working in different areas of society, are all the same when it comes to their spiritual essence and destiny. They are part of a single body, a common root and a common fate. If this higher understanding is affirmed, there is no room for ignorance and the destructive ego to have an effect. This should be the higher goal of the church policies and the governments of all countries who claim to follow Christian spiritual or Yogic values. Until this is fulfilled by affirmation in the church doctrines, teachings and community works, the church cannot claim to uphold Christianity in its truest and most powerful form. Indeed, a person who claims to be a Christian but does not uphold these principles cannot in good conscience consider himself or herself to be a follower of Christianity as Jesus and the Sages of the Old and New Testaments conceptualized it. The idea that God created some human beings who are inherently inferior and others who are inherently superior would point to the concept of God as either cruel and evil if this was done purposely, or limited and imperfect if it was done by mistake.

The story of Noah and his three sons has been used by some groups to justify racism. The deeper implication of the story of Noah and his three sons points to a metaphorical interpretation relating to the mystery of life. It closely resembles the Ancient Egyptian teaching of the Trinity. In Ancient Egypt, the idea of the Trinity was used to explain the origins of Creation. Creation arose as God, the singular essence, differentiated into three aspects. The Supreme Self was known as Neberdjer and the three aspects of the Trinity were Amun, Ra and Ptah, symbolizing the three states of human consciousness and that which transcends them. This teaching will be explored in more detail throughout our study of Christian Yoga.

Conclusion: One World, One Humanity, One Destiny

The animosity and hatred of modern times, caused by the ignorance of the true teachings of the Bible, has led to a situation where social problems have rendered practitioners of religion incapable of reaching a higher level of spiritual understanding. Many people in modern society are caught up in the degraded level of disputes and wars in an attempt to support ideas, which are in reality absurd and destructive in reference to the doctrines of religion. Ironically, the inability of leaders in the church, synagogue or secular society to accept the truth about the origins of humanity comes from their fear of losing control over their followers. Now that modern science is showing that all human beings originated from the same source, in Africa, and that racial distinctions are at least questionable and misleading, it means that those who have perpetrated and sustained racism can no longer use science or biblical teachings to support their evil and ignorant designs. They have no leg to stand on. The following exert was taken from Encarta Encyclopedia 1994, and is typical of the modern scientific understanding of the question of human genetics and race issues.

The concept of race has often been misapplied. One of the most telling arguments against classifying people into races is that persons in various cultures have often mistakenly acted as if one race were superior to another. Although, with social disadvantages eliminated, it is possible that one human group or another might have some genetic advantages in response to such factors as climate, altitude, and specific food availability, these differences are small. There are no differences in native intelligence or mental capacity that cannot be explained by environmental circumstances. Rather than using racial classifications to study human variability, anthropologists today define geographic or social groups by geographic or social criteria. They then study the nature of the genetic attributes of these groups and seek to understand the causes of changes in their genetic makeup. Contributed by: Gabriel W. Laser "Races, Classification of," Microsoft (R) Encarta. Copyright (c) 1994

One of the major problems in society and in the church is that the teachings and scientific evidence presented here has not been taught to the world population at large. Most people grow up accepting the ignorance of their parents who received the erroneous information from their own parents, and so on. Racism, sexism and other scourges of society are not genetically transmitted. They are transmitted by ignorant family members who pass on their prejudices and bigotry's to their children, and so on down through the generations. The cycle of ignorance and strife is thus carried on from one generation to another. A child cannot live in a family and believe in a certain way and act in a certain way if the parents do not allow it. In the same way, the masses of people are like children and the church and government leaders are like the parents. If racism, sexism and other injustices exist, it is because the leaders are not making an effort to lead the masses towards truth and righteousness. Leaders lead in three ways, by example, by words and by influence. The values of truth and righteousness must be part of every aspect of teaching, otherwise they are not good leaders and society will go astray. The leaders of society as well as the leaders of the church must make a concerted effort to engage the struggle against misunderstanding and unrighteousness. Then they will be able to lead society to an enlightened way of relating to other ethnic groups and thereby provide real hope of creating harmony in the human community. Through this harmony it would be easier to cope with the struggles of life and thereby achieve a greater insight into the mystical teachings of Christianity or any other religious path. Anger, hatred, greed and animosity have an adverse effect on the mind. Therefore, those who engage in racism as well as those who do not know how to deal with racists will have a much more difficult time in trying to achieve the kind of mental control and peace which is necessary to progress on the spiritual path. The Bible itself speaks out against any and all forms of egoism, and racism is perhaps the most blatant and destructive form of egoism. In Romans 12:3, above, the followers of Christianity are admonished to take control of one's egoistic tendencies and to practice humility instead of thinking of oneself as superior to others. Instead one must learn to look at others as having been given the same spark of divinity and therefore, all human beings deserve equal treatment, love and compassion. This teaching applies directly to those who try to impose themselves on others (racists, sexists, tyrants, capitalists, etc.). Those who have enough courage to face their fears, prejudices and to approach the scriptures with honesty instead of delusions of superiority and greed will discover forgiveness and inner peace, as well as the true meaning of the scriptural teachings.

DNA and The Spirit

DNA is an abbreviation for "Deoxyribonucleic acid." It is a complex giant molecule that contains the information needed for every cell of a living creature to create its physical features (hair, skin, bones, eyes, legs, etc., as well as their texture, coloration, their efficient functioning, etc.). All of this is contained in a chemically coded form. The Life Force of the Soul or Spirit engenders the impetus in the DNA to function. This in turn leads to the creation of the physical aspect of all living beings (human beings, animals, insects, microorganisms, etc.).

The DNA is what determines if two living beings are compatible with each other for the purpose of mating and producing offspring. If they are not compatible, then they are considered to be different species. All human beings are compatible with each other, therefore, they are members of a single species, i.e. one human race.

Therefore, DNA is an instrument of the Spirit, which it uses to create the body and thereby avail itself of physical existence and experiences. According to mystical philosophy, the soul chooses the particular world, country, and family in which to incarnate in order to have the kind of experiences it wants to experience. This is all expressed in the physical plane through the miracle of DNA.[126]

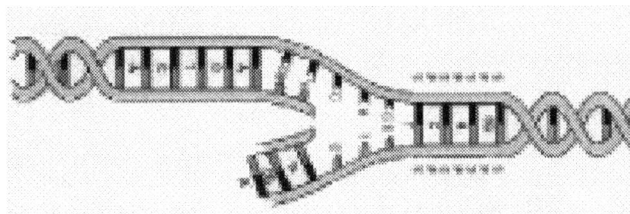

Left: A drawing of a DNA strand.

THE ORIGINS OF PHILOSOPHY

"What is now called the Christian religion has existed among the Ancients and was not absent from the beginning of the human race until Christ came in the flesh from which time the true religion which was already in existence began to be called Christian."

St. Augustine

Saint Augustine (354-430 A.C.E.) was an important Christian theologian and philosopher whose influence helped to shape orthodox Christianity. There are four recognized Christian Fathers of the Latin Church which included *Jerome, Ambrose, Gregory,* and *Augustine.* Of these Augustine is considered to be the greatest. Therefore, his statement is significant in the light of what Christianity became in later years. It is an acknowledgement that Christian philosophy was not new but a reinterpretation of the spiritual wisdom that was already in existence.

The subject of defining knowledge and the nature of existence has been the central issue of the earliest philosophies from around the world. The earliest records of the first civilizations of our time suggest that the prime concerns were of survival, but once this concern was resolved, people were left with the need to understand Creation and their relationship to it. As they observed the movement of the planets and stars they realized that it was possible to predict the movement of heavenly bodies. They related the orderly way of the cosmos to the orderly way of life on earth (plants, animals, elements, etc.) and the orderly factors which govern the existence of humanity and all of nature. In this manner natural laws were studied and understood. Through this study which spanned many thousands of years, certain realizations emerged. The early philosophers discovered that the fundamental laws of existence by which all things in the universe are governed are *Immediate, Universal, Invariable, Evident, Reasonable, Just, Beneficent,* and *Permanent.*[62] Therefore, it was logical to assume that humanity is governed by the very same rules which control every other thing in the universe. So it became important that society should come into harmony with nature in order to not upset the general order of life. They noticed that nothing is destroyed in nature; objects only change form. They observed that all things one day perish, while at the same time life emerges out of death. For example, a new plant grows out of the dead stump of a tree. Animals eat plants and other animals, while mankind eats them all, only to one day die and be swallowed up by the earth in the grave, and then be transformed into earth which provides nutrients for plants, animals and other human beings, in an endless cycle. Thus, they observed that life continually feeds on death in order to exist. Life and death are therefore two sides of the same coin. The early teachers (Sages) of the first places of learning (temples) presented their teachings in a holistic manner. They were careful to maintain the balance in the educational system between the intellectual development and the spiritual evolution of every human being with whom they had contact.

The condition of humanity today is a direct result of the deterioration in values, emphasis on material (intellectual) goals and the denigration of spiritual principles. Teachers and professionals are needed whose inner desire is to help themselves and others learn how to live enriching lives. They need to understand that no academic degrees or material wealth will automatically confer true peace of mind and inner fulfillment (abiding happiness). These spiritual qualities which represent true knowledge and wealth only come from within, from a well-balanced individual. If the lack of ethical values in society is a cause for the absence of self-esteem, inner peace and harmony in its members, then a new form of education, or the rediscovery of a system which worked in the past, along with teachers who are practitioners of virtue and truth, are needed.

In order to provide for the continued development of society and to best serve the needs of humanity as well as themselves, all professionals must be well trained in the psychological aspects of the human being. The psychological and metaphysical implications of religion, the philosophy of human existence, the science of Yoga and modern scientific thought must be mastered. Ancient Mystical philosophy states that greed and moral decay

46

ultimately arise due to the lack of knowledge of one's true spiritual nature (spiritual ignorance). The absence of instruction about who we are and what the universe is creates a void in which negative behavior, greed and a lack of ethics develops. By our own ignorance we either lead ourselves into bad situations in life or leave ourselves open to abuse or control by others who have evil intent.

In ancient Egypt, the entire society was well acquainted with the philosophy of righteous action. It was known as Maat. Maat was seen as the support upon which the society functioned and prospered. The judges and all those connected with the judicial system were initiated into the teachings of Maat. Thus, those who would discharged the laws and regulations of society were well trained in the ethical and spiritual-mystical values of life (presented in this volume), fairness, justice and the responsibility to serve society in order to promote harmony in society and the possibility for spiritual development in an atmosphere of freedom and peace. For only when there is justice and fairness in society can there be an abiding harmony and peace. Harmony and peace are necessary for the pursuit of true happiness and inner fulfillment in life.

This form of education implies the idea of *right thinking* in which life is lived more in accordance with reason, correctness, justice, intuition and truth, rather than for the pursuit of personal gratifications through material gains at any cost. All activities in society should be directed to this lofty but attainable goal. Thus each individual will have an honest possibility to truly become *all that he or she can be* and society will have a real chance to become harmonious and stable.

As the early philosophers progressed in unraveling the secrets of nature, the development of mathematics and writing aided them in their understanding. It enabled the first students of nature to record not only their knowledge about nature, but also their own mental development as they engaged in the contemplation of nature. From here the development of ideas about the inner Self or the Soul emerged as the ancient philosophers began to experience what they called higher forms of consciousness through their practice of spiritual disciplines (meditation, balance of mind, righteousness, reflection on nature, etc.). They observed that beyond the outer forms of nature there is a different existence which defies explanation through any language, because it lies beyond the comprehension of the ordinary person's cognitive ability.

From this understanding there developed a need for a new science or practice which could lead the ordinary human being to live in harmony with nature and to evolve in conscious awareness. The practices of Yoga and Mystical Religion thus emerged.

Ancient Mystical Philosophy

Ancient Mystical Philosophy is the precursor of Religion and Yoga. It is the higher intellectual process which led Sages to question the nature and origin of their existence. Ancient Mystical Philosophy is a way to intellectually understand the process of existence, the reason for life, and the means to master it through intuitional wisdom. In this process of maturing consciousness, intellectual wisdom and knowledge gradually become intuitive.[59] This process leads to greater and greater expansion of the mind and eventually to complete psychological liberation from worldly attachments. Thereby, one achieves a level of psychological experience which is completely peaceful and transcendental. This lofty goal initially inspired Sages and Saints of ancient times to use symbols and myths to express these ideas. Later on whole bodies of mythical literature were developed to further express and elaborate these ideas. This became the basis for religious myths and spiritual scriptures. Eventually they created more detailed literature to intellectually explain the myths and symbols. These came to be known as secret (mystery) writings and holy scriptures. The first of these writings were the Ancient Egyptian hieroglyphs. The following quotation gives us a view from an ancient writer who was a hermetic philosopher in the time of the Ancient Egyptians, Greeks, Romans and early Christians. It illustrates the true goal of philosophy, which is to discover that which is real and transcendental in human experience and not just to possess knowledge of a worldly nature.

"The many do confound philosophy with multifarious reasoning... by mixing it, by means of subtle expositions, with diverse sciences not easy to be grasped such as arithmetic, and music, and geometry. But pure philosophy, which doth depend on Godly piety alone, should only so far occupy itself with other arts, that it may appreciate the working out in numbers of the fore-appointed stations of the stars when they return, and of the course of their procession...know how to appreciate the Earth's dimensions, qualities and quantities, the Water's depths, the strength of

Fire, and the effect and nature of all these...give worship and give praise unto the Art and Mind of God."

A German anthropologist by the name of Adolf Bastian (1826-1905) was one of the first modern researchers to notice that there are recurring themes throughout the varied societies of the world. He called these recurring concepts *"Elementary Ideas."* He further noted that the elementary ideas are manifested in different societies based on their culture and geographic circumstances. He termed these manifestations *"Folk Ideas."* This very idea is present in the statement, *"Truth is One, but Sages speak of it in different ways,"* found in the Indian *Upanishads* (800 BCE).

The main elementary idea which has had a profound effect on humanity as a whole is the understanding of the ultimate reality of existence. The stark difference between the Eastern and Western views on this point has had far reaching effects in the areas of inter-cultural relations and coexistence. Beginning with the Aristotelian thinking (philosophy of Aristotle) from ancient Greece, with its predilection for rational-logical-linear reasoning which was adopted and further developed by Muslim [73] and Western[58] scientists, a definite trend toward discounting other philosophical viewpoints emerged which do not conform to those parameters. It is easy to see how studies which focus on folk differences can conclude that there are various different religious views. Taking it a step further, the mind will develop the idea that one of those ideas must be correct and the others incorrect. An egoistic view will develop with the assumption is that "my" religion is correct and all others are incorrect. However, if it were possible to focus more on the common elementary ideas instead of on the folk differences that separate us, our understanding of the basic function of religion and its universality would emerge. We would even discover that the various differences between religions are only superficial.

Ancient Mystical Philosophy states that "Creation" has not been "Created," that "Creation" is in fact a mental manifestation, and that all mental manifestations are emanations of the Supreme Being. Further, it states that we (our souls) are not only manifestations of the "Creator," but that we are the "Creator"—as the Creator alone exists. With respect to the Roman Catholic interpretation of religion these statements may seem heretical. However, while some Roman Catholic biblical scriptures definitely contradict this ancient model of existence, a detailed study of other biblical scriptures reveal a philosophical view that is similar to Ancient Mystical Philosophy. We will see that not only do these statements make sense in terms of the ancient Christian scriptures of Gnostic Christianity, but the same teachings also appear in the Christian Bible as well in John 10:30, Jesus says he and the Father are one.

In studying Ancient Mystical Philosophy from the Ancient Egyptian and the Far Eastern (India) point of view, life is not at all what we perceive it to be. In fact we will see that we are not who we believe ourselves to be. Indeed we are not individuals, alone in the universe; we are "one" with the Creator. Further, as modern physics studies are confirming, the universe is not really as it appears. What is called inert matter is not inert at all. In fact, the entire phenomenal world is also not what it appears to be. There are other dimensions and other world systems besides our own. In short, anything that can have a name or form is an illusory representation of the true reality whose underlying essence is as modern physics would say, "intelligent energy," or as mystical philosophy would say, "Pure Consciousness, The Self."

With a purified mind attained through the disciplines of Yoga (mystical philosophy), it is possible to transcend the "physical reality" and attain the higher vision of existence, that is, to become Enlightened. As the teachings become "intuitionally" understood, the unconscious is cleansed of the "wrong" thinking to such a degree that a "new" vision is experienced. Those who attain this higher vision will live on in it after the death of the body because they will discover their "real" identity which is immortal and eternal. In the final years of his life, Albert Einstein attempted to construct a mathematical model which showed the universe to be a unified whole. It was called the "Unified Field Theory." This idea evidently emerged from his transcendental mystical experiences which had somehow led him to intuitively "know" the theory of relativity and other important principles by which modern physics is today understood. Einstein admitted having ecstatic mystical experiences where everything, including his body and mind, were united in one whole. Thus, he experienced glimpses of Cosmic Consciousness and stated that spirituality must be affirmed along with science. These are the highest teachings of Ancient Mystical Philosophy. Once their ramifications are truly understood, a new comprehension of life and existence emerges. This means that even though one experiences a feeling of "participating" in the world as an ordinary human being, there is now the possibility that this "world" that has been known all throughout life is not the "Absolute Reality." There is something beyond it. This concept of the Absolute reality is embodied in the idea of *Pa Neter (Pa Ntr)* of the

Ancient Egyptians, *Ntu* of the Yorubas, *Amma* of the Dogon, *Brahman* of Hinduism and Vedanta, the *Tao* of Taoism, the *Dharmakaya* of Buddhism, *The Kingdom of Heaven* of Christianity, *Kether* of the Kabbalah, the *Great Spirit and Quetzalcoatle* of Native Americans, and *Allah* of the Muslims.

The understanding of these teachings allows the mind to be free from craving worldly things and instead to love all things and people equally, since they are all understood to be manifestations of the Creator, the Absolute, one's very Self: Pure Consciousness. Thus, Ancient Mystical Philosophy could have a profound effect on world peace if its study and practice were to become more widespread.

These teachings are the writings of Masters, those who were able to control their minds and bodies in such a way as to ascend to great psychological and psychic heights. Spiritual teaching is usually handed down from teacher to student, in a tradition which spans thousands of years. These teachers or "seers" attained higher levels of communion with Cosmic Intelligence, the Pure Consciousness which underlies all things and then imparted their understanding of this state of consciousness and the means for attaining it to their disciples. Upon realizing this state, these spiritual masters discovered the nature of their own existence and the fact that they, along with the rest of humanity, nature and the universe, are one with that ultimate reality. The Sages realized that even though there are many names and forms in creation, all that can be seen is not only a part of God, the all-encompassing being, but in effect, is God. Nothing else really exists. All is one in God.

The Sages came back from the lofty heights of their achievement to assist others in attaining the beatific visions and the ever-present peace that cannot be disturbed by worldly occurrences. The Sages said that the heights they attained were obtainable by all human beings who possess the desire, will and knowledge to pursue and understand the truth of their inner being. This truth is not in books, but in the innermost heart of every human being.

The teachings are not for everyone, however, since not all humans are spiritually sensitive and psychologically mature enough to control their lower nature (body and ego-mind) and its desires. Many prefer to believe what others who are ignorant have told them or to follow the superficial rituals and traditions which they have learned in church. Others prefer to believe there is nothing beyond ordinary mortal human existence, thinking: *"This is all there is to life and when I die, that will be that."* The Enlightened Sages call this the state of "ignorance."

Those who are beset by ignorance will not discover the deeper essence of Creation because, as we shall see, Creation itself and existence are essentially a mental process. They are based on and sustained by Consciousness. Thus, a person requires intuitional understanding to unravel the mysteries of life. If a person's capacity for intuitional understanding is impaired by ignorance and worldly desires, the mind will not be able to fathom the transcendental vision of Cosmic Consciousness. The mind follows the desires of the heart (unconscious mind). The heart pursues that in which it believes. Therefore, at some point you must begin to desire to become enlightened, otherwise, since the mind survives the death of the body, you will continue to live on from life to life in a continuous state of ignorance, oblivious of your deeper, true nature. Your soul will continue to experience many lifetimes filled with alternating episodes of pleasure and pain, until the desire for worldly experiences is transmuted into spiritual aspiration for self-discovery. They who can control the mind will have a greater opportunity to attain immortality, not of the body, but of the true essence, the ultimate reality that is God: Pure Consciousness, one's deepest Self. When this occurs, then the cycle of birth and death (reincarnation) which is caused by ignorance will be ended for good. Reincarnation was one of the tenets of early Christianity. However in later times this teaching was excluded from the church canon. Though our journey into Christian Yoga we will explore the teachings of reincarnation in more detail as we move forward.

The Purpose of Religion: Religion as a Yoga Philosophy

As one can ascend to the top of a house by means of a ladder or a tree or a staircase or a rope, so diverse is the ways and means to approach God, and every religion in the world shows one of these ways.

—Paramahamsa Ramakrishna (1836-1886)
(Indian Sage)

Religion without myth not only fails to work, it also fails to offer man the promise of unity with the transpersonal and eternal.

THE MYSTICAL JOURNEY FROM JESUS TO CHRIST

—C. G. Jung (1875-1961)
(Western Psychiatrist-Philosopher)

As stated earlier, the term religion comes from the Latin word roots *"RE"* which means *"BACK"* and *"LIGON"* which means *"to hold, to link, to bind."* Therefore, the essence of true religion is that of linking back, specifically, linking its follower's souls back to their original source: God (Supreme Being, Divine Self, The Divine, etc.). Although their souls have come from the universal, all-pervading consciousness, God, human beings have forgotten their origin and therefore wander the earth without knowledge of their true divine nature. Religion is supposed to be a process of assisting men and women to reconnect with the "Creator," God. The human entity (soul) has been deluded into believing that it is composed of a mind and body that will exist for one lifetime. The delusion is believing that when they die, they will cease to exist forever. This is the view held by the majority of Christians today. Some people claim to believe in God and an afterlife, but this belief is shallow due to deep-rooted ignorance. Thus, they are unable to live lives of complete inner peace and harmony based on their belief. Actually, true religious movement is not really a process of re-connection so much as re-membering one's true identity to which one has always been connected. It is like recovering from amnesia.

Although religion in its purest form is a Yoga system, the original intent and meaning of the scriptures are often misunderstood, if not distorted. If religions were devoid of corruption and properly understood and practiced, most would provide a suitable system to bring their followers to spiritual enlightenment. It is a well known fact to religious scholars that the original scriptures of the Western Bible include teachings which closely follow the Ancient Egyptian Mysteries-Yoga system, the Indian philosophical Yoga Vedanta system and the Buddhist philosophical Yoga system. At the Nicean council of Bishops around 325 A.C.E. and later church councils, the doctrine of self-salvation was distorted to the degree that the masses of people were convinced that they needed a savior as a "go between" to reach God. A new religious sect, Orthodox Catholic Christianity, was thus created by the Nicean council under the direction of the Roman Empire, and shortly thereafter the destruction of all other philosophies, religions, and doctrines within the vast Roman Empire was decreed. It was at this time that references to reincarnation and the ability of each individual to become a Christ were either deleted or misrepresented in the biblical scriptures.

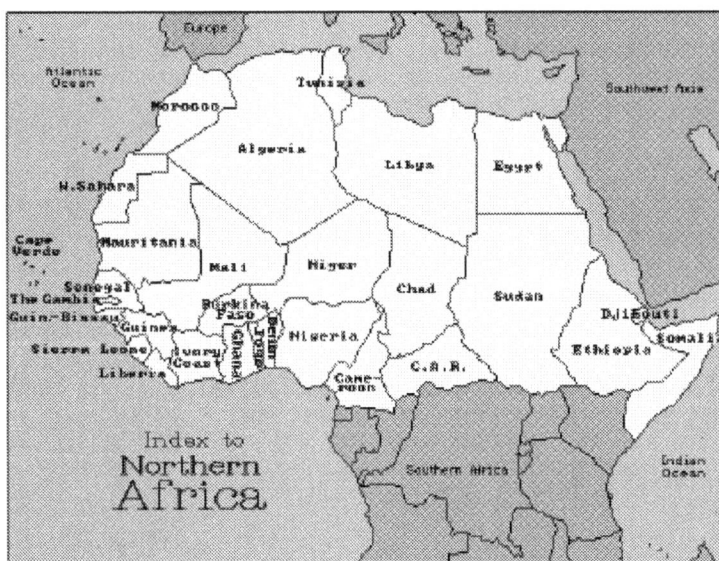

Above: Map of North Africa. Ancient Egypt is located in the northeastern corner of the continent of Africa.

50

CHAPTER II THE ANCIENT EGYPTIAN ORIGINS OF JUDAISM

ANCIENT ORIGINS: WHO WERE THE ANCIENT EGYPTIANS?

hristianity was partly an outgrowth of Judaism, which was itself an outgrowth of Ancient Egyptian culture and religion. So who were the Ancient Egyptians? From the time that the early Greek philosophers set foot on African soil to study the teachings of mystical spirituality in Egypt (900-300 B.C.E.), Western society and culture was forever changed. Ancient Egypt had such a profound effect on Western civilization as well as on the native population of Ancient India (Dravidians) that it is important to understand the history and culture of Ancient Egypt, and the nature of its spiritual tradition in more detail.

The history of Egypt begins in ancient times. It includes the Dynastic Period, the Hellenistic Period, Roman and Byzantine Rule (30 B.C.E.-638 A.C.E.), the Caliphate and the Mamalukes (642-1517 A.C.E.), Ottoman Domination (1082-1882 A.C.E.), and British colonialism (1882-1952 A.C.E.) as well as modern, independent Egypt (1952-). Ancient Egypt or Kamit is a civilization that flourished in Northeast Africa along the Nile River from before 5,500 B.C.E. until 30 B.C.E. In 30 B.C.E. Octavian (who was later known as the Roman Emperor, Augustus) put the last Egyptian King, Ptolemy XIV, a Greek ruler, to death. After this Egypt was formally annexed to Rome. Egyptologists normally divide Ancient Egyptian history into periods: The Early Dynastic Period (3,200-2,575 B.C.E.); The Old Kingdom or Old Empire (2,575-2,134 B.C.E.); the First Intermediate Period (2,134-2,040 B.C.E.); the Middle Kingdom or Middle Empire (2,040-1,640 B.C.E.); The Second Intermediate Period (1,640-1,532 B.C.E.); the New Kingdom or New Empire (1,550-1,070 B.C.E.); the third Intermediate Period (1,070-712 B.C.E.); the Late Period (712-332 B.C.E.); the Nubian Dynasty (712-657 B.C.E.); the Persian Dynasty (525-404 B.C.E.); the Native Revolt and re-establishment of Egyptian rule by Egyptians (404-343 B.C.E.); the Second Persian Period (343-332 B.C.E.); the Greco-Roman Period (332 B.C.E.-395 A.C.E.); the Byzantine Period[I] (395-640 A.C.E) and the Arab Conquest Period (640 A.C.E.). The individual dynasties are numbered, generally in Roman numerals, from I through XXX. The period after the New Kingdom saw greatness in culture and architecture under the rulership of Ramses II. However, after his rule, Egypt saw a decline from which it would never recover. This is the period of the downfall of Ancient Egyptian culture in which the Libyans ruled after The Tanite (or XXI) Dynasty. This was followed by the Nubian conquerors who founded the XXII dynasty and tried to restore Egypt to her past glory. However, having been weakened by the social and political turmoil of wars, Ancient Egypt fell to the Persians once more. The Persians conquered the country until the Greeks, under Alexander, conquered them. The Romans followed the Greeks, and finally the Arabs conquered the land of Egypt in 640 A.C.E to the present.

However, the history which has been classified above is only the history of the "Dynastic Period." It reflects the view of traditional Egyptologists who have refused to accept the evidence of a predynastic period in Ancient Egyptian history contained in Ancient Egyptian documents such as the *Palermo Stone, Royal Tablets at Abydos, Royal Papyrus of Turin,* the *Dynastic List* of Manetho and the eye-witness accounts of Greek historians Herodotus (c. 484-425 B.C.E.) and Diodorus (Greek historian died about 20 B.C.E.). These sources speak clearly of a predynastic society which stretches far into antiquity. The Dynastic period is what most people think of whenever Ancient Egypt is mentioned. This period is when the pharaohs (kings) ruled. The latter part of the Dynastic Period is when the Biblical story of Moses, Joseph, Abraham, etc., occurs (c. 2100? -1,000? B.C.E.).[II] Therefore, those with a Christian background generally only have an idea about Ancient Egypt as it is related in the Bible. Although this biblical notion is very limited in scope, the significant impact of Ancient Egypt on Hebrew and Christian culture is evident even from the biblical scriptures. Actually, Egypt existed much earlier than most traditional Egyptologists are prepared to admit. The new archeological evidence related to the great Sphinx monument on the Giza Plateau and the ancient writings by Manetho, one of the last High Priests of Ancient Egypt, show that Ancient Egyptian history begins earlier than 10,000 B.C.E. and may date back to as early as 30,000-50,000 B.C.E.

It is known that the Pharaonic (royal) calendar was in use by 4,240 B.C.E. This certainly required extensive astronomical skills and time for observation. Therefore, the history of Kamit (Egypt) must be reckoned to be extremely ancient. Thus, in order to grasp the antiquity of Ancient Egyptian culture, religion and philosophy, we will briefly review the history presented by the Ancient Egyptian Priest Manetho and some Greek Historians.

[I] Eastern Roman Empire after the break from Rome.
[II] Outside of the Bible there is no evidence of the birth of Abraham, Joseph, Moses, etc. Therefore, the dates are uncertain.

THE MYSTICAL JOURNEY FROM JESUS TO CHRIST

Diodorus Siculus (Greek Historian) writes in the time of Augustus (first century B.C.):

Below: relief of an Ancient Egyptian man. Taken from the tomb of Rameses III.
C. 1194 B.C.E.

"Now the Ethiopians, as historians relate, were the first of all men and the proofs of this statement, they say, are manifest. For that they did not come into their land as immigrants from abroad but were the natives of it and so justly bear the name of autochthones (sprung from the soil itself), *is, they maintain, conceded by practically all men..."*

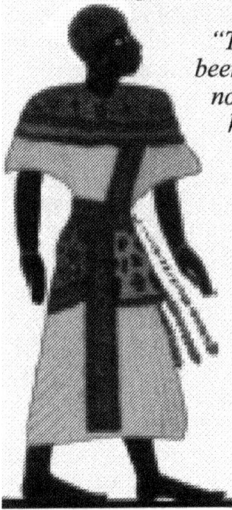

"They also say that the Egyptians are colonists sent out by the Ethiopians, Osiris having been the leader of the colony. For, speaking generally, what is now Egypt, they maintain, was not land, but sea, when in the beginning the universe was being formed; afterwards, however, as the Nile during the times of its inundation carried down the mud from Ethiopia, land was gradually built up from the deposit...And the larger parts of the customs of the Egyptians are, they hold, Ethiopian, the colonists still preserving their ancient manners. For instance, the belief that their kings are Gods, the very special attention which they pay to their burials, and many other matters of a similar nature, are Ethiopian practices, while the shapes of their statues and the forms of their letters are Ethiopian; for of the two kinds of writing which the Egyptians have, that which is known as popular (demotic) *is learned by everyone, while that which is called sacred* (hieratic), *is understood only by the priests of the Egyptians, who learnt it from their Fathers as one of the things which are not divulged, but among the Ethiopians, everyone uses these forms of letters. Furthermore, the orders of the priests, they maintain, have much the same position among both peoples; for all are clean who are engaged in the service of the Gods, keeping themselves shaven, like the Ethiopian priests, and having the same dress and form of staff, which is shaped like a plough and is carried by their kings who wear high felt hats which end in a knob in the top and are circled by the serpents which they call asps; and this symbol appears to carry the thought that it will be the lot who shall dare to attack the king to encounter death-carrying stings. Many other things are told by them concerning their own antiquity and the colony which they sent out that became the Egyptians, but about this there is no special need of our writing anything."*

The Ancient Egyptian texts state:

*"Our people originated at the base of the mountain of the Moon,
at the origin of the Nile river."*

🦅◗⸗ (Ancient Egyptian Hieroglyphic text)

"KMT"
"Egypt," "Burnt," "Land of Blackness,""Land of the Burnt People."

KMT (Ancient Egypt) is situated close to Lake Victoria in present day Africa. This is the same location where the earliest human remains have been found, in the land currently known as Ethiopia-Tanzania. Recent genetic technology, as reported in the new encyclopedias and leading news publications, has revealed that all peoples of the world originated in Africa and migrated to other parts of the world prior to the last Ice Age 40,000 years ago. Therefore, as of this time, genetic testing has revealed that all humans are alike, having had the common origins in Africa. The earliest bone fossils which have been found in many parts of the world are those of the African Grimaldi type. During the Ice Age, it was not possible to communicate or to migrate. Those trapped in specific locations were subject to the regional forces of weather and climate. Cooler climates required less body pigment, thereby producing lighter pigmented people who now differed from their dark-skinned ancestors. After the Ice Age when travel was possible, these light-skinned people who had lived in the northern, colder regions of harsh weather during the Ice Age period moved back to the warmer climates of their ancestors. There they mixed with the people who had remained dark-skinned, producing the Semitic colored people. "Semite" means mixture of skin color shades. The portrait of an Ancient Egyptian man (left) comes from an Ancient Egyptian Tomb.

Therefore, there is only one human race which, due to different climactic and regional exposure, changed to a point where there seemed to be different "types" of people. Differences were noted with respect to skin color, hair texture, customs, languages, psychological and emotional makeup due to the experiences each group had to face and overcome in order to survive. This has been previously addressed under the section "Conclusion: One World, One humanity, One destiny."

From a philosophical standpoint, questioning the origin of humanity is unnecessary when it is understood that _ALL_ come from one origin which some choose to call the "Big Bang" and others "The Supreme Being." In any case the ancient record reflects the known origins of humanity. They also show that even in ancient times, the differences between human beings, including racial difference, gender differences, etc., were understood to be only on the surface. They also relate how in ancient times the Egyptians and Indians shared a common history and culture.

Historical evidence shows that Ethiopia-Nubia, Egypt and India had a common population and shared culture.

"Ancient Egypt was a colony of Nubia - Ethiopia. ...Osiris having been the leader of the colony..."

"And upon his return to Greece, they gathered around and asked, "tell us about this great land of the Blacks called Ethiopia." And Herodotus said, "There are two great Ethiopian nations, one in Sind (India) and the other in Egypt."

Recorded by Diodorus (Greek historian 100 B.C.)[64]

The origins of Greek mythology and philosophy can be found in Ancient Egypt. This fact was recorded by several Greek Historians of the ancient world.

> Solon, Thales, Plato, Eudoxus and Pythagoras went to Egypt and consorted with the priests. Eudoxus they say, received instruction from Chonuphis of Memphis,* Solon from Sonchis of Sais,* and Pythagoras from Oeniphis of Heliopolis.*
>
> –Plutarch (Greek historian c. 46-120 A.C.E.)
*(cities in Ancient Egypt)

> 35. "Almost all the names of the gods came into Greece from Egypt. My inquiries prove that they were all derived from a foreign source, and my opinion is that Egypt furnished the greater number. For with the exception of Neptune and the Dioscuri, whom I mentioned above, and Juno, Vesta, Themis, the Graces, and the Nereids, the other gods have been known from time immemorial in Egypt. This I assert on the authority of the Egyptians themselves."
>
> –Herodotus (The Histories)

The History of Manetho

Manetho was one of the last Ancient Egyptian High Priests who retained the knowledge of the ancient history of Egypt. In 241 B.C.E. he was commissioned to compile a series of wisdom texts by King Ptolemy II, one of the Macedonian (Greek) rulers of Egypt after it was captured and controlled by the Greeks. One of Manetho's compositions included a history of Egypt. However, Manetho's original writings were destroyed by the subsequent rulers of Egypt. Therefore, the accounts of his writings by the Greeks who studied his work constitute the current remaining record of his work, and some of the accounts differ from each other in certain respects. According to the _Armenian Version of Eusebius,_ this history of Manetho included the following periods:

1- **The Gods** - This period was the genesis. It began with the emergence of the great Ennead or Company of gods and goddesses headed by Ra, the Supreme Being. This period lasted 13,900 years. The God, Ra himself, ruled over the earth.

2- **The Demigods** - After the Gods, the Demigods[I] ruled the earth for 1,255 years. Then came a descendent line of royal rulers for 1,817 years followed by 30 rulers in the city of Memphis for 1,790 years. These were followed by another set of royal rulers for 350 years.

3- **The Spirits of the Dead** - After the period of the Demigods came the Spirits of the Dead. This period lasted 5,813 years.

The total number of years outlined above is 24,925 years. This period was then followed by the Dynastic Period which is the only period of Ancient Egypt of which most people have knowledge (c. 5,000 B.C.E.-30 B.C.E.).

[I] Offspring of a Deity (a god) and a mortal human being.

According to *The Old Chronicle* (from Syncellus), Manetho groups 30 dynasties (a succession of rulers from the same family or line) of rulers in Egypt within 113 generations in a period covering 36,525 years.

The Company of Gods and Goddesses of Anu

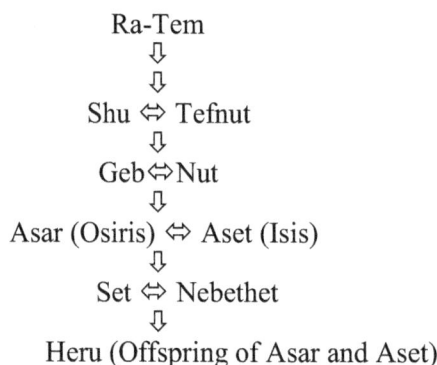

Ra-Tem
⇩
⇩
Shu ⇔ Tefnut
⇩
Geb⇔Nut
⇩
Asar (Osiris) ⇔ Aset (Isis)
⇩
Set ⇔ Nebethet
⇩
Heru (Offspring of Asar and Aset)

————————

The ten gods and goddesses in the cosmological scheme of creation.

The Ancient Egyptian religion (*Shetaut Neter*) provides the first "historical" record of Yoga philosophy and mystical religious literature. The diagram above comes from the cosmological teachings given in the Ancient Egyptian city of Anu (Greek Heliopolis) in c. 36,000 B.C.E.

The idea of creation given above refers to an original Supreme Being from which nine divinities (Company of gods and goddesses, the Ennead) arose. The mystical meaning behind the number nine is that the spirit (The Self - Ra-Tem) differentiates itself into nine divisions, which include the Self or Supreme Divinity along with four pairs of opposites (Shu-Tefnut, Geb-Nut, Asar-Aset, Set-Nebethet) which together constitute eight principles of creation and form the basis of the greatest Ancient Egyptian Epic, the Ausarian Resurrection Myth. The Ancient Egyptian concept of the Ennead (nine gods and goddesses) is expressed in the Ancient Egyptian hieroglyphic symbol ꟾ, meaning *Divinity,* written nine times: ꟾꟾꟾꟾꟾꟾꟾꟾꟾ. Thus, from the original state of singularity, the Self, God, expresses in the form of the eight qualities of nature which are uniform throughout the phenomenal world existing in time and space. The same principle of "nine" is found in the *Sri Yantra* of India, which is a diagram depicting the origin of creation and its separation into pairs opposites which constitute the phenomenal universe. In Christianity the number nine has found expression in several areas. One of the most notable being the *Novena* ritual practiced in the Roman Catholic tradition. The Novena refers to nine days of private or public prayer. The custom of worshiping for nine days was also a Roman custom. The parentalia novendialia was a nine-day observance celebrated by the ancient Romans in honor of deceased family members. The custom was officially adopted by Christianity during the 17th century, although its prototype is sometimes seen as the period of time the disciples of Jesus spent in prayer prior to the descent of the Holy Spirit (see Acts 1). Private novenas are frequently made in honor of the Virgin Mary. Perhaps the best-known liturgical novena is in honor of the Holy Spirit, celebrated as a preparation for Pentecost Sunday.[I] Although the practice can appear superstitious, it is considered a legitimate devotional aid to extended prayer. Another famous festivity is the nine days of Mother[II] Worship practiced in India, where God is worshiped as mother (i.e. The Goddess).

There are two great Enneads in the mythology of Ancient Egypt. One has been espoused by the theology of the city of Anu in Ancient Egypt (above), and the other was espoused by the city of Memphis. The profound wisdom within these cosmological teachings and their relevance to Christianity will become evident as we explore the symbolism of the gods and goddesses which comprise them throughout this work.

More on The Dynastic Period of Ancient Egypt

The Dynastic Period was full of ups and downs, because during this time, there were several attacks from outsiders who sought to conquer Egypt. In general, the intermediate periods are times when outside forces from Asia were partially successful in achieving some control over Egypt or when the pressure caused a temporary internal breakdown of the government, but not the culture. Ancient Egyptian culture re-emerged out of the adversity like a phoenix finding new birth in the Old, Middle and New Kingdom periods.

[I] A Christian festival commemorating the descent of the Holy Ghost upon the disciples.

[II] Worship of the goddess and her wisdom.

As we have seen, Ancient Egyptian civilization extended far into antiquity. The Pre-dynastic Period is the time which saw the construction of the Great Pyramids and the Sphinx. Thus, the Predynastic Period extends from possibly c. 36,000 B.C.E. to c. 5,500 B.C.E. Most traditions from around the world speak of a worldwide flood which wiped out all civilizations on earth. This phenomenon is supposed to have occurred around the year 10,000 B.C.E. This flood myth is also the basis of the story of Noah's Ark in the Bible. The dating of the flood is based on the archeological evidence surrounding the Ancient Egyptian Sphinx. This shows that the Sphinx must be older than 12,000 years since 10,000 B.C.E. is the latest period when rainfall and other water sources would have been sufficient enough in Lower Egypt (Nile Delta) to cause the kind of water damage that is found on the Sphinx. Thus, the Ancient Egyptian Pre-dynastic Period extended to the time prior to and after the flood.

In conjunction with Ancient Egypt, another ancient civilization must be mentioned: Atlantis. Atlantis, in the tradition of antiquity, is a land and advanced civilization which is said to have existed prior to the "flood" and to have been engulfed by the ocean as the result of an earthquake. The first recorded accounts of Atlantis appear in two dialogues by Plato, the "Timaeus" and "Critias." According to the account in Timaeus, the island was described to the Athenian statesman, Solon, by an Egyptian priest, who told him that Atlantis was larger than Libya and Asia Minor combined. The priest also said that a highly advanced civilization existed on Atlantis at about the 10th millennium B.C.E. Further, the priest related that the nation of Atlantis had conquered all the peoples of the Mediterranean except the Athenians. Solon and other Athenians had no previous knowledge of this ancient land.

It is evident that there is more about history that is not known than is known. Therefore, history should be studied with an open mind and never considered to be absolute, since the winds of time have taken all evidence of many civilizations that existed in the past. The important point here is that Ancient Egyptian civilization emerged first out of the cataclysmic flood period and resurrected an advanced society and religious systems from the distant past which it then spread around the world in order to civilize it for the good of all humanity. This is why scholars from all countries were accepted in the Ancient Egyptian University Temples. Some Egyptian Pharaohs even sponsored and financed temples abroad which taught mystical philosophy as well as other disciplines. One such effort was put forth by the Ancient Egyptian King, Amasis, who financed the reconstruction of the famous Temple of Delphi in Greece, which was burnt down in 548 B.C.E.[44]

When the Roman Empire took control of Egypt, the Egyptian religion spread throughout the Roman Empire. However, when Christianity took hold in Rome, the Ancient Egyptian religion and other mystical religions became an obstacle to the Christian Church which had developed divergent ideas about spirituality, and also to the Roman government which sought to consolidate the empire under Rome. Ancient Egyptian religion served to refer people to Egypt as well as to individual spiritual practice. Therefore, it was politically expedient to close all mystical religion temples. At the end of the fourth century A.C.E. the Roman emperor Theodosius decreed that all religions except Christianity were to be stopped and all forms of Christianity besides that of the "Byzantine throne" would also cease to exist. During this time The Temple of Isis (Aset) at Philae[I] in Upper Egypt (deep south of Egypt) temporarily escaped the enforcement of the decree. That Temple of Isis is the location of the last known hieroglyphic inscriptions, dated at 394 A.C.E. Also, the last demotic[II] inscriptions there date to 452 A.C.E. It was not until the sixth century A.C.E. that Emperor Justinian entered a second decree which effectively stopped all mystical religious practices in the Roman empire. This means that not only were the Mystery-Yoga schools and temples to be closed, but also all forms of Christianity which did not agree with the style of Christianity espoused in Rome were to be abolished. Therefore, the Gnostic Christians were persecuted, their churches rededicated to Roman Catholicism and much of their writings were destroyed. Thus, it is evident that the Ancient Egyptian teachings were being practiced and taught well into the Christian era.[III]

The Ancient Egyptian Creation Myths and Their Relationship to Christianity and Gnosticism

Bible - Genesis   1
   2 And the earth was without form, and void; and darkness [was] upon the face of the deep. And the Spirit of God moved upon the face of the waters.

The idea of the primeval waters, and the original primeval Spirit which engendered life in it, occurs in several myths from around the world. It occurs both in the Jewish Bible as well as in Hindu mythology. However, the earliest record of the idea of the primeval waters occurs in the Pre-dynastic culture of Ancient Egyptian religion. This Pre-dynastic (10000-5500 B.C.E.), pre-Ausarian (Osiris) myth spoke of a God who was unborn and undying, and who was the origin of all things. This Deity was described as un-namable, unfathomable, gender-less and

---

[I] Island of the time of Re (Ra).

[II] Later form of the hieroglyphic system.

[III] Year 0 through 452 A.C.E. and later.

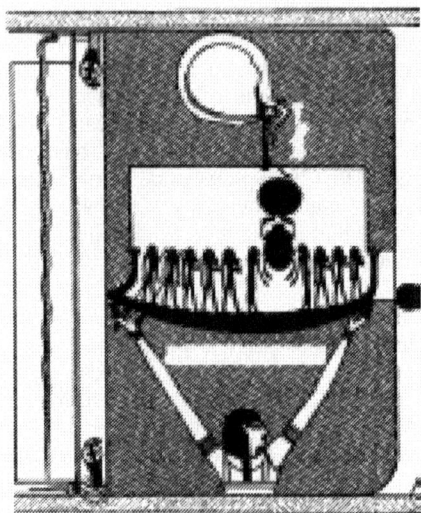

without form, although encompassing all forms and being transcendental. This being was the *God of Light* which illumines all things, and thus was later associated (in Dynastic times) with the Sun in the form of the deities, *Ra* or *Tem,* with *Heru* (Horus) who represents *that which is up there* and *the light,* and finally *Aten.* Tem or Temu was an Ancient Egyptian name for the ocean which is full of life giving potential. This ocean is likened to the deep and boundless abyss of consciousness of the Supreme Deity from which the phenomenal universe emerged. Tem was analogous in nature to later deities such as the Babylonian *Tiamat,* the Chaldean *Thamte,* the Hebrew *Tehorn,* and the Greek *Themis.*

The story related in the Ancient Egyptian *Papyrus of Nesi Amsu* is that this primeval God laid an egg in the primeval *chaotic* waters from which the God him/herself emerged. This primordial God who emerged out of the waters created or emanated Ra, the Sun or Life Force, Djehuti (Ţehuti), the carrier of the **Divine Word** or creative medium, and Maat, the principle of cosmic order and regularity. The underlying emphasis was on the fact that all of these, including human beings and the phenomenal world, are in reality emanations from that same Primeval Ocean. This means that there is one primordial essence for all things, be they plants, humans, gods and goddesses, etc. Other Ancient Egyptian stories tell of how the creator masturbated and engendered life within himself. Another myth tells of how Ra emerged from the ocean on a boat. The boat's movement on the water engenders Creation and sustains it. The term "chaotic" has been used to describe the state of matter prior to the creation of the universe. This term is not exactly correct in conveying the meaning intended however. This meaning is different from the commonly expressed meaning of chaos which implies disorder, confusion and turmoil. The term chaos above refers to the primeval ocean in its undifferentiated, formless state. The Primeval Ocean has its own essential being which is beyond human understanding since human beings can only conceptualize between order and disorder. It is difficult to conceive of that which is beyond order and disorder, and yet that is what the metaphor really means. Still another Ancient Egyptian creation story tells of how Ra gave birth to Nut (the heavens) and Geb (the earth), and that they were locked in a sexual union until Ra commanded Shu (air/space) to separate them. This separation constitutes creation or the coming into existence of the phenomenal universe. These similes, once again, point to the fact that creation did not come from "nowhere" and just simply begin to exist, but that it came out of God and, as such, is part of God even at present.

The primeval Egyptian creation myth is similar in many respects to the Creation story from the Indian mythology associated with the *Laws of Manu* in which Manu, a Sage-Creator God of the Indian Hindu-Vedic tradition, recounts a process of Creation in which the Self Existent Spirit (God) felt desire, and wishing to create all things from his own body, created the primeval waters (Nara) and threw a seed into it. From the seed came the golden cosmic egg. The Self-Existent Spirit developed in the egg into Brahma (Purusha, the singular original essence) and after a year of meditation, divided into two parts (male and female). The Ancient Egyptian and Hindu Creation stories originate in the far reaches of antiquity (5,500 B.C.E. and 3,000 B.C.E. respectively). Their similarity to each other hints at their common origin.

Almost exactly like one of the Ancient Egyptian creation myths, the original Jewish Bible and texts also express the Creation in terms of an act of sexual union. *Elohim* (Ancient Hebrew for gods/goddesses) impregnates the primeval waters with *ruach,* a Hebrew word which means *spirit, wind* or the verb *to hover.* The same word means *to brood* in Syriac. Elohim, also called El, was a name used for God in some Hebrew Scriptures. It was also used in the Old Testament for heathen gods. Thus, as the Book of Genesis explains, Creation began as the spirit of God "moved over the waters" and agitated those waters into a state of movement. In Western traditions the active role of Divinity has been assigned to the male gender while the passive (receiving) role has been assigned to the female gender. This is in contrast to the Southern and Eastern philosophical views where the passive role is assigned to the male gender, and the active role to the female.

Below: The Ancient Egyptian Creation. God rises from the Primeval Ocean to give form to Creation out of the chaotic waters.

Western Christian thinking holds that God and Creation exist as separate realities. Mystical Christianity and Yogic understanding is that Creation and God are one and the same since God transcends Creation while also expressing as Creation. Since God is all that exists, God is also the spirit and the primeval waters at the same time. Therefore, God interacts with him/herself and emanates Creation out of him/herself as well as into him/herself. The term him/herself is used to signify that the Supreme Being is neither male nor female, but encompasses them both (androgyny). So within this teaching of the creation of the world lies the latent idea that Creation and God are one and the same in a mysterious unexplained way. The original Jewish Creation idea, upon which the Christian understanding of Creation is based, also has a latent reference to the femaleness of the primeval waters and the maleness of the Spirit of God which impregnates it through the teaching of ruach. It was not until later times that the male gender took on prominence in Christianity and the female gender was supplanted and almost forgotten.

At the beginning of the Dynastic Period (5,500 B.C.E.), two of the most powerful mystery myths which came to prominence early in Ancient Egyptian mythology were the Ausarian (Osirian) Resurrection and Memphite Theology, which concerned the gods Osiris and Ptah, respectively. Both of these incorporated the qualities of the primeval wisdom inherent in the original theology, but in a form which was more easily grasped by the minds of the new society, which was now a mixture of native Africans and Asiatics. The forms of the Supreme Being (Osiris and Ptah) were now depicted in anthropomorphic images. Three major theologies in total emerged from the original. All incorporated the same idea of a Supreme Being who emerges from a primeval, formless essence. Also, each system of theology used a Trinity to convey spiritual teachings in reference to the Divine nature of humanity. These important Trinities are *Ra-Asar-Heru, Ptah-Sekhmet-Nefertem* and *Amen[1]-Ra-Ptah.* They are most similar to the concept of *The Father-Son-Holy Ghost* of Christianity and the Hindu Trinity of *Brahma-Vishnu-Shiva.* The main difference between the Christian Trinity and the Ancient Egyptian and Hindu trinities is that the Egyptian and Hindu formulation incorporated the female element into the theology as female goddesses or aspects which are complementary to the male deities in the Triad, whereas the Christian Trinity only emphasized the male element of the Divine. This exclusion of the female element is a notable feature of occidental culture which expresses itself in all levels of Western society. The Ancient Egyptian Trinities include the female element directly into the theology of the Trinity itself. In the following Ancient Egyptian Trinities, the female deities are in italics: Amen, *Mut* and their child Khons., Ptah-*Sekhmet*-Nefertem, Heru-*Hathor*-Harsomtus (Horus the Younger), Khnum-*Anukis*-Satis, and the most popular, Asar-*Aset*-Heru (Osiris-Isis-Horus). All of these include the father, mother and child element. The child element relates the Trinity to human beings. Human beings are seen as the offspring of the union of the Supreme Being (Spirit-male essence) and Creation (Matter-female essence), the product of the male and female essence of God. The Christian Trinity refers only to God in the male gender and excludes women and human beings altogether. Though the character of Jesus is supposed to be a reference to humanity, in Orthodox Christianity he has come to be thought of as separate and distant from Creation and from humanity, except through relationship with the church. While the Ancient Egyptian Trinity gives the idea that God is within the human being and in Creation, the Orthodox Christian idea implies that God is separate and different from Creation and humanity.

This dramatic shift from the abstract theology of the primeval ocean with an inscrutable Supreme Being to a concrete theology with deities that are physically depicted and accepted as personalities who existed in fact rather than metaphorically, typifies the effect of occidental culture on the religion and philosophy. This predisposition towards concretization and crystallization of ideas, images and concepts is antithetical to the central purpose and direction of religion and to yogic thinking. It is a movement towards objectification rather than towards a mystical and metaphorical or symbolic understanding. The Western view is more in line with segmentation and linear thought, accenting differences. Most importantly, it is a way of thinking which encourages the emergence of the individual ego and also intensifies it. Ego simply means the acknowledgment of a separation between the self and others (individuality) rather than seeing one's self and others as being one, connected. In religious terms, the understanding of the underlying unity of creation becomes lost as the belief emerges that the individual is a separate and distinct entity apart from nature and God, which are themselves separate and distinct. This is the main difference between orthodox religion and mystical religion.

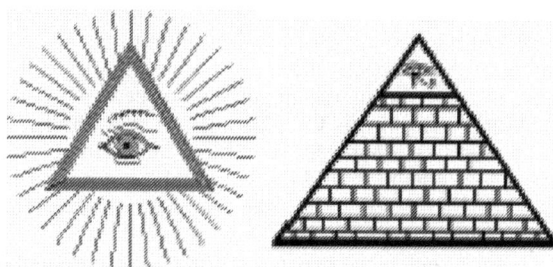

Above left: The Christian symbol of the Trinity.
Above right: The Ancient Egyptian symbol of Heru, The Supreme One, in his house (Pyramid).

The Ancient Egyptian teachings in the religious myths of Amun, Asar and Ptah provide a uniting view of Divinity, Creation and humanity. The theologies concerning Amun and Ptah maintain the universal, underlying essence of the phenomenal world and are highly philosophical and psychological. The Ausarian mystery also maintains the same teaching, but in a less intellectual manner. It is specifically directed towards assisting the

---

[1] Other spellings include *Amun, Amen, Amon, Amonu, Amunu*

aspirant in breaking down the barriers which separate her/him from the truth of their own being. It presents a highly developed myth which is designed to evoke devotional feeling towards the Divine in the form of Osiris, thus allowing the unity of the soul and the Divine (Osiris) to occur in conscious fact. Through initiation into the teachings of the myths and their underlying meanings, and through the practice of ritual identification of the aspirant with the Divine, all-encompassing God, in this case Osiris, the aspirant is led to achieve the state of mystical communion with the Divine in much the same way as Christian mystics would later describe mystical experiences of union with Christ.

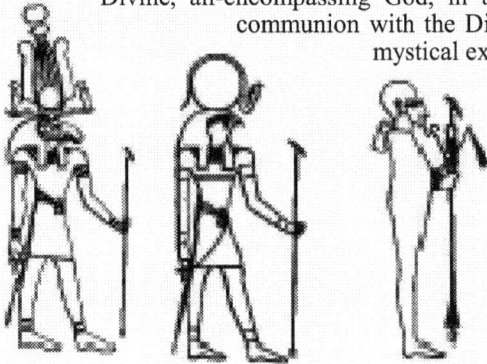

Left: The Ancient Egyptian Trinity of AMUN-RA-PTAH.

The Ausarian Resurrection, Its Historical and Mystical Implications

According to tradition, Asar (Ausar, Asr - Osiris) and Ast (Aset - Isis) were the first King and Queen of Ancient Egypt (c.12,000-10,000 B.C.E.). They taught the people agriculture, established a code of laws and taught all to worship the gods and goddesses as well as the Supreme Being, Ra. One version holds that one day, Asar's brother, Set, became jealous of Asar and killed him.

Right: A map of Northeast Africa, Asia Minor and India, showing the three main locations of the use of the ancient Egyptian Ankh symbol and also the geographic area where Asar traveled and spread the teachings of mystical spirituality (Yoga) which later became associated with Christianity in the Middle East, Rome and Greece, and Vedanta - Yoga in India.

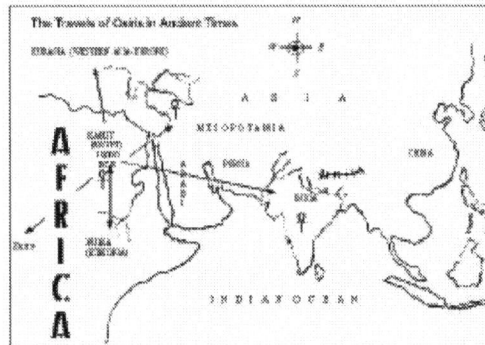

? Cain and Able in the Christian Bible, about a man who murders his brother, has a precursor in n mythological scriptures. Set, who represents the personification of evil forces and negative hatred and greed (the blinding passion that clouds the intellect), plotted in jealousy to usurp the l to kill Asar. Set secretly got the measurements of Asar and constructed a coffin. Through e to get Asar to "try on" the coffin for size. While Asar was resting in the coffin, Set and his nd then dumped it into the Nile river.

its way to the coast of Syria where it became embedded in the earth and from it grew a tree with oma. The King of Syria was out walking and as he passed by the tree, he immediately fell in it aroma, so he had the tree cut down and brought to his palace and cut into the form of a Djed et is the symbol of Asar's back. It has four horizontal lines in relation to a firmly established, straight column. The Djed column is symbolic of the upper energy centers (chakras) that relate to the levels of consciousness of the spirit. Aset, Asar's wife who is the personification of the life giving, mother force in creation and in all humans, went to Syria in search of Asar. Her search led her to the palace of the Syrian King where she took a job as the nurse of the King's son. Aset then told the king that Asar, her husband, is inside the pillar he made from the tree. The King graciously gave her the pillar and she returned with it to Kamit (Kmt, Ancient Egypt).

Upon her return to Kmt (Egypt), Aset went to the papyrus swamps and remained in hiding from Set. She blew air into Asar's nostrils and revived him. This portion of the story is similar to a verse related in the books of Genesis and Job in the Christian Bible as God uses breath to engender life.

Genesis 2
7 And the LORD God formed man [of] the dust of the ground, and breathed into his nostrils the breath of life; and man became a living soul. {of the dust...: Heb. dust of the ground}

Job 33
4 The Spirit of God hath made me, and the breath of the Almighty hath given me life.

THE HISTORY AND PHILOSOPHY OF MYSTICAL CHRISTIANITY

Aset then laid over Asar's dead body and conceived a son, Heru (Horus), through the spirit of Asar with the assistance of the deities Djehuti and Amun. One evening, as Set was hunting in the papyrus swamps, he came upon Aset, Asar and the new born child. In a rage of passion, he dismembered the body of Asar into fourteen pieces and scattered the pieces throughout the land. In this way, it is Set, the brute force of our bodily impulses and desires that "dismembers" the higher intellect of a human being. Under the influence of Set (anger, greed, egoism, etc.), instead of oneness and unity we see multiplicity and separateness which give rise to egoistic (selfish) and violent behavior. Thus, the Ancient Egyptian character of Set is the prototype of the Jewish, Christian and Islamic "Satan." While Set was in a rage, the Great Mother, Aset, fled and went into hiding to a place where she could raise Heru. Then she once again set out to search, now for the pieces of Asar, with the help of Apuat (Anubis) and Nebthet (Nephthys).

After searching all over the world, they found all of the pieces of Asar's body, except for his phallus which was eaten by a fish. A similar story occurs in Hindu mythology in relation to the god Shiva. In Eastern Hindu-Tantra mythology, the God Shiva, who is the equivalent of Asar, also lost his phallus by castration in one story. In Ancient Egyptian and Hindu-Tantra mythology, the loss represents seminal retention in order to channel the sexual energy to the higher spiritual centers, thereby transforming it into spiritual energy. The loss of the phallus represents the cutting of sexual desire which distracts a person from discovering spiritual reality. This retention feeds the soul instead of becoming expressed in the world. In short, it represents cutting off of the desire for worldly pleasure in favor of spiritual realization. Aset, Anubis, and Nephthys "re-membered" all the pieces except the phallus which was eaten by a fish. Asar thus regained life in the realm of the dead. The sacred fish which ate the phallus of Asar was also related to the pilot fish which guide the Boat of Ra. The Ancient Egyptian reverence for the fish influenced the Christian reverence for the fish[1] which became one of the most popular symbols of Jesus. This is one of the important mystical meanings behind Jesus' feeding of five thousand people with bread and fish in Mark 6:30 and 8:1. The practice of celibacy allows a person to develop inner spiritual energy in such abundance that great works, which benefit the masses, can be performed.

One version of the story states that the child Heru was conceived after Asar had lost his phallus. Since the body of Asar was dead and lacking a phallus, Heru, therefore, was born from the union of the spirit of Asar and the life giving power of Aset who represents supreme love and devotion to the Divine. In this manner, the spirit of Asar was resurrected and given life through the son, Heru, and becomes the deity who presides over the fate of souls. This is similar to Christianity in that Jesus is seen as the incarnation of the spirit of God, the Father. Like Jesus, Heru was born as a result of a union of a woman and the spirit of God (Asar). Therefore, Ancient Egypt also provides the prototype for the Christian Virgin Birth teaching. Heru represents the union of spirit and matter, and the renewed life of Asar, his rebirth or resurrection. When Heru became a young man, Asar, in spirit form, encouraged him to take up arms (vitality, wisdom, courage, strength of will) and establish truth, justice and righteousness in the world by challenging Set, its current ruler. During the battle, Set injured the Eye of Heru (intuitional vision) and rendered him powerless against Set's evil might (egoism, anger and hatred). Heru left the scene of the battle in order to contemplate his situation. The deities Djehuti and Hetheru came to help him. Through the magic of right reasoning from Djehuti and the power of sexual sublimation from Hetheru (Hathor), Heru regained strength (spiritual energy, faith and will power) to face Set again. Heru was able to wrest (gain control over) the testicles of Set and thus take away his power of brute force and egoistic impulsiveness. In achieving this control over Set, Heru was able to control the lower self. The injuring of Heru and the subsequent time spent in solitude and reflection represent the stage of asceticism which implies celibacy and control over the senses in order to curb the externalized nature of the mind. The "battle" between Heru and Set is said to have lasted for three days. This is the same amount of time which was assigned to the resurrection of Jesus and to other saviors such as the god Attis.

Asar represents the human soul. The soul is an emanation from the Divine Spirit of God. It incarnates in the realm of time and space and becomes intoxicated with the sense pleasures of creation. Asar is equivalent to the idea of Tem arising from the primeval waters after willing to evolve the universe and create order in those chaotic waters. The lack of vigilance which caused his being tricked into the coffin of Set implies that Asar forgot himself and allowed his passions to control him. This is the predicament of every soul which incarnates in the realm of time and space and forgets its primeval origin. However, Asar is resurrected by righteousness, wisdom, devotion and supreme love, the qualities represented by Aset.

The idea of the primeval ocean and the absolute transcendental reality is inherent in the Ancient Egyptian Theban mythology concerning the god Amun and in the Memphite Theology relating to the god Ptah. It is equivalent to the Indian Vedantic teaching concerning the deities Brahman and Narayana. All of them are considered to be infinite, transcendental and unfathomable in their absolute aspects. From a mystical point of view, this metaphor of the ocean also refers to the mind and its underlying consciousness. What is considered normal human consciousness is always

---

[1] See front cover.

59

in a state of motion due to thoughts. Thoughts objectify the subtle matter of consciousness (Genesis 1:1-2). If those thoughts were to be somehow calmed, a new vision of reality would emerge in the mind that is not distorted by the wave-like thoughts. This attainment of a restful state of mind undisturbed by thoughts is achieved through the understanding of the myth and the practice of its teachings in day to day life, along with meditation on the true nature of the soul.

Heru eventually regained rulership of Egypt and thereby redeemed his father. In so doing, Heru reestablished the correct position of the Divine (Asar) and achieved control over the elements of the lower self as symbolized by Set (anger, hate, greed, lust, unrest, segmentation, etc.).

Putting the pieces of Asar back together again refers to integrating the personality of the spiritual aspirant to a degree where the true Self is discovered. An ordinary human being is not aware of his/her true nature because they are constantly in a state of worry or preoccupation over some thought about the past, present or future. Essentially, their awareness of the true Self has been killed by the demon of anger, hatred, greed, fear, insecurity, lust, etc. Egoism (Set), in the form of these base emotions and the thoughts they engender, has effectively chopped up their sense of universality. When the thoughts are recognized to be merely waves in the ocean of consciousness and the mind is calmed through the practice of yoga, wisdom and meditation, the mind assumes its unruffled state, which then produces a clear image of the true Self. This is the redemption and resurrection of our true Self and it is the resurrection referred to by the Ausarian myth and the Gnostic Christian mysticism. It does not refer to the resurrection of the physical body at the end of time in some future *Armageddon* as asserted by the orthodox Roman theologians. It is, however, a resurrection in consciousness which is to occur while one is alive and existing in a physical body. The term Armageddon comes from the Hebrew term *har megiddo*, or "hill of Megiddo." In the Bible book of Revelation 16:16, the hill of Megiddo is the place where the final battle between the forces of God and the demonic kings of the earth will be fought at the end of the world. Thus, a mythological understanding of the battle as being between the lower and Higher Self in every human being as was taught by the Ancient Egyptian Mystery system, was transformed into a battle between cosmic forces that would someday bring an end to the world. This tradition has led Zoroastrians, Jews, Muslims, and Christians to adhere to a doctrine of fear based on an impending doom.

In Ancient Egyptian religion the process of resurrection or spiritual enlightenment is as follows. Through the practice of *Maat* or virtuous actions and the constant remembrance of the divine essence of the individual self as being one with the Divine (Asar), the aspirant is gradually led to identification with Asar, the all-encompassing and transcendental Self. This remembrance is the main objective of the mystery rituals and practices in the religion of Asar and Aset. This process involves the identification of the aspirant with the Divine through ritual offerings to the Divine as the true Self, and to personal reference of the individual self as the Divine as well. In other words, the aspirant is treated as the Divinity who has been dismembered and who is reconstituting him/herself in order to regain the primordial state of consciousness. The name of the aspirant is changed to Asar as an understanding that the aspirant, like all things, is a manifestation of the Divine Self. Since all is the Divine (Asar), then all is to be named Asar. Thus, instead of Judy, the aspirant now becomes Asar Judy.

The Christian Eucharist and the Eucharist of the Ancient Egyptian Mysteries

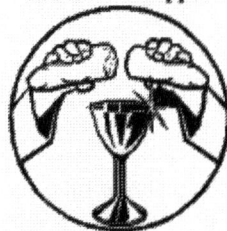

The Lord's Supper

The Eucharist is perhaps the most highly regarded ritual of Christianity. It is regarded as a sacrament. A sacrament is a visible form of invisible grace. Grace is the divine good which is bestowed on people by God in the form of prosperity, happiness, and spiritual enlightenment. In some churches, the bread or host is seen as the sacrament itself. The sacraments are any of the traditional seven rites that were instituted by Jesus and recorded in the New Testament which confer sanctifying grace.

In the Ancient Egyptian Pyramid Texts (c.5,000 B.C.E.), the rituals performed by the aspirant involve accepting the ritual offerings of loaves of bread, cakes, wine, beer and other articles, which represent the "Art" or ritual offering *Eye*. The *Eye* refers to the intuitional vision of Heru in his victorious aspect, vanquisher of Set. This *Eye* signifies intuitional knowledge of the Self. In the texts the aspirant is continuously admonished to "receive" the Eye and to consume it as the essence of Heru and Asar. In doing so the aspirant can assume his/her true nature. Thousands of years later, the early Christians used the ritual in much the same way. The Christian Host is supposed to be understood as a medium to join with the Divine in the form of Christ. In this sense, the ritual of the Eucharist represents the open performance of the Ausarian mystery for the masses of Christians all over the world, even though they are not aware of its origin or deeper meaning.

The mystery play of the Ausarian Resurrection refers a mystical transformation that is to occur within the innermost heart of the individual rather than a ritual to be participated in out of custom or social duty. It is this mystical union with the Divine which bestows the true knowledge of the Self. This was the knowledge which the Sages of Ancient Egypt, as well as their Gnostic descendants who created the Gnostic Christian Gospels, were trying to convey. This form of knowledge or Gnosticism is the mystical experience itself, and not the intellectual knowledge which can be acquired through the scriptures or the practice of rituals. Therefore, it is this mystical experience of union with the Divine which is at the heart of all mystery religions and Yoga philosophies. In the mass ritual of the Christian Church, when a person receives the bread and wine of the Eucharist, they are supposed to be feeling and understanding that they are receiving the Divine within themselves and thus becoming Divine as well.

The following selections from the Ancient Egyptian Pyramid Texts (below-left) illustrate the significance of the Eye and its identification with the offering of wine and bread of the Christian Eucharist (below-right).

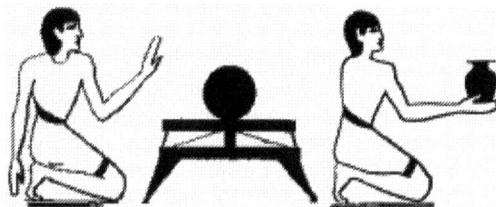

Ancient Egyptian priests offer the traditional bread and wine of the Eucharist ritual to Asar (Osiris).

Utterance 28
O Osiris Unas, Horus has given you his Eye; provide your face with it.
O Osiris Unas, take the Eye of Horus which was wrested from Set and which you shall take to your mouth, with which you shall split open your mouth— WINE.
Utterance 89
O Osiris Unas, take the Eye of Horus which Set has pulled out—A LOAF.
Utterance 93
O King, take this bread of yours which is the Eye of Horus.

From the Christian Bible:

Matthew 26:
26. And as they were eating, Jesus took bread, and blessed [it], and broke [it], and gave [it] to the disciples, and said, Take, eat; this is my body.
27 And he took the cup, and gave thanks, and gave [it] to them, saying, Drink ye all of it;
28 For this is my blood of the new testament, which is shed for many for the remission of sin.

It is important to understand that the eucharist ritual is the central rite of the Catholic mass or church service. It re-enacts the Last Supper of Jesus and his disciples before he was crucified. It has important mystical symbolism which is of the most advanced practice of religion.

Through various arguments and similes, mystical philosophy shows that the phenomenal world is in reality an expression of the underlying Divine essence. Modern physics calls this essence energy, while mystical philosophy would call it Consciousness and religion, God. Nevertheless, philosophy is the discipline which trains the mind to become introspective and discerning of reality versus unreality. Mystical experience is the perfection and consummation of that practice, and is itself the absolute proof of the existence of the divine, transcendental state of consciousness. Therefore, those who refute the mysteries without undergoing the disciplines leading to transformation from a conditioned state of mind (concepts) will continue to remain oblivious to that which lies beyond the phenomenal world of time-space-causation which ordinary human consciousness is aware of exclusively.

The strong influence of the Ausarian Mystery was felt in later cults and mystery religions in the Near East under various names. Hippolitus quotes a Naasene source in the following: *"Hail Attis, gloomy mutilation of Rhea. Assyrians style thee thrice-longed-for Adonis, and the whole of Egypt calls thee Asar, Samothracians, venerable Adam; Haemonians, Corybas; and the Phrygians named the at one time Pappa, at another time God... or the green Ear of Corn that has been reaped."*[103]

Attis was a mystery religion imported into Rome around 204 B.C.E. The goddess *Cybele* begot Attis by eating an almond or pomegranate. Thus, she conceived Attis as a "virgin" as Aset had conceived Heru and as Mary would conceive Jesus. Like Jesus, Attis' birthday is also on December 25th, and his passion was celebrated on March 25th, exactly nine months prior to the birthday on the winter solstice. Again, like Jesus, Attis was a sacrificial victim who was slain and eaten in order to save humankind. He was eaten in the form of bread by his worshipers, and he then resurrected as the "High God."[21\111] The dates of Attis' death and resurrection are the same as those of Heru, and later Jesus. Thus, there is synchronicity within the myths with regard to the idea of the resurrection of the soul, since the passion and death is only a hint of the rebirth which will occur "nine months" later.

In metaphorical terms, the passion of Asar, Jesus and Attis and the passion plays related to their mysteries are referring to the ordinary unenlightened state of human consciousness which is led, due to its own lower nature, to repeated reincarnations (births and deaths) which include untold suffering and pain. The true aim of the mystery is for the initiate to assume the role of the victorious divinity and realize that she or he is in reality "The High Divinity." This is what Jesus meant when he said "I and the Father are One" and "Know ye not that ye are gods?" When this realization has dawned and become rooted in the mind of a human being, the cycle of births and deaths (reincarnations) ends, and they resume their true state of being, free from the bonds of nature and ignorance.

Theban Theology and The Triad of Creation

The form of religious practice which came to prominence in the city of Thebes, Egypt, is referred to as Theban theology. It centers around the deity of Amen or Amun within the Ancient Egyptian Trinity of Amun-Ra-Ptah. Amun symbolizes the hidden aspect of existence, the underlying essence of phenomenal reality and the witnessing consciousness which underlies all. In much the same way that modern physics would say that energy underlies all objects, Amun or pure conscious awareness underlies all objects in the physical world, as well as the mind itself. Amun is the hidden and secret aspect of the Trinity while Ra and Ptah symbolize the physical expression of it as mind and physical nature, respectively. In this sense, existence is formed of a Trinity of consciousness wherein there is a conscious witness of creation (*Amun*), a medium of vision or sight represented by *Ra*, and the physical objects of creation which are being seen, represented by *Ptah.*[1]

This theology contains valuable information about the triad of human consciousness which is also contained in the idea of the Christian Trinity. Most Christologists believe that he doctrine of the Christian Trinity was stated in early Christian creeds to counter beliefs such as Gnosticism which followed the idea that each individual is a manifestation of, and indeed one with, God. However, this is only partially true. Upon closer examination we see that the teaching of the Trinity was not introduced by the early Christians, but merely adopted by them in a limited form. The term *trinitas* first appears in the 2nd century A.C.E in the Christian literature. It was first used by Tertulian, a Latin theologian. The concept was developed through the course of the debates which sought to determine the nature of Christ (Christology). It was not until the 4th century that the Orthodox Roman Christian Fathers finally formulated the complete doctrine, which taught that there was co-equality between the persons *God (Father)-Son-Holy Ghost* of the Christian Godhead. St. Augustine's influential work in the 4th-century, *De Trinitate,* meaning "On the Trinity," (written c. 400-416 A.C.E.), compared, in a limited sense, the three-in-oneness concept of God with corresponding features in the human mind. He suggested that the Holy Spirit could be understood as a mutual love between Son and Father.

Matthew 28:19

19 Go ye therefore, and teach all nations, baptizing them in the name of the Father, and of the Son, and of the Holy spirit: {teach...: or, make disciples, or, Christians of all nations}

The passage above is the only place where the threefold character of Divinity is alluded to in the Bible. This is why the debates arose many years after the compilation of the books included in the Bible. Those who included this passage either did not understand its true meaning or if they did, they did not explain it, so it was necessary for subsequent church Fathers to formulate a doctrine to explain it. Since by this time the mystical practitioners of Christianity and of other religions in the Roman Empire were persecuted, if not murdered or otherwise silenced, the deeper meaning of this teaching was thus, lost to them. The following verses give an indication as to the ideas associated with the Holy Spirit.

Genesis 1

2 And the earth was without form, and void; and darkness [was] upon the face of the deep. And the Spirit of God moved upon the face of the waters.

Luke 1:15

15 For he shall be great in the sight of the Lord, and shall drink neither wine nor strong drink; and he shall be filled with the Holy Spirit, even from his mother's womb.

---

[1] Theban theology represents a vast topic of Ancient Egyptian teaching which is fully explored in the book *Egyptian Yoga Volume II: The Supreme Wisdom of Enlightenment.*

THE HISTORY AND PHILOSOPHY OF MYSTICAL CHRISTIANITY

The biblical statements above illustrate the Orthodox Christian view that God made creation and human beings through the power of the Holy Spirit. This is a teaching that was already expressed previously in the Ancient Egyptian Trinity. In a sense this idea corresponds with ancient mystical philosophy because the phenomenal world, including human beings, did emerge from the Supreme Divinity through a vehicle of three fold nature. However, on a more subtle level, this is only the elementary understanding of the philosophy behind the Trinity. The church fathers could not explain the nature of this Trinity in the deeper mystical sense referring to human consciousness and the physical universe. Their insistence on each character of the Trinity as being "equal" was also incomprehensible. So they fell back on the notion of blind faith saying that there is a mystery behind the Trinity and that believing in it was the duty of a true Christian. This seemingly complicated Triune notion of Divinity, along with church corruption and persecutions of other nations and religions, opened the door to alternative religions such as Islam and the later Protestant movements.

The Gnostics Christians, and later the Sufis[1], on the other hand, claimed that the phenomenal world is nothing but the Kingdom of Heaven itself and further, that the essence of every human being, the innermost Self, is one with God. They emphatically stated that the individual must acquire the knowledge which helps him or her to discover this essential truth which is masked by the ignorance of the mind. At the heart of this ignorance is the notion of the human ego. In order to discover one's innate oneness with the Supreme Being, one must discard one's individuality and be absorbed (in consciousness) into the Divine in a mystical sense. This is the deeper implication of Matthew 22: 37-38:

Matthew 22

37 Jesus said to him, Thou shalt love the Lord thy God with all thy heart, and with all thy soul, and with all thy mind.
  38 This is the first and great commandment.

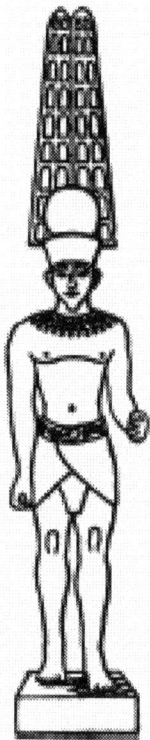

Left: The Ancient Egyptian god Amun (Amen) in the anthropomorphic (with human features) form.

The church fathers staunchly opposed this view, stating that there would be a bodily resurrection and that each individual person (ego) would join God in heaven if they lived righteously. What is really meant here is that each individual would somehow come back to life at the end of time and go to live in a spiritual world where they would be able to see Jesus and God on a throne and live happily ever after alongside them. The mystical understanding of the Gnostics, Ancient Egyptians, Buddhists, Taoists and Vedantins was and is that the world and indeed the entire universe, including human beings, is that Supreme Being and that to truly come to know that Being is to become "like unto it." When you learn something, it becomes a part of you. In a manner of speaking, when you discover Divinity, you become Divine. Traces of the mystical path may still be found in the present day orthodox Christian Bible. Three of the most important mystical passages come from the Gospels of John and Luke. They are rarely discussed in reference to their profound mystical meaning for each individual Christian follower.

John 10
30 *I and [my] Father are one.*
34 Jesus answered them, *Is it not written in your law, I said ,Ye are gods?*

Luke 17
20. And when he was asked by the Pharisees, when the Kingdom of God should come, he answered them and said, The Kingdom of God cometh not with observation
21 Neither shall they say, Lo here! or, lo there! for, behold, *the Kingdom of God is within you.*

A similar passage occurs in the Old Testament, Psalms 82:6, *I have said, Ye [are] gods; and all of you [are] children of the Most High.* In the passages above from the New Testament, Jesus is unequivocally stating that all of us individual human beings, male and female, are as he is. In reality, we are all Divine beings who are actually one with the Supreme Being and not separate entities. In addition, we are also one with all objects in Creation. In yoga texts, the example of the ocean and its waves is given. While each individual wave is different in appearance, what sustains them all is the ocean itself. Each wave (persons, objects), though on the surface appearing to be separate from other waves (objects and other persons) around it, is in reality of the same essence as all the other waves. In the same way Creation, all human life, animals and inanimate objects, arise in and is sustained by the ocean of divine consciousness, God. The problem of those who are ignorant of their true Self is

---

[1] Islamic mystics.

that they believe themselves to be separate from God, humanity and nature. They have not delved into the depths of their own being to discover their oneness with all Creation. This idea of separation gives rise to ego-consciousness. In turn, ego-consciousness, with its constant agitation due to desires, passions and ignorance of its essential nature, perpetuates the feeling of separation in every human being, the "I, me, mine, them, us, you" attitude. As a result, people spend their entire lives trying to acquire objects, situations and relationships with other people believing that this will make them feel whole and complete, and thus happy and peaceful. However, this sense of completeness which bestows true everlasting peace and happiness (bliss) can only come from understanding their own true nature as the all-encompassing Self. When this is realized, all cravings cease. Will the ocean crave for a wave when it encompasses that wave? However, not realizing this, the masses of people engage in a futile struggle to fulfill their ego-based desires thinking that somehow, one day they will find peace and happiness in the world of objects (waves). This is like trying to throw a stick up at the sky with the intent of hitting it. No matter how much you desire it and no matter how much effort you put into the attempt, you cannot succeed in the end.

Thus, we see that Orthodox Christianity was developed by those who advocated, however unwittingly, the path of egoism, while the mystics promote the path of egolessness as a way to find God. This distinction is crucial to the understanding of mystical and non-mystical philosophy. Egoism leads to experiences of alternating pain, pleasure, happiness, disappointment, etc., driving the soul to reincarnate again and again in the world of time and space, in a futile search for fulfillment. This is known as the "cycle of birth and death."

The path of egolessness leads the human being through a gradually increasing feeling of expansion and peace. In this state of consciousness, one realizes one's true self to be all-encompassing, immortal and infinite. This is why Jesus placed so much emphasis on humility, living in peace, providing selfless service to all human beings and universal love.

Matthew 22
36 Master, which [is] the great commandment in the law?
37 Jesus said to him, Thou shalt love the Lord thy God with all thy heart, and with all thy soul, and with all thy mind.
38 This is the first and great commandment.
39 And the second [is] like it, Thou shalt love thy neighbor as thyself.
40 On these two commandments hang all the law and the prophets.

These factors are essential features of Yoga in India as well as in Ancient Egypt. These practices lead to an effacement of the ego. During the time of the formation of the Christian religion, Gnosticism represented a religious movement which included numerous sects, and was widespread by the 2nd century A.C.E. Gnostic Christianity promised salvation through a special knowledge of God revealed through a direct mystical experience. As these sects incorporated many tenets of Orthodox Christianity, Gnostic Christianity was a serious competitor of early Orthodox Christianity which condemned it as heresy, meaning deviation from church dogma. Gnostic Christianity was condemned along with *Arianism*. Arianism was a theological stance, considered heretical to Christianity, and based on the teachings of Arius (c. 250-336 A.C.E.). Arius taught that Christ was a created being, and not divine. Therefore, since Jesus the Son had a definite beginning, as opposed to God who is beginning-less, he (Jesus) is mortal, and as such can have no direct knowledge of God. Arianism was officially condemned at the Council of Nicea (325 A.C.E.). It is interesting to note that this very idea of Arianism was an outgrowth of the Docetist Gnostic philosophy, and the same philosophy was also contained in the Ancient Egyptian texts such as the *'Egyptian Book of Coming forth by Day'* and the *'Papyrus of Nesi-Khensu'* in the following statements:

"God cannot be seen with mortal eyes...
God is invisible and inscrutable to Gods as well as men."
"Soul to heaven, body to earth."

However, the idea here is not that God cannot be known to humans, but that God cannot be known from the standpoint of the human ego concept of Self. God can be known if the personal ego self concept is transcended, but cannot be known through ordinary human consciousness which sees all things as separate from God and works through the medium of the limited mind and senses. The misunderstanding of this teaching led to much strife between Gnostic Christians and the Orthodox Christian community which sought to establish a dogma rooted in a concrete, ego-consciousness based reality rather than a mystical, transcendental one of the Gnostics. The emphasis on concrete physical reality in the church, rather than transcendental or mystical consciousness led to repudiation of all mystical religions and mystery cults by the Orthodox Church leadership. The Orthodox Christian groups gravitated towards government and social positions while the Gnostics moved away from these, seeing them as worldly endeavors. Thus, the Orthodox Christians gradually converted many Roman government officials and gained the favor of the government, and eventually the exclusive right to profess and practice Christianity. The desire of the church leaders to consolidate control over their domain created a climate which allowed for abuses and persecution to occur. Anyone who opposed the church for any reason risked being called a heretic.

Corruption of various church leaders was another effect of the ego dominance over the church. Corrupt church fathers hoarded wealth and created animosity towards anyone who did not agree with church dogma. It is no surprise then, that the confusion over doctrines and the well-documented corruption of church leadership led to the separation of the Western and Eastern churches, the emergence of Islam, and later to the emergence of Protestantism. Later, the same problem led to the even greater proliferation of church denominations and divisions in modern times. These divisions prompted the ecumenical movement in the twentieth century. In its early centuries, the Christian Catholic Church was undivided, but over time rifts emerged between Gnostics and the orthodox, and between the Western Church, Eastern and Egyptian churches. These were mostly the result of strong differences in beliefs as outlined above. Ecumenism, or the ecumenical movement, is the open recognition that the church is not united and an attempt to express the unity of the past in an effort to bring all Christians closer together. The term *ecumenical* originates in a Greek word *oikos*, which means "household," and is closely related to the word *oikoumene*, which means "the inhabited world." Thus, the term ecumenism is used by modern day Christian denominations with the hope of bridging the gaps that separate them. In essence, it suggests the ideal of a whole, worldwide community of God.

Many Orthodox Church fathers were afraid to let go of what they considered to be a concrete reality created by God. This view of the world caused them to develop feelings of possessiveness and further hardened their egoistic attachment to historical events, wealth and political power rather than to mystical thinking, openness, tolerance and understanding. Christian philosophy developed in the church as an intellectual philosophy which was created at church councils rather than a mystical religion which was revealed through mystical experience (seers, prophets, Saints and Sages). In this manner, the texts which were originally written by those who had authentic mystical experiences came to be included in the Bible cannon only after being altered and reworked to suit the opinions of the church leadership.

The church fathers remained antagonistic towards the path of mysticism, in part, because they feared giving up their hold on the power of the church which they gained through control of the Roman Empire, but they were also afraid of giving up their personal individuality. Therefore, Christian philosophy developed as a dualistic teaching which was directed towards a distant God rather than an immanent (residing in nature and in the human soul) Divinity. The theme of the underlying unity between God and Creation was well developed in the Ancient Egyptian theological system of the city of Memphis. It said that Creation (including human beings) is an emanation of the mind of God, and is therefore, one with God. This is the highest mystical interpretation of Creation. The Gnostic teachings of Jesus from the Gospel of Thomas in reference to the Kingdom of Heaven is in exact agreement with this Ancient Egyptian idea, but the Orthodox Church repudiates these as blasphemy or as an abomination.

JUDAISM AND ANCIENT EGYPTIAN RELIGION

The earliest record of the Hebrew people comes from an Ancient Egyptian temple inscription which describes them as a tribe of nomadic peoples in one of the subject territories of the Ancient Egyptian realm (Cannan). However, they are not referred to as slaves, but as one of the many groups which the Egyptians had conquered in the area. This misconception about the slavery of the Jews in Egypt has been promulgated throughout history based on the writings of the Bible. Yet there is no evidence that the Hebrews were slaves except in the writings of the Bible. Further, here is no evidence that the Hebrews were used as slave laborers to construct the great pyramids at Giza. In fact, their construction occurred long before the reputed birth date of Abraham, who is supposed to be the first Jew. While there is no factual evidence to support it, biblical scholars believe that Abraham may have lived around 2,100 B.C.E. According to the most conservative dating by modern Egyptologists, the pyramids were constructed in the Old Kingdom Period (2,575-2,134 B.C.E.).

Even though there is some evidence to show that the Hebrews were a splinter group of Egyptians and that the Jewish religion is based on Ancient Egyptian Religion, they were also influenced by Mesopotamian religions as well. The Hebrew language and culture were influenced by the Babylonians.[1] It was eventually submerged by Aramaic. Aramaic is a biblical Semitic language, the original language of parts of the Old Testament. After the Babylonian captivity of the Hebrews, it was the common written and spoken language of the Middle East (Southwest Asia) until replaced by Arabic. However, minor dialects persist. After the destruction of the second Temple at Jerusalem in A.C.E. 70, the use of Hebrew almost totally ceased. With the use of Hebrew by poets and

---

[1] Babylon, an ancient city of Mesopotamia located on the Euphrates River.

rabbis,[1] Hebrew became a literary and even holy language, used in the performance of synagogue services only. In the 18th century, Hebrew was revived and used in secular circles. In 1948, when the state of Israel was founded, Hebrew was declared the official national language.[117]

It must be clearly understood, however, that the reemergence of the Hebrew language does not mean that the modern day Jews understand all of the meanings of the Hebrew words or certain terms, etc. Most Bible scholars admit this point. They have succeeded in regaining much of the lost language, and with it much of Hebrew culture, but there will always be some nuances of the language which will remain lost. In any case, to the extent that it is possible, the language provides a cultural identity which allows those who can learn it to access ancestral mythological roots. However, if any language or culture is used as a means to develop cultural identity and set one group apart from others, this is an egoistic reason, based on adherence to myth and tradition as opposed to universal religious experience that will lead to conflicts, repudiation and self-centeredness at the individual level, as well as the national level. Nations, borders, languages, culture and governments are abstractions that people create. They are not separate realities in nature. Nature does not recognize borders or culture, only people make these distinctions, often based on ignorance and misunderstanding. Saints and Sages do not recognize languages and customs as real divisions between peoples. When a person identifies himself or herself with nationalistic policies or philosophies, they become instruments of that policy or philosophy. They lose their individual free will. When religion is used to promote nationalistic policies or philosophies it is no longer religion, but an instrument for promoting the egoistic desires of people. This will invariably lead to the subjugation of one group of people by others.

The Jewish story of the birth of Moses was told in the birth of Sargon I many years before.

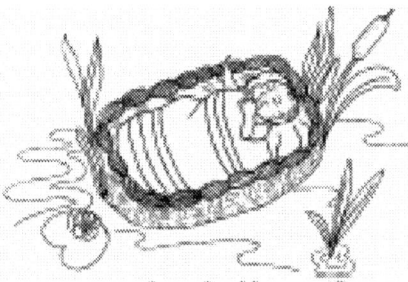

When people become deluded and feel they belong to a certain group or culture with particular customs, language and opinions, they begin to separate from others. The separation is emotional, philosophical, etc., but it is not real otherwise. This is not a desirable situation from a spiritual point of view. Culture and language should not be seen as a person's identity. A human being cannot transcend the world as long as he or she holds onto the idea that he or she is of a particular group or other ("I am German," "I am American," "I am Spanish," "I am Jewish," "I am Christian," etc.). While living in a culture, a spiritual aspirant should assert: "I am a spirit living as a German man," "I am a spirit living as an American woman," "I am a spirit living as a Spanish man," etc. Likewise, a person should not identify with a particular religion either. A spiritual aspirant should assert: "I am practicing this religion to lead me to enlightenment. I might have been born as a Hindu or a Muslim in a previous incarnation, but now I am a Christian and I will use its wisdom to lead me to God, the goal of all religions." This attitude promotes harmony, understanding and peace between religions. This atmosphere of peace will allow for the exchange of spiritual wisdom between them. This exchange will lead to greater spiritual awareness and evolution instead of strife, distraction and unrest between them.

According to the biblical tradition, at about 1400? B.C.E., the Hebrews were in Egypt, serving as slaves. A Jewish woman placed her son in a basket and allowed it to float downstream where the Egyptian queen found it and then adopted the child. The child was Moses, the chosen one of God, who would lead the Jews out of bondage in Egypt. Moses was taken in by the royal family and taught all of the wisdom related to rulership of the nation as well as religious wisdom in reference to running the Egyptian Temples. He was being groomed to be king and high priest of Egypt. This is why the Bible says he was knowledgeable in the wisdom of the Egyptians (Bible: Acts 7:22 and Koran C.144-(Verses 37 to 76)-). A story similar to the birth of Moses, about a child being placed in a basket and put in a stream which was later found by a queen, can be found in Zoroastrian mythology as well.[58] Also, the Semitic ruler, Sargon I, was rescued in the same manner after he was placed in a basket and sent floating down a river. Sargon I reigned about 2335-2279 B.C.E. He was called Sargon, The Great. He was one of the first known major Semitic conquerors known in history. He was successful in conquering the entire country of Sumer. Sumer is an ancient country of south western Asia, which corresponds approximately to the land known as Babylonia of

---

[1] Rabbi, (Hebrew "my master"). Since the Middle Ages, the Rabbi was the individual responsible for religious education, guidance, and services in the synagogue. His position is based on his learning, but entails no special privileges. His duties include interpreting Jewish law and guiding the spiritual lives of people. Originally applied to scholars and teachers of the law; used in New Testament as a title of respect in addressing Jesus Christ. [117]

biblical times. Babylon was an ancient city of Mesopotamia which was located on the Euphrates River about 55mi (89km) South of the present-day Baghdad. Sargon created an empire stretching from the Mediterranean to the Persian Gulf in c.2350 B.C.E.

At around 1200? B.C.E. Moses led the Hebrews, who were by this time in reality people of Egyptian blood, out of Egypt into the Sinai desert where he was given the Ten Commandments by God. Moses subsequently wrote the Pentateuch[I] and gave these teachings to the people. Under the rulership of Joshua, the Hebrews gained control over the land of Palestine where they continued to mix with other Canaanites, who were themselves descendents of the Ethiopians and relatives of the Egyptians. Under the rulership of King David (circa 1000-961 B.C.E.), the Hebrews became a local power. David's son, Solomon, ruled from around 961 to 922 B.C.E. and was famed for his wisdom, which very closely follows the Ancient Egyptian teachings of Sage Amenemope. Solomon commissioned the building of the first Jewish[II] temple in Jerusalem.

Following Solomon's passing, the kingdom was split into two realms. These were Judah and Israel. According to the Old Testament, the Hebrews had been subdivided into 13 tribes. Ten of these were incorporated into Israel and the other three were incorporated into Judah. The Old Testament describes a story of how King Ahab of Israel (c. 869-850 B.C.E.) married Jezebel and allowed the introduction of the worship of Phoenician Gods. The prophet Elijah denounced the king and called on the Hebrew people to repent.

At around 721 B.C.E. the Assyrians conquered Israel. The tribes there disappeared. This led to the mythical stories related to the "Ten Lost Tribes." The Hebrews who had become part of Judah also became subject to the Assyrians rule. Then they were driven into exile and experienced the Babylonian Captivity. In 586 B.C.E., King Cyrus the Great of Persia allowed them to return to Jerusalem,[III] where they rebuilt the temple. However, they continued to be subjects of the Persian Empire and later became subjects of the empire of Alexander the Great (c. 300 B.C.E.). The Maccabees[IV] revolted during the 2nd and 1st centuries B.C.E. and restored Hebrew independence for some time. However, the Hebrews, not long after, became subjects of the Roman Empire, a subjugation which continued well after the death of Jesus.

So it is clear to see why, at the time Jesus would have lived, the Jewish people would have been eager to see a liberator who would free them from domination by other peoples. However, at the time when Jesus would have been preaching, there is every indication that he was ignored by the majority of the Jewish population, who were searching, not for a spiritual liberator which Jesus was, but for a great warrior and conqueror like King David. In the year 66 A.C.E., the Jews staged a revolt against Rome, but after four years (70 A.C.E.) they were defeated by the Roman legions. At that time Jerusalem was destroyed, dispersing the Jews. It was not until 1948 that the new state of Israel was formed in the Middle East after so many centuries.

We have seen how the character, Moses, played an important part in the creation of Jewish religion and how the Bible itself acknowledges that the new religion (Judaism) sprang forth out of Ancient Egypt as Moses learned the wisdom of the Egyptians (Acts 7:22), created the Pentateuch which in turn gave rise to the Jewish laws and scriptures (Torah[V]). Another correlation between Judaism and Ancient Egyptian religion is the format of daily worship which in Ancient Egypt consisted of a service at dawn, one at midday and another at sunset, commemorating God who manifests as the Trinity Khepri-Ra-Tem and sustains Creation. The Jews apparently adopted this triune format of worship and practice it to this day. Later in our journey we will see how the Ten Commandments and the Laws given by Moses can be traced to the Ancient Egyptian *Book of Coming Forth By Day* and the Wisdom Texts.[VI]

Acts 7
22 And Moses was learned in all the wisdom of the Egyptians, and was mighty in words and in deeds.

[I] The first five books of the Hebrew Scriptures.

[II] The term "Jewish" means specifically those tribes that accepted the god Yahweh as their deity.

[III] Jerusalem (Hebrew Yerushalayim; Arabic al-Quds) is the largest city and capital of Israel. Jerusalem is held to be a holy city for three of the world's major religions: Judaism, Christianity, and Islam.

[IV] The Maccabees were a family of Jewish rulers and patriots in the 2nd and 1st centuries B.C.E., and more correctly known as the Hasmonaeans, from Hashmon or Hasmon, the name of an ancestor. The title of the Bible Books (1 Maccabees and 2 Maccabees) is derived from the nickname of the military leader Judas, or Judah Maccabeus and is part of the Old Testament for Roman Catholics and Orthodox Christians.

[V] The entire body of religious law and learning including both sacred literature and oral tradition.

[VI] Wisdom teachings given by Ancient Egyptian Sages upon which the entire philosophy and religion of Ancient Egypt is based.

So the question now arises, if Ancient Egypt had such high culture and social advancement in spiritual practice and mystical philosophy, why was it necessary for Moses to lead the people who were following Judaism out of Egypt? The following historians and writers from ancient times provide some clues to answer the previous question.

"In the reign of Apis, the son of Pharonaeus, a portion of the Egyptian army deserted from Egypt and took up their habitation in...Palestine...These were the very men who went out with Moses."
-Eusebius (260?-340? A.C.E.)[I]

"This region (Judea[II]) lies toward the north; and it is inhabited in general, as each place in particular, by mixed stocks of people from Egyptian and Arabian and Phoenician tribes...But though the inhabitants are mixed up thus, the most prevalent of the accredited reports in regard to the temple at Jerusalem represents the ancestors of the present Judaeans, as they are called, as Egyptians.

Moses, namely, was one of the Egyptian priests, and held a part of Lower Egypt, as it is called, but he went away from there to Judaea, since he was displaced with the state of affairs there, and was accompanied by many people who worshipped the Divine Being."
-Strabo (63? BC-A.C.E. 24?)[III]

"The Jews were a tribe of Egyptians who revolted from the established religion."

-Celsus, Aulus Cornelius
(Roman writer, 1st century A.C.E.)

Many people misunderstand the word "slavery" as it is used in history. The slavery that was practiced in ancient times CANNOT be compared to that which was practiced by the European nations in reference to Africans or Native Americans. The European form of slavery was characterized by egoism, racism violence, brutality, degradation, mis-education, mistreatment and all manner of atrocities and injustices. In ancient times, people found themselves as slaves as a consequence of losing a war or incurring a dept, for example, but they were not kidnapped as part of an organized slavery business and forced to give up their religion and customs. Slaves were part of the family of the master, and might even marry into the family. The children could be born free. This form of slavery is described in the Bible (Exodus 21 1:11). However, the European form of slavery was based on racism, the idea that one race is superior to another, and was intended to be a permanent situation. This form of slavery upheld ignorant notions of superiority, inferiority, segregation and anti-miscegenation. The perpetuators of the European slave trade were in no way sanctioned by any teaching that can be found in the Bible. They were not Christians at all, and no negative judgement should fall on Christianity in its true practice because of their actions.

It must also be clearly understood that historically, the Jewish people do not appear as anything other than a tribe or sect of Ancient Egyptians who were under the control of the Ancient Egyptian government during the time when the Egyptian civilization encompassed south west Asia (Syria, Palestine, Iraq, Turkey, etc.). This is not a far-fetched notion since Herodotus (c.484-425 B.C.E.), the Greek historian, considered the Chaldeans, a group who lived as far into the Middle East as the area that is modern day Iraq,[IV] to be Egyptians as well. The term "Hebrew" means "those who pass from place to place." They were considered as an inconsequential group of wanderers. They were enslaved by most of the great empires of the Middle East at one time or another. The Hebrews had no permanent place to live or permanent homeland in ancient times, as their own name attests, except possibly the land of Egypt. However, Egypt was so permeated by the ancient Shetaut Neter (Ancient Egyptian Religion and its gods and goddesses), that Judaism would not have survived there beyond cult status. Hence, the need for an exodus. Further, although the Jewish religion has been erroneously linked with the idea of race or ethnicity, the term "Jew"[V] does not connote a

---

[I] (Citing the Greek philosopher, Polema) Eusebius of Caesarea (also called Pamphili) (260?-340?), Christian theologian, most learned man of his age; 'History of the Christian Church', most important ancient record of church; called Father of Church History; chief figure at Council of Nicaea (from Compton's Encyclopedia)

[II] Judea (or Judaea, or Judah), a Greek and Roman name for s. Palestine; in time of Jesus part of province of Syria and also kingdom of the Herods; in Roman times southernmost division of Palestine, Israel.[123]

[III] Greek historian and geographer who was born in Amasya, Pontus (now in Turkey). He explored the Nile with the expedition of Aelius Gallus, a Roman prefect of Egypt.

[IV] Also the area where Abraham came from.

[V] **Jew** (joō) *n.* **1.** An adherent of Judaism as a religion or culture.[115]

racial, ethnic or genetic relationship. It is a religion which was developed around the Hebrew culture. The Hebrews shared the same history of wandering in ancient times with other Semitic[I] nomads, and not all Hebrews, who were living in Palestine, were Jews.

Below left: The Hindu god Indra. Below right : The Hindu god Vishnu

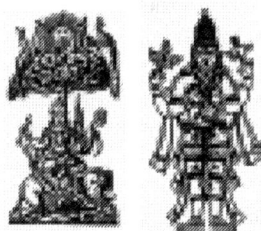

Many times in the emergence of new mythologies, the founders or followers of the new system will create stories to show how the new system surpasses the old. The story of Exodus is such an example. Moses went to Mount Sinai to talk to God and brought back Ten Commandments. At the time that Moses was supposed to have lived (1200?-1000? B.C.E.), Ancient Egypt was the most powerful culture in the ancient world. However, it was also on a social and cultural decline from its previous height as the foremost culture in religious practice, art, science, social order, etc. So it became necessary for a small group who left Egypt, that were themselves Egyptians, to legitimize the inception of the new theology by claiming to have triumphed over the mighty Egyptians with the help of their new "true God" who defeated the "weak Gods" of Egypt. This triumphant story would surely bring people to convert to the new faith since up to that time the Ancient Egyptian gods and goddesses had been seen not only as the most powerful divinities, but also as the source of all other deities in other religions. So in effect, by saying that the Jewish God "defeated" the Ancient Egyptian God by freeing the Jews, it is the same as saying that a new, more powerful religion is to be followed. This form of commencement for a spiritual tradition is not uncommon.

In India, the emergence of Hinduism saw a similar situation as the one that occurred between the Jews and Ancient Egyptian Religion. In a later period (c. 800 B.C.E.), the earlier Vedic-Aryan religious teachings related to the God, Indra (c. 1,000 B.C.E.), were supplanted by the teachings related to the Upanishadic and Vaishnava tradition of Vishnu worship which includes the devotion to God in the form of the Vishnu avatars Rama and Krishna. The Vaishnava tradition was developed by the indigenous Indian peoples to counter the religion imposed on them by the Vedic Aryans. In the epic stories known as the Ramayana and the Mahabharata, Vishnu incarnates as Rama and Krishna, respectively, and throughout the stories it is related how Vishnu's incarnations are more powerful than Indra, who is portrayed as being feeble and weak. Some of the writings of the Upanishadic Tradition,[II] the writings which supercede the Vedic Tradition, contain specific verses stating that they supersede the Vedas. One such statement can be found in the Mundaka Upanishad and another in the Brihadaranyaka Upanishad. A similar situation occurred with the emergence of Buddhism. The story of Buddha's struggle to attain enlightenment, the inceptive and most influential work of Buddhist mythology, relates how he strived to practice the austere paths of Hinduism. He practiced renunciation of the world and all sorts of penances and asceticism, even to the point of almost starving to death. Then he discovered a "new" path, The Middle Path, and for a long time it was held to be superior to Hinduism by many. It found a great following in China and Tibet, as well as the countries of Indo-China. The Indochinese peninsula includes a small part of Bangladesh, most of Myanmar (Burma), Thailand, Cambodia, and parts of Malaysia, Laos, and Vietnam. Currently in the west, Buddhism is rarely related to its roots in Hinduism and Yoga philosophy. Upon close examination, the roots of the teaching of the middle path along with the other major tenets of Buddhism can be found in the Upanishadic Tradition,[III] especially in the Isha Upanishad.

In this area of study, an important figure from Mesopotamia is Hammurabi. Hammurabi lived around 1792-1750 B.C.E. He was king of Babylonia in the first dynasty. He expanded his rule over Mesopotamia and organized the empire by building wheat granaries, canals and classified the law into the famous Code of Hammurabi. The divine origin ascribed to the Code is of particular interest to our study. Hammurabi can be seen receiving the Code in a bas-

---

[I] Of or pertaining to the Semites, especially Jewish or Arabic. 2. Pertaining to a subfamily of the Afro-Asiatic language family that includes Arabic and Hebrew.[115]

[II] Any of a group of philosophical treatises contributing to the theology of ancient Hinduism-Vedanta Philosophy, elaborating on and superseding the earlier Vedas.

[III] Spiritual tradition in india based on the scriptures known as the Upanishads. It is also referred to as Vedanta Philosophy, the culmination or summary of the Vedic Tradition whish is itself based on the scriptures known as the Vedas.

relief in which he is depicted as receiving the Code from the sun-god, Shamash, in much the same way that Moses would later receive the Ten Commandments from God. This mode of introducing a teaching or new order, by claiming it to be divinely ordained, is in reality an attempt to impress on the masses of people the authenticity, importance and force with which the new teaching must be followed. Like Moses, Hammurabi created the laws himself, wishing to institute a new order for society. Whether or not they were divinely inspired relates to the degree of communion they were able to achieve with the Divine Self, God. This they could only ascertain for themselves. People tend to follow a teaching when they believe that it is inspired by God even if they cannot know for certain in their minds, they feel they somehow "know" in their hearts or they are urged, by passionate preachers, to have faith. However, if people are fanatical instead of introspective and sober, they may follow the teachings of an ignorant personality and even follow them blindly, to their death.

The idea that the Jews are more powerful than the other groups by virtue of their god is also reflected in the Bible verse in Genesis 9:26-27:

> 26 And he said, Blessed [be] the LORD God of Shem; and Canaan shall be his servant. {his servant: or, servant to them}
> 27 God shall enlarge Japheth, and he shall dwell in the tents of Shem; and Canaan shall be his servant. {enlarge: or, persuade}

In the Bible itself there is an attempt to show that the main Jewish ancestors comes from the blood-line of Shem" (Genesis 11:10-26). This is done in an effort to follow up on the idea given in Genesis 9:26-27, that the Canaanites should be serving the Jews. These Biblical statements, like "be fruitful and multiply" (Genesis 1:28) and other "commands" of God are in reality mandates or directives written into the Bible for directing the goals and objectives of the Jews. They are similar to political edicts, and acted to reinforce a particular agenda for the masses of people to believe in and pursue. They give a purpose and meaning to the lives of the Jews but they are not to be understood as spiritual edicts to be followed literally. They were written for a certain time and purpose which is several thousands of years removed from the present. It is notable that if Noah was angry with Ham, why did he not curse Ham? Instead he cursed Canaan. This is because the land of Canaan was the place where the Hebrews had always lived as wanderers and some of them were the writers of the Bible scriptures. They always longed to have a homeland in Canaan and the scriptures of the Old Testament are therefore directed at rallying people together in a movement towards conquering the land of Canaan and its people. The early Jews wanted to live in Canaan (Palestine) and not in Ethiopia (Ham). Judging from the times they were recorded, the clear implication is that the inhabitants of the land of Canaan, who were not followers of Judaism, were to be conquered by the Jews and used by them for their survival.

In the Bible, the book of Exodus is so called because it relates the departure of the Jewish people out of Egypt. It is traditionally ascribed to Moses. Most modern scholars believe that its present form was compiled by members of the Jewish priesthood sometime around 550 B.C.E. Some sections (20:23-23:33) are believed to be of even greater antiquity. Some believe that they may have originated in pre-Mosaic times. It is very likely that this section along with Chapters 25-31, in which God describes to Moses the proper way to arrange the Tabernacle and its furnishings as well as the ritual and dress of the priests, is in part the "wisdom of the Egyptians" which is referred to in Acts 7:22.

Ancient Egypt and the Exodus

The Bible book of Exodus recounts how the Jews left Egypt and escaped bondage in order to seek a new life and their own homeland. In popular tradition, the story of Exodus has come to be associated with the Ancient Egyptian Pharaoh Rameses (Ramses). Many Bible scholars and theologians promote the idea that he was forced to let the Jews go just as the Bible recounts. However, records of this Pharaoh's activities are much earlier than the ascribed date for the life of Moses (1200?-1000? B.C.E.).

Some scholars have suggested that Moses may have lived in the 14th century, others have suggested the 12th. They base these figures on the writings of the Bible. The dating of the original Bible scriptures is based on comparisons of its grammar to other writings of the period. This method is inexact. Nevertheless, many Egyptologists have accepted this criterion when dating Ancient Egyptian events, using the Bible sometimes as the only source. This is of course unacceptable, especially in the light of the Ancient Egyptian writings which contain a more complete history as well as the dating of the Sphinx.

Also, there were several Ancient Egyptian kings who went by the name Rameses. The Ramses' kings were so powerful that it is virtually inconceivable that any kind of exodus story or defiance from nomadic groups would have been allowed without any records at all in the Egyptian inscriptions. Pharaoh Ramses II (1279-1212 B.C.E.), the son of Seti I, ascended the throne of Egypt and became the third ruler of the 19th Dynasty. Ramses III (reigned 1182-1151 B.C.E.) was the king of Egypt in the 20th Dynasty. He was a great military leader who saved the country from invaders several times. It was not until after the rule of Ramses III that Egypt went into a sharp decline due to the weak rulers,[I] invasions and internal corruption. During the reign of the Ramses' Kings, there is no record of an exodus by the Jews or by any other group. However, it would have still required divine intervention to neutralize the Ancient Egyptian forces. If this had occurred, some record would certainly have survived somewhere either in official records or in private (unofficial) writings such as the papyri or graffito, much of which survives to this day.

There are many Ancient Egyptian records which have been found. They are private and graffito type records which expound on many other topics such as politics, the economy, sex, gossip, etc.

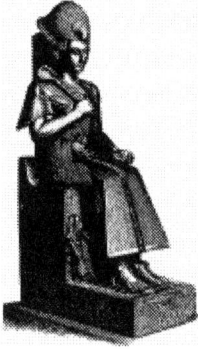

The word "Rameses" appears four times in the Bible books Genesis, Exodus and Numbers.

Left: Rameses II ("Rameses the Great" c. 1,290-1,224 B.C.E), recognized as the most powerful Ancient Egyptian king of his time.

Genesis 47:11
11 And Joseph placed his father and his brethren, and gave them a possession in the land of Egypt, in the best of the land, in the land of *Rameses*, as Pharaoh had commanded.

Exodus 12:37
37. And the children of Israel journeyed from *Rameses* to Succoth, about six hundred thousand on foot [that were] men, besides children.

Numbers 33:3
3 And they departed from *Rameses* in the first month, on the fifteenth day of the first month; on the next day after the passover the children of Israel went out with an high hand in the sight of all the Egyptians.

Numbers 33:5
5 And the children of Israel removed from *Rameses*, and encamped in Succoth.

As can be readily surmised from the passages above, the word Rameses refers to the land of Egypt and not to a particular king. The power of the Rameses kings was so great at that time (c. 1,307-1,070 B.C.E.) that the entire land of Ancient Egypt was referred to as Rameses by foreigners.

If understood in an allegorical sense, with the wisdom of Yoga, the story of Exodus is not to be seen as an historical teaching, but as a metaphor relating to the awakening of the soul and the journey towards enlightenment which requires a movement away from ignorance and unrighteousness. Ancient Egypt, which was held to be the light of the world in regard to religion, art and civilization by all ancient cultures, was portrayed in Exodus as a decadent society. In mythical terms, the Jews escaped the bondage to what they saw as spiritual ignorance. From their point of view, all religions except theirs was ignorant and abominable. It was necessary to denigrate Ancient Egyptian Religion in order to promote Judaism and set it apart from Shetaut Neter (Ancient Egyptian Religion). There is no evidence to show that the Ancient Egyptians worshipped idols in the time of Moses or at any time previous to that. During his time the Ancient Egyptian religion was seen as the highest achievement in spirituality by other countries and even seven hundred years later the same was reported by the Greek historians and philosophers such as Pythagoras, Herodotus, Diodorus, Plato and Iamblichus.[127] Thus, it is more likely that the creators of Judaism sought to pit Judaism against Shetaut Neter in order to garnish the prestige and preeminence of Ancient Egypt religion and culture.

[I] Weak in morality and managerial skills.

Ancient Egypt, Sumeria and Judaism

Many scholars have pointed to Ancient Sumer in Mesopotamia as the seat of civilization. Further, they have tried to show some important similarities between Sumerian religion and Judaism. However, as we have seen, the origins of Ancient Egypt go farther in antiquity than any other civilization. Also, the borders of Ancient Egypt spanned from Ethiopia to the Ganges river in India, and beyond, in the time of Asar (Predynastic Period), and from Ethiopia to the head of the Euphrates river in Southwest Asia, an area including Syria, Babylon, Mitanni, Assyria, Cyprus and Phoenicia, in the time of Pharoah Djehutimes III (Thutmosis III) in 1479 B.C.E. though the reign of Pharoah Amenhotep IV (Akhenaton). Under Ramses II, Palestine (Canaan) remained part of Egypt (c. 1,200 B.C.E.), but later on it was lost to invaders under weaker rulers. Later, under the Ptolematic[1] kings, Egypt regained control of Palestine and southern Turkey (330 B.C.E.-30 B.C.E.). This means that Ancient Egypt controlled Mesopotamia and the Biblical lands during various periods in history.

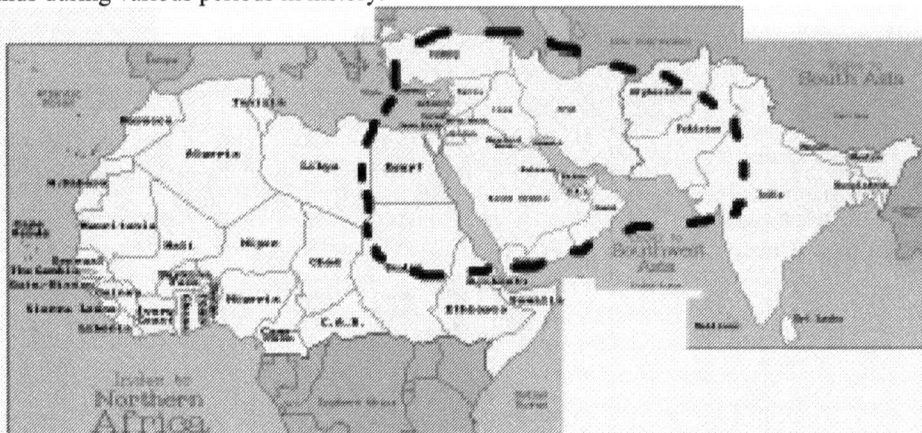

Above: Ancient Egyptian borders in Ancient times.

"And upon his return to Greece, they gathered around and asked, "tell us about this great land of the Blacks called Ethiopia." And Herodotus said, "There are two great Ethiopian nations, one in Sind (India) and the other in Egypt."

Recorded by *Diodorus* (Greek historian 100 B.C.)[64]

Thus, the similarities between Ancient Egyptian religion and other religions are not likely due to the influence of the other religions on Ancient Egypt, but rather the other way around. Sumerian religion is believed to have influenced Judaism. However, a brief study of Sumerian religion reads almost exactly like Ancient Egyptian religion in its basic respects. Sumer was known as the southern region of ancient Mesopotamia. This area was later known as the southern part of Babylonia and today it is known as south central Iraq. Like Ancient Egypt, it was an agricultural civilization and flourished there during the 3rd and 4th millennia B.C.E.

---

[1] Descendants of Ptolemy, a general of Alexander the Great, who took control of Egypt after Alexander died.

SUMERIAN RELIGION[75/117]	ANCIENT EGYPTIAN RELIGION
A- The Sumerians believed that the universe was ruled by a pantheon of divinities comprising a group of living beings, human in form, but immortal and possessing superhuman powers. They believed these beings to be invisible to mortal eyes. They controlled and guided the cosmos in accordance with well-laid plans and duly prescribed laws.	A- The Ancient Egyptian Religion was headed by a pantheon as well. It was comprised of Ra or Pa-Neter, the Supreme Being, and from him emanated the neteru or gods and goddesses. They were depicted with human forms but were symbolic of unseen cosmic principles.
B- The Sumerians recognized four leading deities. They were known as gods of creation. These gods were An, the god of heaven, Ki, the goddess of earth, Enlil, the god of air, and Enki, the god of water. Thus, heaven, earth, air, and water were considered as the four major constituents of the universe.	B- The main gods and goddesses of the Ancient Egyptian pantheon of the city of Anu were: Shu- Air Tefnut- Moisture Geb- Earth Nut- Sky, Heaven
C- It was held that the act of creation was accomplished through the utterance of the divine word. The deity doing the creating had only to make plans mentally and then pronounce the name of the thing to be created.	C- Creation was accomplished by God in the form of Neberdjer, by uttering his own name. God could create by merely thinking it into existence. The same creative word teaching was adopted by the Greeks and the Christians (John 1:1 - *In the beginning was the Word, and the Word was with God, and the Word was God.*).
D- To maintain the universe in harmonious and continuous operation and to avoid conflict and confusion, the gods brought the "me" into being. It was a set of unchangeable and universal rules and laws or laws that all beings were required to obey.	D- In order to maintain the universe God instituted Maat. Maat is the principle and philosophy of cosmic order, justice, righteousness and harmony which all nature follows. All human beings were required to practice Maat in order to live in harmony with nature and each other, and to reach the eternal abode to live with God after death.
E- Each of the important deities was the patron of one or more Sumerian cities. Large temples were erected in the name of the deity, who was worshiped as the divine ruler and protector of the city. Temple rites were conducted by many priests, priestesses, singers, musicians, sacred prostitutes, and eunuchs. Sacrifices were offered daily.	E- The cities of Ancient Egypt were known as Nomes. Each had a patron deity. Many temples survive to this day. Daily rituals were performed by priests and priestesses.
F- The Sumerians believed that human beings were fashioned of clay.	F- The Ancient Egyptians believed that God in the form of Knum, fashioned human beings on a potter's wheel.
G- When human beings die, it was believed, their spirits descend to the netherworld.	G- When human beings die they go to the Duat (netherworld) where they are judged in accordance with their deeds while on earth.

Many people have come to interpret the stories contained in the Bible as historical facts instead of as mythic metaphors for spiritual education, such as the incident when Moses saw a vision of God as a burning bush. Moses' vision of the burning bush symbolizes the fire of knowledge that burns in a mind that is purified with devotion and wisdom related to the Divine. When Moses asks God his name, God tells him that his name is Yahweh or Jehovah. There is much confusion over the pronunciation and meaning of that name among Jewish and non-Jewish scholars.

The translation is often given as "I am" or "The Existing One," the proper name of the Hebrew God. Jehovah is an erroneously transliterated form of the term which appears in the Masoretic Hebrew text. Much like the Ancient Egyptian scripture, the word Jehovah originally consisted of the consonants *JHWH* or *JHVH*, with the vowels of a separate word, *Adonai* (Lord). What its original vowels were is a matter of speculation. Because of an interpretation of such texts as Exodus 20:7 and Leviticus 24:11, the name came to be regarded as too sacred for expression. The scribes, in reading aloud, substituted "Lord" and therefore wrote the vowel markings for "Lord" (*Adonai*) into the consonantal framework JHVH as a reminder to future readers as to the desired pronunciation. The older interpreters explain the verb in a metaphysical and abstract sense: The "I am" of scripture is "He who is," the absolutely existent.[75] The teaching of how Moses parted the Red Sea refers to the separation of the mind from confusion. It means the blossoming of the intellect that allows a person to see clearly what is truth (real) and what is untruth (unreal). Also, the crossing of the sea implies crossing over the ocean of ignorance and discovering the truth (God) which lies beyond. The story of the parting of the sea occurs in two Ancient Egyptian myths prior to the biblical story of Moses: The story of the Book of Djehuti and the story of the Pharaoh and the lost jewel.

Like the Pharaoh Akhenaton (c.1379-1362 B.C.E.), who lived earlier than the Ramses' kings, Moses was attempting to reform a religion which focused too much attention on rituals related to many gods and goddesses, and too little acknowledging the Supreme Being which is above them. While many people in modern times consider Judaism to be a monotheistic religion, it originated out of a polytheistic history. Also, upon closer examination, it will become clear that what most people call monotheism is in reality an extreme form of idolatry. This theme will be developed further throughout the study of Christian Yoga in the following sections of this volume. The early polytheism of the Hebrews is evinced by the fact that *Yahweh* (*JHWH*) was originally considered to be <u>one</u> of the *Elohim* ("the goddesses and the gods"). The Elohim of Judaism can be equated to the *neteru* or gods and goddesses of Ancient Egypt. Thus, Moses sought to create an entirely new culture based on the same ideal as that of Ancient Egypt, but in the process of creating this new religion the image of Ancient Egyptian culture and religion was impugned in the Torah and in the Biblical traditions. Moses and the Jewish tradition succeeded in surviving the test of time. However, this was due less to the power of the teaching than to the staunch and tenacious traditions and rituals upholding the Jewish idea of monotheism and the covenant as exclusive, historical events instead of as metaphorical ones. These ideas in Judaism, developed by the priesthoods, which advocated rituals that promoted segregation and the prohibition from marrying those from other faiths has also led to racial segregation in modern times. These traditions became part of Jewish culture over time and formed the basis of the idea in many people's minds that the Jews are a racial class or a separate ethnic group. This same idea was instrumental in creating ethnic animosity against Jews. They were seen as a rival group who banded together to increase wealth amongst themselves and control the economy. They were also seen by other religious groups as spiritual elitists who consider themselves as chosen people who follow the "real" God while others are following "idols" and "lies."

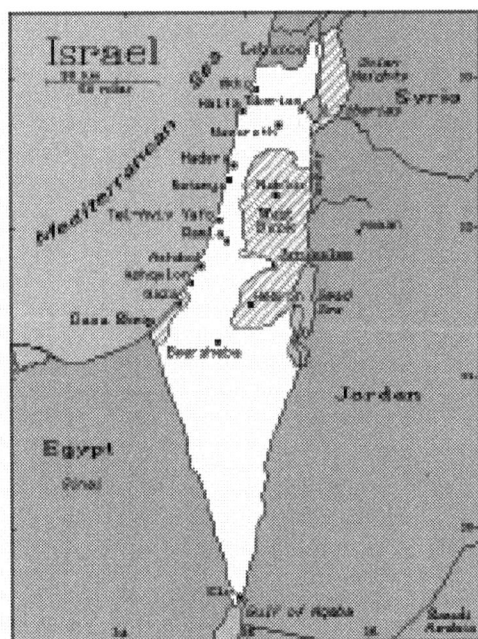

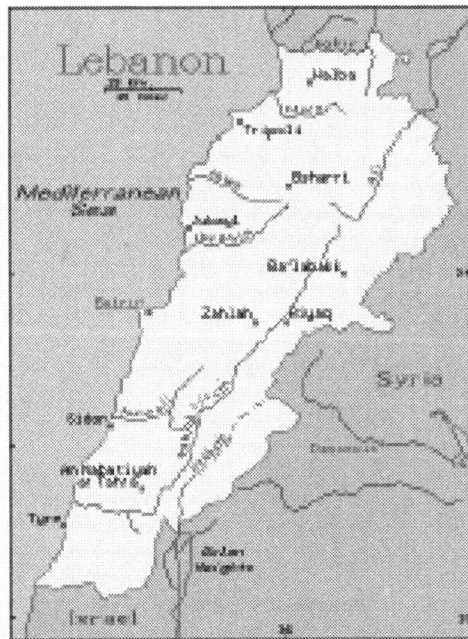

Below left:
The Modern state of Israel.

Below right:
Lebanon.

In mystical terms the name Jehovah relates to the self-existent Supreme Being which is the reality behind all things. Thus, Judaism represents an attempt to go back to that essential truth which is at the heart of all religions, which they had adopted from Ancient Egypt. As we will see, this idea was always and continues to be the central teaching of Ancient Egyptian and Indian religion and Yoga philosophy. Therefore, it cannot be said that Moses was an innovator in religious thought, but that he attempted to reinterpret some of the preexisting religious symbolism into a new system. The story of Exodus also shows the student of religion and yoga some of the pitfalls of orthodox religion. Orthodox religion uses a specific language relating to certain images and symbols which contain a particular relationship to a "special" group of people, whereas yoga philosophy is universal and applies to all forms of spirituality. This is why the yogic aspects of religion can be easily seen and understood by a yogi who studies any religion, but a person who is involved with orthodox religion cannot easily see the religious points in yoga or even see points of commonality in other religions besides their own. However, if that person is highly advanced and has discovered that the goal of all religions and mystical philosophies is one and the same, then they will see commonality in all forms of worship. They will have a universal, inclusive point of view and not an exclusive, closed minded point of view.

JUDAISM IN ETHIOPIA

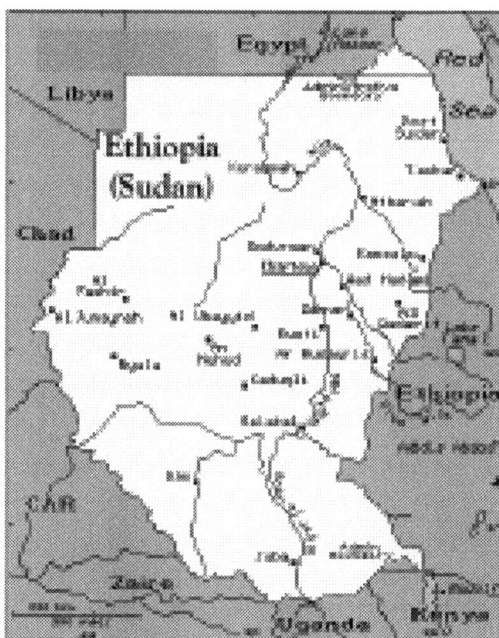

In ancient times (1500-600 B.C.E.) Ethiopia had been an independent country, which spawned the creation of Ancient Egypt.

Judaism has a long history in Ethiopia which begins prior to the early period of Christianity (100-500 A.C.E.). The name Falasha is Amharic for "exiles" or "landless ones.[I]" This is similar to the term "Hebrews" meaning "those who pass from place to place." The Falashas themselves refer to their sect as Beta Esrael ("House of Israel"). The Falashas are a native Jewish sect of Ethiopia. The origin of the Falashas is unknown, but one Falasha tradition claims to trace their ancestry to Menelek (Menelik), who was the son of King Solomon[II] of Israel and the queen of Sheba.[III] Some scholars place the date of their origin before the 2nd century B.C.E. since the Falashas are unfamiliar with either the Palestinian or Babylonian Talmud (post-biblical developments of Judaism).

Interestingly, the Hebrew Scriptures are unknown to the Falashas. The Bible of the Falashas is written in what is classified as an archaic Semitic dialect, known as Gecez. Thus, the religion of the Falashas is a modified form of Mosaic Judaism, unaffected generally by post-biblical developments. The Falashas retain animal sacrifice. They celebrate scriptural and non-scriptural feast days, although the latter are not the same as those celebrated by other Jews. One of the Falasha non-scriptural feast days, for example, is the Commemoration of Abraham. The Sabbath regulations of the Falashas are stringent. They observe biblical dietary laws, but not the post-biblical rabbinic regulations.

[I] Recall that the original Hebrews of the Bible Old Testament tradition were nomadic wanderers.
[II] Solomon (c. 974-c. 937 BC) In the Old Testament, third king of Israel, son of David by Bathsheba. During a peaceful reign, he was famed for his wisdom and his alliances with Egypt and Phoenicia. The much later biblical Proverbs, Ecclesiastes, and Song of Songs are attributed to him. He built the temple in Jerusalem with the aid of heavy taxation and forced labor, resulting in the revolt of N Israel.[126]
[III] Sheba: Ancient name for a kingdom which flourished in S Yemen (Sha'abijah) at around the 1st century B.C.E. It was once renowned for gold and spices. According to the Old Testament, its queen visited Solomon.

75

Among the Falashas, marriage outside the religious community is forbidden. Monogamy is practiced. Marriage at a very early age is rare, and high moral standards are maintained. The center of Falasha religious life is the masjid, or synagogue. The chief functionary in each village is the high priest, who is assisted by lower priests. Falasha monks live alone or in monasteries isolated from other Falashas. Rabbis do not exist among the Falashas.

In ancient times, Ethiopia had been an independent country which spawned the creation of Ancient Egypt.[I] In those ancient times, the Ethiopians and the Egyptians recognized the same supreme Divinity under the names Asar, Amun, Ptah, etc., as well as the manifestations of God in the form of gods and goddesses. At one time Ethiopia was ruled by Egypt and at another time (Nubian Dynasty period, 712-657 B.C.E.) it became allied with Egypt and even ruled over Egypt. When Egypt was finally taken over by Coptic Christianity after the Roman edicts which outlawed all other religions except Christianity, Ethiopia also converted to Coptic Christianity, but several Ethiopian groups adhered to the Ancient form of Judaism, independent of other Jews in the Diaspora. The kingdom of Aksum[II] flourished from the 1st–10th centuries A.C.E., reaching its peak about the 4th century. Coptic Christianity from Egypt was introduced to Ethiopia around the 4th century, and began to decline in the 7th century as Islam expanded into Ethiopia. The Arab conquests isolated Aksum from the rest of the Christian world.

The experience of the Falashas in Ethiopia points to the differences between the form of Judaism that has been developed in western countries (America, Europe and Israel) and that which existed prior to the developments of the Talmudic tradition in the last 1,700 hundred years or more. The Talmudic traditions, which form the basis of popular modern Judaism, are a product of the rabbinical tradition which has sought to explain the original teachings given in the Old Testament. Before Coptic Christianity spread to Ethiopia, Judaism was already present. Since Ethiopia was the only African nation to maintain its independence throughout history, including the period of the European slave trade and the African colonization period, its Christians, and the Copts in Egypt, also kept alive the oldest form of non Roman-Catholic Christianity.

During the 10th century, a kingdom emerged in Ethiopia that formed the basis of Abyssinia (former name of Ethiopia). It was reinforced in 1270 with the founding of a new dynasty. Although it remained independent throughout the period of the European colonization (enslavement) of Africa, Abyssinia suffered civil unrest and several invasions from the 16th century on, and was eventually reunited in 1889 under Menelik II, with Italian support. In 1896 Menelik put down an invasion by Italy. They claimed he had agreed to make the country an Italian protectorate.[126] The next events in the history of Ethiopia led to the development of a new religious idea which traced its origins to the early followers of Judaism in Ethiopia. This new religious idea was Rastafarianism.

Under Haile Selassie I, a few Falashas rose to positions of prominence in education and government, but reports of their persecution followed the emperor's ouster in 1974. In 1975 they were recognized by the Chief Rabbinate as Jews and allowed to settle in Israel. More than 12,000 Falashas were airlifted to Israel in late 1984 and early 1985, when the Ethiopian government halted the program. The airlift resumed in 1989, and about 3,500 Falashas emigrated to Israel in 1990. Nearly all of the more than 14,000 Falashas remaining in Ethiopia were evacuated by the Israeli government in May 1991.[75] Since that time the Israeli government has instituted a program to assimilate the Falashas. This program has come under fire by many critics. One aspect of the program separates Falasha youths from their families and indoctrinates them into the modern religious traditions as well as the political doctrines related to Palestine and the relations with the surrounding Arab countries.

Rastafarianism and the Judeo-Christian Religion

Rastafarianism is another development which should be noted in our study of the history of the modern Judeo-Christian tradition. It is a philosophy that developed in the 1930's and centered in Jamaica (Caribbean). Rastafarians see themselves as the true Israelites, the "chosen people" of the Bible. Ethiopia is seen as the Promised Land, while all countries outside Africa are seen as Babylon or the place of exile. As a custom, many Rastafarians do not cut their hair, citing biblical injunctions against this practice. So instead they wear it in long dreadlocks which are often covered in woolen hats displaying the Rastafarian colors, red, green, and gold. The food restrictions are very strict. No pork, shellfish, salt, milk, or coffee are allowed.

One reason why Rastafarianism is notable is that it is a religion that originated in the Caribbean. It is partly based on some of the ideals of Marcus Garvey and on the emperor of Ethiopia. Marcus Garvey had called on black people to return to Africa and set up a black-governed country there. When Haile Selassie (Ras Tafari, "Lion of Judah") became the emperor of Ethiopia in 1930, this event was seen as a fulfillment of prophecy. Therefore, some

---

[I] The Ancient Egyptian traditions says that Osiris, the first king of Egypt, was an Ethiopian who led a group of Ethiopian colonizers into northeast Africa (Egypt) and started civilization there.

[II] Aksum, Ethiopia, served as capital of ancient Kingdom of Aksum, which flourished from 1st to 10th century; extended influence over much of Arabian Peninsula; Christianized during 4th century; kingdom ended 1270 with abdication of ruling prince; city today a tourist attraction known for its 126 tall granite obelisks and other antiquities.[126]

Rastafarians acknowledged him as an incarnation of God (Jah), and others regarded him as a prophet. In Rastafarianism, the use of ganja (marijuana) is considered a sacrament. In Rastafarianism there is no church system. By 1990, there were close to one million Rastafarians in the world.

Thus, the philosophy of Rastafarianism is closely associated with the struggle of African peoples to liberate themselves from the slavery and exploitation imposed on them by European countries. The country of Ethiopia, in Africa, became a special focus since it was a symbol of African resistance. This hope also focused on one man, Haile Selassie I.

Haile Selassie I (1892-1975), was the last emperor of Ethiopia and ruled from 1930-1974. Haile Selassie I was born near Harar on July 23, 1892. His original name was Lij Tafari Makonnen. Selassie was a grandnephew of Emperor Menelik II. In 1916 he ousted Menelik's successor, Lij Iyasu, and replaced him with Zauditu, who was the old emperor's daughter. Then he made himself the regent and heir to the throne of the country. When Zauditu died in 1930, Lij Tafari Makonnen succeeded her and took the name Haile Selassie I. This name means "Might of the Trinity." His other titles included Conquering Lion of the Tribe of Judah, Elect of God, and King of Kings.

Rastafarianism traces its roots to the Old Testament. The Old Testament records a visit to Ethiopia by the Queen of Sheba. Its ruling house is said to have descended from King Solomon's son. Modern history dates back to Menelik (reigned 1889-1913), whose line of succession led to Emperor Haile Selassie, who was crowned in 1930. His reign was interrupted by the 1936 Italian invasion, which gained control of Ethiopia. Haile Selassie fled to England and raised an army there. With the assistance of the British troops he freed the country in 1941 and ruled until 1974. Haile Selassie was seen by many as slow in dealing with issues of social injustice and economic crisis due to droughts and famine in the country. A military junta deposed him in 1974 due to many years of unrest in the country caused by social and economic instability. He died in 1975. Followers of the Rastafarian religion believe that he was the Messiah, the incarnation of God (Jah).

While Ethiopia has undergone many struggles since the death of Haile Selassie, Rastafarians still look to Ethiopia and to Africa in general, as the motherland which needs to be redeemed. The struggle of Rastafarians to maintain their identity has seen periods of persecution and outright rejection by other peoples. Also, there are many who don the colors of Rastafarianism but who do not follow its teachings and simply use this religion as a means to remain outside the mainstream of society and use drugs. However, the philosophy of Rastafarianism seeks redemption of Africa, which is commensurate with redemption of its people. Thus, it emphasizes that African peoples should have their own separate identity and not to adopt the religion of the slave masters (European Christianity) which marginalizes the role of African peoples and erroneously portrays them as a cursed inferior people, fit only to be slaves. Recall that the curse upon the ancestors of Ham stems from the misinterpretation of the story of Noah and his three sons by racist slave traders and others who wanted to denigrate African peoples and establish a basis for legitimizing the practice of slavery. Rastafarianism is an effort to establish a positive connection to the Bible as well as an attempt to provide a vision for the liberation of African peoples in the Diaspora. However, as with other traditions which seek to isolate their teachings as exclusive, Rastafarianism cannot be practiced by everyone since, like Judaism, it is strongly tied in with a particular culture. Culture-based religions tend to exclude other cultures and points of view, fomenting unrest and divisiveness between peoples of different backgrounds. This emphasis on culture, history and tradition forces the practitioners of the culture-based religion to keep out and even ostracize others whom come from different cultural backgrounds. Even though it is laudable that people of African descent are striving to raise themselves up from the scourge of slavery, racism and unhealthy dietary practices, it must be understood that true liberation cannot come from culture-based religion itself because this form of religious practice ties people to cultures, rituals, and worldly concepts. All religions need to incorporate Yoga-Mysticism, and in so doing a practitioner will be able to rise above culture differences and thereby truly becomes a source for uplifting all peoples, regardless of their religion or ethnicity. This is why Yoga can help all religions. It is not tied to any specific culture or religious tradition and therefore, can be practiced by anyone, anywhere in the world. If peoples of all religions were to emphasize the Yogic principles within their respective religions there would be an automatic movement towards ecumenism among all faiths.[1] This should be one of the most important ideas to be learned from this book.

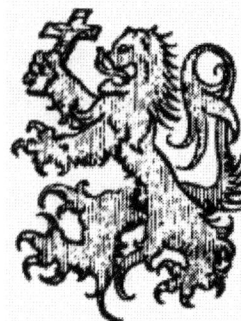

Above: Ras Tafari, "Lion of Judah" symbol from Ethiopia.

---

[1] A movement promoting worldwide unity among religions through greater cooperation and improved understanding.

CHAPTER III: THE ANCIENT EGYPTIAN ORIGINS OF CHRISTIANITY

THE ANCIENT EGYPTIAN ORIGINS OF CHRISTIANITY

As previously discussed, in the time of Abraham, Ancient Egypt was THE civilization of the ancient world. Everyone looked to Egypt for art, culture and religion. The following map shows the extent of the Ancient Egyptian civilization. It extended to encompass the entire area that was later referred to as the Promised Land by the Hebrews, and which today includes Israel, Lebanon, Syria, Iraq, Jordan and Saudi Arabia. Thus, here we find another proof that the original Hebrews, as well as the family of Abraham, the first Jew, were related to Ancient Egypt from the beginning.

The decline of Ancient Egyptian society due to wars, internal corruption, and the normal cyclical decline of civilizations created a spiritual vacuum which elicited a reworking of the *Ausarian* salvation story. The modern day Coptic Christians are ethnic decedents of the Ancient Egyptian culture. The Coptic language and symbolism, such as the painted coffins in the style of Ancient Egyptian burial reliefs along with certain modern traditions in the Coptic Church, clearly show the incorporation of the teachings from the Ancient Egyptian mysteries into Christian Theology.[64] Perhaps the most important example of this is the incorporation of the Ancient Egyptian name *Neberdjer*. Neberdjer means all-encompassing Supreme Being. Asar, Amun, Ptah, Aset and other Ancient Egyptian gods and goddesses were known as Neberdjer. It is from here that the Jewish and Christian idea of God, the all-encompassing Father (God) comes.

Map of the Ancient Egyptian civilization in the time of the Abraham and Moses. It encompasses all of the Holy Land of the Bible.

Matthew - Chap. 2

13. And when they had departed, behold, the angel of the Lord appeareth to Joseph in a dream, saying, Arise, and take the young child and his mother, and flee into Egypt, and be thou there until I bring thee word: for Herod will seek the young child to destroy him.

14 When he arose, he took the young child and his mother by night, and departed into Egypt:
15 And was there until the death of Herod: that it might be fulfilled which was spoken from the Lord by the prophet, saying, Out of Egypt have I called my son.

The quote above from the Christian Bible shows that the early development of Jesus' life took place in Ancient Egypt. In reference to the journey of Jesus into Egypt, the Apocryphal Gospels[113] state that when the Virgin Mary and her son arrived in Egypt, *"there was a movement and quaking throughout all the land, and all the idols fell down from their pedestals and were broken in pieces."* It is further written that the nobles and priests consulted with a certain priest, *"a devil" used to speak from out of an idol."* When they asked him about the meaning of the disturbances he told them that the footsteps of the son of the *"secret and hidden God"* had fallen upon the land of Egypt. They accepted his determination and then set forth to make a figure of this God.

In the earliest Christian Gospels there is an association of the God of Moses and Christianity with the Ancient Egyptian God Amun. Amun was known universally in Egypt and in Palestine as the "hidden Supreme Being." This title was used for Amun exclusively.

> *9. He (Amun) makes Himself to be hidden.*
>
> —From the Ancient Egyptian Hymns of Amun

In the Egyptian Gnostic Gospel of Thomas, verse 109, the same reference is used to designate the nature of the Kingdom of heaven and with it the nature of the Christian Divinity.

> 109 Jesus said, "The Kingdom is like a man who had a [hidden] treasure in his field without knowing it...

Further, from the Bible we also learn the following about Moses:

The Bible Act. 7:22
 And Moses was learned in all of the wisdom of the Egyptians, and was mighty in words and in deeds.

Thus, the Bible itself states that Moses (1200?-1000? B.C.E.), who is reputed to have written the laws and guidelines upon which Jewish, Christian and Islamic society are based, was knowledgeable in all of the "wisdom" and "words" of Egypt; i.e., he was an Ancient Egyptian priest. This is supported by the ancient historians Manetho, the High Priest of the Temple of Aset in Lower (North) Egypt, and Plutarch, Greek author (c. 46-120 A.C.E.), who called him, *"a priest of Aset, a Hierophant (high priest) of Heliopolis."* Philo of Alexandria (Gnostic Jewish philosopher c. 20 B.C.E. - c. A.C.E. 54) also made this point about Moses. They also say that his initiate name was *Osarisiph.* The similarity between the names Osarisiph and Osiris or Asar leads us to reflect further on the link between Ancient Egyptian and Old Testament mythologies and spiritual teachings. The Old Testament stories of Adam and Eve as well as Cain and Abel point us to the same conclusion. Adam and Eve beget Seth, which is the same name as the brother of Asar in Egypt (Seth, Set). Cain murders his brother Abel, just as Set had murdered his brother Asar in Egyptian Mythology.

There are other important links between Christianity and Ancient Egyptian religion. Ancient Egyptian Mythology holds that the first piece of land that was created by God was the Ancient Egyptian city of Anu. In the Ancient Egyptian city of Anu[1] there was a holy well. Egyptian tradition held that the God, Ra,, symbolized by the sun. Creator of the universe and father of Asar, had washed his face in its waters after rising for the first time on this earth out of the primeval ocean. The Christian tradition also holds that the Virgin Mary washed Jesus' clothes in the waters of this same well. The well is also known as the "Virgin's Well," and it is referred to as "Ain ash-shems" or "Well of the sun" by the Arabs.[110]

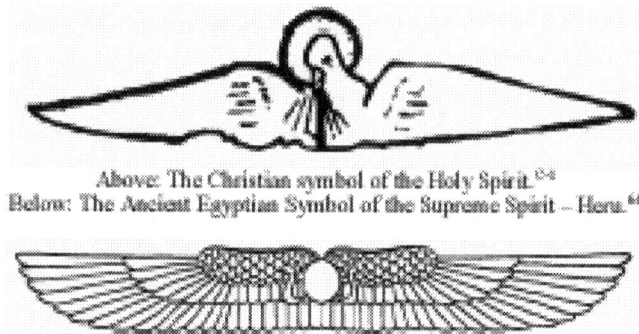

Above: The Christian symbol of the Holy Spirit.
Below: The Ancient Egyptian Symbol of the Supreme Spirit – Heru.

The dove has been an important symbol in Christian iconography from very early times and references to it may be found in the Bible. In John 1:32, it is written: *And John bore testimony, saying, I saw the Spirit descending from heaven like a dove, and he abode upon him.* In this aspect the dove and its wings imply purity and the all-pervasive nature of the spirit of God as well as God-Consciousness itself. The Ancient Egyptian *Winged Disk* of *Ra-Heru* imparts the same idea. *Ur-Uatchit*, the winged disk, is used as a symbol of the sun which pervades over all with its light and spiritual power. In the form of Heru as the Hawk, the bird figure symbolizes purity of intellect which leads to discrimination between that which is real (truth-wisdom-self-knowledge) and that which is not (ignorance-egoism). In the form of a swallow, as the bird of Aset, the bird figure symbolizes intuitional wisdom of the Self.

---

[1] "On" of the Bible and called "Heliopolis" by the Greeks.

The Christian dove is an expression of the divine spirit which not only acts as the source of power which sustains all life but also descends upon human beings to bring enlightenment to them. These functions are akin to the Benu of Ancient Egypt, which was known to the Greeks as the Phoenix. According to legend, the Phoenix is a bird that lived in Arabia. Early Christian tradition (as early as the first century A.C.E.) adopted the Phoenix as a symbol of both immortality and resurrection. However, upon examination of Ancient Egyptian mythology, a more ancient origin emerges. The *Benu* is a mythical bird in Ancient Egyptian Mythology. Its symbolism was transferred to Greece and Arabia in the form of the Phoenix by the early Greek and Asiatic philosophers who studied in Ancient Egypt. According to ancient tradition, the Phoenix would consume itself on a funeral pyre every 500 years, whereupon a new, young Phoenix sprang from its own ashes. Similarly, in Ancient Egyptian mythology, the Benu represented the sun that dies at night only to be reborn in the morning, also alluding to the process of reincarnation and rebirth. The legend of the Phoenix was related by St. Clementin in the first epistle to the Corinthians.

One of the main teachings from Coptic Christianity is found in the Gospel of Thomas. It refers to the Kingdom of Heaven as being *"spread upon the earth."* This teaching also appears in Ancient Egyptian wisdom much earlier than in any other mystical system. The Ancient Egyptian story of the *History of Creation* contains the explanation of the statement used by Jesus.

> Neberdjer, speaks: *"I have done my will in everything on this earth. I have spread myself abroad therein, and I have made strong my hand. I was one by myself, for they [the gods and goddesses] had not been brought forth, and I have emitted from myself neither Shu nor Tefnut. I brought my own name into my mouth as a word of power, and I forthwith came into being under the form of things which are and as the Divine Kheperi. I came into being from out of primeval matter, and from the beginning I appeared as the form of the multitudinous things which exist; nothing whatsoever existed at that time in this earth, and it was I who made whatsoever was made...*[109]

All of these factors of correlation further uncover the origin of Jewish and Christian mythology in Ancient Egyptian mysticism. The Torah means "to teach" in Hebrew. It is, strictly speaking, the first five books of the Old Testament. These are Genesis, Exodus, Leviticus, Numbers, and Deuteronomy. These five books are also called the *Pentateuch*. Moses is generally claimed to be the author of the Torah, having received it through inspiration from God while on Mount Sinai for 40 days and nights. The Torah is kept in an ark in synagogues and is read during the Sabbath services. As a term, Torah may also signify the entire Jewish Bible as well as all customs and laws of Judaism.

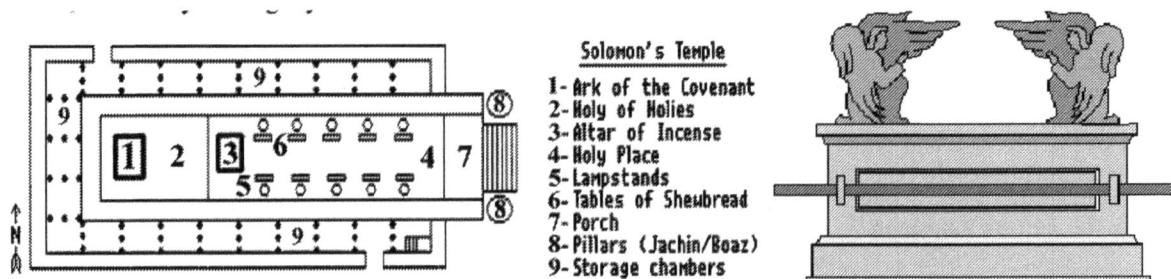

Solomon's Temple
1- Ark of the Covenant
2- Holy of Holies
3- Altar of Incense
4- Holy Place
5- Lampstands
6- Tables of Shewbread
7- Porch
8- Pillars (Jachin/Boaz)
9- Storage chambers

King Solomon built the first Jewish temple which was called "the house of the LORD." The details of the structure of the building as well as its dedication were recorded in 1 Kings: 5-8 and 2 Chronicles: 2-7. According to ancient Jewish tradition, the 'Ark of the Covenant' was a portable wooden chest which was adorned with gold. It contained the two stone tablets on which the Ten Commandments given to Moses by God had been inscribed. The Ark was held as the most sacred shrine of ancient Israel since it symbolized God's covenant with his "chosen people," the Jews. Only the high priest was allowed to look upon it. No one else could touch it. King Solomon built a tabernacle to house the Ark, but it was destroyed in 586 B.C.E. by the Babylonians and no further record of the original Ark remains. In today's synagogues (buildings or places of meeting for Jewish worship and religious instruction), the Holy Ark is a recess or closet in which the sacred scrolls of the congregation are kept.

The Ancient Egyptian religion of Asar also used an Ark. It was used to keep the pieces of the body of the dismembered Asar[I]. There are many surviving pictures and sculptures of the Ancient Egyptian Ark which often show the Ancient Egyptian deities Apuat, and sometimes Sebek, sitting on it in the form of guardians. The measurements given for the Ark are similar in all respects to the stone chest which may still be seen in the "Kings Chamber" of the Great Pyramid in Egypt. It was used for initiation rites and meditation exercises in Ancient Egypt.

[I] See section of this book entitles: "The Ausarian Resurrection, Its Historical and Mystical Implications"

The "Coffined One," the initiate assuming the place of Asar, would be led to achieve greater and greater levels of Enlightenment through the use of special wisdom and meditation techniques along with controlled cosmic and psychic forces harnessed by the pyramid itself. Upon close examination, there are several similarities in the structure of the Jewish temple which coincide with those of the traditional Ancient Egyptian architecture and mythology.

Above: A diagram of the Temple of Amun-Ra at Karnak, Egypt, showing the Pylons (A), the Court (B), the Hypostyle Hall (C), the Chapel of Amun (Holy of Holies - D), the Chapel of Mut (E), the Chapel of Khons (F). At right: Anubis guarding the Ark of Asar from Ancient Egypt.

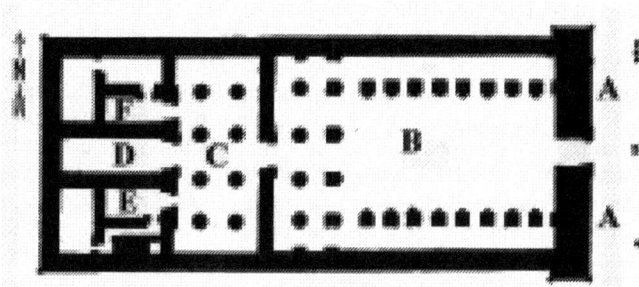

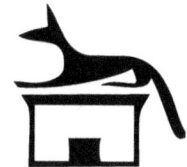

THE ANCIENT AFRICAN ANCESTRY OF JESUS

Jesus of Nazareth (c. 4 B.C.E. - c. 30 A.C.E.) is generally held to be the founder of Christianity. In his late twenties Jesus began to preach the teachings of salvation, and was thereafter referred to as Jesus Christ or Jesus the Christ. The title combines a well-known Hebrew term, Jesus, and a Greek translation of a Hebrew word for messiah, Christ. Thus, the word "Jesus," originally meaning in Hebrew: Joshua, "God is salvation," is combined with "Christ," which comes from a Greek translation for messiah, meaning "anointed one," thus rendering "the anointed savior." The messiah was a prophesied and long expected king and deliverer of Israel. Jesus was supposed to have been born around 4 B.C.E. All that is known of the life of Jesus comes from the study of the four Gospels of Matthew, Mark, Luke, and John, which are the first four books of the New Testament in the Christian Bible along with the newly discovered texts from Egypt and Palestine. There is no other information corroborating his existence and works.

The Gospels contain little information about what Jesus looked like and what occurred in his early life prior to his initiation into the mysteries of mystical religion by John the Baptist. The Christian tradition (writings after the original Christian texts) developed several stories related to the childhood of Jesus, but these were created hundreds of years after the cited death of Jesus. However, there are three important sources which shed some light on these questions. The first is the Bible itself. In the books of Matthew and Luke, the genealogy of Jesus is presented. The story is given of Noah and his three sons: Shem, Ham and Japheth. Each son had his own wife. Noah, his wife, sons and close family relations survived the world flood due to the grace of God, and then they repopulated the earth. The Sumerian story of Gilgamesh contains a section which includes an account of the world flood that resembles the Biblical story very closely. Historians and scholars have therefore speculated that the writers of the Bible were influenced by the Sumerians. According to the Bible in Genesis Chapter 10, the children of Ham populated ancient Africa. Ham became the father of Mizraim (Egypt), Cush (Ethiopia), Phut (Africans in Libya) and Canaan (Palestine). The Ancient Egyptian records verify that all lands from Ethiopia to the Caucasus mountains was under the control of the Egyptian government at several times through history. The entire area was populated by descendents of Ham (Ethiopians, Egyptians and Canaanites). This is the first indication of Jesus' ancestry. Since he was a Canaanite he was a descendent of the bloodline of Ham. However, the Bible is even more specific on this question as we will see.

The Bible describes the origin of humanity in a very metaphorical way. As we will see, the physical appearance of the Ancient Egyptian, Cushite, Colchian and Hebrew people can be verified by the writings of historians who lived in biblical times. The Jewish sages who were creating the Genesis text between the years 1,000 B.C.E. to 100 B.C.E. looked at the neighboring lands (Ethiopia, Egypt, Cannan and South West Asia) along with the peoples, Ethiopians, Egyptians, Canaanites (includes Hebrews) etc. Then they set about to explain how the known nations came into being and how they related to each other. This teaching is set forth in the genealogy of Noah. The word race, as referring to people according to racial classifications (black, white, red, yellow, etc.) does not occur anywhere in the Bible. As we saw earlier, even modern science is recognizing that race classifications are bogus forms of social analysis. They are finding that differences in appearance among people can be accounted for by environmental factors and that genetically speaking, human beings are equal in every respect.[I] However, since the usage of terms such as those used for race classifications are common, they will be used in this section for the sake of clarity in the discussion as it pertains to the understanding of who the Ancient Egyptians and Jews were. In this manner, the study of Christian Yoga will be accurate in using modern terminology, but it should never be assumed that the author agrees with the use of the term "race" as a correct way of classifying human beings. It is crucial to understand the cultural and ethnic relationship between the Ancient Egyptians and Jews in order to gain insight into the deeper mystical teachings that are embedded in Judaism and Christianity. Also, this study will bring light to the question of how race distinctions were adopted by the church and western society and how this notion of race differences came to be used, through the story of Noah, as a means to practice racism in the general society. The purpose of our study is to show that not only is racism based on ignorance, but to emphasize that the Bible scriptures themselves speak on the unity of humanity and of its common origin.

In order to discover the origins of humanity, we will examine the teachings related to the sons of Ham more closely. In the time period when the book of Genesis was written, the three basic groups of people who were observed by the Genesis writers were the Africans, Asiatics and Europeans. The Africans inhabited the area from Africa to the Caucasus mountains which includes the land now called Palestine (ancient Canaan). As discussed, the Ancient Egyptian culture at one time extended to the area covering what is now referred to as the Middle East all the way to India. They were observed to have such similarity in language, customs and physical appearance that the Greek historians of 400 B.C.E. concluded that the inhabitants of that area were all one people. This group included the Ethiopians (Cushites), the Egyptians (descendents of Mizraim) and the Canaanites.

Some notable descendents of the Canaanites were given in Genesis 10-13:18. These were

> *Girgashite or Girgasite*: Descendants of Canaan and one of the nations living east of the sea of Galilee when the Israelites entered the promised land
>
> *Hivite*: 6th generation of descendants of Canaan, the son of Ham, who were living in northern Canaan near Mount Hermon at the time of the conquest.
>
> *Sinite*: A tribe of the Canaanites descended from Canaan inhabiting the northern part of the Lebanon district.
>
> *Heth*: A son of Canaan and progenitor of the Hittites.
>
> *Jesubites*: Descendents of the third son of Canaan who lived in Jebus, the early name of Jerusalem.

The following excerpt comes from the "History" of Herodotus[II]:

> There can be no doubt that the Colchians are an Egyptian race. Before I heard any mention of the fact from others, I had remarked it myself. After the thought had struck me, I made inquiries on the subject both in Colchis and in Egypt, and I found that the Colchians had a more distinct recollection of the Egyptians, than the Egyptians had of them. Still the Egyptians said that they believed the Colchians to be descended from the army of Sesostris. My own conjectures were founded, first, on the fact that they are black-skinned and have woolly hair, which certainly amounts to but little, since several other nations are so too; but further and more especially, on the circumstance that the Colchians, the Egyptians, and the Ethiopians, are the only nations who have practiced circumcision from the earliest times. The Phoenicians and the Syrians of Palestine themselves confess that they learnt the custom of the Egyptians; and the Syrians who dwell about the rivers Thermodon and Parthenius, as well as their neighbors the Macronians, say that they

---

[I] The concept of race has often been misapplied. One of the most telling arguments against classifying people into races is that persons in various cultures have often mistakenly acted as if one race were superior to another. This has no basis in reality. Although, with social disadvantages eliminated, it is possible that one human group or another might have some genetic advantages in response to such factors as climate, altitude, and specific food availability, these differences are small and do not point to racial superiority but to a greater ability to cope with specific environmental conditions. There are no differences in native intelligence or mental capacity that cannot be explained by environmental circumstances, culture or the ability to engage in the development of the sciences or the accumulation of knowledge. Rather than using racial classifications to study human variability, anthropologists today define geographic or social groups by geographic or social criteria. They then study the nature of the genetic attributes of these groups and seek to understand the causes of changes in their genetic makeup.[75]

[II] , a Greek historian who lived around c.484-425 B.C.E.

have recently adopted it from the Colchians. Now these are the only nations who use circumcision, and it is plain that they all imitate herein the Egyptians. With respect to the Ethiopians, indeed, I cannot decide whether they learnt the practice of the Egyptians, or the Egyptians of them- it is undoubtedly of very ancient date in Ethiopia- but that the others derived their knowledge of it from Egypt is clear to me from the fact that the Phoenicians, when they come to have commerce with the Greeks, cease to follow the Egyptians in this custom, and allow their children to remain uncircumcised. I will add a further proof to the identity of the Egyptians and the Colchians. These two nations weave their linen in exactly the same way, and this is a way entirely unknown to the rest of the world; they also in their whole mode of life and in their language resemble one another.

Colchis was an ancient country located on the eastern shore of the Black Sea. It was south of the Caucasus Mountains which are now part of the Republic of Georgia. Colchis was an independent nation until about 100 BC, when it was conquered by Mithradates VI Eupator, king of Pontus. In Greek mythology, Colchis was the home of the princess Medea and the repository of the golden fleece sought by Jason and his Argonauts.[75] This excerpt shows that the peoples of Syria and Palestine were strongly influenced by the culture of Egypt, not just through casual association, but by blood relation, being of the same skin color and practicing the same customs (including circumcision which the Jews adopted) and having similar language. This relationship is one of the reasons why Moses went to such great lengths to separate the Jewish religion from its roots and strong ties to the culture from Ancient Egypt. The Bible itself recounts that when the Jews entered Egypt they numbered seventy. But after 400 years of living in Egypt, their numbers were much higher. When Moses left Egypt in the exodus, there were 600,000 people in his group, all of whom were of direct Egyptian ancestry or mixed Egyptian-Hebrews, like those who had entered Egypt previously. Therefore, they were religiously Jewish, but ethnically Egyptian, steeped in Egyptian culture. Thus, it is clear to see that the Hebrews were more closely related to the Egyptians than even the Colchians or any of the other groups of Canaanites (Girgashite or Girgasite, Hivite, Sinite, Hethians, Jesubites, Phoenicians, etc.)

Herodotus informed us in his writings that even the Colchians[I] appear to be related to the Egyptians because of their customs and physical appearance, being "black skinned." The next group mentioned in the Bible was the Asiatic. The Asiatic peoples were also observed to be of the same language, customs and physical appearance. They inhabited the area from Middle Asia. This group includes the peoples known in modern times as Persians and Iraqis, etc. The last group observed were the European peoples. In ancient times, the Indo-European[II] group of peoples occupied the area of the world known today as Northern Asia, from Scandinavia to Eastern Siberia. As the Indo-European groups and Asiatic groups moved south and west towards India, Africa, Asia Minor and Europe, a convergence and mixture of cultures and ethnic groups began. The focal point was the area of South West Asia which includes Palestine (the Biblical Holy land - Canaan), Saudi Arabia, Jordan, Yemen, Oman, Israel, Turkey, Iran and Iraq. This is why the people of this region are referred to as Semites. However, there is clear indication from the evidence we have seen in the Bible and in history, including the writings of ancient historians which indicate that the early Hebrews and Jews were of Egyptian (African) descent and later became Semitic by mixing with other groups. Thus, it is clear to see that the Bible describes the entire geographical area where the events of the Old Testament took place as being inhabited by the descendents of Ham, the African peoples and Shem, the Asiatics. Many people feel that Ur, the city from which Abraham emerged, was not a member of the Hamitic blood line because the Chaldeans were believed to be Mesopotamians descended from Shem.

The biblical name, "Ur of the Chaldees," refers to the Chaldeans, who settled in the area of southern Iraq about 900 B.C.E. The Book of Genesis (see 11:27-32) describes Ur as the starting point of the westward migration of the family of Abraham to Palestine about 1900 B.C.E. Thus, at the time when Abraham would have lived, the Egyptian civilization was in the Middle Kingdom Period (or Middle Empire 2,040-1,640 B.C.E.). Pharaoh Sesostris I, who reigned 1962-1928 B.C.E., built fortresses throughout Nubia and established trade with foreign lands. He sent governors to Palestine. In ancient times, according to the Egyptian story of Asar (Osiris), the Egyptians ruled all of Asia Minor as far as India and beyond. Due to invasions and wars these lands were ceded to the conquering peoples. But during the Middle Kingdom Period, Palestine was once again controlled by Egypt as it was in ancient times. Thus, during this period the inhabitants of Ur were not Chaldeans, but Sumerians. This points to a discrepancy in the

---

[I] Colchis, ancient country on the eastern shore of the Black Sea, south of the Caucasus Mountains, now part of the Republic of Georgia. Colchis was independent until about 100 BC, when it was conquered by Mithradates VI Eupator, king of Pontus. In Greek mythology, Colchis was the home of the princess Medea and the repository of the golden fleece sought by Jason and his Argonauts.[75]

[II] In·do-Eu·ro·pe·an (in'do-yoor'e-pe'en) Noun1. a. A family of languages consisting of most of the languages of Europe as well as those of Iran, the Indian subcontinent, and other parts of Asia. 1. b. Proto-Indo-European. 2. A member of a group of people who speak an Indo-European language. (American Heritage Dictionary)

Bible, which is most likely due to different writings of different writers from different periods being mixed and faulty editing by the early church councils.

The Gilgamesh Epic is an important Middle Eastern work of literature. It was written on 12 clay tablets in cuneiform about 2000 B.C.E. The Gilgamesh Epic relates the story of its hero, Gilgamesh, and includes the city of Uruk which is known in the Bible as Erech (now Warka, Iraq). The Sumerians created an advanced culture which included the development of cuneiform writing but their country soon fell to outside invasions. There was a brief Sumerian renaissance centered on Ur, which continued until c.1950 B.C.E. when Semitic Amorites overran much of Sumeria. This was the beginning of a long period of instability in Mesopotamia until the first Babylonian Dynasty was founded in 1830 B.C.E., which reached its height with Hammurabi. This date is believed to mark the end of the Sumerian state. Thereafter the Sumerian civilization was then adopted almost completely by Babylonia. The dates for Abraham's departure from Ur are possibly related to this period since there were undoubtedly many migrations out of the area during that time. It is clear to see that Abraham was influenced by Sumerian culture and there is evidence that there was trade between the Sumerians and the Ancient Egyptians.

The land of the Sumerians was called Sumer and was referred to as Shinar in the Bible. The Sumerians, up until recently, have been credited with forming the earliest of the ancient civilizations. However, their origins are obscured in the past. They are not believed to have been Semites like most of the peoples of the region. They apparently spoke a language, which was unrelated to other known tongues. It is believed that they may have come to southern Mesopotamia, the area of Ur, from Persia, or northeastern Mesopotamia before 4,000 B.C.E. However, this is speculation by archeologists. It has also been widely circulated that the Sumerians were the first to create writing and that they influenced Ancient Egyptian culture. As we have seen in our study of ancient history so far, it is unlikely that this is true. In addition, the syllabic signs of Ancient Egyptian Hieroglyphic language did not indicate differences in vowel sounds, as did the Sumerian script. While the Sumerian language has been thought by some scholars to be related to the Ancient Egyptian. The similarities are only due to general correspondences which all pictographic languages have in their original forms. Thus, Ancient Egyptian, Sumerian and Mayan show several similarities but these cannot be used to say that one originates from the other. The Sumerian language is believed to be agglutinative and unrelated to any other known language. The Ancient Egyptian language is related to the Hamitic (African) family of languages.[123]

The biblical scriptures relating to conquering the peoples of the "Promised Land" should not be understood as the conquering of people with different ethnicity, for it has been shown through the Bible itself that the Jews were ethnically related to the Ethiopians, Egyptians and Canaanites. Rather, these passages should be understood as a group of people with one religion, trying to establish it amongst others of their own kind.

According to the Bible, the origin of humanity is described in the book of Genesis. For our present study, we will now focus on the passages found in Chapter 2, verse 8.

8. And the Lord God planted a garden eastward in Eden; and there he put the man whom he had formed.

In Genesis, Chapter 1, the Bible describes how God created the earth. Verse eight, above, is important because after having created the earth itself, God has now created Eden upon it. Eden is defined as a place for human beings to live. This idea carries many implications. One implication is that out of the whole creation, there is a special place for human beings which is presumably most suitable for sustaining life and for providing fulfillment of a person's needs.

Genesis, Chapter 2, cont.
9   And out of the ground made the Lord God to grow every tree that is pleasant to the sight, and good for food[1]; the tree of life also in the midst of the garden, and the tree of knowledge of good and evil.
10 And a river went out of Eden to water the garden; and from there it was parted, and became into four heads.
11 The name of the first [is] Pison: which goest around the whole land of Havilah, where [there is] gold;
12 And the gold of that land [is] good: there [is] bdellium and the onyx stone.
13 And the name of the second river [is] Gihon: the same that goest around the whole land of Cush. {Ethiopia: Heb. Cush}
14 And the name of the third river [is] Hiddekel: which floweth toward the east of Assyria. And the fourth river [is] Euphrates. {toward...: or, eastward to Assyria}

---

[1] The Bible here advocates vegetarianism.

15 And the Lord God took the man, and put him into the garden of Eden to tend it and to keep it. {the man: or, Adam}

NOTE: Strong's Concordance of the Bible defines Eden (05731) {ay'-den} the same as 05730; 1568; Eden= "pleasure" 1) the first habitat of man after the creation; site unknown.

Contrary to the popular or superficial understanding of the phrase, "The Garden of Eden," it does not refer to a place called "Garden of Eden." The text is actually referring to a garden which has been created within this special location on earth called Eden. Four rivers are used to describe the location of this garden in Eden. One river went out of Eden and separated into four rivers to water the garden. The first one, Pison, means "increase."[124] Pison runs through the land of Havilah, a district in Arabia named after a son of Cush (Havilah), located in the northwest part of Yemen.[124] The next river is Gihon. Gihon means "bursting forth."[124] Strong's Concordance of the Bible holds that Gihon was a spring near Jerusalem where the anointing of Solomon as king took place. However, the Bible scripture says that Gihon skirts the land of Cush which is modern day Ethiopia. This description strongly resembles the Nile River[I] which originates deep in the heart of Africa with its source, the Kagera River in Burundi. River Hiddekel means "rapid."[124] It flowed eastward through Assyria according to the Bible (Gen. 2:14). It is now known as the Tigris river. The fourth river is the Euphrates, which means "fruitfulness." [124] Its sources are in the Armenian mountains and it empties into the Persian Gulf. Keep in mind that the area being described was all connected until recently. The present separation is due to the creation of the Suez Canal. This description of the rivers clearly refers to the garden as being located in the area between Ethiopia, in northeast Africa, and the northern part of Southeast Asia at the Armenian and Caucasus mountains. This entire area was said by the Bible to be the land of the descendents of Cush, the son of Ham.

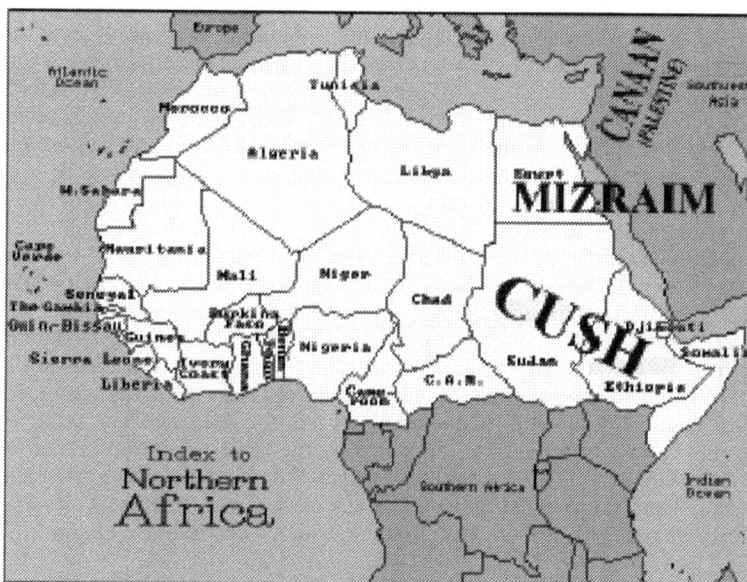

The location of Eden and the Garden of Eden.

According to the Old Testament, Cush became the ancestor of the Ethiopians, Mizraim of the Egyptians, Canaan of the Canaanites, the pre-Israelite inhabitants of Palestine, and Phut of an African people inhabiting Libya (see Genesis 10:1, 6-20). Egypt is referred to several times in the Psalms as the "Land of Ham" (see Psalms 105:23, 24, 27; 106:22), evidently because of the genealogy in Genesis. Psalm 105:24 even confirms that the Jews increased

---

[I] The Nile's southernmost source is the Kagera River in Burundi, which empties into Lake Victoria. From Lake Victoria the river flows through Uganda to Sudan, where the main branch is known as the Mountain Nile. It flows through the vast swamps of As Sudd in southern Sudan and then for the next 500 miles (800 kilometers) is known as the White Nile. The Blue Nile, the largest tributary, joins the White Nile near Khartoum. From Khartoum to Aswan the combined White and Blue Nile are known as the United Nile or simply as the Nile River. Its last major tributary, the Atbarah River, joins it about 200 miles (320 kilometers) north of Khartoum. Farther north the Nile flows in a broad S-bend through the arid Nubian Desert and descends in six cataracts, or waterfalls, before it enters Lake Nasser near the Egypt-Sudan border. As the Nile approaches the Mediterranean Sea north of Cairo, it fans into a broad delta and branches into two major channels Rosetta on the west and Damietta on the east. An extensive network of irrigation canals crisscrosses the delta.Excerpted from *Compton's Interactive Encyclopedia*. Copyright (c) 1994, 1995 Compton's NewMedia, Inc.

their number by mixing with and adding to their numbers with the descendents of Ham. Philologists[1] and ethnologists recognize a distinct North African family of peoples and tongues that they term Hamito-Semitic. Canaan, in the Old Testament, is a designation of the land to the west of the Jordan River, later known as Palestine, and the name of the reputed ancestor of the Canaanites, the original inhabitants of that land, the Hebrew people who later called themselves Jews.[75]

Psalms 105

23   Israel also came into Egypt; and Jacob sojourned in the land of Ham.

24   And he increased his people greatly; and made them stronger than their enemies.

27   They showed his signs among them, and wonders in the land of Ham.

Psalms106

22   Wondrous works in the land of Ham, [and] terrible things by the Red sea.

NOTE: Strong's Concordance of the Bible defines: Immanuel 0410 'el {ale}
shortened from 0352; 1) god, god-like one, mighty one.

The ancestry of humanity and the location of Eden leads to Ethiopia and Egypt, in Africa. This is essentially the same area of the Egyptian civilization in Biblical times. Herodotus, a Greek historian who traveled the area around 484-425 B.C.E.,[117] journeyed through the ancient world, including Asia Minor, Mesopotamia, Babylon, and Egypt. He described the Ethiopians as: "The tallest, most beautiful and long-lived of the human races," "There are two great Ethiopian (Black) nations, one in Sind (India) and the other in Egypt," and "The Colchians, Ethiopians and Egyptians have thick lips, broad nose, wooly hair, and they are burnt (dark) of skin color." The Christian Bible is reputed to have been written over a period of at least 1,000 years, from the time of Moses (1,200?-1,000? B.C.E.) to the end of the Roman Empire (395 A.C.E.). So if the creators of the book of Genesis observed the area described as Eden at the beginning of the creation of the Bible texts and noted the inhabitants as being of African descent, and then five hundred years later, the same is reported by independent eye witnesses (Herodotus, Diodorus, etc.), it must be concluded that the main characters of the Bible, including the Egyptians, Hebrews and Jews, were African peoples and their descendents. Further, this conclusion explains why the teachings of Judaism are so closely related to those of Ancient Egypt. While it is true that at around the time of Jesus the Greeks and Romans had attained control of the areas which had previously encompassed the Egyptian civilization, they would have access to every means of reproducing images of themselves. Therefore, assuming from these images that an accurate depiction of the population is being given would be an erroneous assumption. One only needs to look at the past icons and artwork of Ancient Egypt to see the presence and dominance of the African characteristics of Ancient Egyptian society. One of these pictures was included in Chapter Two of this book in the section entitled: *Ancient Origins: Who Were the Ancient Egyptians?*   In early times the population of Egypt and indeed Canaan as well, were African, dark skinned people. As they mixed with the Asiatics and the Europeans, the general hue of the population became lighter. However, even in the late period of the Ancient Egyptian civilization, just before the Christian era (500 B.C.E.), prominent Greek historians stated that the populations of Ethiopia, Egypt, and the areas now called Palestine and Iraq (where Abraham was born) were all populated by one ethnic group, the Africans. The same was true of India as well. In ancient times the people were described as Ethiopians by the Greek historian Herodotus. However, after mixing with the Indo-Aryans, the Greeks, the Arabs, and the British, the skin tone of the population has changed dramatically from its original state. Thus, the population in Southwest Asia (Iran, Iraq, Syria, etc.) had an African Ancestry. It was not until the Jews mixed with the Greeks, Romans and Aryans that they came to be regarded as part of the "White racial group."

According to the Bible, Ham was the progenitor of the African peoples, Shem was the progenitor of the Asians and Japheth was the progenitor of the Germanic anc Celtic peoples. Genesis 9:27 suggests an understanding by the Bible writers that the people living in modern day Europe were related to the Asiatics where it says: "he (Japheth) shall dwell in the tents of Shem," i.e. in Asia. Europe is in reality not a continent, but a section of Asia and therefore should be referred to as Eurasia.

Genesis 9:27
God shall enlarge Japheth, and he shall dwell in the tents of Shem; and Canaan shall be his
servant. {enlarge: or, persuade}

---

[1] Literary studies or historical linguistics studies.

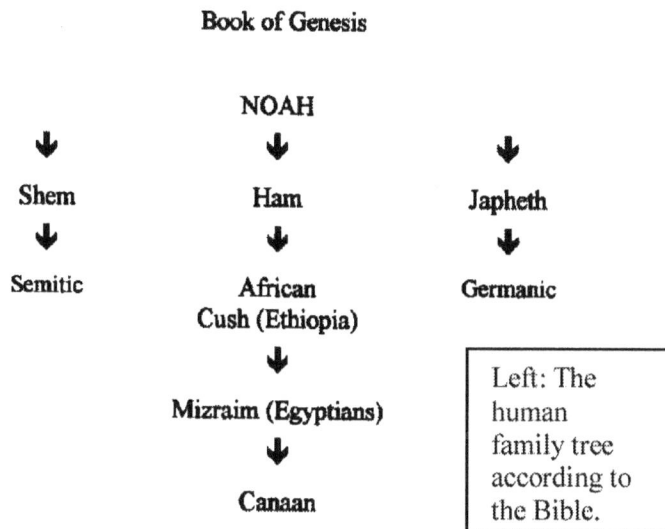

Book of Genesis

```
                    NOAH
   ↓                 ↓                 ↓
 Shem               Ham             Japheth
   ↓                 ↓                 ↓
Semitic           African          Germanic
              Cush (Ethiopia)
                    ↓
             Mizraim (Egyptians)
                    ↓
                 Canaan
```

> Left: The human family tree according to the Bible.

The understanding of Jesus' ancestry is important in understanding the origins and meaning of his teachings. In Matthew, Chapter 1:1-16, the genealogy of Jesus is given. It traces his ancestry all the way back to Abraham who is considered as the patriarch of the Jews. He lived in the ancient city known as Ur, close to the Euphrates river. Ur was situated close to southern end of the Euphrates. In ancient times this was known as the land of the Elamites. Elam[I] was a son of Shem, the son of Noah. Ur means "eternity." It was an area referred to in the Bible as a province east of Babylon and northeast of the lower Tigris.[124] While Shem was considered as the patiarch of the Semitic races of people, one should bear in mind that the appearance of the people in modern times should not be taken as a reflection of the ancient past. For instance, the people who inhabit the land of Egypt today bear little resemblance to the Ancient Egyptians. The reports from ancient historians will assist our study. Herodotus traveled the area in question. He reported that the Elamites were relatives of the Ethiopians:

"They (Elamites) were just like the southern Ethiopians, except for their language and their hair; their hair is straight while that of the Ethiopians in Libya is the crimpest and curliest in the world."[12]

This account points to the ethnic relationship between northeast Africa and Mesopotamia. Other accounts presented earlier in this text showed how the entire area from Northeast Africa to Southern Asia was at one time, in the distant past, ethnically related. Once again, the change in hair texture, from "wooly" to "straight" can be accounted for by environmental factors. However, wooly hair is not necessarily a sign which denotes all Africans. This is one of the great misconceptions that has fostered ignorance in all peoples (white, black, brown etc.).

We learned earlier that this area (Eden) was populated by the descendents of Ham. Therefore, Jesus and all Jews of the time were of African or Africans mixed with Asiatics, but not European as the modern iconography such as that which is promoted in movies or European art suggests. Jesus was, at least in part, a member of the dark-skinned group of Noah's ancestors. This is supported by the Bible itself. In Genesis 38 it is stated that Judah begot Perez by Tamar. Perez (Perets, Perez or Pharez {peh'-rets}) was the twin son with Zarah of Judah by Tamar and an ancestor of two families, of Judah, the Hezronites and Hamulites; from the Hezronites came the royal line of David and Christ. Among his ancestors, one in particular ties him into the line of Ham directly. Matthew 1:5 states that "And Salmon begot Boaz of Rahab." Tamar and Rahab were Canaanite women. As we learned earlier, Canaan was the son of Ham and therefore, he and all of his descendents are part of the Hamitic or African group of peoples if we use the classification system of the Bible. Thus, the blood line of the Bible indicates that Jesus is at least part African in his ancestry. This genealogy therefore supports the descriptions given in Revelation 1, Daniel 7, Ezekiel 8 and by Josephus.

The legends of a curse upon the ancestors of Ham stem from the misinterpretation of the story of Noah and his three sons. According to the canonical Bible texts, Ham saw his father naked and drunk. Because of this, Noah cursed, not Ham, but one of Ham's sons, Canaan. The rabbinical concepts as to how the Africans became black came well after the Jews had left Egypt and had mixed with Europeans. There were many concepts which all sought to somehow show that the occupants of the "Holy Land" were not worthy of this honor. Thus, they set out to discredit the peoples of dark complexion. One such Jewish concept held that Ham had sexual relations in the Ark and violated a rule set forth by Noah. For this reason his seed was cursed with ugliness and darkness (The Midrash Rabbah, Genesis, Noah, Chapter 37.)[125]

The Descriptions of Jesus

In the Bible, book of Isaiah, the ancestry of Mary, the mother of Jesus, was given. It ties Mary directly to the blood line of David.

[I] Elam was a biblical name for an ancient Persian province of Susiana, on the northern coast of the Persian Gulf, or for the north western part of Susiana.

Isaiah 7

> 13 And he said, Hear ye now, O house of David; [Is it] a small thing for you to weary men, but will ye weary my God also?
> 14 Therefore the Lord himself shall give you a sign; Behold, the virgin shall conceive, and bear a son, and shall call his name Immanuel (Emmanuel).

The passage above declares Mary, the mother of Jesus as descendant from the blood line of David. We have seen earlier that the line of David, although strongly related to the line of Shem, Noah's Son and progenitor of the so called Semitic races, it is also mixed with the line of Ham, Noah's son and progenitor of the African so called races. Therefore, while all the Jews in ancient times had an African ancestry due to the intermixing of Abraham, Joseph, Moses and the early Jews with Egyptian women, Jesus has a direct ancestry which can be traced to the Canaanites, the descendants of the Egyptians who were themselves descendants of the Cushites (Ethiopians).

Jesus was, like Moses, a student of the Egyptian spiritual teachings and a promoter of the same mystical philosophy which was practiced in Ethiopia and Egypt since the beginning of humanity. This view is not a supposition. In addition, as we have seen, the Bible itself supports it. The Bible references to God as appearing to seers as having skin the color of "brass" and "amber" and having "wool" for hair etc. closely resemble the description of the Ancient Egyptian God Asar who was known as "The Lord of the Perfect Black" and as the "Black One." Nonetheless, it must be clearly understood that the assertion of Jesus' African ancestry is in the interest of correctness and for the purpose of showing his connection to the culture and mystical philosophy of Ancient Egypt. Indeed he himself affirmed the universality of human beings and through his actions showed that all human beings are related in a way that far surpasses the color of the skin.

Revelation 1

> 14 His head and [his] hairs [were] white like wool, as white as snow; and his eyes [were] as a flame of fire;
> 15 And his feet like fine brass, as if they burned in a furnace; and his voice as the sound of many waters.

Daniel 7

> 9. I beheld till the thrones were placed, and the Ancient of days did sit, whose garment [was] white as snow, and the hair of his head like the pure wool: his throne [was like] the fiery flame, [and] his wheels [as] burning fire.

Ezekiel 8

> 1. And it came to pass in the sixth year, in the sixth [month], in the fifth [day] of the month, [as] I sat in my house, and the elders of Judah sat before me, that the hand of the Lord God fell there upon me.
> 2 Then I beheld, and lo a likeness as the appearance of fire: from the appearance of his loins even downward, fire; and from his loins even upward, as the appearance of brightness, as the color of amber.

The writings of one Jewish Historian, Josephus (AD 37 or 38-circa 101), of Jerusalem concur with the African ancestry of Jesus as he describes Christ as "a man of simple appearance, mature age, dark skin with little hair."

The Personality of Jesus and the Mystical Christ

According to the Biblical story, at around 26 or 27 A.C.E., John (John the Baptist), the son of Zacharias and Elizabeth who was born six months before Jesus, spent 30 years in the desert preparing for his priestly duties and later preaching the word of God. He baptized Jesus in the Jordan River. After a time of solitude and reflection in the desert, Jesus began his own ministry, gathering many followers and disciples around him. He preached to people that they should love God and their neighbors even if they are foreigners or enemies. He taught that salvation depends on true devotion to God's will rather than following the letter of the religious law as prescribed in the Old Testament or through outdated rituals and traditions which had been developed by the Rabbis. These laws had been corrupted by the Jewish church leaders through misunderstanding and greed. This new interpretation of the true practice of religion was expressed in Matthew 12 when Jesus went against the established traditions about the Sabbath.

Matthew 12

> 1. At that time Jesus went on the sabbath through the grain fields; and his disciples were hungry, and began to pluck the heads of grain, and to eat.

2 But when the Pharisees saw [it], they said to him, Behold, thy disciples do that which it is not lawful to do on the sabbath.

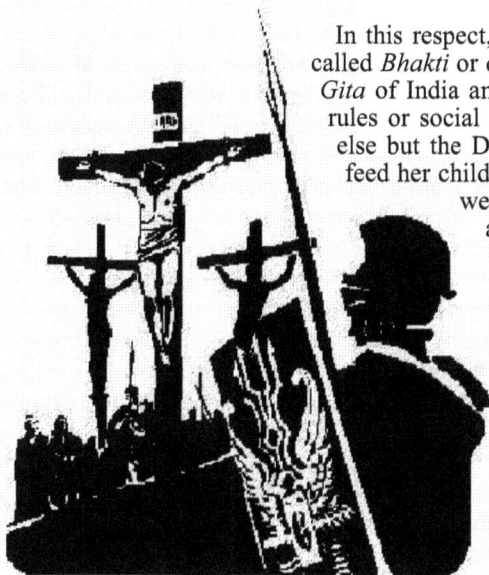

In this respect, Jesus' teaching is closely related to the form of spiritual discipline called *Bhakti* or devotional Surrender to God which was popularized in the *Bhagavad Gita* of India and in the Ausarian mysteries of Ancient Egypt. Devotion transcends rules or social conventions. True devotion towards the Divine means forsaking all else but the Divine, just as a mother may forsake rules about stealing in order to feed her child. The rules imposed by the Pharisees and those of the Old Testament were designed for keeping a certain kind of order in society. Naturally, at some point in the spiritual movement there is a time where social convention and the needs of the spiritual aspirant diverge. When this point arises, the aspirant must know how to live in the world while not being involved in it. In this manner, social conventions are upheld for the good of those who need society for their spiritual evolution while, at the same time, the aspirant moves towards detachment and freedom from society.

Jesus' growing number of followers caused a group in the Jewish priestly hierarchy in the Temple in Jerusalem to fear him as a reformer who would expose their greed and spiritual immaturity. Jesus knew of their plots against him, and so he gathered his main disciples for a Last Supper. At this occasion he instituted the sacrament of Holy Communion, which later became the ritual of the Eucharist Christian Sacrament. Later that night he was arrested by agents of the Jewish priests who were in league with the Roman officials. Then he was denounced before Pontius Pilate, the Roman governor, on the charge that he claimed to be king of the Jews. The standard practice of the Roman government was to seek out and execute any leaders of protest or revolt movements in their provinces or captured territories. Jesus was crucified by Roman soldiers on a hill outside the city wall. He died and was buried after suffering for three hours. On the third day after his death, his tomb was found empty. After that, Jesus appeared to his disciples on nine occasions and forty days after his resurrection he ascended into heaven. His followers then began their own ministries to take his teachings to all peoples around the world.

Many Christians worship Jesus Christ as the Son of God, who lived as a man in order to bring God's message to the troubled world. They also believe he is one with God (see John 10:30), that he is at the same time truly Divine and truly human. It is believed that by his preaching and the sacrifice of his death and his resurrection, he revealed for all humankind the way to live righteously and find eternal life. The term "Son of God" was first applied to the king of Israel because he was regarded as having been chosen by God to lead the people. (2 Sm. 7, 14, Ps 2, 7). It is also used to denote the faithful Israelite. When used as a reference to Jesus, it relates his kingly nature as the Messiah as well as his faithfulness as an Israelite, but also as the actual offspring of God (Mt. 4, 1-11). In Ancient Egypt, every pharaoh (king) was referred to as the "Son of God" because they were seen as Heru, the son of Asar (Osiris) who looks after the people and protects them. The pharaoh was seen as the special chosen one of God, as stated in the following verse from the Ancient Egyptian Instructions of Meri-ka-ra:

"From a million men God singled him (the pharaoh) out.
A goodly office is kingship..."

While there is no direct evidence that any one person called *"Jesus"* ever existed except in the Gnostic texts and the New Testament, there is ample substantiation of the Christian story from a psycho-mythological perspective. It is more likely that the role ascribed to a personality called Jesus was a composite based on mystery religions which also included resurrection and savior themes. This idea is supported by the inclusion of various preexisting elements from ancient religions into the Christian myth. There were many sect leaders of the Jewish and non-Jewish groups who were variously called *"Teacher of Righteousness,"* *"Master"* and so on, along with known prophets of the time who traveled widely and had also claimed to be the *"messiah"* and called themselves or were referred to by others as *"the Son of God."*

At the time when the Roman General, Titus, conquered the city of Jerusalem (after 30 A.C.E.), there was no evidence of a sect of Jesus. However, the Romans brought to an end various local Jewish customs which included human sacrifice. Therefore, while the reformers of Jewish religion, such as those who called themselves *messiah*s were pushing for changes, their teachings would have been repudiated by others whose positions in society, government and the economy would have been threatened by reform. Those who would have had the most to lose were the Roman authorities and the traditional Jewish religious leaders, both of whom would have viewed any successful sect as a threat to their authority and control over the Jewish people. The study of the period surrounding the early development of Christianity reveals one thing for certain: Jesus was not the first nor the only slain Jewish cult leader to claim to be the Messiah; there were several.

In the time when Jesus would have taught, the Jewish people lived in Egypt and Palestine. They were all under the domination of the Roman Empire, especially after the destruction of the Jewish Temple in c. 70 A.C.E. There were four main sects of Judaism. These comprised what is referred to as the "Jewish People" or followers of the Jewish religion who were, culturally speaking, Hebrews. The sects were: *Pharisees, Sadducees, Essenes* and the *Zealots*. Each of these groups affected the development of the Jewish scriptures and undoubtedly had members who claimed to be Messiahs.

A- The Pharisees emphasized strict interpretation and observance of the Mosaic law (Old Testament) in both its oral and written form. In Christian times the term came to be known also as a hypocritically self-righteous person because of Jesus' teaching given in Matthew 23:13 which denounces the Pharisees for not practicing the teachings correctly due to greed, the desire to remain in power over the people and ignorance, adhering to the letter instead of the spirit of the laws and rituals, which obstructs others from doing so either. The origins of the Pharisees can be traced to the second century B.C.E.

B- The Sadducees were a priestly, aristocratic Jewish sect founded in the second century B.C.E. that accepted only the written Mosaic law. This group ceased to exist after the destruction of the Temple in 70 A.C.E.

C- The Essenes were a Jewish religious sect, which existed in Palestine from the 2nd century B.C.E. to the end of the 1st century A.C.E. The members of the sect lived in communal groups, isolated from the rest of society. Sharing all possessions in common, they stressed ritual purity and were stricter than the Pharisees in their observance. A secrecy developed about the sect, and they shunned public life as well as temple worship. The Dead Sea Scrolls were probably their work.[117]

D- The Zealots were members of a Jewish movement of the first century A.C.E. that fought against Roman rule in Palestine as incompatible with strict monotheism.

Christianity thus developed as a new sect of Judaism. It sought to bring forth the deeper teachings which had been lost by the other sects due to infighting, corruption and misunderstanding of the true meaning of the scriptures. The first converts to Christianity, the majority of whom were most often non-Roman peoples, the poor, slaves, the politically oppressed and women of ancient times, saw Christianity not only as a spiritual liberator, but as a philosophy which would lead them to liberation from the social oppression of the Romans as well.

As both the canonical and Gnostic Gospels were written, two distinct views developed with reference to the story of Jesus. The orthodox community held that Jesus was a real historical character who physically died and was resurrected. The other, from Gnostic Christianity, held that Jesus story was a metaphor, a symbol of the human soul that takes on human form and forgets whence it came. It becomes identified with its physical body and thus suffers the joys and sorrows of the body until death comes. The time of the resurrection refers to the resurrection of the spirit through the realization of wisdom which leads to Enlightenment–not to bodily resurrection. The former idea became the central doctrine of the Orthodox Christian Church while the latter became the theme of the Gnostic Christians. The *"Apostles Creed"* promoted by the Orthodox Catholic Church affirmed the historicity of the life of Jesus rather than its metaphorical, metaphysical and universal principles.

The Apostles Creed:

I believe in God, the Father Almighty, Creator of heaven and earth, and in Jesus Christ, His only son, our Lord; who was conceived by the Holy Ghost, born of the Virgin Mary...suffered under Pontius Pilate, was crucified, died, and was buried.

THE HISTORY AND PHILOSOPHY OF MYSTICAL CHRISTIANITY

Below: How Jesus may have appeared in ancient times.
Drawing by Asar Oronde Reid.

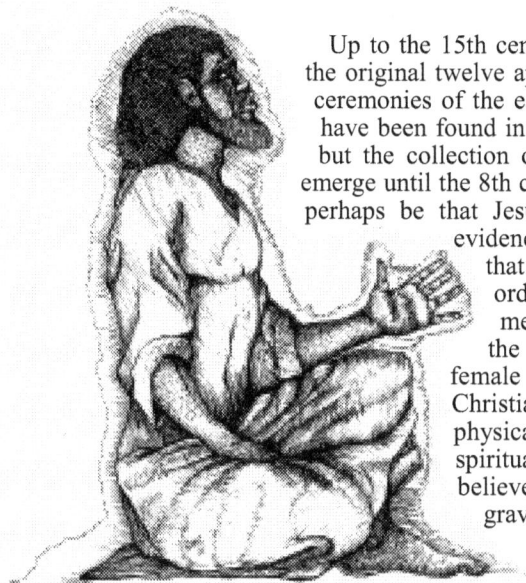

Up to the 15th century, it was widely believed that the creed had been established by the original twelve apostles. However, modern scholarship has traced it to the baptismal ceremonies of the early church, hundreds of years after Jesus' time. Similar statements have been found in the writings of Irenaeus and Tertulian in the 2nd and 3rd centuries, but the collection of statements which is now called "The Apostle's Creed" did not emerge until the 8th century A.C.E. The only possibly historical part of the statement may perhaps be that Jesus *"suffered under Pontius Pilate."* However, there is historical evidence that there were many who were slain by the Roman authorities at that time as trouble-makers or cult leaders who opposed the established order. The rest is myth and metaphor. It should also be noted that the meaning of the word "Jesus" also signifies "savior," and that some of the Gnostic groups had female leaders (saviors) and exemplified the female aspect of the Divine. The main difference between Orthodox Christianity and other religions seems to have been the insistence on a physical resurrection from the dead. While other religions proclaimed a spiritual transformation of some kind, the Orthodox Christians fervently believed and still believe in a mysterious bodily resurrection from the grave.

There are many writings from the time during which Jesus would have lived in existence today. At the time (100 B.C.E.-100 A.C.E.) there were many chroniclers among the Jews who lived in the land which was then called Canaan (today-Israel, Palestine). It is known from the writings that there were two major Jewish groups, those who lived in Galilee in the North and those who lived in Jerusalem in the South. As it occurs today, the inhabitants of the two regions noted each others regional differences as to dress, accent, customs and ideas. The Jerusalemites saw the Galileans as country folk, while they saw themselves as city dwellers. In the writings of the time there were several wandering prophets and others claiming to be messiahs, but there is no mention of a Jesus of Nazareth. In fact, no reference to a particular person called Jesus of Nazareth occurs until almost one to two generations later in the writings of the canonical Christian and Gnostic Christian Gospels. Therefore, they were not written by anyone who saw Jesus or knew him in person.

Who was Jesus of Nazareth? The two-thousand year old Christian story tells of a man who was born to poor Jewish parents with the grand destiny of saving all humanity. The story also tells us that Jesus was the son of a mortal woman who was impregnated by God. While Jesus is the focus of this work, it is extremely important to have a clear understanding of what religion is and how it is to be studied. Otherwise, this simple but profound story will continue to be a source of confusion. Therefore, we must first begin by understanding the relationship between religion, society and human development. Also, we must have a clear understanding of the events which occurred prior to and during the development of Christianity in order to determine the origins of the story and discover its place in history.

Christology is the branch of Christian theology that is concerned with the person of Jesus Christ. Christology attempts to explain the soteriology (saving work) of Christ by first explaining who the person (Jesus) was. For those who have a devotional view towards God and Jesus Christ, it may be sufficient just to believe that Jesus was a divine personality who had some higher relationship to God and who acts as an intercessor between them and God. However, in a comprehensive, integral spiritual movement, certain intellectual questions must be answered because Divinity is to be worshiped not only emotionally, but also intellectually, through one's actions, and ultimately with one's entire being in order to enhance the total spiritual movement. This idea is emphasized in the following passages which are the cornerstone of Christian philosophy:

Matthew 22
36 Master, which [is] the great commandment in the law?
37 Jesus said to him, Thou shalt love the Lord thy God with all thy heart, and with all thy soul, and with all thy mind.
38 This is the first and great commandment.
39 And the second [is] like it, Thou shalt love thy neighbor as thyself.
40 On these two commandments hang all the law and the prophets.

Verse 22:37 is particularly important to every aspirant because it points to the exact method of practicing the teachings. How is it possible to devote all of one's being to God? What does this mean? Should one throw away all possessions and become a monk or nun? Should one cease all activities in the world and leave all contact with civilization? These questions became the subject of intense debates among the early Orthodox Church fathers since they had, in effect, begun to develop a new religion based on their own ideas instead of following the ancient mystical tradition that gave birth to Christianity and held the answers to these important questions. Mystical teachings of the Ancient Egyptian religions such as the cult of Aset (Isis) and Asar (Osiris) were handed down from teacher to disciple in an unbroken tradition for several millennia. When the Orthodox Roman Church set out to destroy all other religions with the might of the Roman armies, they were actually severing their own link to the authentic mystery teachers of the time. Priests and priestesses of the mystery religions from all over the Roman empire were executed and their temples desecrated or destroyed, leaving the true meaning of the teachings which had been inscribed in stone or other media open to debate and wide interpretation. Therefore, the argument over the personality of Jesus was a source of great conflict in the early church, and it continues to be a source of conflict among the Church leadership even today. This point is of such importance that it will be discussed further in reference to initiation and the initiatic form of education.

The personality of Jesus is described in an objective manner in the New Testament. In Mark 8-27:29, Jesus asks his disciples: *"But who do you say that I am?"* The reply to this question is critical to our understanding of Christian philosophy as a whole because this understanding will govern and direct our religious thoughts and aspirations. If our thoughts are in error, it is possible that through frustration and our own misunderstanding, we may lead ourselves astray or lose our faith completely. If we understand Jesus as the only historical personality who is to be called *"Christ,"* a Godlike personality who is separate and above us, then our direction will be toward seeking "the Christ" who is "somewhere" outside of ourselves to come and save us. This is the view which is most prominently put forth in the New Testament of the Bible.

27. And Jesus went out, and his disciples, into the towns of Caesarea Philippi: and by the way he asked his disciples, saying to them, Who do men say that I am?
28 And they answered, John the Baptist: but some [say], Elijah; and others, One of the prophets.
29 And he saith to them, But who you say that I am? And Peter answereth and saith to him, Thou art the Christ.

However, if we understand Jesus as a guide, a mentor who is showing us the way to our own *Christhood*, we will seek the Christ within us. This is the message of the Gnostic Christian Gospels. The understanding of "Christ" and of Christian life is a personal quest which we must realize within ourselves as opposed to a search for someone or a deity who will save us. From a psychological perspective, it is our own Christhood which saves each one of us. The passage below from the *Gospel of Thomas* contains a different interpretation of the New Testament statement from Mark (above). It directs our search for Christ away from Jesus "himself" and back to ourselves. It leads us to understand that when we have realized the Christhood within ourselves, we are to be considered as "equals" to Jesus himself.

14. Jesus says to his disciples: "Compare me and tell me whom I am like." Simon Peter says to him: "You are like a just angel!" Matthew says to him: "You are like a wise man and a philosopher!" Thomas says to him: "Master, my tongue cannot find words to say whom you are like!" Jesus says: "I am no longer thy master; for you have drunk, and you are inebriated from the bubbling spring which I have measured out."

The previous passage from the Gospel of Thomas also gives direct insight into the deeper implications of the following verse from Matthew 12:24-25, wherein it is implied that all who attain such wisdom (Enlightenment) are equals.

24 The disciple is not above [his] teacher, nor the servant above his lord.
25 It is enough for the disciple that he should be as his teacher, and the servant as his lord. If they have called the master of the house Beelzebub, how much more [shall they call] them of his household?

The Orthodox Christian doctrine holds that Christ has two distinct natures, one Divine and one human. These two are distinct, yet joined in one *person* and one *substance*. One of the principal divergent understandings of Christ was found in Arianism. The Orthodox Christian Churches of Rome and Constantinople opposed Arianism and sought to stop its spread. Arius, a native of Libya in North Africa, neighboring Alexandria, Egypt, developed a teaching which was later called Arianism. Arius' teaching held that God is unbegotten and without beginning. Therefore, the Son, the Second Person of the Trinity, cannot be considered in the same sense as God because he (Jesus) is begotten. According to this view, the Son did not come from the Divine substance of the Father. This means that he did not exist with God from all eternity, but was created later like nature and all other creatures. Further, the Son exists, as all other things in creation, by the will of the Father. The teachings of Arius were condemned at the first Council at Nicea in 325. Arius was banished from Christendom, but his teaching gained strength to the point where he was recalled out of exile. However, over a period of time the teaching was finally defeated in later Councils when opponents who supported the Nicean resolutions gained strength again and were able to emphasize the orthodox teachings and exclude divergent views.

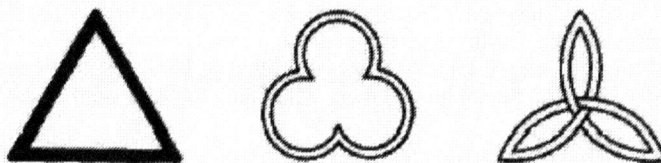

Above: Christian symbols of the Trinity.

As introduced earlier, the idea of the Trinity was well understood in Ancient Egypt since it originated there. The teaching spread to neighboring countries where it found strong adherents in Libya, Syria and Ethiopia (Sudan). However, during the emergence of Christianity, there developed a misunderstanding over the true intent of the religion as a result of conflicts between the early church fathers. There was a conflict between those who followed the non-dualistic view from Egypt and India, which held that the Trinity is an emanation of the single Supreme Essence, and those who followed the Aristotelian-rational, dualistic view of Europe and Zoroastrianism from Persia.

At the mythological religious level, the Trinity may be viewed as three personalities. This portrayal shows the three personalities as manifestations of God as expressed in time and space, as well as in Creation and all life. This is the elementary view, the view of the masses and of those who are less spiritually sensitive and mature. As the understanding of religion develops, the aspirant must begin to understand the Trinity in a much more profound sense. It is to be viewed in its transcendental form. The Trinity is in reality one being, and every element of it, Father, Son, and Holy Spirit, has the same underlying essence, which is the transcendental Supreme Being that is beyond the three.

This more profound understanding is reached by those who, through intense spiritual practice, are able to move beyond the ritualistic and mythological aspects of religion. In so doing, one discovers that the Trinity is like a mask that covers the underlying essence of all existence. When the mask is uncovered, there is no more Trinity, merely one essence which is nameless, formless and transcendental. Further, when you, as the spiritual aspirant, remove your own egoistic mask, you will discover that your underlying essence is one and the same as that of the Trinity. For indeed the Trinity is a symbol of cosmic and human egoism. This understanding will be explored in more detail in Section III. For now you must keep in mind that the ritualistic and mythological levels of religion are presented as a dualistic teaching to aid the spiritually immature follower because the ordinary mind operates almost exclusively in dualistic terms. It is oblivious to anything outside of its dualistic concept of existence. However, if the correct movement is promoted with the correct guidance, the spiritual aspirant will be led to understand the non-dualistic aspects of spirituality and discover the nature of the Transcendental Self.

First we will explore the myth of Jesus as a human personality with a distinct ego, and then we will discover the transcendental Jesus who is beyond human categories of thought and must, therefore, be experienced intuitionally with the heart rather than intellectually with the mind. When a human being is truly able to apply his or her mind completely on the Divine, such as the description given in Matthew 22:37, they can transcend the mind itself into the realm of intuitional spiritual realization, i.e. Christ Consciousness. Then there is a realization that the non-dualistic view of Jesus Christ represents an all-encompassing view of creation and of human consciousness which transcends the individual human ego and lifts us into the realm of resurrection and immortality.

With this understanding we will see that the conflicts within the early church were the result of different levels of comprehension between the elementary advocates of dualism and the advanced advocates of non-dualism who originated their teaching with the wisdom they gained from the Ancient Egyptian tradition. The teaching of non-dualism is expressed in the statement: *"The Kingdom of the Father is spread upon the earth and men do not see it!"* from the Gospel of Thomas. It points to the non-dualistic nature of creation which is not perceived by spiritually immature people due to their inability to overcome the dualistic view of themselves and of nature. The teachings of Jesus are directed toward abolishing this dualism and liberating the soul from the underlying cause of duality: misunderstanding. Thus, correct understanding of Christianity and of mystical Christian practice allows the ordinary human being to be freed from the ignorance of the mind, to wake up to the greater reality. This is the essence of Christian Yoga.

CHRISTIANITY AND THE ANCIENT EGYPTIAN RELIGION

The symbol of the *Lamb* alone or the *Ram*, who was the leader of the herd, sometimes stood alone as symbols of Christ. Some of the scriptures of the Bible gave impetus to these symbols. The same symbols were of prime importance in Egyptian mythology since the lamb was also a symbol of Heru and the Ram was a symbol of *Amun* or *Amen*, the High God, and also of *Knum*, the creator of men, who fashions them on the potter's wheel.

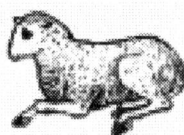

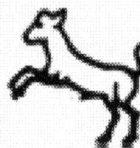

At left: The lamb, a symbol of Jesus.   Right: The lamb of Ancient Egypt

John 1

29. The next day John seeth Jesus coming to him, and saith, Behold the Lamb of God, who taketh away the sin of the world.

John 6

56 He that eateth my flesh, and drinketh my blood, dwelleth in me, and I in him.

The story of Jesus Christ, *The Good Shepherd,* is similar to that of the Ancient Egyptian God Asar, who, along with the Egyptian god Djehuti (later known as Hermes by the Greeks), was also known as the *"Good Shepherd."* In Hindu mythology the equivalent teaching is expressed in relation to the god Krishna. He was known as Govinda or cowherd. Asar was also symbolically eaten and assimilated by the aspirants who wished to become *"one with him."* In the same way, Jesus exhorted his followers to eat his flesh and drink his blood. The statement above from John 6 points to the mystery of the Eucharist. The profound history and meaning of this ritual will be discussed in a separate section later on.

The Lord's Prayer given by Jesus in Matthew 6:9: *(Our Father who art in heaven...)* is very close to a prayer to the Ancient Egyptian God, *Amen*, which begins *O Amen, O Amen, who art in heaven...*[72/114] Amen was the High God of Egypt, the Hidden immanent and panentheistic source underlying all things and all phenomena. Another Ancient Egyptian hymn reads as follows: *O Amen, O Amen, O God, O God, O Amen, I adore thy name, grant thou to me that I may understand thee; Grant thou that I may have peace in the Duat, and that I may possess all my members therein...*

The Jews were saved from certain death due to starvation twice. According to the Bible, the first time Jews were saved from death was when Ancient Egypt became the refuge for Abraham from the famines of the Near East. Then later, according to the story of Joseph in the Bible, the Jewish people survived the droughts and famine of Cannan by seeking refuge once again in the land of Egypt. The extension of asylum to Jesus along with his family in Egypt during the time of persecution, at his birth and his subsequent upbringing there, further explains the similarity to the Egyptian savior character of Heru, who is known for *walking on water* just as Jesus is said to have done in Matthew 14:26. Heru and Jesus share several titles. Like Jesus, Heru was the symbol of:

*"The resurrection and the life," "The anointed one," "The WORD made flesh," "The KRST (Christ)," "The WORD made TRUTH," "The one who comes to fulfill the LAW," "The destroyer of the enemies[1] of his father" "The one who walks upon the water of his Father"*61

---

[1] ENEMIES: ignorance, lies, deception, too much talking, covetousness, depravity, selfishness, etc.

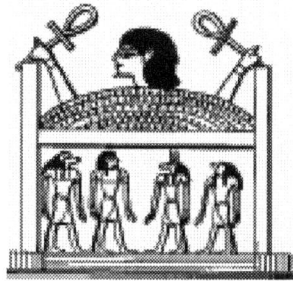

Above left: Asar (Osiris) rising from the tomb.
Above right: Jesus rising from the sepulcher.

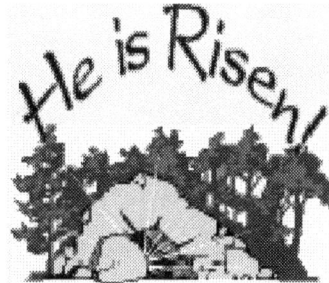

One important correlation between Jesus and Heru is the date of the celebration of the holidays surrounding them. The birthday of Heru in Ancient Egypt was celebrated on December 25. This date is three days following the winter solstice (around Dec. 21), when the sun begins to rise again toward its summit towards the equator. It reaches this summit at the summer solstice, which occurs around June 21st. in the early Christian era the birthday of Jesus was changed from January 6 to December 25 by later Christian authorities.

Another significant correlation is the Christian myth surrounding the story of the three kings who traveled to the site of the birth of Jesus. The story of the birth of Jesus tells of how three kings from the east traveled to see the new-born baby Jesus. It is said that a star guided them to the birthplace. The star Sirius was held to be specially important in Ancient Egyptian culture and religion because its rising announced the flooding of the Nile River, which was the source of all sustenance. There are three stars in the Orion constellation which point almost directly to Sirius. Sirius is associated with Aset, the mother of Heru and Aset as well as Heru were the prototypes for the Christian story of Mary and Jesus as will be shown throughout our journey. Also, there is an Ancient Egyptian relief which shows three gods bringing gifts to Aset. It will be discussed in more detail later on in this volume. Thus, the story of the three kings in the Christian myth is in reality a metaphor to describe the three stars in the Orion constellation. These in turn relate to the relationship of the three aspects of the human personality towards the Self. The movement of the three towards the one symbolizes the rising light of salvation which is being born on the winter solstice of life, from the Ancient Egyptian goddess Aset, mother, mentor, council and teacher of Heru, who is the prototype of Mary, mother, mentor, council and teacher of Jesus.

The birth of Jesus, attended by the three kings.

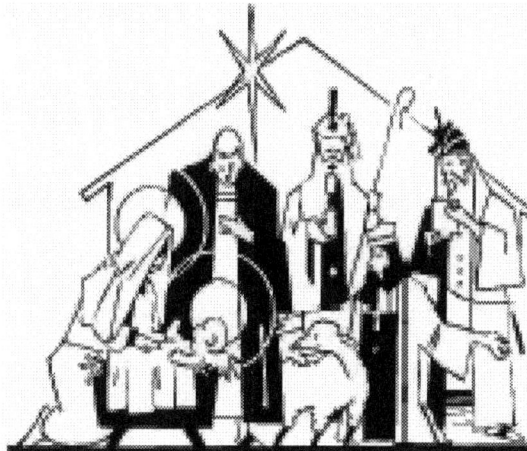

Below: The Ancient Egyptian Annunciation and birth of Heru, attended by three gods (wise men).

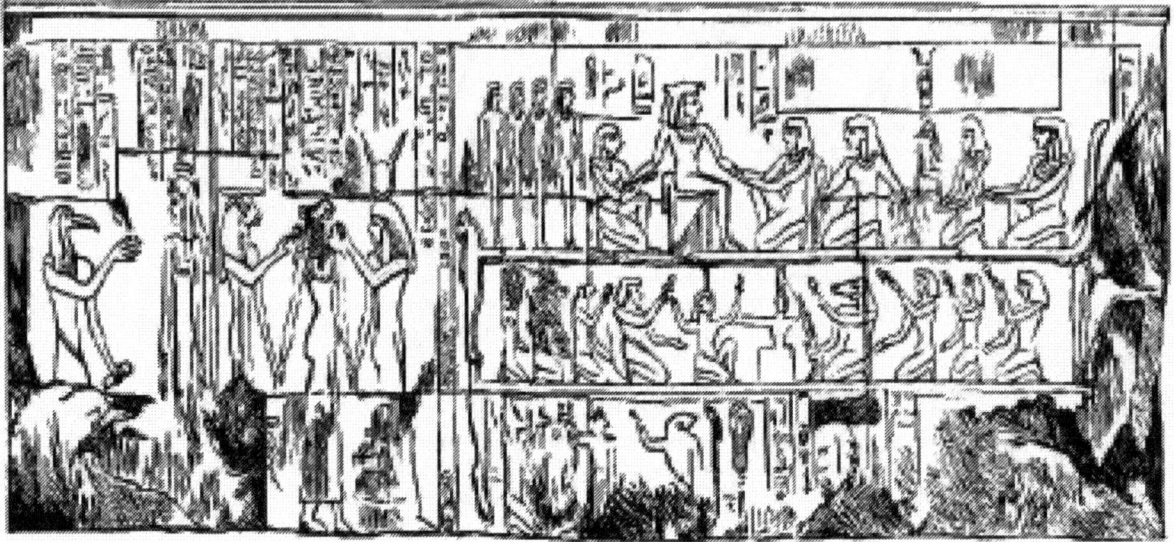

The deeper significance of the Ancient Egyptian Relief:

The origins of the transcendental themes of Christianity reach far into Ancient Egyptian antiquity. In the New Testament Book of Matthew 1:20-23, the story of the Annunciation, Conception, Birth and Adoration of the child, Jesus, is presented. It tells how the "angel of the Lord" appears to Joseph, informing him that his wife Mary is pregnant by the Holy Spirit of God. The figure above is a drawing of the image engraved in the Holy of Holies or *Mesken,* in the temple of Luxor (5,500-1,700 BCE). In the first scene (A) at left, the god Tehuti, the transmitter of the *word* (logos), is depicted in the act of announcing to queen Mut-em-Ua (who has assumed the role of Aset) that she will give birth to the child who will be the righteous, divine heir (Heru). In the next scene (B) Knum (Khnum, Kneph), the ram headed god (also associated with Amun), along with Hathor, provide her with the Life Force (Spirit) through two Ankhs. In this same scene (B), the virgin is pictured as becoming pregnant (conceiving) through that Spirit. In the following scene (C), the mother is being attended to while the child is being supported by nurses. The next scene (D) is the Adoration wherein the child is enthroned and adored by Amun, the hidden Holy Spirit behind all creation, with three men behind him (Amun) who offer boons or gifts with the right hand (open facing up) and eternal life with the left (holding the Ankh).

This set of scenes attests to the deeper significance of the virgin birth mystery. Every mother is a goddess and every child is a product or mixture of Creation or physical nature and the spirit of God. Through this metaphor, we are to understand that each human being has a divine origin, heritage and birthright. Therefore, it is clear to see the meaning of the Christian statements: *"I and [my] Father are one." "Jesus answered them, 'Is it not written in your law that ye are gods?,'"* from John 10:30 and 34, respectively.

Considering the correlations described above it would be natural for the Egyptian decedents, the *Copts,* to accept Christianity in general, and Gnostic Christianity in particular, as their "new" faith. The existence of the Coptic Library of Gnostic Gospels known today as the 'Nag Hammadi Library' should therefore be no surprise. There are most likely several other volumes of ancient writings to be uncovered. With this view, it may be possible to see the newly discovered Coptic manuscripts of Nag Hammadi, Egypt, as a fourth intervention on behalf of Egypt to save Christianity and the Jewish faith by preserving the wisdom of early Christianity which the Orthodox Christian Church sought to destroy 1,700 years ago.

THE EVOLUTION OF THE CROSS

✠

The Latin Cross

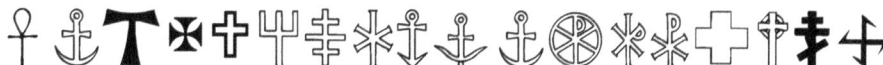

The Latin Cross

Other important cross variations used by the Christian Church throughout history.

The Christian Cross is an example of a symbol which was assimilated hundreds of years after the proposed death of Jesus. It was previously considered as pagan and was resisted by the early Catholic Bishops, until it was eventually changed from its original form as the Egyptian *Ankh Cross,* ☥, to its present form. As previously discussed, Jesus' death had originally been reported as having occurred by crucifixion on a tree and not on a cross (Acts 5:30; 1 Peter 2:24). In Acts, Jesus was said to have been slain and hung on a tree. In 1 Peter, it is stated that he (Jesus) *"bore our sins in his body on the tree."*

When Jesus was crucified by the Romans he was not crucified alone. There were two other men who were also condemned to death. They were indeed criminals. Thus, there were three crucifixions at the same time. At one point during the crucifixion, the Roman soldiers mocked Jesus and one of the criminals at his side also turned to him and mocked him (Luke 23 36:43). The other one, however, turned to Jesus and asked for forgiveness. Jesus granted him absolution, showing that even a sinful person such as a criminal, can be redeemed by faith and righteous action (turning towards the Divine). The mystical symbolism of the three crucifixions can be related to the three states of the human personality. Now we will discuss the three major personality types and how they relate to the passion of Jesus on the cross. For simplicity we will use the analogy of a video cassette player to understand the mind.

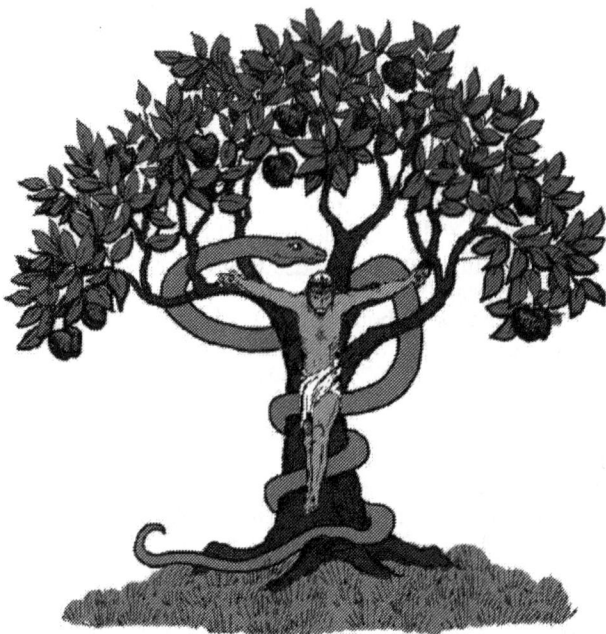

The DULL Personality is lethargic, lazy, depressed, full of anger, vengeful, covetous, hateful, greedy, self-destructive, suicidal, a meat eater, etc. How did they get this way? They poisoned their mind for so long that the light of the soul barely shines enough to keep them alive. They have entertained thoughts like, "The world is cruel," "I hate life," "I don't believe in God," "To hell with you and everybody," "If you don't care about me then I don't care about you," and so on. They have desired so many things and have been frustrated so much that they hate the world and themselves, so they strike out in the hope of hurting the world and ending their own pain. Their enjoyment is when others are suffering and when they suffer as well. Smoking, drugs and alcohol are forms of suffering. Even though they feel good at the time they are used, in reality these are intense forms of pain from a Yogic point of view. In reality they are a call for help because an advanced human being does not have any need for depending on petty things of the world or on drugs to escape the world. A true human being is a master of the world, a king or queen. Anyone else is merely a child from a spiritual point of view. This personality is like a video machine that has stopped playing the movie of life and has begun to chew up the video tape. It has seen so many scenes of violence, hatred, destruction and fear that it has pulled back from life and wants to self-destruct. This personality is like a person that cannot even stop and reason that smoking is bad. If you tell them this truth they will even want to fight with you. This is because they are so degraded that the prospect of losing even the poison is unbearable. What does this say about a system that promotes meat and tobacco, knowing that it is purposely addictive and poisonous? The world has unrighteous people who are ready and waiting to exploit others. They are driven by spiritual ignorance, hatred and greed (egoism), the same as anyone else. Should you play into their hands and give yourself over as a sacrifice to their greed? They will receive their consequences so do not resent them. Resentment leads to negativity, and it is therefore against truth and righteousness. If you succeed in turning your life around you will deprive them of their desire to exploit you and they will suffer economically. Eventually they will have to pay for their own mistakes. The Dull personality is the criminal who mocked Jesus.

"Be free from resentment under the experience of being wronged,"

"Do not conspire against others. God will punish accordingly. Schemes do not prevail; only the laws of God do. Live in peace, since what God gives comes by itself."

—Ancient Egyptian Proverbs

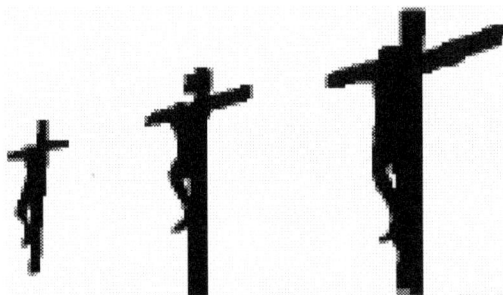

Above: Jesus and the two thieves being crucified.

The AGITATED Personality is the person who is anxious, with uncontrolled thoughts, unable to calm down, loves spicy or salty foods, etc. The mind is always racing from one thought to the next, from one scheme to the next, and is always full of delusions and haunting memories. They think that they will get over on the world and make the big score. They constantly have to be into something and hate to be alone with their thoughts. This personality is like a video machine that is constantly playing one movie after another. They are constantly involved in movement physically, but especially mentally, never allowing themselves a moment of introspection. If there is a brief period of introspection, the mind is too weak to do what is right. This is like a smoker who knows that smoking is bad but cannot stop himself.

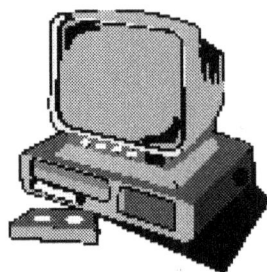

This personality is constantly on a roller-coaster ride of emotions, sometimes joyous and at other times angry or sorrowful. They are constantly elated over some prospect or depressed over some prospect. They anticipate the future, yearning for what they desire and if it does not come they become angry, resentful and frustrated. They have not learned to weather the stormy seas of life's ups and downs, and they have no anchor to hold on to. So they are tossed about by the winds and rough seas of life. They therefore, never discover true peace, what the Ancient Egyptians called *HETEP* and the Indian yoga tradition calls *SHANTI*. They never discover the bliss of the inner self except in brief moments when their pressure is released through sexual activity or in the perception of having acquired some object (including persons or relationships) they wanted. How long does the pleasure last when you get something you wanted or after a sexual encounter? Since the disease of agitation is still in the mind, the release of tension is only temporary and the cycle repeats itself even up to the time of death and beyond. Like a drug addict you must constantly seek that thing you want to fulfill your desires, but you are always frustrated since no object in the world has the capacity to fulfill anyone's desires. Most people never discover the reason why they always end up running into the wall of frustration after they acquire an object, and therefore live their lives in a constant but fruitless search for fulfillment through objects. After death their desires push them to more frustrations, and so they experience a lesser hell than the DULL personalities, but it is still hell nonetheless.

24 His disciples said to Him, "Show us the place where You are, since it is necessary for us to seek it."
He (Jesus) said to them, "Whoever has ears, let him hear. There is light within a man of light, and he (or "it") lights up the whole world. If he (or "it") does not shine, he or "it") is darkness."

—Gospel of Thomas

Therefore, you must realize that the world cannot bring you true peace and fulfillment. Only you can do that. How? In order to become a lucid personality you must integrate your personality by keeping your balance of mind. Trust in God and know that all happens for a reason. Know that if you reach for God you will not be disappointed because God is the only truth and never ending reality. God is not here today and then gone tomorrow, like the transient objects of the world (including people). God is accessible, but only for those who seek. Otherwise, you are on your own and you don't stand a chance on your own.

> 31 Therefore be not anxious, saying, What shall we eat? or,
> What shall we drink? or, With what shall we be clothed?
> 32 (For after all these things do the Gentiles seek:) for your
> heavenly Father knoweth that ye have need of all these things.
> 33 But seek ye first the Kingdom of God, and his righteousness;
> and all these things shall be added to you.
>
> —Matthew 6

The agitated personality is like that video machine that plays a mixture of action movies, love story movies, comedy shows, etc., constantly. It becomes caught up in the emotions of the shows that it plays, and cries when there is a sad movie and laughs when there is a funny movie, and is always anticipating when it will be able to play the next movie or show. It develops a preference for action movies and hates sad shows, or vice versa. This video machine has forgotten its true nature and has become completely caught up in the emotions and feelings of the movies. It remains confused and lost, never finding true peace and happiness because it is looking for it in the movie, and not in realizing the true nature, the tape deck, which is never really affected by the emotions or actions in the movies that it plays. Every human being's soul is like that tape deck. The constant playing of movies (dramas of human life) has made the soul forget its true nature. This is why yoga prescribes the practice of meditation, devotional worship and reflection on the teachings. These practices help you to remember the truth by giving you a break from the world and the ego with its desires and activities. The Agitated personality is represented by the criminal who led a life of sin but who also had some spiritual aspiration and turned to Jesus.

> 60 <They saw> a Samaritan carrying a lamb on his way to Judea.
> He (Jesus) said to his disciples, "(Why does) that man (carry) the lamb around?"
> They said to him, "So that he may kill it and eat it."
> He said to them, "While it is alive, he will not eat it, but only when
> he has killed it and it has become a corpse."
> They said to him, "He cannot do so otherwise."
> He said to them, "You too, look for a place for yourself within the
> Repose, lest you become a corpse and be eaten."
>
> —Gospel of Thomas

The LUCID Personality is balanced in pain and in pleasure. He or she knows that the world is a changing arena of ups and downs, so therefore there is no reason to fret about life since whatever happens or does not happen is God's will. It is a good thing for things to be set up this way because if the world was "perfect," according to the ego's standards, who would seek the Divine? Even though the joy of Enlightenment, God, the Kingdom of Heaven, Buddha Consciousness, etc., is a billion times greater that the worldly pleasures of human beings, people would continue to pursue worldly pleasures and continue to be deluded. They would not care about anything else if there was no adversity in life. Such is the power of sense pleasure which deludes the mind of human beings. For no matter how good your situation is, no matter how many millions, houses, cars, relationships, etc., you have, it will all end someday and you will feel pain and sorrow.

> 111 Jesus said, "The heavens and the earth will be rolled up in your
> presence. And one who lives from the Living One will not see death."
> Does not Jesus say, "Whoever finds himself is superior to the world?"
>
> —Gospel of Thomas

The way to develop the lucidity in your mind which will lead to spiritual awakening is to seek that which is not changing, that which is of even greater wealth, and that which you can take with you after death: ENLIGHTENMENT, THE KINGDOM OF HEAVEN. Looking at Jesus' crucifixion with the other two persons as a metaphor, Jesus represents the lucid personality while the other two men being crucified represent the dull and agitated aspects of the personality. While they are on the cross they curse Jesus and mock him. But later on one of them turns towards him and asks for forgiveness and to be admitted into the Kingdom of Heaven. The physical personality of Jesus is the Lucid personality. At the point where they were all crucified, there was a final separation from mortal existence and therefore, Jesus henceforth manifested as Christ in full glory, transcending all physicality. In essence, he left the three aspects of the personality behind. Thus, the crucifixion scene provides a profound teaching in reference to the personality and the process of purifying the personality. By turning towards Christhood and in effect acting as Christ, it is possible to become like Christ and attain salvation by moving away from dullness and agitation and turning the personality towards lucidity, clarity, peace and universal love, and thereby moving into the transcendent, going beyond all aspects of personality.

The Christian Crosses and the Mystical Ankh Cross

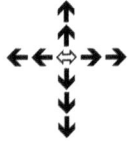

Above: The possible directions of spiritual evolution as symbolized by the cross.

Greeks from the early Christian times said that the Egyptian *Ankh*, ♀ , was "common to the worship of Christ and *Serapis* (Greek name for Asar). In Roman times, Saint Helena (c. 255-330), the mother of Roman Emperor Constantine-I (Constantine the Great) became a Christian around the time her son became emperor of Rome. Early church historians relate many stories about Helena. One of the stories was that Helena inspired the building of the Church of the Nativity in Bethlehem. Later tradition says that she founded the true cross on which Christ died. This was the *Tau Cross,* **T**, which resembles the Druid crosses. The *Maltese Cross,* ✠, was related to gods and goddesses of Malta before it was adopted by Christianity. One of the most important symbolic references of the Christian cross or "Latin Cross," ♱, is that its vertical axis symbolizes the vertical movement of spiritual discipline (self-effort) which implies true transformation in all areas (mental, spiritual, physical) of life. The vertical movement pierces the horizontal axis of the cross, a symbol of time and space (lateral movement, reincarnation, stagnation, etc.). Other important crosses used by the Christian church were: Early crosses, ⚚ ⳨ ⳩; Anchor crosses, ⚓ ⚓ ⚓; Monograms of Christ, ⊕ ✳ ✸; Greek cross, ✚; Celtic cross, ☨; Eastern cross, ☦; Craponee Swastika cross, ⛨ (similar to the Indian and Persian swastika, 卐). Originally, the swastika symbol was an ancient sign used to denote the manner in which spiritual energy flows. It was not until the Nazi party of Germany adopted it in 1935 that the symbol was used for promoting hatred, racism, murder and greed. Prior to this time it was an ancient cosmic or religious symbol used by the Vedic-Aryans, Hindus and Greeks. The Nazi movement led to the killing of more than six million people who were following the Jewish faith. This is known as the Jewish Holocaust. The Swastika continues to be used today by various hate groups (Dull state of personality) which seek to establish white supremacy. The Swastika is formed by a cross with the ends of the arms bent at right angles in either a clockwise or a counterclockwise direction, denoting the form of energy being manifested.

Early Christianity mimicked preexisting religions which also included slain saviors. In other religions saviors such as *Asar (Osiris),*[I] *Odin*[II] and *Zeus,*[III] were slain, their deaths symbolizing the new life to come in the Spirit. Like other mystery religions, Gnostic Christianity understood the tree or cross symbol as being metaphorical. It referred to a symbolic meaning and not a historical one. In one aspect, the cross symbol refers to matter, which is composed of elements. In relation to Christian mythology, it specifically referred to the human body, into which all souls incarnate.

When the soul manifests itself in human form, it is as if coming down from the subtle Spirit state to the gross state of physical matter (Genesis 1:1-2). From the realm of infinity and eternity it is coming down to the realm of limitation and finite existence in time and space. In essence, all human souls are crucified on the cross of matter (time and space) when they become born into a human body and they identify themselves with that body as who they are (ego-consciousness), instead of their Higher Soul essence. However, in the process of spiritual aspiration, when the Soul remembers its essential nature, the physical body is symbolically crucified on the tree of life, leaving the Soul free to experience eternity. This crucifiction allows for the resurrection of one's higher nature, Christ, which now becomes established in one's personality. One attains Christhood, the Kingdom of Heaven, Enlightenment when this spiritual awakening (resurrection) occurs. This is the true second birth. of being "born again" to the higher truth.

[I] Asar, God of the dead and of resurrection in Ancient Egypt.

[II] Odin, one of the principal gods in Norse mythology. He was a war god.

[III] In Greek mythology, the chief of the gods (Roman Jupiter).

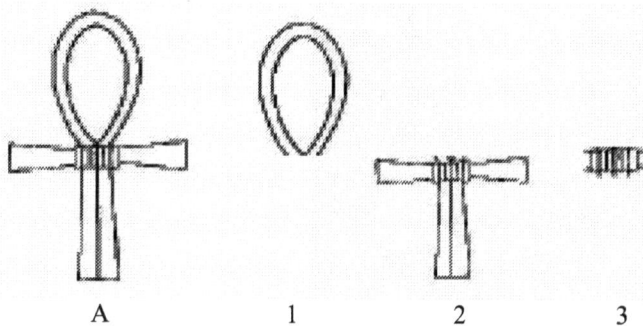

The Parts of the Ankh

A. The Ankh refers to life in the form of a human being. 1- Above: The Shen Ring: eternity, feminine principal, womb, magnetically charged. 2- Above: The Cross: That which is temporal, time-space principal, phallic principal, electrically charged. 3- Above: The Ankh Knot: That which holds the two principals together, (eternity-temporal, immortal-mortal, spirit-body) creating the human being.

"Involvement in a form is the beginning of the death of life. It is a straightening and a limiting; a binding and a constricting. Form checks life, thwarts it, and yet enables it to organize. Seen from the point of view of free moving force, incarceration in a form is extinction. Form disciplines force with a merciless severity."

"Evil is simply misplaced force. It can be misplaced in time, like the violence that is acceptable in war is unacceptable in peace. It can be misplaced in space, like a burning coal on the rug rather than the fireplace. Or it can be misplaced in proportion, like an excess of love can make us overly sentimental, or a lack of love can make us cruel and destructive. It is in things such as these that evil lies, not in a personal Devil who acts as an Adversary."

As the two preceding proverbs from the Kabbalah suggest, time and space, in and of themselves, are not evil. However, when the spirit becomes identified with the limited concept of time and space by developing a dependency on physical objects for happiness and by developing a longing for pleasures of the senses, evil in the form of egotistical, self-centered behavior emerges. The spirit falls, as it were, to earth. In essence, every soul that turns away from its Divine essence is Lucifer, the devil. In Christian mythology, Lucifer is an angel of light who has been beguiled by the forms of matter, time and space. From a psycho-mythological perspective, every soul who lives in a state of "separation" from or forgetfulness of its Divine nature lives in its own "hell."

Isaiah 14
12 How art thou fallen from heaven, O Lucifer, son of the morning! [how] art thou cut down to the ground, which didst weaken the nations!

So as we have seen, the passion of Jesus is a symbol of the passion experienced by every soul which comes into physical form only to suffer human existence and die a painful death as the body grows old, becomes sick and finally dies. The spirit is symbolically crucified on the cross of time and space when it enters into physical form. The task, then, is to return to the primordial state of consciousness prior to the involvement in matter, time and space. For these reasons the Gnostic Christians distinguished between the *physical* body of Jesus of Nazareth and the *spiritual* Christ which is ultimately separate from all physical phenomena. While appearing on the surface to be a dualistic philosophy, a deeper understanding of Gnostic Christianity reveals the wisdom behind the teaching. This Gnostic understanding was called *Docetism*. It led to the orthodox denunciation of its followers as *heretical*. The Docetist doctrine, from the Greek meaning "to seem," held that Christ did not have a material human body but rather, that he was a "phantasmal" human and that his birth, death, and other earthly manifestations were merely illusions. This belief was regarded as one of the first Christian heresies. Docetism reached a height in 2nd century Gnosticism. Serapion, the bishop of Antioch (190-203), was the first to use the name "Docetist." Docetism was condemned officially at the Council of Chalcedon (451 A.C.E). The debate over the correct cross and doctrine which Christianity should follow leads us now into the discussion of the conflicts of the early Christian Church.

101

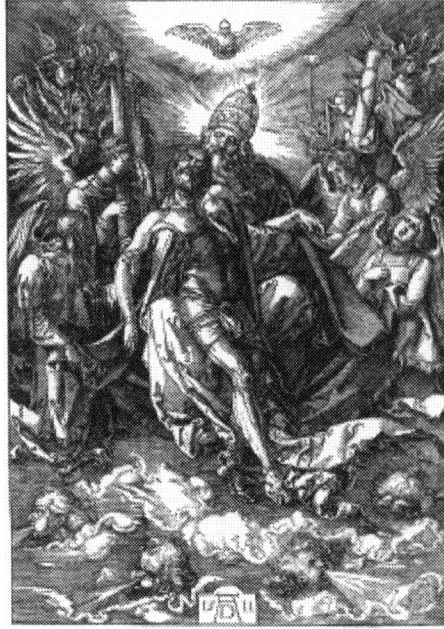

Above: The Holy Trinity, by Albrecht Dürer (1511 A.C.E.)

The reader will note that several depictions of Jesus have been used in this book. This is because the author wishes to convey the diversity of ways in which Jesus has been conceptualized by various cultures. The images are alright for the purpose of engendering a devotional feeling in the spiritual aspirant as long as they do not come to be regarded as absolute realities, as if Jesus actually looked in some particular way or other. Also, images are dangerous if they are used by cultures that espouse superiority over other cultures and their religions. Then the images take on a function that is not only idolatrous but sinister as well.

CHAPTER IIII: HOW OTHER SPIRITUAL TRADITIONS INFLUENCED CHRISTIANITY

OTHER SAVIORS OF THE ANCIENT WORLD

Many attempts have been made to root the story of Jesus in history rather than allowing it to remain as a myth. It has been suggested by Celsus[I] and the Talmudic tradition[II] that the idea for Jesus came from a man by the name of *Jesus ben Pandera.*[21] The story holds that he lived 50-100 years prior to the birth of the supposed Jesus of Nazareth and was the son of a Roman soldier named Pandera (or Panthera) and a Jewish prostitute. Jesus ben Pandera was called a holy man. He worked miracles, foretold of the world's end, healed the sick and was eventually executed. It is possible that the name "Pandera" was associated with *Pandora,*[III] the first woman, or with *Dionysus,*[IV] the son of *Pan,*[V] whose totem animal was the panther. The root of all the words is *Pan.* This root links them mythological. Dionysus was also a savior who performed miracles and was revered through many festivals in many countries of the ancient world. *Appolonius of Tyana*[VI] was another important figure who existed at the time of Jesus' proposed birth. The important factor here is that there is ample evidence in the writings of the time about Appolonius and his life. He was said to have performed miracles, healed the sick and foretold the future. He studied philosophy and the teachings of the Gnostic mystery schools of Greece and then traveled to India and Egypt where he was instructed by Sages. He returned to Rome and preached salvation and resistance against injustice. Thus, it is believed by some scholars that the story of Appolonius and that of other mythic gods and saviors such as Heru of Egypt and Mithra of Persia have been woven into the Christian story along with their festivals and rituals. Much in the same way, the Islamic tradition assimilated the previously pagan *Ka'bah*[VII] (Kaaba) which is today the holiest Islamic shrine in the city of Mecca.

Another prototype of the crucified savior comes from the Greek mythology surrounding *Orpheus.* In Greek mythology, Orpheus was considered to be a fine poet and musician. He was the son of Calliope, the muse[VIII] of epic poetry, and the husband of Eurydice. After Eurydice died, Orpheus descended into the Underworld to rescue her. He was initially successful but lost Eurydice when he disobeyed the command from Hades not to look back at her. Like Jesus and other crucified saviors, Orpheus' body was destroyed (crucified). Orpheus appears on a cylinder seal from around 300 A.C.E. as a crucified savior. These crucifixions are all metaphors relating that body identification must be destroyed in order that our spiritual consciousness may come forth.

THE ANCIENT EGYPTIAN AND INDIAN BACKGROUND OF CHRISTIANITY

Much of the philosophy inherent in the Gnostic Christian texts which will be compared in this work bears a direct resemblance in meaning, as well as in the form, to the teachings of India and Ancient Egypt. Similar ideas, stories, parables and similes are used to convey the spiritual ideas. The indication of a link between different cultures is compelling when there are similarities not only in the ideas conveyed, but also in the scriptural and/or allegorical forms used as well as the plots and themes of the myths. The conviction of Moses that "God is one" (De 6:4) occurs in Egypt much earlier than anywhere else in our history. In the Ancient Egyptian texts, God is described as,

---

[I] Celsus, Aulus Cornelius (1st century A.C.E.), was a Roman encyclopedist and author of a comprehensive work covering several topics.

[II] The Talmud is a collection of 63 books of writings of the ancient rabbis, which were written around the 5th century A.C.E. They are concerned with Jewish life and express teachings through parables and legends. The Talmud includes legendary accounts of the Jewish people as well as codes of law, therefore, the study of the Talmud is important to the Jewish faith.

[III] Pandora, in Greek mythology, first woman. She was made by Zeus' orders for revenge against Prometheus, who had created man and stolen fire from heaven for man. Pandora was endowed with charm as well as with guile. She was sent to Prometheus' brother Epimetheus, and brought with her a box that she had been forbidden to open. When she opened it all the evils of the human race flew out. Hope remained at the bottom of the box. [117]

[IV] Dionysus, in Greek mythology, the god of fruitfulness and wine, the son of Zeus and Semele. Women in orgiastic and secretive rites worshipped him. [117]

[V] Pan: In Greek mythology, the god of flocks and herds (Roman Sylvanus), shown as a man with the horns, ears, and hoofed legs of a goat, and playing a shepherd's panpipe (or syrinx). [126]

[VI] Tyana refers to North Turkey.

[VII] In Mecca, Saudi Arabia, an oblong building in the quadrangle of the Great Mosque, into the NE corner of which is built the Black Stone declared by the prophet Mohammed to have been given to Abraham by the archangel Gabriel, and revered by Muslims. All Muslims face toward the Ka'aba when they pray, and it is the focus of the hajj (pilgrimage). [126]

[VIII] *Greek Mythology.* Any of the nine daughters of Mnemosyne and Zeus, each of whom presided over a different art or science. [115]

"𓂋𓏏𓏤𓅆 𓂋𓏏𓏤𓅆 𓅃𓏤 𓈖 𓅃𓏤," "Only One, Without a Second!" Also, the idea of the flood by which God destroys civilization occurs in the Theban Recession of the *Book of Coming Forth By Day* which tells the story of how Asar intended to blot out all humankind by a flood.

One Gnostic Christian text in particular, the *Gospel of Thomas,* seems to be directly linked to India and Egypt. In the years between 50 -70 A.C.E., there were already Christians in *Kerala* and *Malabar*, India. In *The Acts of Judas Thomas,* an ancient Syriac work, the apostles cast lots among themselves after the ascension of Jesus in order to determine where they should go to preach the Gospel. Thomas drew India, and it is said that he started Christian Churches there which were said to have flourished with believers, and still do today.

It is very possible that Thomas would have found as many eager followers in India as there were in Egypt since the Gnostic form of Christianity has many similarities to the philosophy of Buddha, which at the time had become the leading religious faith in India and the rest of Asia. Further, Gnostic Christianity contained an element of religious, economic and social equality, which partly explains the fervor of its adherents around the world who were oppressed by archaic and corrupt religious and governmental organizations of the time. This would also explain why Gnosticism survived longest in the Eastern countries and in Upper Egypt (interior of Africa). Those areas were farthest away from the persecutions of the Roman Catholic sect, which according to Gnostic accounts, was setting itself up as the only true religion.

In India, five to six hundred years before Christianity, Buddhism had caused a renaissance of sorts. The Brahmanic system of castes, female subjugation and racism through the institutionalized doctrines of the Brahmin (religious) caste had taken its toll on the masses of India in much the same way as corruption and social decline had occurred in Egypt at the end of the Dynastic Period (350 B.C.E.). The ideas inherent in Buddhism such as Karma, (the law of cause and effect and reincarnation), *Maya*, (Cosmic Illusion) and *Buddhi* (Intellect) existed in the Vedantic and Yogic scriptures of India prior to the formalization of the Buddhist religion. However, the spiritual system developed in the sixth century B.C.E. by Gautama, the Buddha, represented a reform as well as a refinement of the older teachings which were already widely accepted. Especially emphasized was that God, the ultimate reality, alone exists and that everyone is equally able to achieve oneness with that reality. Buddhism also placed important emphasis on non-violence which certainly became a central part of Christian doctrine. In the same sense that Buddhism proclaims that everyone can have *Buddha Consciousness* (or *Buddha Nature*) and thus become a Buddha, Gnostic Christianity affirms that everyone can achieve *Christ Consciousness* and thus become a *Christ*. One more important similarity between Christianity and India is the correlation between the birth stories of Jesus and Krishna. This similarity will be explored in the following section.

The Birth Stories of Heru, Jesus, Krishna, and Buddha

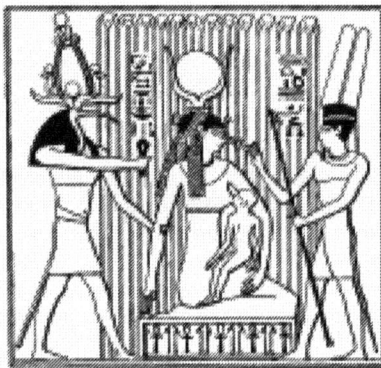

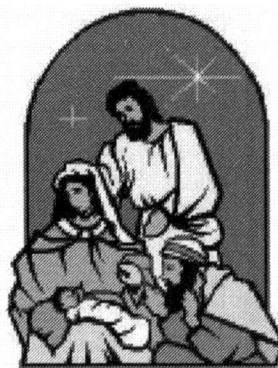

Above left: The Humble Birth of Jesus in the manger
Above right: The Humble Birth of Heru in the papyrus swamps

According to Christian mythology, Jesus is the incarnated Son of God. His birth is symbolic of the birth of spiritual aspiration in every human being. Therefore, Jesus' birth is a very auspicious occasion for mystically symbolic reasons. In ancient times, the birth of Heru from Egypt was also on December 25th. Therefore, Jesus and Heru have much in common. When Jesus was born, the prevailing king, Herod, sought to kill him since it had been prophesied that the "savior" had been born. So he ordered that all male children born around that time should be killed (Mat. 2:16). Mystically, this points to the anguish which is associated with incarnation as well as the death of worldly consciousness, as symbolized by the children who died, when Christhood is born in the heart. The way to spiritual evolution is by dying to the world or more accurately, killing off one's worldly desires. Almost exactly the same events occurred at the time of the birth of Krishna in India, six hundred years before the story of Jesus. When Krishna was born, his uncle tried to kill him by murdering all the male children born at that time. In Ancient Egypt the savior, Heru, was also persecuted at the time of his birth by his evil uncle, Set. The perilous nature of the births of Jesus, Krishna and Heru points to the common origin of their stories as well as the common goal of their incarnations, to deliver the world from oppression and unrighteousness and show the way to enlightenment. The birth of the savior means that from the glorious realm of the Father (God), the soul incarnates into the realm of good and evil, time and space, wherein it experiences pain and sorrow. The danger and flight surrounding the births of these saviors symbolize the persecution that a spiritual aspirant experiences upon treading the spiritual path, which is contrary to the worldly philosophy of life that advocates seeking sense pleasures, fame, fortune, etc. Worldly people seeks to impose these on everyone by force through the media, peer pressure, and the ignorance of family members who ignorantly follow what they were taught by their parents. All three saviors were born in humble surroundings (Jesus in a manger, Krishna in a prison cell where the evil king had his parents imprisoned, and Heru in a swamp). The humble births symbolize humility and effacement of the ego. Thus, the births of Jesus, Krishna and Heru are metaphors for the commencement of spiritual life in every aspirant, which must be characterized by an attainment of sincerity and humility.

The deity Heru of Ancient Egypt is the prototype for the Gnostic savior Jesus, as well as Krishna and Buddha of India. In reality, Heru is none other than the innermost heroic character which lies deep within the heart of everyone. In the same manner as Jesus says that he is within anyone who is in him, Heru represents the same principle which is also evident in the Krishna and Buddha myths.

John 15
     5 I am the vine, ye [are] the branches: He that abideth in me, and I in him, the same bringeth forth much fruit: for without me ye can do nothing without me.

The following statement by an Egyptian initiate affirms his identity with Heru:

"My heart (mind-memory) is with me and it shall not be taken away, for... I live by truth, in which I exist; I am Heru who is in the heart, that which is in the middle of the body. I live by saying what is in my heart...I have committed no sin against the gods.[45]

The following statements are encountered throughout Egyptian mythology in reference to the symbolism of Heru. These statements are also encountered in Christian mythology in reference to the symbolism of Jesus Christ.

"The resurrection and the life," "The anointed one," "The WORD made flesh," "The KRST," "The WORD made TRUTH," "The one who comes to fulfill the LAW," "The destroyer of the enemies of his father," "The one who walks upon the water of his Father.[64]

The following statements from the Bhagavad Gita impart the same wisdom in reference to the presence of the "Savior" in the form of Krishna as being within oneself and in Creation.

Gita: Chapter 7, Jnana Vijnana Yogah—. The Yoga of Wisdom and Realization

Below: Krishna and his mother Yashoda.

9. I am the pure fragrance in earth, I am the effulgence in fire, I am the life in all living beings, I am the austerity in the ascetics.

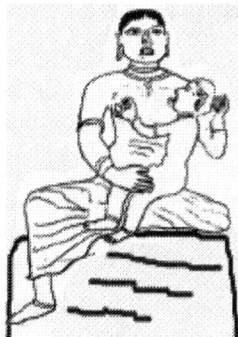

Gita: Chapter 13 Kshetra-Kshetrajna Vibhag Yogah—. The Division of Field and The Knower of The Field

15. That Brahman is within and outside of all beings; He is that which is the moveable as well as the immovable. Because of subtlety, He is not known (through The senses); He is distant (for the ignorant) and very near too (for the wise).

Lord Krishna is a God form or symbol in the Indian Hindu mythological system who represents an incarnation of the Supreme Being, Brahman. Literally translated, the name "Krishna" means "Black" or "The Black One." Therefore, Lord Krishna and Asar (Asar) both were known as "The Black One." Krishna of India and Heru of Egypt have equivalent symbolism in that they show, through their myths, what is correct action that leads the way to salvation. The blackness symbolizes the infinite depths of consciousness, the womb from which all creation arises (human thoughts as well as the universe).

Like Heru, Krishna was viciously pursued from the time of his birth by his uncle, the king, who also usurped the kingdom from the rightful heir. Krishna's uncle, Kamsa, was afraid because he knew that Krishna was prophesied to be the righteous king who would end the injustices of the existing king. When the evil King Kamsa, Krishna's Uncle, foresaw that Krishna would assume the kingship and defeat him, he ordered that all male children born around the same time as Krishna be killed (this part also parallels the story of Jesus exactly).

Like Heru, the eyes of Krishna represent the Sun and the Moon, duality unified into one whole. Krishna was born from a virgin mother as were Heru and Jesus, to fight the forces of evil on earth. As with Heru, he contained the entire Universe in his essence. Heru, Jesus and Krishna are symbols of the Christ in each of our spirits. Our soul is entombed in our physical bodies and constantly engaged in a battle of opposites (duality): good-evil, light-dark, ying-yang, positive-negative, prosperity-adversity, desire-self-control, etc. This is the endless battle which goes on in the realm of time and space, the earth, intermediate and heavenly realms (physical, astral and causal worlds).

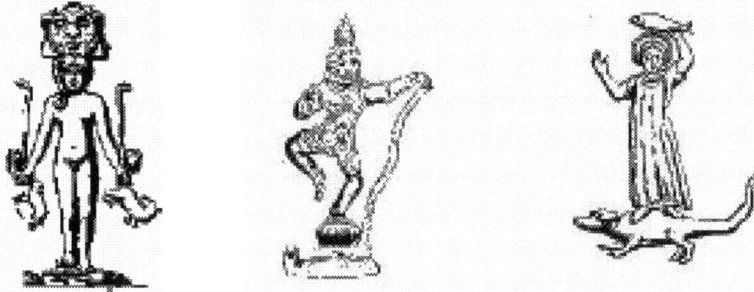

At far left: Heru as a child and master of nature. Center: Krishna as a child and master of nature. Right: Jesus as a child and master of nature.

The story surrounding the birth of a savior was never intended to be understood in a factual or literal sense. This is because there is something more important, beyond the actual facts themselves, which the Sages of ancient times sought to convey. Interestingly enough, just like orthodox Christians believe in the biblical scriptures literally rather than metaphorically, many in the Hare Krishna organization[1] similarly believe in the literal interpretations of the scriptures with respect to the birth and life of Krishna. Thus, just as the Orthodox Christians believe that in order to be saved they must go through Jesus, the Hare Krishnas also emphatically believe that to be saved one must go through Krishna. The saviors' birth stories refer to a message or messages about the qualities or ideas about the savior and the savior's mission. Principally, we are to understand that a savior is a metaphor for a transcendental reality, a principle which lies within each of us. It is we, our deeper Self, who incarnates, so to speak, and it is we who are persecuted by the world with its endless attempts to force us to conform, because of our desires and attachments. We are weakened by our own egoism and thereby give up our freedom and succumb to the transient and unfulfilling joys and sorrows, negativity and illusions of the world. But it is also we, who through our own intellect expanded by wisdom (understanding the teachings) and self-effort (righteousness actions based on truth) directed toward the Divine, will effect our own salvation and transcend the ego and thereby the world as well.

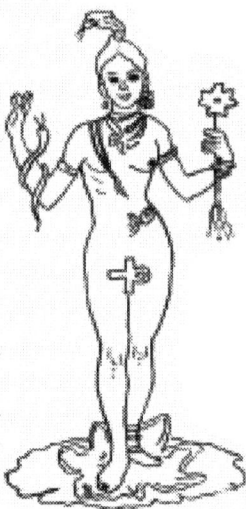

In Indian Samkhya philosophy, the Moon represents the mind and the Sun represents God, the Supreme Being. In Kemetic (Ancient Egyptian) philosophy, the Moon is a symbol of the god Thoth (Tehuti-Hermes), the god of Wisdom (intellect, higher mind-purified mind) and the Sun represents the god Ra as well. Thus, the Self (God) reflects the light of consciousness onto the human mind just as the sun reflects light on the Moon. Heru and Krishna each symbolize the combination of the Moon and the Sun. Thus, the implication is that in order to become one with the universe such as Heru or Krishna, the following change in consciousness must occur: The mind (intellect) must merge with the Cosmic Mind (God). This change in consciousness may be effected by turning the thoughts of the mind to God as opposed to the objects of the world or shifting one's perception of worldly objects and seeing them as expressions of God instead as separate, self-existing realities. As the moon is a reflection of the sunlight, the human mind is a reflection of the cosmic mind: God. Therefore, by changing one's consciousness, one's awareness of reality, one may find the balance between the two opposites and thereby become the master of the two. In Christian mythology, Jesus represents the unitary vision of life which sees all as being part of one family and one source. Thus, Heru, Krishna, Buddha and Jesus are the primary expressions of the highest potential of the soul.

At left: The modern Indian portrayal of the Ancient Indian androgynous divinity,

---

[1] Hare Krishna, a Hindu sect, also known as the International Society of Krishna Consciousness, that first became popular in the United States and Canada in the 1960s and 1970s. Hare Krishnas teach devotion to Krishna as a means of gaining enlightenment, and practice chanting of holy words known as mantras.[117]

Ardhanari. Ardhanari is half male and half female, and uses the Ancient Egyptian and Christian Gnostic symbol of the Ankh to denote the female side with the loop and the male side with the cross. The Ankh symbol contains mystical symbolism in reference to the complementary nature of the male and female aspects of Creation as well as within every man and woman. This is why the Gospel of Thomas (below) admonishes that everyone must become one again. Jesus' reference to "Above and Below" also shows the connection to the Ancient Egyptian teachings of the god Djehuti (Hermes).

> "As above, so below; as below, so above."
>
> -From the Kybalion, a Hermetic Text

The teaching related to the androgynous nature of the spirit can be found in the Gospel of Thomas:

> Jesus said to them, "When you make the two one, and when you make the inside like the outside and the outside like the inside, and the above like the below, and when you make the male and the female one and the same, so that the male not be male nor the female; and when you fashion eyes in the place of an eye, and a hand in place of a hand, and a foot in place of a foot, and a likeness in place of a likeness; then will you enter [the Kingdom]."

THE PHILOSOPHY OF BUDDHA (C. 600 B.C.E.)

There are two major forms of Buddhism, one of which is further divided into two branches. All forms of Buddhism developed from the original teachings given by Gautama and other Sages. Gautama was an Indian prince who became disillusioned with the world. He discovered that all life ends in sorrow due to death and that all the activities that people pursue in the world in search of happiness are in reality leading them towards pain and disappointment. So he set out to discover the meaning of life and the means to attain freedom from the pain and sorrow of life. The major Buddhist sects developed at various times through history out of the original monastic form. They are listed in the following time-line:

Buddha and other Sages and Saints
1200 B.C.E-600 B.C.E

Hinayana, "The Small Vehicle" (also known as Theravada)
Monastic form of Buddhism c.600 B.C.E.

Mahayana "The Large Vehicle"
Buddhism of the lay population living in society. c.150 B.C.E.-100 A.C.E.

Tibetan Buddhism
Branch of Mahayana differing mainly in the development of and accent on the Tibetan Book of the Dead.

Zen Buddhism
Branch of Mahayana differing mainly in the form of meditation practice.

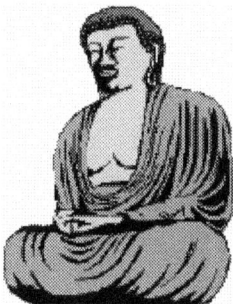

Buddha: The Enlightened one

The Buddha or *"The Enlightened One"* developed a philosophy based on ideas which existed previously in India in Jain philosophy and the Upanishads. In much the same way as the term Christ refers to anyone who has attained "Christhood," the term Buddha refers to any one who has attained the state of Enlightenment. In this context there have been many male and female Christs and Buddhas throughout history.

Buddha recognized that many people took the teachings to extreme. Teachings such as reducing one's Karma by reducing one's worldly involvements or of non-violence which stressed not harming any creatures were understood by some (*Jainism*) to mean not to physically move so as not to step on insects or not breathing in without covering the mouth so as not to kill microorganisms. Others felt that they should not talk to anyone or interact with others in any way. These teachings were taken to such extremes that some aspirants would remain silent so long as to lose their capacity to speak at all.

Prior to Buddha, other teachings such as those of the "Brahmins," (followers of the teachings related to Brahman) the *Samnyasa* or renunciates, and the Jains followed the idea that one was supposed to renounce the apparent reality of the world as an illusion. Some of these teachings were taken to extremes wherein some followers would starve themselves to the point of death believing it would lead them to spiritual enlightenment. Others became deeply involved with the intellectual aspects of philosophy, endlessly questioning, "Where did I come from? Who put me here? How long will I need to do spiritual practice? Where did Brahman (God) come from?," etc. Buddha saw the error of the way in which the teaching was understood and set out to reform the religion.

Buddha emphasized attaining salvation rather than asking so many questions. He likened people who asked too many intellectual questions to a person whose house (lifetime) is burning down while they ask, "How did the fire get started?" instead of first worrying about getting out of the house. Further, Buddha saw that renouncing attachment to worldly objects was not necessarily a physical discipline, but more importantly, it was a psychological one and therefore, he created a philosophical discipline which explained the psychology behind human suffering and how to end that suffering, a philosophy emphasizing "BALANCE" rather than extremes. In essence, he recommended a "Middle Path" which leads to Enlightenment. He recognized that extremes cause mental upsets because one extreme leads to another. Therefore, mental balance is the way to achieve mental peace and serenity, which will allow the transcendental vision of the Self to emerge in the mind. The following segment from the *Isha Upanishad* shows that a balanced approach or *"middle path"* to a spiritual discipline was already addressed as being desirable for spiritual growth. Buddhism later represented an accent or emphasis on this feature of the doctrine:

To darkness are they doomed who devote themselves only to life in the world, and to a greater darkness they who devote themselves only to meditation.
Life in the world alone leads to one result, meditation alone leads to another. So we have heard from the wise. They who devote themselves both to life in the world and to meditation, by life in the world overcome death, and by meditation achieve immortality. To darkness are they doomed who worship only the body, and to greater darkness they who worship only the spirit.

This Buddhist Yogic psychological discipline became the Noble Eight-fold Path which was later adapted by the Indian Sage Patanjali and developed into the eight major Yoga disciplines of Classical Indian Yoga.

The "Middle Path" is also the central feature of Maat Philosophy from Ancient Egypt. It was referred to as "Keeping the Balance." See the book "The Wisdom of Maati" by Dr. Muata Ashby.

Summary of Buddhist Philosophy

<u>The Setting in Motion of the Wheel of the Law</u>:

The Noble Truth of Suffering is:

The reason for all suffering is participation in the world process:

One is unhappy because one invariably expects to find happiness in worldly things. Thus, one develops feelings of desire for things and fear of losing them. All life is sorrowful. Even pleasurable moments are sorrowful because they set us up for disappointment later on at some point.

The Noble Truth of the Cause of Suffering:

The cause of suffering is Ignorance (Avidya).
You have a fundamental misconception about reality. There is no other single hindrance such as this hindrance of IGNORANCE, obstructed by which mankind for a long, long time runs on, round and round in circles (Ittivutaka).

The Noble Truth of the End of Suffering:

The End of Suffering is **NIRVANA** ("Mind without Desires" Contentment — Enlightenment).

Nirvana, or Nibbana, is the indescribable state attained by enlightened Sages and Saints. In Buddhism, Nirvana is the extinction of craving; in Hinduism, it is the home of liberated souls united with the divine and in Jainism, it is the place of liberated souls. Upon death, Enlightenment is completed in the state of Parinirvana. From a psychological perspective, Nirvana is the psychological position where one is indifferent to elation, desire for things or the fear of their loss. The way to Nirvana is the basis of Buddha's teaching.

The Noble Eight-fold Path:
The Noble Eight-fold Path is the practical means to disentangle the knot of ignorance and illusion.

1- Right Understanding is learning how to see the world as it truly is.

2- Right Thought is understanding that thought has great power on oneself
and others, and that whatever one focuses on gains more life; one becomes it.

3- Right Speech is knowing what to say, how to say it, when to say it, and
when to remain silent.

4- Right Action: Guidelines for controlling one's behavior and allowing
calmness of mind to pursue Enlightenment:
1. Not intentionally taking the life of any creature.
2. Not taking anything which is not freely given.
3. Not indulging in irresponsible sexual behavior.
4. Not speaking falsely, abusively or maliciously.
5. Not consuming alcohol or drugs.

5- Right Livelihood is making a living in such a way as to benefit oneself
and all other beings.

6- Right Effort is determination and perseverance in one's spiritual discipline
to transcend one's lower nature.

7- Right Mindfulness is learning how to be aware of everything that one
does at all times, not acting automatically, reacting to events as an animal.

8- Right Meditation is a way to transcend into higher forms of
consciousness including: "The four stages with form" and "The four stages without form." These
comprise successive levels of introvertedness: Joy, Equanimity, and Mindfulness.

At the level where Buddha Consciousness is reached, it is now possible to live and participate in the world though remaining completely detached from it. This concept is that of the Bodhisatva who, out of compassion, helps others on their spiritual journey to achieving Buddha Consciousness. This philosophy is known as: *"Joyful participation in the sorrows of the world."* This philosophy is not unlike Jesus' compassion for the world by willingly submitting to the pain of life in order to show the path to the Kingdom of Heaven through selfless service and humanitarianism. The Yoga system of Patanjali and the Philosophy of Buddha represent the many paths to union with the Divine which may be used integrally according to the psychological makeup (character) of the individual.

The Buddhist Wheel of disciplines.

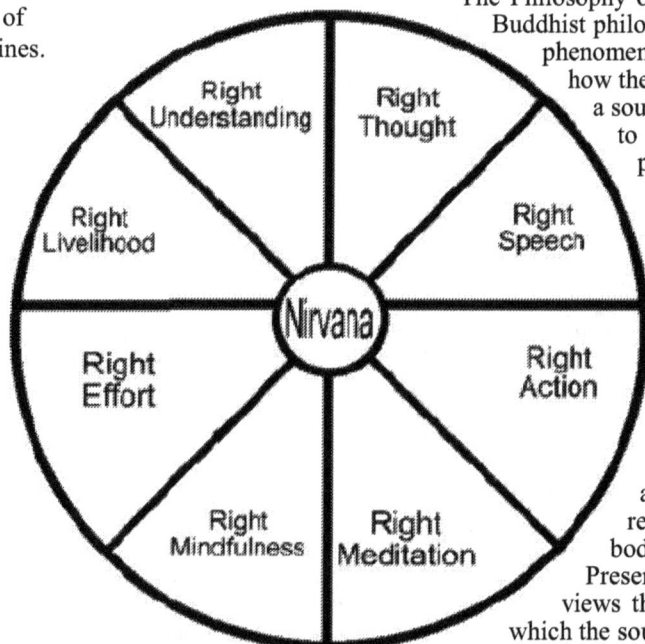

The Philosophy of "Nothingness" was extensively espoused by the Buddhist philosophers of India. Their attempt to explain what the phenomenal universe is began with an attempt to explain how the universe developed. It was assumed that there was a source that produced the universe. This philosophy led to the belief that the entire universe came from a primeval, ultimate void called *Shunya.* Therefore, Buddhist disciplines are directed toward emptying the human mind of that which prevents the perception of that ultimate reality which is the source of all creation. This Buddhist discipline was directed toward the eradication of the superficial elements of the human being which block her/his perception of ultimate existence. The root of human spiritual obstruction is said to be the sense of individualism. From this individualism emerges egoistic desire. Upon reflection, you will discover that everything you are, is related to your mental ideas which all reference you to a specific time and place, your body, your relatives, your society, your country, etc. Present day Eastern philosophy (and early Christianity) views these elements as superficial garments of the soul, which the soul clings to, due to ignorance. When these elements are given up, the practitioner of this spiritual discipline goes beyond them and discovers the "nothingness" out of which the universe arises. This nothingness was erroneously assumed by some to be a kind of non-existence.

At another level of understanding, this nothingness is a state of consciousness wherein there is no mental movement caused by thoughts. In reality the void refers to the absence of concepts in the mind. This state renders the mind undifferentiated, uncolored and free. In effect, the mind can be trained to let go of thinking and classifying objects. When this occurs there are no more concepts in the mind and therefore, it is said to be void of concepts. When all of the concepts which have been learned by the mind through many lifetimes and the egoistic desires based on those concepts are dropped, then there arises the awareness of the Absolute. There is supreme calm and peace. Since thoughts are created by desires, the main aim of Buddhist philosophy is to end desires so that the human being may be able to discover his/her true Self as being one with the source of creation. Further, all the planets, matter, living beings, and even the individual human ego is discovered to be an emanation from that source. Hence the term *Nirvana* (Nir-vana), *without-desire* (craving), is used to denote this ultimate state of oneness with the source of creation.

One important difference between Buddhism and the other Hindu religions is that Buddhism does not advocate worshipping Buddha, whereas most other religions do advocate worshiping a deity. However, Buddha is to be paid homage and to be emulated through the practice of Buddhist teaching. This practice will lead to one discovering one's own essential "Buddha Nature." So if a person is interested in a psychological spiritual discipline rather than a religious based system of deities, Buddhism offers less images of deities on the surface. However, the Mahayana form of Buddhism offers many "Buddhas" which can be equated to deities. They symbolize various aspects of consciousness and various aspects of Buddhist philosophy.

Jesus and Buddha

In much the same way that there were no written Christian texts or personal imagery of Jesus until several decades after his the death, there were no written Buddhist texts or images of the Buddha until several decades after his death. The devotional aspect of Buddha developed extensively through the *Mahayana* sect which catered to the masses of the people, unlike the *Hinayana* sect which was comprised of those who wished to completely renounce the world (monks) to devote their complete attention to spiritual realization.

There are many close similarities between Christianity and Buddhism. One of the most striking is the *"refuge doctrine"* which is found in both Christianity and Buddhism. The idea behind the refuge doctrine is that through the practice of placing one's trust, troubles, joys and sorrows in the hands of the deity, our own minds will be unburdened and exclusively directed towards the deity. The peace which can be gained from this way of living is immense. Through the increasing levels of peace and healing which can be gained, increasing levels of spiritual sensitivity are attained. This idea is strongly expressed in the following Christian statements:

Matthew 11
    28 Come to me, all [ye] that labor and are heavy laden, and I will give you rest.
    29 Take my yoke upon you, and learn from me; for I am meek and lowly in heart:
         and ye shall find rest to your souls.

The message of devotion is also an integral part of Buddhist philosophy in the following credo:

        I go to the Buddha for refuge.
        I go to the doctrine for refuge.
        I go to the monastic order for refuge.

The Buddhist aspirant is admonished to take refuge in the *Buddha* (one's innate *Buddha Consciousness*), the *Dharma* (Buddhist spiritual discipline), and the *Sanga* (company of enlightened personalities). Jesus also exhorted his followers to bring him their troubles "and He will give them rest."

The concept of refuge in the Divinity is also found in the Gita, Chapter 9:

32. O Arjuna, those who take refuge in Me, whether men born in a lowly class, or women, or Vaishyas, or Shudras, even they are sure to attain the highest goal.

The preceding statements are very important for spiritual as well as social reasons because all three spiritual personalities, Jesus, Buddha and Krishna, are not only trying to free us from our ignorance about ourselves, but also the erroneous notions about the social order which is fraught with injustices such as racism (caste system), economic disparity and sexism. Worry and preoccupation with worldly affairs are one of the principal obstacles to spiritual movement, therefore, one of the quickest paths to spiritual evolution would be by relieving one's burden by taking refuge in something greater than one's small and helpless human ego.

THE HISTORY AND PHILOSOPHY OF MYSTICAL CHRISTIANITY

After the downfall of Ancient Egyptian religion due to the edicts from the Roman Catholic church, Christian missionaries were sent out to all parts of the Roman Empire and the land south of Egypt was converted to Christianity. This land was known as Kush in Biblical times and currently it is known as Ethiopia and the Sudan. In an Ethiopian text from the Christian period in Ethiopia called *"The Bandlet of Righteousness,"* also known as "An Ethiopian Book of the Dead," the refuge teaching also appears. This book represents a partial adaptation of an Egyptian book, *The Ancient Egyptian Book of Coming Forth By Day,* to the Christian doctrine. It emphasizes acting righteously and knowing the secret names of the Divine, which when uttered, will allow a person to pass safely through portals and to avoid pitfalls and suffering in hell after death. So it represents an evolution from the Ancient Egyptian neteru (gods and goddesses) which were previously followed in Ethiopia to the use of Jesus and the angels as symbols and icons of spiritual teaching. However, the format, style, theme and procedure outlined in the text is wholly Ancient Egyptian in character. The manner in which the names or words of power can be obtained is through becoming righteous.

> O Holy Trinity, I, your servant Walda Michael, take refuge in each of your Names, and in the Names of the angels, and of your priests so that the foul spirits and the hosts of Diabolos may not approach me on my right hand, or on my left, or before me or behind me, wheresoever I may be...

The refuge teaching may also be found in the Koran:

> 7:200 If a suggestion from Satan assail thy (mind), seek refuge with Allah; for He heareth and knoweth (all things).
> 113:1 SURA 113. Falaq, or The Dawn. In the name of Allah, Most Gracious, Most Merciful. Say: I seek refuge with the Lord of the Dawn...
> 114:1 SURA 114. Nas, or Mankind. In the name of Allah, Most Gracious, Most Merciful. Say: I seek refuge with the Lord and Cherisher of Mankind...

The temptation episodes of the Christian, Islamic and Buddhist stories are essentially equal mystically. They relate to the temptations a human being experiences due to attachments to the world of sensual pleasures. In order to overcome them, it is necessary to seek refuge or assistance from the Divine essence within the heart. Therein lies the strength to overcome the weakness of the mind and body. Jesus' experience of Enlightenment after his baptism (initiation) by John the Baptist and his subsequent meditation and fasting period in the wilderness left him weakened. It was at this time that he was tempted or tested by the devil.

The Indian Bodhi Tree (the Buddhist Tree of Life and enlightenment.)

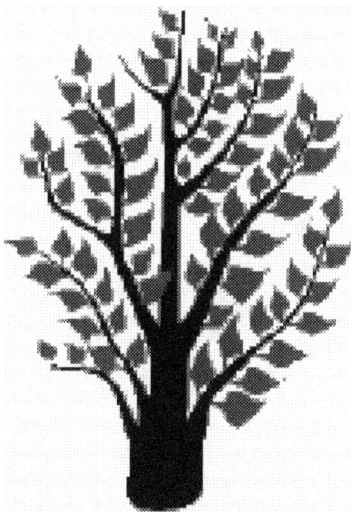

Luke 4

3 And the devil said to him, If thou art the Son of God, command this stone that it be made bread.
4 And Jesus answered him, saying, It is written, That man shall not live by bread alone, but by every word of God.
5 And the devil, taking him up upon a high mountain, showed to him all the kingdoms of the world in a moment of time.
6 And the devil said to him, All this power will I give thee, and the glory of them: for that is delivered to me; and to whomever I will I give it.
7 If thou therefore wilt worship me, all shall be thine.
8 And Jesus answered and said to him, Get thee behind me, Satan: for it is written, Thou shalt worship the Lord thy God, and him only shalt thou serve.
9 And he brought him to Jerusalem, and set him on a pinnacle of the temple, and said to him, If thou art the Son of God, cast thyself down from here:
10 For it is written, He shall give his angels charge over thee, to keep thee:
11 And in [their] hands they shall bear thee up, lest at any time thou dash thy foot against a stone.
12 And Jesus answering said to him, It is said, Thou shalt not tempt the Lord thy God.
13 And when the devil had ended all the temptation, he departed from him for a season.

The first temptation in verse #3 was with satisfaction of the pleasures of the body in the form of food and by implication, sexuality as well. This temptation corresponds to the mastery over the first and second Chakras or Energy Centers of the Kundalini-Serpent Power consciousness levels as described in Kundalini or Serpent Power Yoga. The second temptation in verses #5-8 was two-fold. It consisted of power to rule over others and indulgence in worldly pleasures by worshiping and identifying with the desires of the body rather than keeping one-pointed attention towards the Divine (*the Lord thy God*) as the only reality. Jesus instead asserted his rulership over Satan, the lower self, or the human desires and frailties. This temptation corresponds to the mastery over the third Chakra of the Serpent Power.[I] The third temptation in verses #9-12 was the enticement of Jesus to use his spiritual powers for his own gain and to satisfy his own desires, thereby altering the divine plan and order of the universe. If Jesus had acceded to use his spiritual powers for his own purposes he would be no better than ordinary human beings who constantly seek to achieve specific ends in the world of time of space by manipulating other people and situations to their own advantage. Therefore, those people are incessantly distracted and concerned with the loss or gain of worldly possessions and pleasures. Jesus transcended the ego-self-consciousness, and therefore was acting to fulfill the divine plan. In effect, Jesus is now the manifestation, medium and fulfillment of the divine plan. He was the Christ with Christ Consciousness, and the personality of Jesus with the ordinary consciousness had ceased to exist. This temptation corresponds to the mastery over the fourth through the sixth Chakras of the Serpent Power.

Buddha had tried many forms of spirituality, from extreme asceticism to intensive study of the teachings. He did not succeed in his quest for enlightenment so he decided to try one more time. He decided to sit in meditation for as long as it would take to attain enlightenment or die trying. He meditated for forty-nine days and forty-nine nights under the Bodhi Tree and attained enlightenment on the fiftieth. However, Buddha underwent a similar test upon completing intense austerities and fasting just before reaching Enlightenment. *Mara*, the Lord of desire, tempted Buddha by offering him worldly power and empires. Secondly, he told Buddha that he should not forsake the religion of his forefathers (Brahmanism) and that he should carry out his duties to society as king, and then become saintly in his old age. This was the test of attachment. Very often when a spiritual aspirant seeks to discover the transcendental truth, he or she comes into conflict with his/her previously developed ego-based attachments and thought processes with respect to society. There emerges a pull from the old thoughts and feelings to conform and acquiesce. If there is acquiescence to the desires and attachments of the mind with respect to finding happiness through society, the individual becomes enslaved like an animal is enslaved by its own limited condition. Spiritual strength involves determining what is true and then being able to live in accordance with that truth no matter what the world says, and the truth is that true, lasting and undisturbed happiness and peace cannot be found in the world. In reality, it is not the world that is the problem, but one's expectations from and attachments to the world as a source of true happiness. Thus an aspirant must develop detachment, a way of looking at and interacting with the world without expectation of becoming truly happy as a result of anything that may or may not happen. Then Mara sent his daughters to tempt Buddha. They represented *Lust, Thirst, and Delight.* They tried to entice him with sensual pleasures and rebuked him for abandoning his family and society. They painted a perfect picture of family life and of kingship in his mind without showing the illusoriness and pain of human relationships, and the ultimate end of human life which is death and the loss of all material wealth that is gained. Buddha saw through the illusion and was therefore unaffected by it. Mara then sent an army against him, but Buddha saw through all of these as illusions, as being minor appearances in the vast ocean of consciousness which is eternal and immortal, so he was incapable of experiencing fear.

Duties to society and ritualistic practices of religion are for those who need guidance in their life, not for those who have found the calling to the Divine. Even though they uphold righteous laws for the benefit of society, true spiritual seekers recognize that their allegiance is to the calling and not to any development or rule created by human beings in the world of human experience. This temptation corresponds to the mastery over the third Chakra of the Serpent Power. Buddha had transcended his identification as the ego and the body. He was one with Buddha Consciousness, so he was unmoved by the temptations of the body (lust, thirst, attachment, delight in sensual pleasures). These temptations correspond to the mastery over the first and second Chakras of the Serpent Power. He knew that the pleasures that most people seek through family life are the same pursuits that lead to painful outcomes later. Children, spouses and material wealth are the greatest sources of sorrow because they inevitably lead one to experience mental upset, discord and worry, even though they seem to be the source of delight in the beginning. Also family members which are so dear will eventually die, causing more intense pain and sorrow. Perhaps most importantly, knowing the true nature of all human beings and objects in creation as being the divine immortal Self makes desire for family relationships and sentimental attachments an absurd and unnecessary exercise in vanity and egoism. When one discovers that one is united with the universe through the experience of enlightenment, there is no need or desire to experience ordinary human relationships. Everyone is understood to be your kin, your child, your brother, sister, etc. So the idea of creating a family or entering into worldly entanglements to satisfy the egoistic desires of the mind or body becomes null and void.

Buddha's realization that his true Self transcended all events in time and space made the illusory army of Mara ineffectual. This army is the same one that manifests in ordinary human consciousness as fear, uncontrolled thoughts, worries and desires. They prevent the experience of true mental peace because they constantly put pressure on the mind to compel it to actions even when it does not agree with them. Thoughts and worries can only be experienced when there is identification with the mind-body-ego concept of self. When the identification shifts to

---

[I] See the book "The Serpent Power" by Dr. Muata Ashby.

the all-encompassing Divine Self, all events in time and space are transcended and nullified. They become like passing clouds which are viewed by the vast sky as passing developments which do not affect it in any way. This temptation corresponds to the mastery over the fourth through the sixth Chakras of the Serpent Power. In the same way that Jesus underwent a spiritual transformation, Buddha underwent a transformation from identification with his ego personality as Siddhartha Gautama, his original name, to Buddha, *the Enlightened One*. In much the same way that Christ is a title and not the name of a specific personality, the term Buddha is also a title for those who have transcended ordinary consciousness and who have attained illumination of intellect (Buddhi).

Upon his success in attaining Enlightenment through his own discovery of the *middle way* which repudiated the extreme austerity of the Brahmins, Buddha converted Brahmin ascetics to his system of Yoga and charged them with the mission to spread the word, just as Jesus would in Palestine hundreds of years later. Buddha told his disciples: *Go ye then through every country, convert those not yet converted.*[106] Similarly, in Matthew Chapter 10 of the Bible we read:

5. These twelve Jesus sent forth, and commanded them, saying, Go not into the way of the Gentiles, and enter ye not into [any] city of the Samaritans:
6 But go rather to the lost sheep of the house of Israel.
7 And as ye go, proclaim, saying, The kingdom of heaven is at hand.
8 Heal the sick, cleanse the lepers, raise the dead, cast out demons: freely ye have received, freely give.

Another similarity to Christianity is that the Buddhist hierarchy which developed centuries after the passing of Buddha gradually rejected the vows of renunciation which Buddha proclaimed. When Buddhism was adopted by the royalty of India, it spread throughout the country and became the dominant form of religion. However, this position of prominence and power caused a conflict in the minds of Buddhist leaders. The original doctrines of Buddha were transformed into teachings which led to the practice of partial disciplines rather than strict adherence to the *Dharma* or spiritual discipline as set down by Buddha. New Buddhist sects arose, and with them, the idea of attaining *Nirvana* through extinction of desire and ego-consciousness was transformed into an idea of personal immortality, and the experience of sensual pleasures after death in the astral plane or heaven. In this sense, the program of transcendence of the ego was substituted for an egoistic concept of spirituality. This is similar to what occurred in the early years of Roman Catholicism. The Church Fathers gradually moved away from a mystical interpretation of Christianity and formed a religious doctrine based on a bodily resurrection from death, leading to one's existence in heaven at the right hand of the Father. The same predicament was experienced in Islamic countries during the years immediately following the death of Muhammad (also Mohammed).

The wisdom teachings do not preclude the possibility of owning material goods or ruling of countries (power). However, they do caution that those who propose to carry out these actions should strive to give prominence to the mystical aspects of reality and to always remember that there is no true rulership or ownership from an absolute perspective, since all things are composed of and ultimately dissolve into the Divine Self. This point is made clear in scriptures such as *The Bhagavad Gita, The Yoga Vasistha,* and *The Ausarian Resurrection* which tell of mighty rulers and royalty who were righteous and followed the path of yoga, and even became Enlightened while ruling their countries with moderation and wisdom. They were able to do this because they maintained a vision of selfless service, detachment and dispassion while performing their duties. The story of Queen Chudala and King Shikidwaja in the Yoga Vasistha is such an example.[87] They ruled while practicing yoga and keeping company with Sages who guided them.

The pressures of secular life, due to one's previous conditioning and attachments, cannot be underestimated. These pressures operate at a subconscious level wherein their force drowns the light of intellectual and spiritual reasoning. Eventually the subject finds him/herself justifying or excusing unrighteous behaviors which in turn intensify ego consciousness and lead to further entanglements in the world of desires and mental agitation. All of this draws the mind away from divine realization and closer to egoistic concepts, desires and activities which end in disappointment and frustration. For those who are firmly established in their identification with the transcendental Self, there is no conflict with worldly activity since it is not done for the ego, but for the good of all. When enlightened people operate in the world they use their resources for the good of humanity and not solely for personal gain. For those who are not established in their Higher Self, there is a constant struggle to remain balanced and focused on the spiritual discipline. The answer is to spiritualize all of your worldly activities. This can be successfully accomplished by maintaining a constant awareness of the activity of the mind (mindfulness) at all times and not identifying with any egoism (desires, emotions or thoughts which do not affirm the oneness of humanity and creation) which may arise. This exercise of constant awareness is gradually perfected with practice and by keeping regular company with those who are established in the Higher Self (Sages) or advanced disciples so as to remain focused on the teachings of the spiritual discipline.

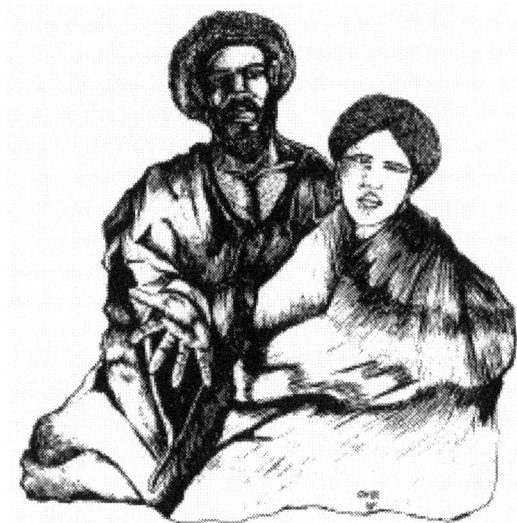

Above: Jesus and Mary Magdalene, by Asar Oronde Reid

CHAPTER V: THE ORIGINS AND HIDDEN MEANING OF THE BIBLE

THE COMPILATION OF THE CANONICAL GOSPELS

The subject of the creation of the New Testament and the Bible as it is known today takes us back to the 3rd century B.C.E. when the *Septuagint* was created. The Septuagint is the name given to the ancient Greek translation of the Hebrew scriptures as they existed at the time. Before this time the books which today constitute the Old Testament had not been compiled nor was Christianity created. The Jewish leaders had been debating for hundreds of years as to which books should be included as canonical Jewish texts. Here once again Alexandria, Egypt and the mystical philosophy of Ancient Egyptian Religion played an important part in the consolidation of Jewish theology.

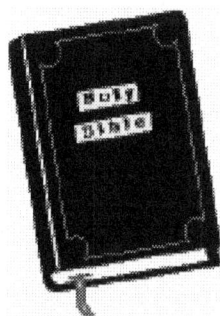

Above Left: The Bible   Above Right: The Torah

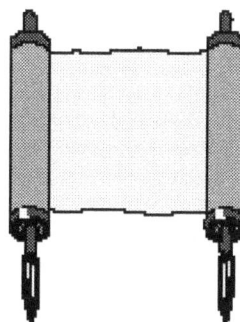

The term "Septuagint" comes from the Latin *Septuagint* or *seventy* - LXX. The number seventy refers to the seventy (or seventy-two) translators who were appointed by the Jewish high priest to render the Hebrew scriptures into Greek at the request of the Hellenistic-Egyptian emperor Ptolemy II.

The Torah or the five books of Moses—Genesis though Deuteronomy—were translated into Greek to serve the needs of the Greek-speaking Jews outside of Palestine who were no longer able to read their scriptures in the original Hebrew. The translation of the other books of the Hebrew Old Testament and the addition of new Jewish books and parts of books, known as the Apocrypha, constituted the final production of the Greek Old Testament. This became the Bible of the early Christian Church. Thus, the Septuagint, rather than the original Hebrew text, became the Old Testament of the Christian Bible of the early Christian Church.

Later, the Jewish religious authorities rejected the Christian Old Testament which was based on the Septuagint. They preferred to use only the scriptures which were more ancient and which were originally written in Hebrew. Therefore, the Jewish Bible took form as the *Torah* or body of Jewish literature including the *Pentateuch* or first five books of the Hebrew scriptures and the accepted literature of religious laws and teachings of Judaism. It is important to realize that both the Jewish and Christian Old Testaments were not written by one person or even a group of people. Modern scholarship now concludes that the writings were compilations which were created over a period of over one thousand years and which underwent extensive editing. Modern scholarship has revealed, through linguistic analysis, handwriting analysis and scientific analysis such as x-ray and other technology, that the writing styles of the books differ, showing varied authorship and various changes or re-writes to the original fragments which survive.

The compilation of the canonical New Testament centers around an important theologian called Paul. In the New Testament, Paul is considered to be the first Christian evangelist and theologian. His original name was Saul. He was born in Tarsus[I] of Jewish parents. He became a Pharisee as well as an educated Roman citizen. Pharisees were members of an ancient Jewish sect that emphasized the strict interpretation and observance of the Mosaic law. Saul became a well-known Christian persecutor. However, he underwent a major spiritual transformation due to a vision of Jesus he received while en-route to Damascus to persecute Christians. After his conversion to Christianity, Paul became a zealous disciple. He declared that Jesus was the Messiah and that he was sacrificed to atone for all the sins

---

[I] Tarsus or ancient Cydnus, is a city of southern Turkey, on the Tarsus River, near the Mediterranean Sea.

of mankind. His many epistles,[1] which recounted his travels throughout the Roman empire as he set up Christian Churches, were letters written to the Corinthians, Romans, Philippians, Hebrews, and others whom he had indoctrinated with the Christian theology. Through the letters, he attempted to maintain contact with the churches he had set up and attempted to give them some inspiration and encouragement in the face of persecution. These epistles became a central part of Christian literature and thus, make up an integral part of the New Testament of the Christian Bible.

The process by which the Hebrew and Christian scriptures were created is extremely important. It must be understood that their creation was certainly influenced by Enlightened Sages, as well as editors and others who used the scriptures and created new ones for their own purposes over a large period of time. Every writer knows the importance of an editor. Very often once a work is completed it undergoes a rigorous process of rewriting which serves to mold or sculpt it into the final work of art will become. While working with the author, the editor(s) may revise and/or rearrange certain elements until the ideas of the author are well-illustrated through the text. If the author is not present to explain or clarify the meaning or able to control the production of the work, it may turn out to be something completely dissimilar to the original intent of the author.

When the Roman emperor, Constantine, decided to consolidate the canonical books of the Christian Bible, his political, economic and military power controlled which versions would be admitted and which would be excluded. His political influence was felt as he associated with the Orthodox Catholic Christians and controlled the way in which the judicial system permitted or outlawed a particular religious faith. His economic power was instrumental in the financing of the version of the Bible he wanted. No other Christian sects had the resources of the Roman Empire to mass-produce Bibles which required many scribes. His military power was significant because he and his successors had control over the armies of Rome and therefore, were able to enforce their laws and decrees.

Thus, it must be understood that the scriptures presently constituting the canonical Bibles of the Roman church should be considered equally with all other contemporary scriptures written by those who considered themselves as part of the Christian faith.

THE HINTS OF A SECRET TEACHING IN THE TRADITIONAL BIBLE

Since the time of the origins of Christianity, there has been a controversy over the authenticity and authority of the teachings given by the Orthodox Catholic Church. There was one important personality who shaped the orthodox view. This was Ireaneus. Ireaneus (140?-202? A.C.E.) was a Christian Bishop and a Father of the Church. He was born in Asia Minor. In his childhood in Asia Minor, he heard the preaching of St. Polycarp (69?-155?) who was said to be the disciple of St. John and to have known the other disciples of Jesus. This association gave him authority in the church. Interestingly, it also shows that the Orthodox Church valued the teacher-disciple relationship in much the same way as the Ancient Egyptian Religion did prior to Christianity, and the Yoga of India continues to do today. At about the year 180, he wrote an important work against the Gnostic view. It was known as "Against the Heresies." The Orthodox Catholic view was typified by the strong efforts of Bishop Irenaeus who fought vehemently to discredit the Gnostic Christian sects which vied with his own for the right to promulgate the teachings. He declared that the Apostles are:

...like a rich man {depositing money} in a bank, placed in the church {Orthodox Catholic} fully everything that belongs to truth: so that every one, whoever will, can draw from her the water of life.[94]

Thus, according to Irenaeus, a true Christian believes *"the one and only truth from the apostles, which is handed down by the church."* Any other teaching or source of Christian wisdom was to be considered *"heretic."* Thus, we have the beginnings of the orthodox movement within Christianity. Irenaeus' discourses claimed a proprietary hold on what is true Christianity. This form of thinking developed into the driving force of the church and dominated its development throughout history.

Yet, in the traditional versions of the Bible, there are hints of a hidden and secret teaching which was given to the few, which lends support to the idea promoted by the Gnostics that they were the custodians of *"secret teachings given by Jesus himself,"* hence the titles, *Apocryphon* (secret Book) *of John* and *Secret Book of James*, etc. The Gnostics also claimed to have teachings which surpassed even those of the apostles since they were obtained by *"direct experience"* of the Divine. These teachings were to be imparted only to the spiritually mature. It is easy now to understand why the orthodoxy fought against the Gnostics. If one can obtain spiritual insight by direct experience of the Divine, where does this leave the church and its authority? Is it even necessary? Logically, if you got the

---

[1] A letter written by an Apostle, one of the 12 disciples chosen by Christ to preach the Gospel.

teaching in a direct line of discipleship, your teaching is the correct one provided that it is imparted properly and understood properly. However, this was never stated in the early Christian texts. It was a later development. Actually, the Gnostic texts suggest that the "direct experience" is higher than any scriptural teaching. This view is in line with the mystical sciences of Ancient Egypt and India. When a student attains Enlightenment after receiving direct teaching from an Enlightened Sage or Spiritual Preceptor, that student also has direct access to the truth. Further, they are equally able to espouse the teachings and even to introduce new teachings or modernize the teachings as the need arises. Therefore, this form of spirituality is in complete opposition to the basic Orthodox Church system. Still, the Bible contains references to hidden teachings. The following passages are examples of the allusions to the secret teachings in the Bible canon.

Mark 5:37
37 And he permitted no man to follow him, except Peter, and James, and John the brother of James.

Mark 9:2
2 And after six days Jesus taketh [with him] Peter, and James, and John, and leadeth them up upon a high mountain apart by themselves: and he was transfigured before them.

Mark 13:3
3 And as he sat upon the mount of Olives opposite the temple, Peter and James and John and Andrew asked him privately…

Mark 14:33
33 And he taketh with him Peter and James and John, and began to be greatly amazed, and to be very heavy…

Luke 8:51
51 And when he came into the house, he allowed no man to go in, except Peter, and James, and John, and the father and the mother of the maiden.

Acts 1:13
13 And when they had come in, they went into an upper room, where abode both Peter, James, John, Andrew, Philip, Thomas, Bartholomew, Matthew, James [the son] of Alphaeus, Simon Zelotes, and Judas [the brother] of James.

Compare the passage from Mark 9:2 to the following passage from the Bhagavad Gita in which Krishna speaks to his disciple, Arjuna, in confidence:

Gita: Chapter 4, Jnan Vibhag Yogah—The Yoga of Wisdom

3. You are my friend and devotee. Therefore, I have declared the same ancient Yoga to you, which is a supreme secret.

Gita: Chapter 9, Raja Vidya Raja Guhya Yogah—The Yoga of Royal Knowledge and Royal Secret

1. I will declare to you who are devoid of caviling,[1] the greatest secret in the form of the indirect and direct knowledge of Brahman, knowing which you will attain freedom from the evil of the world-process.

2. This knowledge is the king of all knowledges, the king of all secrets, the best among all purifier, fit to be realized directly by (intuition), of highest merit, very easy of attainment, and yet imperishable.

The *Gospel of Thomas* goes further than the Bible in that it does not only state unequivocally that there is a secret teaching given by Jesus, but also that this teaching is only to be given to those who are *"worthy"* of it.

62. Jesus said: "It is to those who are worthy of my mysteries that I tell my mysteries...

These *mysteries* are the main issue of Gnosticism, and were at the heart of the controversy between early Orthodox Christian and Gnostic Christian sects. Therefore, a detailed study of the mysteries, their history and practice is essential to understanding both Orthodoxy and Gnosticism.

---

[1] **cav·il** (kăv/əl) *v.* **cav·iled** also **cav·illed, cav·il·ing cav·il·ling, cav·ils cav·ils**. *--intr.* **1.** To find fault unnecessarily; raise trivial objections. *--tr.* **1.** To quibble about; detect petty flaws in. **--cav·il** *n.* A carping or trivial objection. **--cav/il·er** *n.*

THE TEN COMMANDMENTS AND THE PRECEPTS OF MAAT

The similarity between the Ten Commandments, along with the other rules and regulations given to Moses by God in the other books of the Old Testament and the 42 Laws of Maat from Ancient Egypt further unveils the close association between Jewish and Ancient Egyptian religious morality. A simple comparison of the following biblical scriptures to the more Ancient Egyptian ones uncovers the ancient pre-Christian origins of the norms of ethical conduct. A life of ethical conduct was and is the first essential step in the practice of spirituality. The reader will also notice that one of the main teachings of Jesus, to love thy neighbor (non-violence), already existed in both the Ancient Egyptian scriptures and in the Old Testament, long before the birth of Jesus. The following list of commandments comes from the Old Testament of the Bible, the book of Exodus. The subsequent text comes from the Book of Leviticus, which contains segments of the additional laws given to Moses by God. You may directly compare these to the 42 Laws or Precepts of Maat by looking up the specific law to which it corresponds. Simply look for a number in parenthesis, ( ), after the Bible text. This is the number of the specific Precept of Maat from the list which follows after the text of Leviticus.

The Ten Commandments

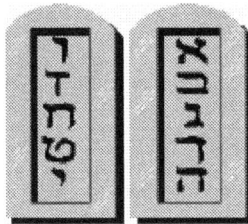

Exodus 20 3:17
    1. Thou shalt have no other Gods before me. (Neberdjer and Pa-Neter philosophy of Ancient Egypt)
    2. Thou shalt not make to thee any graven image. (Neteru philosophy of Ancient Egypt)
    3. Thou shalt not take the name of the Lord thy God in vain (38)
    4. Remember the Sabbath day, to keep it holy. (21)
    5. Honor thy father and thy mother. (Contained in the wisdom texts of Ancient Egypt.)
    6. Thou shalt not kill. (The ancient Hebrew: Thou shall not commit murder.) (5)
    7. Thou shalt not commit adultery. (19)
    8. Thou shalt not steal. (4), (8)
    9. Thou shalt not bear false witness against thy neighbor. (17)
  10 Thou shalt not covet thy neighbors house, thou shalt not covet thy neighbors wife, nor his male servant, nor his female servant, nor his ox, nor his donkey, nor any thing that [is] thy neighbors. (41)

Leviticus 18

  22 Thou shalt not lie with mankind, as with womankind: it [is] abomination. (27)

  26 Ye shall therefore keep my statutes and my judgments, and shall not commit [any] of these abominations; [neither] any of your own nation, nor any stranger that sojourneth among you...(22)

Leviticus 19

  11. Ye shall not steal (2), (4), neither deal falsely (7), neither lie (9) one to another.

  12 And ye shall not swear by my name falsely, neither shalt thou profane the name of thy God: I [am] the Lord. (32), (42)

  13 Thou shalt not defraud thy neighbor, neither rob [him]: (4), (41)

  15 Ye shall do no unrighteousness in judgment: thou shalt not respect the person of the poor, nor honor the person of the mighty: [but] in righteousness shalt thou judge thy neighbor. (31)

  17 Thou shalt not hate thy brother in thy heart...(20), (42)

18 Thou shalt not avenge, nor bear any grudge against the children of thy people, but thou shalt love thy neighbor as thyself: I [am] the Lord. (28)

30. Ye shall keep my Sabbaths, and reverence my sanctuary: I [am] the Lord. (8), (21)

33 And if a stranger shall sojourn with thee in your land, ye shall not oppress him. {vex: or, oppress}

34 [But] the stranger that dwelleth with you shall be to you as one born among you, and thou shalt love him as thyself; for ye were strangers in the land of Egypt: I [am] the Lord your God. (29)

35 Ye shall do no unrighteousness in judgment, in length, in weight, or in volume. (6)

Leviticus 20
13 If a man also shall lie with mankind, as he lieth with a woman, both of them have committed an abomination: they shall surely be put to death; their blood [shall be] upon them. (27)

Leviticus 22
32 Neither shall ye profane my holy name; but I will be hallowed among the children of Israel: I [am] the Lord who hallow you... (38)

NOTE: A more detailed comparison between Jewish moral teachings and the teachings of Maat from Ancient Egypt is presented in Chapter 8 of this book.

The first two commandments (1. Thou shalt have no other Gods before me and 2. Thou shalt not make to thee any graven image) are an attempt to separate the new Jewish religion from the religion of Ancient Egypt. Since the Ancient Egyptian religion was seen as polytheistic by those who did not have higher understanding, it was assumed to be a confusing hodgepodge of differing idols. However, a deeper study of Ancient Egyptian religion reveals that at no time was polytheism promoted or espoused. The practice of making graven images of God was also never practiced in Ancient Egypt. What was engraved on walls and inscriptions were the wisdom teachings related to God as they manifest in Creation. This is referred to as the Medu Neter (Nedjer). The Medu Neter extols the mythology related to the neteru. Neteru are the cosmic forces which constitute and sustain Creation and human existence. These were symbolized as gods and goddesses. The idea of a nameless, formless, indefinable, inscrutable supreme being occurs first in Ancient Egypt. The name for this concept was a reference to the "Divinity of Light" and later the terms "Neberdjer" or Pa-Neter were used. *Pa-Neter* means "The Supreme Being" (see precept #38 and 42 below) as opposed to *neteru*, which means the emanations from the Supreme Being. It is comparable to the "I am that I am" or "Yahweh" (Jehovah) of the Hebrews and "Brahman" of the Hindus. Thus, it is clear that the ten commandments are an attempt at a reinterpretation of the wisdom teachings of Ancient Egypt, albeit with some areas of incomplete understanding of Ancient Egyptian religious philosophy.

The teachings related to honoring one's parents were a very important ethical and social aspect of Ancient Egyptian life. Therefore, we find precepts related to this issue in the Ancient Egyptian Wisdom texts, the writings upon which the forty-two precepts of Maat are based.

From the Instructions of Sage Ani:

> Libate for your father and mother,
> Who are resting in the valley (deceased)...
>
> Double the food your mother gave you,
> Support her as she supported you...

The 42 Laws or Precepts of Maat were the basis of Ancient Egyptian philosophy at least 2,000 years before Christianity. They were declarations which the initiate was to utter upon being judged by the gods and goddesses as being righteous or not. The judgement is symbolized by the scales of balance where the heart[1] of an individual is weighed against the feather of Maat. Maat is the goddess of truth. There is a god or goddess (guardian angel or patron saint in Christian terminology) who presides over each precept of Maat. An individual is judged by how they were able to follow the Precepts. If the heart is light, meaning that they kept the laws, they can answer affirmatively ("I have not done so and so") and thereby discover God. If they cannot answer affirmatively they will experience hellish conditions. Either way an individual's fate is not determined by some God "up" there but by himself or

---

[1] Will be explained further in the next section.

herself, by means of his or her actions while alive. The scales in Ancient Egypt very closely resemble the Christian symbol called *DIIS Manubus* meaning "To the spirit of the blessed."

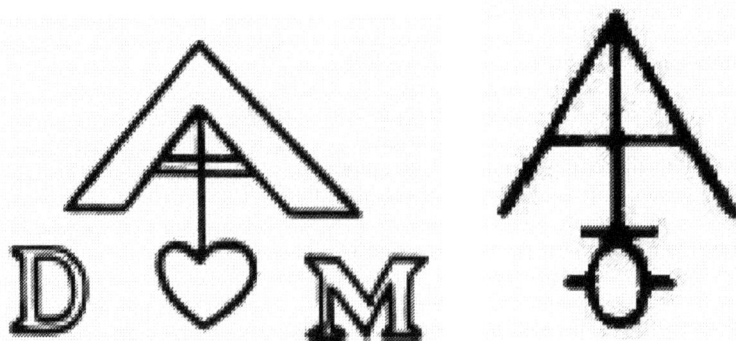

Far left: The Ancient Egyptian Hieroglyph symbolizing the Judgement of the Heart on the Scales of Truth.
 Right: The Christian Symbol: DIIS Manubus: To the spirit of the blessed.

The following is a composite summary of "negative confessions" from several Ancient Egyptian *Books of Coming Forth by Day*. They are often referred to as "Negative Confessions" since the person uttering them is affirming what moral principles they have not transgressed. In this respect they are similar to the Yamas or ethical restraints of India. While all of these books include 42 precepts, some specific precepts varied according to the specific initiate for which they were prepared and the priests who compiled them. Therefore, I have included more than one precept per line where I felt it was appropriate to show that there were slight variations in the precepts and to more accurately reflect the broader view of the original texts.

(1) "I have not done iniquity." Variant: Acting with falsehood.
(2) "I have not robbed with violence."
(3) "I have not done violence (To anyone or anything)." Variant: Rapacious (Taking by force; plundering.)
(4) "I have not committed theft." Variant: Coveted.
(5) "I have not murdered man or woman." Variant: Or ordered someone else to commit murder.
(6) "I have not defrauded offerings." Variant: or destroyed food supplies or increased or decreased the measures to profit.
(7) "I have not acted deceitfully." Variant: With crookedness.
(8) "I have not robbed the things that belong to God."
(9) "I have told no lies."
(10) "I have not snatched away food."
(11) "I have not uttered evil words." Variant: Or allowed myself to become sullen, to sulk or become depressed.
(12) "I have attacked no one."
(13) "I have not slaughtered the cattle that are set apart for the Gods." Variant: The Sacred bull – (Apis)
(14) "I have not eaten my heart" (overcome with anguish and distraught). Variant: Committed perjury.
(15) "I have not laid waste the ploughed lands."
(16) "I have not been an eavesdropper or pried into matters to make mischief." Variant: Spy.
(17) "I have not spoken against anyone." Variant: Babbled, gossiped.
(18) "I have not allowed myself to become angry without cause."
(19) "I have not committed adultery." Variant: And homosexuality.
(20) "I have not committed any sin against my own purity."
(21) "I have not violated sacred times and seasons."
(22) "I have not done that which is abominable."
(23) "I have not uttered fiery words. I have not been a man or woman of anger."
(24) "I have not stopped my ears against the words of right and wrong (Maat)."
(25) "I have not stirred up strife (disturbance)." "I have not caused terror." "I have not struck fear into any man."
(26) "I have not caused any one to weep." Variant: Hoodwinked.
(27) "I have not lusted or committed fornication nor have I lain with others of my same sex." Variant: or sex with a boy.
(28) "I have not avenged myself." Variant: Resentment.
(29) "I have not worked grief, I have not abused anyone." Variant: Quarrelsome nature.
(30) "I have not acted insolently or with violence."
(31) "I have not judged hastily." Variant: or been impatient.
(32) "I have not transgressed or angered God."

(33) "I have not multiplied my speech overmuch (talk too much).

(34) "I have not done harm or evil." Variant: Thought evil.

(35) "I have not worked treason or curses on the King."

(36) "I have never befouled the water." Variant: held back the water from flowing in its season.

(37) "I have not spoken scornfully." Variant: Or yelled unnecessarily or raised my voice.

(38) "I have not cursed The God."

(39) "I have not behaved with arrogance." Variant: Boastful.

(40) "I have not been overwhelmingly proud or sought for distinctions for myself (Selfishness)."

(41) "I have never magnified my condition beyond what was fitting or increased my wealth, except with such things as are (justly) mine own possessions by means of Maat." Variant: I have not disputed over possessions except when they concern my own rightful possessions. Variant: I have not desired more than what is rightfully mine.

(42) "I have never thought evil (blasphemed) or slighted The God in my native town."

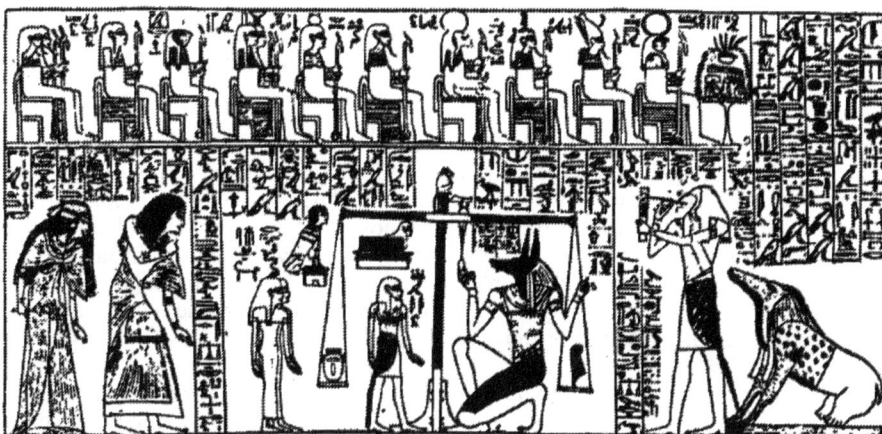

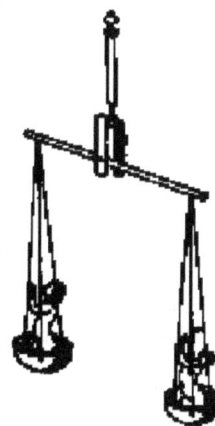

Above left: The Scales of Maat from the Kenna Papyrus.
Above Right: The scales of Christian mythology. In Christian art, the archangel Michael is frequently portrayed holding a pair of scales. One of his responsibilities is to weigh the soul of the dead.[C-1]

THE SIGNIFICANCE OF THE PRECEPTS OF MAAT

At the time of death or prior to death, the heart (consciousness, Ab) of the human being is weighed against truth, symbolized by the feather of Maat. Here our divine faculties of reason and moral rectitude and our ability to practice the precepts while on earth are judged. Below: The Scales of Maat in the Ancient Egyptian Judgement scene from the *Book of Coming Forth By Day* (Book of the Dead).

In the Hall of Maati, the heart and internal organs of the deceased are judged by the 42 judges (gods and goddesses) who are each in charge of one regulation. All 42 regulations or virtuous guidelines for living make up the basis for the 42 "negative confessions." If one lives righteously, one will be able to say that one has NOT committed any offense. Upon uttering these words, the deceased takes on a new name. For example, instead of Lisa Williams, it is now Asar Lisa Williams.

The objective of life is to become "light of heart." That is to say, one should live a life that is free of stress and which promotes mental peace. When this is possible, the mind relaxes and reveals the divine nature of the soul. If the heart is weighed down by egoism due to a life of worry, lies, frustration, and desire, the heart will be judged as heavier than the feather. Instead of moving forward to join with Asar (God), the deceased, in this case, Asar Lisa Williams, is sent back to the world in the form of an animal if her acts were very sinful or she will undergo reincarnation into a human form to again try to become "light of heart."

If the heart of Asar Lisa Williams is found to be lighter than the feather or of equal weight, it signifies that she has lead a virtuous life and has mastered the *knowledge and wisdom of every god* (all of which are aspects of the one God, meaning she has mastered all 42 precepts) and that she is fit for a new life. Asar Lisa Williams is ready to transcend this world onto the next realm of existence. She is ready to journey back to meet Cosmic Asar, who represents Cosmic Consciousness, her own Higher Self (God).

Asar Lisa Williams, through her own virtuous life, is allowed to take or fashion a new, glorious body, to live in eternity as one with Asar (God). Thus, Asar Lisa Williams, the individual human soul, meets and joins with Asar (God), the Supreme Being. This is the attainment of Enlightenment or the Kingdom of Heaven. This signifies that our own nature is that of universal consciousness. What was separated only by ignorance is now re-united, re-membered. It is only due to ignorance and to distraction in the world of seemingly desirable objects that we think we are individual human beings with bodies which are mortal. In reality, we are immortal and eternal beings who are one with the universe and each other. Through ignorance, fueled by egoistic desire, we have come to believe that the human existence is all there is. Through the process of living the teachings of Maat or in the case of Christianity, the Commandments and Beatitudes (given by Jesus), the mind can be lightened to such a degree that it allows the soul to behold its true nature unclouded by the passions and desires of the mind.

The objective of all mystical religions and philosophies is to achieve this realization before the time of death. To realize this even before death, it is necessary to live in a virtuous manner, learning the lessons of human existence and uncovering the veil of ignorance which blinds us from the realization of our essential nature. We must therefore master the knowledge and wisdom of every "god," every precept.

Anubis (god of discernment between reality and illusion) and Djehuti (god of reason and truth) oversee the scales of Maat. They judge the condition of the Heart (Ab) and determine its level of spiritual achievement. This is also symbolized by the Ammit monster, devourer of hearts, who, according to the Ancient Egyptian *Kenna* papyrus, determines those who are the advanced spirits and worthy of salvation (those who have developed their higher consciousness centers: selflessness, peacefulness, universal love, etc.), symbolized by the fourth through seventh rings or levels of consciousness, and those who have not progressed beyond their base animal natures (lower consciousness centers: fear, attachments, egoistic desires, anger, hatred, etc.), symbolized by the lower three rings. The unrighteous are symbolically devoured by the Ammit monsters (demon).

As in the *Kundalini Chakra* system of India, those who achieve no higher than the level of the third Energy Center or Chakra are considered to be people on the same level of consciousness as animals. They are mostly concerned with satisfying the pleasures and desires of the senses (food, sex, controlling other people) and, therefore, will have to reincarnate in order to further evolve beyond this stage. Upon reincarnating, they will once again have the possibility of confronting situations which will afford them the opportunity to perform correct action and thus, to change. Correct action leads to correct feeling and thinking. Correct feeling and correct thinking lead to a state of consciousness which is unburdened. This is the goal— to unburden the mind so that consciousness, the soul, may be revealed in its true appearance. When this occurs the soul is discovered to be one with God and not individual and separate. One realizes that the Kingdom of Heaven is within oneself. This is the highest realization of all mysteries, yogas and religious systems.

The Egyptian *Book of Coming Forth By Day* is a text of wisdom about the true nature of reality and also of *Hekau* (chants, words of power, utterances) to assist the initiate in making that reality evident. These chants are in reality wisdom affirmations which the initiate recites in order to assist him or her in changing the consciousness level of the mind. The hekau themselves may have no special power except in their assistance to the mind to change its perception through repetition with understanding and feeling in order to transform the mind into a still and centered state. Through these affirmations, the initiate is able to change his/her consciousness from body consciousness ("I am a body") to Cosmic Consciousness ("I am God"). This form of affirmatory (using affirmation in the first person) spiritual discipline is recognized by Indian Gurus as the most intense form of spiritual discipline. However, there must be clear and profound understanding of the teachings before the affirmations can have the intended result. It is also to be found in the Bible and in the Gnostic Gospels as we will see. Compare the preceding statements in the Indian Upanishads and the Christian Bible to the following Ancient Egyptian scriptures (*Metu Neter,* Sacred Speech) taken from the *Egyptian Book of Coming Forth By Day* (c. 10,000-5,000 B.C.E.) and other hieroglyphic texts:

From Indian Yoga wisdom:	From the Bible:	From Ancient Egypt:
"Aham brahma asmi" - I Am the Absolute	On the name of GOD: *"I Am That I Am."*(The Bible, Exodus 3:14) Jesus speaks of his own origin and identity: *"I and the Father (GOD) are ONE."* John 10:30	*Nuk Pu Nuk. ("I Am That I Am.")* In reference to the relationship between GOD and Mankind: *Ntef änuk, änuk Ntef. ("He is I and I am He.")*

The 42 declarations of purity have profound implications for the spiritual development of the individual as well as for society. They may be grouped under three basic ethical teachings, *Truth, Non-violence* and *Self-Control*. Under the heading of self-control, three subheadings may be added, *Balance of Mind or Right Thinking Based on Reason, Non-stealing* and *Sex-Sublimation*. The principles of Maat are very similar to the principles of Dharma of India.

The Ancient Egyptians included elaborate scrolls with the mummies of the dead. These were known as the Books of the Dead. The early Coptic Christians also included a Book of the Dead and mummified their dead in keeping with the Ancient Egyptian traditions. The book consisted of sheets of papyrus inscribed with Gnostic Christian texts such as the gospels. Many of these Books of the Dead can be found in the British Museum. One of the surviving books, (Oriental #4919 (2), contains a copy of the Apocryphal letter of King Abgar to Christ and the first words of each of the four Gospels.

Maat Principles of Ethical Conduct	Hindu Dharma Principles of Ethical Conduct (From the *Manu Smriti*)
• **Truth** (1), (6), (7), (9), (24) • **Non-violence** (2), (3), (5), (12), (25), (26), (28), (30), (34) • **Right Action- Self-Control (Living in accordance with the teachings of Maat)** (15), (20), (22), (36) • **Right Speech** (11), (17), (23), (33), (35), (37) • **Right Worship** (13), (21), (32), (38), (42) • **Selfless Service** (29) • **Balance of Mind - Reason – Right Thinking** (14), (16), (18), (31), (39) • **Not-stealing** (4), (8), (10), (41) • **Sex-Sublimation** (19), (27)	• Firmness. • Forgiveness, forbearance. • Control of Senses. • Non Stealing. • Purity of body and mind. • Control of mind. • Purity of Intellect. • Knowledge. • Truthfulness. • Absence of anger.

There is one more important factor, which is inherent in the Precepts of Maat that must receive special mention. Generally when people are ignorant of the greater spiritual realities and caught up in the emotionality of human life, they tend to look for something to blame for their miseries. They want to find a cause for the troubles of life and the easiest way to do this is to look around into the world and point to those factors around them, which seem to affect them, be they people, situations or objects. In Chapter 125 of the *Book of Coming Forth By Day*, the use of the word *nuk* ("I") is emphasized with a special connotation. The spiritual aspirant says continually "I have..." He or she does not say "You have allowed me" or "The devil made me do it" or "I wanted to, but I couldn't" etc.

There is a process of responsibility wherein the spiritual aspirant recognizes that he or she has the obligation to act righteously and, in so doing, to purify their own heart. Spiritual practice can succeed only when you assume responsibility for your actions, thoughts, words and feelings. If you constantly blame your adversities on others or on situations, etc., you will be living life according to ignorance and weakness. True spiritual strength comes from leaning upon the Self within for spiritual support and well being, rather than upon external situations, people or objects, even though the help itself may come in the form of external situations, people or objects.

Thus, within the teachings of Maat can be found all of the important injunctions for living a life, which promotes purity, harmony and sanctity. While these may be found in other spiritual traditions from around the world, seldom is the emphasis on non-violence and balance to be found. In Christianity, Jesus emphasized non-violence and in Hinduism and Buddhism, the discipline of *Dharma*, composed of *Yamas and Nyamas*, which are moral (righteous) observances and restraints for spiritual living, emphasizes non-violence. These are the restraints *(Yamas)*: Non-violence, Abstinence from falsehood (Truthfulness), Non-stealing, and Abstinence from sex-pleasure. These are the ethical observances *(Nyamas)*: Purity, Contentment, Austerity, Study of scriptures (and -repetition of *Mantra*-chanting*)*, and Surrender to God.

The Ancient Egyptian, Hindu and Buddhist traditions were the first to recognize the power of non-violence to heal the anger and hatred within the aggressor as well as the victim. When this spiritual force is developed it is more formidable than any kind of physical violence. Therefore, anyone who wishes to promote peace and harmony in the world must begin by purifying every bit of negativity within themselves. This is the only way to promote harmony and peace in others. Conversely, if there is anger within you, you are indeed promoting anger outside of yourself and your efforts will be unsuccessful in the end.

THE EFFECT OF ZOROASTRIANISM ON WESTERN RELIGIONS

Zoroastrianism is a religion originated by Zoroaster, a Sage who is believed to have lived in the 6th century B.C.E. Zoroastrianism became the state religion of Persia in the period from 229-652 A.C.E. Zoroastrianism viewed the world as divided between the spirits of good and evil, God and nature. The main doctrine of Zoroastrianism came to mean that there is a God who exists in fact, separate from humankind and from nature in a particular physical location. Zoroastrians worship *Ahura Mazda* as the Supreme Deity. Ahura Mazda is all light and all goodness. As soon as Ahura Mazda appeared though, another god appeared, *Angra Mainyu*, (Ahura Mazda's shadow), the Lord of Darkness. In a fit of jealousy he cast darkness upon the light. Therefore, the creation of the God of light, nature, exists in a state of mixture.

According to Zoroastrian doctrine, the human soul, which is essentially light, is also mixed with darkness by virtue of its association with the body. Thus, in order to achieve salvation, one must consciously, and with intention, reject the bad and adhere to the good. Hence, the idea emerges that we must not come into harmony with nature, the works of humanity, and the body and its desires, because these are part of the "darkness" that pull a human being away from blessedness. Instead, we must constantly fight to subdue our physical nature and our outer nature, the environment. Neither is to be respected and accepted, instead one is to despise and repudiate them for being the vehicle of darkness. The terms "Good God," "Good religion" and the "goodness of man" became central to the Zoroastrian doctrine. While there is no notion of original sin, Zoroastrians believe that every individual is responsible for his/her part in the cosmic struggle of good and evil. Zoroastrians also believe in a savior who will come and usher in the victory of the forces of good against the forces of evil, and then establish a golden age for the

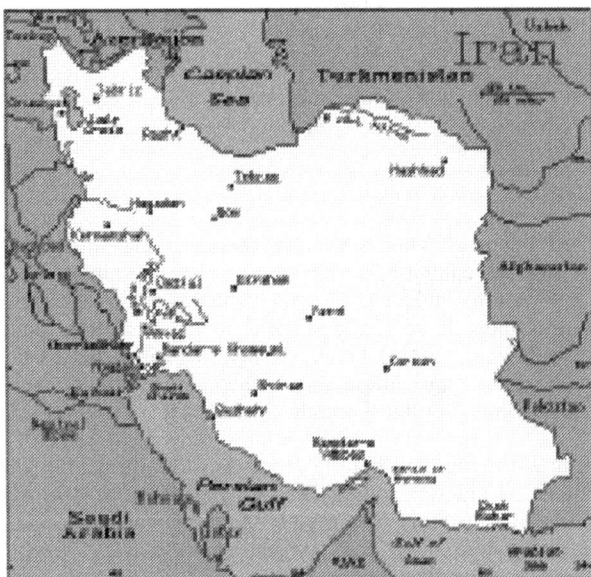

righteous as the following Zoroastrian quotation suggests:

Powerful in immortality shall be the soul of the follower of Truth, but lasting torment shall there be for the man who cleaves to the Lie.

Left: Persia - Modern day Iran.

It must be remembered that truth, from the Zoroastrian point of view, is not to be compared with the mystical truth of the Gnostics. The Zoroastrian ideal is complete faith in a dualistic universe, which is governed by forces of light (good) and forces of darkness (evil). The mystical understanding sees duality only as a manifestation of the transcendental Self in time and space due to ignorance. However, upon transcending time and space, through enlightenment, duality is discovered to be an illusion. The Zoroastrian dualistic point of view sees and affirms only the reality of time and space. If it recognizes anything above time and space it ascribes dualistic concepts to that as well. Thus, the dualistic concept offers no final resolution to the question of existence since one duality inevitably leads to another in an endless chain of causality. The Latin term for this kind of philosophical argument is *regresus ad infinitum* or "regressing to infinity." If there is a "good God" and a "bad God" then they both thwart each others will, but if the good one will win out one day then it must mean that the bad one is not so bad or not a god at all! The reasoning just presented points to the fallacy of dualistic thinking. Duality is an aspect of the human mind and its weak concepts about nature. When the ignorance of the mind is purged then the non-dualistic reality of the universe emerges. This is called Gnosis by the Christian Gnostic mystics.

The language and scriptures of Zoroastrianism have been found to be extremely similar to the language and scriptures of the Indo-European Aryans who invaded eastern Asia (Europe) and southern Asia (India) between 1,700 and 1,300 B.C.E. Therefore, it is likely that Zoroaster was an Aryan Sage or strongly influenced by Aryan dualistic philosophy. In much the same way as occurred in India and Europe, the Aryan views of ritualism and the worship of a God in fact who resides somewhere outside and apart from man and creation were transferred to Mesopotamia. Zoroastrian ideas contrasted with the Gnostic, Egyptian and Dravidian (pre-Aryan culture in India) understanding of God as being within nature and the human heart. The Zoroastrian ideas were introduced to the Semitic groups who lived in the Near East and became a strong religious belief which profoundly influenced other religious movements of Asia minor including Judaism with its God, Yahweh, who is all good in the writings of Moses (Torah). See Exodus 7: 13-14

> Exodus 7
> 13. And he hardened Pharaoh's heart, that he hearkened not to them; as the LORD had said.
> 14. And the LORD said to Moses, Pharaoh's heart [is] hardened, he refuseth to let the people go.

In the book of Exodus, of the Old Testament, God tells Moses to confront Pharaoh and ask him to let the Jews leave Egypt. At one point Pharaoh agreed, but then had a sudden change of heart which was prompted by God as well. So it must be asked why did God harden Pharaoh's heart if he wanted to let the Jews leave? This wonderful situation in Jewish mythology points to the universal aspect of God who is operating through the duality of human experience and through nature itself. It is a recognition that the same Supreme Being that is behind the evil people is also behind the good people as well. But how can God be good and bad at the same time? The answer is that God is in reality neither good nor evil, just as the sun cannot be said to be good or evil. It sustains life on earth and makes it possible for people to act in evil ways or good ways according to their inclinations based on their ethical character, a product of their level of spiritual evolution. God sustains Creation and it is human beings who act in evil or righteous ways in accordance with their desires. However, God is there for all who wish to discover him/her while nature, the school of hard knocks, is there to guide wayward souls on their journey though life by means of trial and error, tribulations, frustrations and disappointments, as well as short lived successes and fleeting pleasures.

Zoroastrian philosophy would say that good and evil are separate and distinct entities contending for control of the earth. Zoroastrians believe that at 1,000 year intervals, a savior, born of a virgin, comes to earth, at which time the dead are raised. At this time the heavenly forces engage in a battle against the demonic or evil forces.[84] Prior to the advent of Zoroastrianism, the Ancient Egyptians held that the God Djehuti would incarnate to restore unrighteousness in the world whenever necessary. Heru exemplifies another expression of this same idea. Similarly, in Indian philosophy, the god Vishnu incarnates at regular intervals to relieve the world from evil. The stories of his incarnations are recounted in the Ramayana-Yoga Vasistha and the Mahabharata. In Buddhist scriptures, there is a story of *Kalki Avatara*, a savior who will come to earth to destroy evil and announce the end of the earth. The number 1,000 also appears in Hinduism where Indian Sages stated that a day of the god Brahma (the creator of the world) lasts 1,000 years. Likewise this same idea appeared in the Bible, Psalms 90:4. It states that *1,000 years are like a day in the sight of God*. These idea transferred to the New Testament Christian faith in the notion that Jesus would return in the year 1,000. Thus, at the end of each millennium, 1,000 years intervals after the death of Jesus Christ, Christians enter into a panic about the coming end of the world.

Zoroastrianism has important correlations to the Indo-European Vedic Aryans. The Zoroastrian god Ahura of the Seven Chapters, has wives, called Ahuranis. They are comparable to the wives of the Hindu-Vedic god, Varuna. Varuna's wives (Varunanis), are the rain clouds and waters of Creation. Ahura is possessor of Asha, as Varuna is custodian of Rta ("Truth" or "cosmic order" = Asha = Old Persian. Arta). In Zoroastrian mythology, the sun is the "eye" of both deities, and the name of Ahura is at times joined to that of the god Mithra. In a Hindu Veda, the names of Mithra and Varuna are similarly joined. The Zoroastrian Seven Chapters also revere Haoma (Hindu-Vedic, Soma), a divinized plant yielding an intoxicating juice. The worship of ancestors and nature spirits and other deities (for example, the fire god, called Agni by the Hindus) likewise have Vedic correspondences.[75] Thus, it is widely accepted that Zoroastrian mythology is an extension of Vedic Aryan mythology which entered into India, China and eastern Europe with the invading hoards of Indo-Europeans from North Asia (modern day Russia-Siberia).

Clearly, there are almost exact correlations between Zoroastrianism, early Mesopotamian mythology, Judaism of the Old Testament and Christianity in reference to the dualistic view of divinity and of spiritual life in general. So Judaism and Christianity appear to be an amalgam of Ancient Egyptian and Mesopotamian traditions. Thus, while there is a strong mystical philosophy which underlies Christianity from the African (Egyptian) and Indian influence, it is also true that much of the dualistic thinking in Christianity originated from the influences of Mesopotamian religion and the Aryan religion from north Asia. While Judaism still expects a savior, Christians accepted Jesus as the savior and Lucifer as the lord of darkness (the devil).

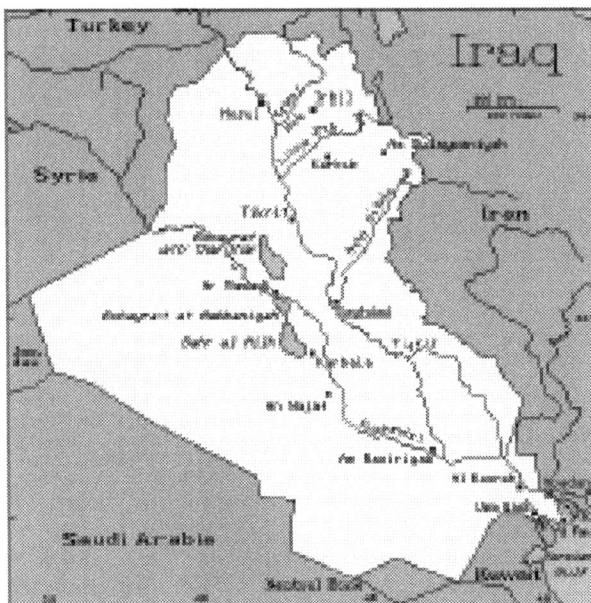

Left: The land of the Zoroastrians.

From the Bible: Revelation 20:5

5 But the rest of the dead lived not again until the thousand years were finished. This [is] the first resurrection.

The belief in the return of Jesus was so strong that in the year 1,000 A.C.E. all of Christendom was stricken by panic due to the expectation of the return of Jesus. When the millennium came and went, the disconcerted nobles who had donated their lands and property to the church in order to receive redemption and absolution fought to get their fortunes back.

In the Book of Genesis, Abraham, whom the Jews consider as the first Jew, lived in the city of Ur in Southern Mesopotamia. The city of Ur was founded in 4,000 B.C.E. by Sumerians. According to the Bible, Abraham migrated westward to Palestine with his family at about 1,900 B.C.E. The ruins of Ur are approximately located midway between the modern city of Baghdad, Iraq, and the Persian Gulf, on the edge of the al-Hajar Desert and south of the Euphrates River. The site of Ur is known today as Tell al-Muqayyar, Iraq. In the times of Abraham, this was the same area where Zoroastrian and Indo-Aryan beliefs were strongest. According to Jewish belief, God made a covenant with Abraham, that if he would keep God's laws and serve him above all others, that he, Abraham, would be the father of many peoples and that those peoples would be given *"the entire land of Canaan."* As previously discussed, with this statement, the idea of a *"promised land"* was born along with the sanction of God to acquire it.

Genesis 17
    8 And I will give to thee, and to thy seed after thee, the land in which thou art a stranger, all the land of Canaan, for an everlasting possession; and I will be their God.

Having established the covenant, Abraham and his family moved to Egypt in order to escape the famines which struck Persia and Canaan during that time.

Genesis 12
    10. And there was a famine in the land: and Abram (Abraham) went down into Egypt to dwell there; for the famine [was] grievous in the land.

As previously discussed, by the time Moses is said to have led the Jewish people out of Egypt the small family of Abraham had become an entire community, a nation of people who had been previously living in Egypt. Therefore, the Jews that left Egypt were indeed Egyptians who elected to follow Moses with his particular teaching which was a variation of the Ancient Egyptian religion blended with Zoroastrian ideas. They are heretofore referred to as *"the people"* or *"the children of Israel."*

Exodus 13
    16 And it shall be for a token upon thy hand, and for frontlets between thy eyes: for by strength of hand the LORD brought us forth out of Egypt.

Exodus 20
    22. And the LORD said to Moses, Thus thou shalt say to the children of Israel, Ye have seen that I have talked with you from heaven.
    23 Ye shall not make with me gods of silver, neither shall ye make to you gods of gold.
    24 An altar of earth thou shalt make to me, and shalt sacrifice on it thy burnt offerings, and thy peace offerings, thy sheep, and thy oxen: in all places where I record my name I will come to thee, and I will bless thee.

Other influences of Zoroastrianism on Christianity by way of its impact on early Judaism included the adoption of the virulent dislike for all other religions and sects, along with the idea of purgatory which became part of the church dogma around the seventh century. While there is no historical evidence that any person by the name of Abraham ever existed, the mythological correspondences between the Jewish, Zoroastrian and Vedic stories suggests that there is a common origin to them.

ISLAM AND CHRISTIANITY

In the sixth century A.C.E., the Jewish and Zoroastrian influence continued through Mohammed in a new direction. Mohammed was an ordinary man who became a practitioner of monastic meditation. In his early life he followed the Arab religions, but broke away from these when he had a series of visions. Out of these insights he developed the teachings of Islam, and these developed into the religion of the Muslims.[I] The teachings of Islam are compiled in the *Koran* or Islamic Holy scripture. Mohammed accepted the teachings of the Old Testament in his creation of the new religion (Islam). Having originated out of the Old Testament tradition, which itself has its roots in Ancient Egyptian religion, the Islamic tradition (600 A.C.E.) picked up on the Old Testament teachings about Egypt and portrayed the same negative view as the following verse from the Koran attests. However, in the same manner that the Jews denigrated Ancient Egypt for the sake of promoting Yahweh, the Muslims disparaged Egypt for the sake of promoting Allah, the Supreme Being in Islamic tradition.

C.102.-(Verses 71-92)-Allah works in His world — in mercy for his servants, and in just punishment for those who do wrong. Thus was it in Noah's story, for he worked unselfishly for his people, though rejected of them. So it was with Moses, He preached to Pharaoh and the Egyptians, but most of them preferred falsehood and pride to the Truth of Allah, and perished. Even Pharaoh's confession of Allah at the last was too late, as his life had been spent in luxury, pride, and oppression.

It is notable, in the quotation above, that the Koran acknowledges that the God of the Jews is also the God that Islam recognizes as Allah. The following *Suras* or statements from the Koran show the similarity of ideology between Judaism, Orthodox Christianity and Islam on the question of the acceptance of Abraham (A), the idea of one God (B), and Jesus (C).

(A)
2:122 Section 15. O Children of Israel! Call to mind the special favor which I bestowed upon you, and that I preferred you to all others (for My Message).
2:123 Then guard yourselves against a day when one soul shall not avail another, nor shall compensation be accepted from her, nor shall intercession profit her, nor shall anyone be helped (from outside).
2:124 And remember that Abraham was tried by his Lord with certain Commands, which he fulfilled: He said: "I will make thee an Imam[II] to the Nations." He pleaded: "And also (Imams) from my offspring!" He answered: "But My Promise is not within the reach of evildoers."
2:125 Remember We made the House a place of assembly for men and a place of safety; and take ye the Station of Abraham as a place of prayer; and We covenanted with Abraham and Ismail, that they should sanctify My house for those who compass it round, or use it as a retreat, or bow, or Prostrate themselves (therein in prayer).

(B)
2:163 And your Allah is One God: There is no god but He, Most Gracious, Most Merciful.

(C)
4:171 O People of the Book! Commit no excesses in your religion: Nor say of Allah ought but the truth. Christ Jesus the son of Mary was (no more than) an apostle of Allah, and His Word, which He bestowed on Mary, and a Spirit proceeding from Him: So believe in Allah and His apostles. Say not "Trinity": desist: It will be better for you: For Allah is One God: Glory be to Him: (Far Exalted is He) above having a son. To Him belong all things in the heavens and on earth. And enough is Allah as a Disposer of affairs.

5:76 They do blaspheme who say: Allah is one of three in a Trinity: For there is no god except One God. If they desist not from their word (of blasphemy), verily a grievous penalty will befall the blasphemers among them.

[I] A believer in or adherent of Islam.
[II] **i·mam** also **I·mam** (ĭ-mäm/) *n. Islam.* **1.a.** In law and theology, the caliph who is successor to Mohammed as the lawful supreme leader of the Islamic community.[115]

6:19 Say: "What thing is most weighty in evidence?" Say: "Allah is witness between me and you; this Koran hath been revealed to me by inspiration, that I may warn you and all whom it reaches. Can ye possibly bear witness that besides Allah there is another god?" Say: "Nay! I cannot bear witness!" Say: "But in truth He is the One God, and I truly am innocent of (your blasphemy of) joining others with Him."

9:31 They take their priests and their anchorites to be their lords in derogation of Allah, and (they take as their Lord) Christ the son of Mary; Yet they were commanded to worship but One God: There is no god but He. Praise and glory to Him: (Far is He) from having the partners they associate (with Him).

14:52 Here is a Message for mankind: Let them take warning therefrom, and let them know that He is (no other than) One God: Let men of understanding take heed.

16:51 Section 7. Allah has said: "Take not (for worship) two gods: For He is just One God: Then fear Me (and Me alone)."

21:108 Say: "What has come to me by inspiration is that your God is One God: Will ye therefore bow to His Will (in Islam)?"

Many of the statements above consist in delineating the differences between Islam, Christianity and Judaism, whereby the prophet Muhammad chastises the Christians for believing in a prophet (Jesus) as God, and as God in the form of a Trinity. Other statements are emphatic admonitions to the effect that Allah is the only God, and that he is one and alone. Further, that anyone who does not know this and who dies unbelieving will not be saved.

These statements and belief systems were adopted by honest believers and also by unscrupulous opportunists who saw a chance to wage war on other peoples. This was a driving factor which fueled the rapid expansion of Islam throughout the Middle East leading to "holy wars" which expanded the Islamic conquests to encompass North Africa, Spain, South Eastern Europe, Turkey, Persia, Arabia and Western India.[77]

Islam's conquest of Persia around the seventh century led to the decline and near disappearance of the Zoroastrian religion in Persia. In the same manner that the Christian Church had adopted several ideas and symbols which had been previously labeled as "heretical," such as the cross, Islam adopted and accepted the teachings from the Old Testament and the worship of the *Ka'bah,* which had previously been a ritual worship center of many so called pagan gods in Mecca.

Even though the three major western world religions (Christianity, Islam, Judaism) share several common beliefs such as the same monotheistic and anthropomorphic belief in one God and the basic beliefs of the ancient Hebrew scriptures that are found in the Old Testament of the Christian Bible and in the Jewish Torah, the accent on *Folk* differences at the lower stage of religion (myth) has been instrumental in fueling the fires of discontent and animosity between them.[76]

Islam came to prominence at a time (c. 600 A.C.E.) when the Christian Church was in conflict due to corruption, invaders from Europe (Vikings, Vandals, Celts, Visigoths, etc.), internal disagreements and the loss of faith in church doctrine which was seen as ineffective and unfulfilling by many. The many prophecies which never came true and the disregard of the church leaders for the teachings of Jesus in favor of conquest and personal or church enrichment fostered a climate of unrest and discontent with the church.

Islam offered a new direction to those disillusioned by the Christian Church. This way was even more so grounded in the world of human activity, as it emphasized less mysticism, more action in the world, more ritualistic exercises and blind obedience rather than dogmas related to celibacy, asceticism, renunciation, humility, etc., which though espoused by Christian leaders, were misunderstood and ignored by many of them. Islam offered a polygamous lifestyle, as well as a warlike and hostile attitude towards nature. It also promoted the pursuit of fulfillment of sensual pleasures while on earth as opposed to hoping to experience heavenly enjoyments after death, a doctrine heavily promoted by the Christians. Rather than effacement of the ego self-concept, the form of Islam which developed after the passing of the Prophet Muhammad encouraged the pride of Islamic culture and the pursuit of glory through establishing supremacy over the known world. Islamic conquests would eventually encompass North Africa, Spain, Turkey, South-East Europe, the Near East and India.

Ironically, Muhammad, the founder of Islam, was opposed by other Arab leaders in the earlier stages of the development of his "new" religion in much the same way as Jesus was repudiated by the religious leaders of his time. Muhammad was forced to flee into Egypt and Ethiopia where he and his followers further developed Islamic philosophy. In this manner, Muhammad gained from the Gnostic Egyptian religion and culture. He also married an Ethiopian woman.

The word *"Islam"* means to *"surrender."* In its religious application, Islam refers to *"surrendering to the will or the law of God."* Muhammad said he had been given the word of God by the Angel Gabriel in a revelation. Thus, the origin of Islam is rooted in Jewish and Zoroastrian mythology. The major tenets of Orthodox Islam are:

1- *There is only one God, unitary and omnipresent. God is separate from creation and manages it from afar.*
2- *The plurality of Gods or the extension of God's divinity to any person is strongly rejected.*
3- *God created nature through a primordial act of mercy, lest there would be only nothingness.*
4- *God governs creation. All areas of creation were given laws to follow. The following of these laws creates perfect harmony. The breaking of them creates disharmony. Since there are laws, there is no need for miracles. The Koran is the highest miracle which no man will match.*
5- *The ultimate purpose of humanity is to serve God in order to reform the earth.*
6- *God has four functions: Creation, Sustenance, Guidance, Judgment.*
7- *After death, those who lived by the laws will go to the Garden (Heaven); those who did not will go to Hell.*

Allah is the Muslim (A believer in or adherent of Islam - Koran 22:78) name for the Supreme Being. The term provides insights into the origins of Islamic theology. It is a contraction of the Arabic word al-llah or "The God." The word and the idea existed in the Arabian tradition before Islam. In this mythology there was a limited form of monotheism which was practiced. Even though other lesser gods were recognized, the pre-Islamic Arabs also recognized Allah as their Supreme God. So the Islamic and Jewish traditions have polytheistic backgrounds from which they selected one divinity to represent a Supreme Being above the others. Thus, upon closer examination, the Jewish and Islamic traditions have much in common with Ancient Egyptian religion which is composed of a Supreme Being (Pa Neter) from which the gods and goddesses (neteru) emanate. It is also notable that the term Allah meaning "The God" is exactly the same as the Ancient Egyptian term Pa-Neter which means "The God," and "Supreme Being." The following statements from Ancient Egyptian mystical philosophy denote a remarkable concordance with the Islamic teachings.

The number given in parenthesis denotes the Islamic tenet (above) to which the Ancient Egyptian philosophy corresponds.

(A) Ancient Egyptian philosophy: God is "Only One Without a second." (1)

(B) Plurality means: "Consisting of more than one choice." While Ancient Egyptian religion appears to consist of many gods and goddesses, in reality they are only symbols referring to the one Supreme Being. This form of religious practice was the basis of Ancient Egyptian religion and the religion of other nations, but was misunderstood over a period of time. However, before the emergence of Islam, the Arab peoples were in contact with and at one time governed by the Ancient Egyptians, and were thus exposed to their religion. The reverence of the Jews and the Muslims for a single supreme God is in agreement with Ancient Egyptian religion. However, the manner of worship and the understanding about who that Divinity is was changed by the Jews and Muslims. In Ancient Egyptian Religion, God is not separate and far away from Creation. God is Creation itself and the force, which sustains all life. (2)

(C) God created the universe by uttering the first thought and sound and brought order out of the preexisting void. (3)

(D) Maat (cosmic principle of truth, order, righteousness and harmony) is the means by which God governs the universe. (4)

(E) Ancient Egyptian Proverbs: "Give thyself to The God, keep thou thyself daily for The God; and let tomorrow be as today." "What is loved by God is obedience; God hateth disobedience." (5)

(F) In Ancient Egyptian Religion, God is the Creator in the form of Khepri, the Sustainer in the form of Ra and the Destroyer in the form of Tem. The first teaching related to a judgement of the soul as well as heaven and hell occurs in the Ancient Egyptian Religion. However, God does not judge. Every human being is the judge of himself or herself on the day of judgement because it is their own actions lead them to experience hellish or heavenly conditions after death. The coveted goal is to go to heaven (Pet) and to meet God and become one with God. (6)

The Islamic tradition believes in a final judgement. It is believed that on the Day of Judgment, all humanity will be gathered by God. All individuals will be judged according to their deeds alone. Those who "succeed" will go to the Garden (heaven), and those who "lose" will go to hell.

As stated earlier, the religion of Islam is in agreement with the existence of Abraham and Jesus and there is special veneration for the Virgin Mary. While there are only seventeen references to the Virgin Mary in the Christian New Testament, she is mentioned thirty-four times in the Quran (Koran). Muslims believed that she would conceive miraculously, and that God sent angels to tell her the good news. This tradition follows the New Testament closely; see the passages below from the Quran.

> "Behold!" the Angels said: 'O Mary God hath chosen thee above the women of all nations."
> (Quran 3:42)

> The Angels proceeded: "O Mary! God giveth thee glad tidings of a word from Him: his name will be Jesus, the son of Mary, held in honor in this world and the Hereafter and (of the company of) those nearest to God. He shall speak to the people in childhood and in maturity." (Quran 3:46)

> Upon receiving this news, although a good piece of news, Mary in her innocence, was shocked. Mary responded: "O My Lord! How shall I have a son when no man hath touched me?" The Angel replied: "Even so: God critter what he willeth: When He decreed a Plan, He but saith to it, 'Be' and it is." (Quran 3:47-48)

Muslims believe that Jesus was a prophet of Allah and that he performed miracles. However, they believe that he was only preparing the way for Muhammad, the prophet and founder of the Islamic faith. The following passage from the Koran illustrates the Islamic view.

> 61:6 And remember, Jesus, the son of Mary, said: "O Children of Israel! I am the apostle of Allah (sent) to you, confirming the Law (which came) before me, and giving Glad Tidings of an Apostle to come after me, whose name shall be Ahmad. " But when he came to them with Clear Signs, they said, "This is evident sorcery!"

Islam in America: Malcolm X and The Nation of Islam

In the 1950's and 60's, a movement called the Nation of Islam came to its peak in the United States of America. The Black Muslims are a United States religious movement that is officially called the Nation of Islam. It was founded in Detroit in 1930 by W. D. Fard. The group's origins are founded in two Black self-improvement movements known as the Moorish Science Temple of America, which was founded in 1913 by Prophet Drew Ali, and the Universal Negro Improvement Association, which was founded in 1914 by Marcus Garvey. When Ali died, the leadership of his movement passed to Wallace D. Fard. In 1930 Fard founded a temple in Detroit which was later known as a mosque. This event is regarded as the actual beginning of the Nation of Islam. Mr. Fard used many names including: Walli Farad and Master Farad Muhammad. He was also called God, Allah, or the Great Mahdi by some Black Muslims. The branch of the Nation of Islam in Chicago was founded in 1933. After Mr. Fard's mysterious disappearance, the leadership of the group went to the leader of the Detroit temple, Elijah Muhammad, who then moved to Chicago.

The Muslims adhere strictly to the Koran's moral codes. They saved many people by turning them away from a life of drug addiction, crime and lack of education. The moral codes they adhered to included abstaining from alcohol, drugs, gambling, and smoking. One of the criticisms of the group was that women are subservient to men. The Muslims maintain their own schools, farms, and businesses, living as independently as possible from the larger society. In the 1960s, Malcolm X carried the Muslim message to a larger, more sophisticated audience.

Malcolm became a member of the Nation in the 1950's and turned away from a life of crime. In the Nation of Islam he was taught that white people are devils. The actions of many whites during the period of slavery and the practices of discrimination, lynching, etc., seemed to support this view. This philosophy, while giving African Americans an alternative to the racist philosophy of America which promoted the idea of the inferiority of blacks and the superiority of whites, also served to widen the rift between blacks and whites. When Malcolm traveled abroad and discovered that there were white Muslims and other white people who were against racism, and who stood for righteousness, he began to teach that righteousness, rather than race, should be the standard for judging others. He was suspended from the church in 1963 after which he turned away from the doctrines of hatred and racism and sought to bring forth a new vision through a purer form of Islam. He founded a new church, the Muslim Mosque in 1963 and in 1964 he converted to Islam as practiced by the Muslims in Mecca. Malcolm discovered that he doctrines which formed the basis of the Nation of Islam were different from those of Orthodox Islam as practiced in the Middle East. He was assassinated in 1965 by members of the Nation of Islam due to his rift with the group, and in particular with Elijah Muhammad. However, as in the death of Dr. Martin Luther King, the circumstances of Malcolm's death and the statements of the assassins lead to the strong suspicion that the government was partly responsible as instigators of the animosity between the parties and facilitators of the actual assassinations. Elijah Muhammad died in 1975 and was succeeded by his son Wallace, who called for radical changes in the movement, including the welcoming of whites into the movement and the promotion of women to leadership positions. He stressed strict Islamic beliefs and practices.

Formerly called the Nation of Islam, after 1975 the group was officially known as the American Muslim Mission and as the World Community of Al-Islam in the West. Its members refer to themselves as Bilalians. Its leaders advocate economic cooperation and self-sufficiency and enjoin a strict Islamic code of behavior governing such matters as diet, dress, and interpersonal relations. Members follow some Islamic religious ritual and pray five times daily. In the late 1970's a dissident faction emerged. It, led by Louis Farrakhan, assumed the original name, Nation of Islam, and reasserted the principles of black separatism.[75/115]

The Origins of Esoteric (Mystical) Islam: Sufism (c. 700 A.C.E)

As stated earlier, Orthodox Judaism was, in great part, an outgrowth of Ancient Egyptian Religion Christianity was an outgrowth of Judaism and Ancient Egyptian Religion, and Islam was an outgrowth of Judaism and Christianity. Jewish mysticism (Kabbalism or Cabalism), Christian mysticism (Gnostic Christianity) and Islamic mysticism (Sufism) can be seen as outgrowths of Shetaut Neter (Ancient Egyptian Mysticism). *Sufism* or mystical Islam emerged in the Middle East within 100 years after Islam became established there as a dominant religious doctrine. The name "*Sufi*" comes from "Suf" which means "wool." The name Sufi was adopted since the ascetic followers of this doctrine wore coarse woolen garments *(sufu)*. Sufism represented a turning away from the egocentric doctrines of orthodox Islam and Catholicism and a reaffirmation of the mystical traditions which had preceded them. In this sense, Sufism has much in common with Gnostic Christianity, Indian Vedanta and the Ancient Egyptian Ausarian Mysticism.

To the followers of Orthodox Islam, Sufism has almost always been regarded as heresy since its main goal is to lead the Sufi follower to have *"Mystic Knowledge of God."* Sufism is based upon the fundamental Islamic tenets of living in harmony with others but beyond these ideas, the Sufis also hold that:

A- God, as creator of the universe, transcends it.
B- God cannot be expressed in words.
C- The inner light (one's own soul-spirit) is a sufficient source of religious guidance.
D- The Universe and God are actually one.
E- Since humans are part of creation, a human being can, through mystical discipline, become one with God.
F- The Sufi mystic is described as a pilgrim on a journey following a path of seven stages:

> 1- Repentance
> 2- Abstinence
> 3- Renunciation
> 4- Poverty
> 5- Patience
> 6- Trust in God
> 7-Acquiescence to the will of God

G- As in Ancient Egyptian Mysticism, Christian Mysticism and the Bhakti Yoga of India, some Sufis practice devotion by employing the energies of love and directing them solely toward the Divine (union with God). Through rituals such as reading, listening to poetry, other works of literature, and devotional dancing (the *Whirling Dervishes*), an ecstatic mental-emotional feeling develops which can be used to sublimate and direct psychic (spiritual) energy to becoming attuned to and attaining union with the divine forces.

The following passage from Philo of Alexandria[I] gives an impression of the worship of God in the form of Devotional Love ["heavenly love"] as he attempted to introduce it to Orthodox Christianity according to his own knowledge and experience in the mystery schools of his time.

> "Now they who betake themselves to this service [of God do so], not because of any custom, or on someone's advice and appeal, but carried away with heavenly love, like those initiated into the Bacchic[II] or Corybantic[III] Mysteries, they are a-fire with God until they see the object of their love.[63]

H- Sufism incorporates teachings in reference to the subtle spiritual body which may be compared to the Egyptian teachings of the "Pillar of Asar" and the four levels of the Serpent Power (Energy Centers in the body), and the Chakras of the Indian Kundalini Yoga. These are:

The Energy Centers:

Sufi	Egyptian	Indian
The Teacher	Ikh	Sahasrara
The Mysterious center	Sekhem	Visuddha
The Secret Center	Kheper	Anahata
Center of the Self	Ob	Manipura

Historical evidence and Sufi Mystic literature clearly show that Sufi followers had relationships (cultural, ethnic and social ties) with Egypt, the Essenes (Jewish tribe of Jesus) and the Hindus and Buddhists of the Far East. Thus, it is not surprising that the energy center system of Sufism is closely related to the Uraeus Serpent Power and Tantric Kundalini mystical yoga systems of Egypt and India, respectively.

WHAT IS THE PHILOSOPHY OF GNOSTICISM?

Romans 12

> 2 And be not conformed to this world: but be ye transformed by the renewing of your mind, that ye may prove what [is] that good, and acceptable, and perfect, will of God.

The use of the word transformation in this statement above from the Bible seems to imply that the desired spiritual movement in a Christian follower is much more than an ordinary change in the mind. What is this *"transformation"* and does the Bible provide the information necessary in order to achieve the desired transformation? What is this renewing of the mind? The detailed study of these points and a profound understanding of their meaning is essential to the correct practice of Christian spirituality. The correct practice of Christian spirituality will lead every human being to discover the answers to the questions just asked above. However, before we can even attempt to answer these most profound questions, we must first understand what the questions are leading us to understand, and then the answers will become obvious. Having information and having knowledge (Gnosticism) are not necessarily the same thing. There are two forms of knowledge: direct and indirect. Indirect knowledge is something you learn and are convinced of intellectually. This is gained by studying the scriptures and hearing the discourses from the Sages and Saints. Direct knowledge on the other hand, is something you experience. It is something which requires no thinking or intellectual reflection to be understood... it is "knowing-experiencing" knowledge as opposed to learning or "thinking" knowledge. Gnosis therefore means intuitional knowledge. Intuition is defined as "the faculty of knowing as if by instinct, without conscious reasoning."[115] One may learn about a flower by reading, but one does not become the flower or experience the flower through that information. To know

---

[I] Philo Judaeus, or Philo of Alexandria (c. 20 BC - c. AD 54), Jewish philosopher living in Egypt. Attempted to blend the theology of the Jewish scriptures with Egyptian-Hermetic, Gnostic, and Greek philosophy.
[II] Bacchic: pertaining to Bacchus and bacchanalia; drunken; jovial; n. drinking song. Bacchus:
In Greek and Roman mythology Bacchus is the god of fertility (related to Dionysus) and of wine. His rites (the Bacchanalia) were orgiastic.
[III] Frenzied. A corybant was a priest, votary or attendant of Cybele (Cybele- Phrygian mythology, an earth-nature goddess, identified by the Greeks with the Greek goddess Rhea and honored in Rome.). corybantic, adj. pertaining to wild and noisy rites performed by these; n. wild, frenzied dance.[126]

something intuitionally is in effect, to become it within one's consciousness. In order for Gnosis to occur, it is necessary to become "identified" with the object of study. One may accomplish this through concentrated thought and meditation on that object to the exclusion of all other objects. However, there are millions of individual objects in the universe. To become one with each of them would take at the very least, millions of life times. The simpler way is to achieve supreme wisdom by identifying (becoming one in consciousness) with God, the source, sustenance and substratum of all objects in existence. Becoming one with or merging with God is therefore the same as becoming one with all existence, having all knowledge, all power — omnipresent, omniscient, omnipotent, etc.

Below: A Gnostic symbol used to represent the Trinity.

All of our information about the world is information we have been told or gathered by our senses which are especially made to gather information from the physical realm, to the extent that they can. Human senses are very limited. This limited information forms the basis of what we believe to be "real" and "true." This process of learning with the use of the senses and the mental processes constitutes our "psychological conditioning" into certain modes of behavior and certain beliefs. This is the process of the formation of the limited human intellect. However, if our senses were designed differently, for example, if we had the eyes of an owl, the canine sense of smell, or the hearing of a bat, our perceptions of the world would be quite different. Our perceptions would lead to different beliefs about what the world is and therefore, our experiences would be quite different. Similarly, if we could see things (matter) the way a particle accelerator or an electron microscope sees it, we would live in a world of pure energy held together by magnetic forces which are unseen.

Below: The Ancient Egyptian symbol adopted by early Christians.

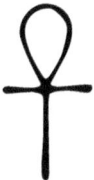

Due to their limitations, the human senses miss a whole other reality which lies beyond ordinary sense perceptions. The "Absolute Truth" (God) which underlies all things in the "physical" realm cannot be sensed with the ordinary senses, designed only for the physical world, nor with the mind which is conditioned to believe in duality and multiplicity. Therefore, in order to know the truth, that is, to have Gnosis or experiential, intuitional knowledge of the transcendent and divine essence of anything, we must be able to connect with its divine essence. Any other essence that may be gathered by the use of senses or other information gathering devices will only be a distortion of the truth, an illusion. In order to perceive the "Absolute," non-changing truth, we must become one with that Absolute Truth. To do this is to become God-like, even while still alive as the Ancient Egyptians would say.

"Gods are immortal men, and men are mortal Gods."

"Men and women are to become God-like through a life of virtue and the cultivation of the spirit through scientific knowledge, practice and bodily discipline."

Ancient Egyptian Mystical Aphorisms

The most important tenet of Gnosticism is that the true way to know God is by looking within, and not out, because our deepest self is God, regardless of sex, race, creed, or religion. Therefore, in order to know God, it is necessary to become God and the way to this exalted mystical experience is to cleanse the mind and body of negative feelings, emotions, thoughts and most of all, ignorance about one's true nature. This can be accomplished through the practice of the teachings and through the practice of meditation on the Divine.

Jesus said: "If you bring forth what is within you, what you bring forth will save you. If you do not bring forth what is within you, what you do not bring forth will destroy you.[91]

The same idea is one of the themes taken up in Chapter 4, Jnan Vibhag Yogah— The Yoga of Wisdom of the Bhagavad Gita:

35. Having known this (wisdom), O Arjuna, you will never enter into delusion again. You will behold all beings within your very Self, as well as in Me.

The "knowing" of the Self within was at the core of the Ancient Egyptian Mysteries as well. The following verse from the Egyptian Book of Coming Forth By Day is the point where the initiate or disciple begins to discover a new world within him/herself:

"I know my Heart, I have achieved power over it, I have achieved the power to do what pleases my Ka (spirit), I will remain aware in my Ab (heart-mind), my Ba (soul) will not be fettered or restrained at the entrance of the West, I will be able to come and go as I please.[45]

The two statements which follow, come from the teachings of *Hermes Trismegistos*. Hermes is the Greek name of the Ancient Egyptian God, Thoth[I] or Djehuti, one of the most important characters in Egyptian mythology and philosophy.

"The race is never taught, but when God willeth it, its memory is restored by the Creator. You will see within yourself the Simple Vision brought to Birth by the compassion of God; no one can be saved before Rebirth. [63]

"To Know God, strive to grow in stature beyond all measure; conceive that there is nothing beyond thy capability. Know thyself deathless and able to know all things, all arts, sciences, the way of every life. Become higher than the highest height and lower than the lowest depth. Amass in thyself all senses of animals, fire, water, dryness and moistness. Think of thyself in all places at the same time, earth, sea, sky, not yet born, in the womb, young, old, dead, and in the after death state.[63]

Thus, knowing or Gnosis means the absolute knowing. That is, knowing that which upon knowing all other things are also known. Therefore, all practices of Gnosticism as with other mystery systems are directed to aiding in the discovery of the transcendental reality behind all things and that lies within oneself.

From the Gospel of Thomas:

3. "When you know yourselves, then you will be known, and you will know that it is you who are the sons of the living Father. But if you do not know yourselves, then you will be in a state of poverty!"
81. Jesus says: "I am the All, and the All has gone out from me and the All has come back to me. Cleave the wood: I am there; lift the stone and thou shalt find me there!"

GNOSTIC CHRISTIANITY AND CHINESE TAOISM

Above: the Chinese symbol of cosmic balance: Ying-Yang. Below: the Ancient Egyptian symbol of cosmic balance: Heru-Set.

From the Gospel of Thomas:

55. "If they ask you: 'What sign of your Father is in you?' tell them: 'It is a movement and a rest.'"

The statement above is most significant in that it shows a conception of God, the "Father," and hence the "Kingdom of the Father" as a realm governed by "movement and rest." The very same spiritual principle has found extensive exposition in Hinduism and Shaktism of India and the Tantrism of Ancient Egypt through the teaching that God is the spirit, the motionless vivifier of creation while the female element is the visible aspect of creation when the spirit is in motion. In Indian terms from *Samkhya* philosophy, Brahman, (God), the *Absolute Reality* behind all phenomena, is the formless, timeless, infinite nature of consciousness when at rest and Prakriti (Shakti-Maya), or nature, is consciousness when in motion. Ancient Egyptian Mythology holds the same symbolism. In Memphite theology the god Ptah is seen as the Supreme Spirit who creates all by his mental will. When Ptah creates, his consort, *Sekhmet,* vivifies Creation. Sekhmet is the goddess of the cosmic life force energy known as *Sekhem.*[II] When human consciousness only experiences consciousness (creation) in motion, it is said to be caught in the state of ignorance, deluded by *maya* (cosmic illusion), and thus must practice yogic disciplines in order to quiet the mind to "realize" Brahman (motionless), the Absolute which transcends creation. This is why there is prime emphasis given to the development of peace of mind in all spiritual teachings around the world. Statement sixsteen from the *"Tao Te Ching"* gives a deeper insight into the meaning of the word *"rest."*

SIXTEEN

Empty yourself of everything.
Let the mind rest at peace.
The ten thousand things rise and fall while the Self watches their return.
They grow and flourish and then return to the source.
Returning to the source is stillness, which is the way of nature.
The way of nature is unchanging.
Knowing constancy is insight.

[I] Greek name for the Ancient Egyptian God.
[II] In Indian mysticism the Life Force energy is called Prana or Shakti. In Chinese Taoism the Life Force energy is called Chi.

Not knowing constancy leads to disaster.
Knowing constancy, the mind is open.
With an open mind, you will be openhearted.
Being openhearted, you will act royally.
Being royal, you will attain the divine.
Being divine, you will be at one with the Tao.
Being at one with the Tao is eternal.
And though the body dies, the Tao will never pass away.

In China, the philosophy of *Taoism* developed the idea of movement and rest to a very extensive degree. Since the experience of rest and movement are the expressions of duality in human consciousness, Taoism advocates, as Jesus did, that the disciple or aspirant must unite the male and female aspects of her/himself. That is to say, that we must try to see with our inner perception, the single essence behind the apparent multiplicity of the world, *"The ten thousand things."* At this point, the aspirant is said to have achieved or realized the *"Tao"* or *"The Way of Nature,"* oneness of consciousness with the absolute reality behind the multiplicity of the world, the *"Self"* which is *"stillness."*

Historical evidence shows that the early Chinese dynasties (Shang Dynasty c.1,523 B.C.E.- c.1,927 B.C.E. and Chou Dynasty c.770 B.C.E.-c.221 B.C.E.) were culturally linked to India, North East Africa and the area now referred to as the Middle East. This is supported by ancient Middle Eastern inscriptions and historians which explain how Asar, at the time he ruled Egypt, extended the Egyptian culture to the farthest reaches of Asia. The Egyptian word for Eternal Spirit is *"Shen."* In the Chinese Mystical Philosophy, Shen also means Eternal Spirit.

The *"Tao Te Ching"* (c. 600 B.C.E.) was a spiritual text which appeared in China around the same time as the teachings of Buddha (c.550 B.C.E.). The Tao or *"The Way,"* is a philosophical exposition of Chinese mystical philosophy. It was the first place outside of Egypt where the teaching of the Supreme Being was expressed as an idea of a "way" or manner of manifestation. In Ancient Egypt the exact term used to refer to religion was, 𓂋𓏤𓈖𓏏𓊹, Shetaut Neter, meaning "The Hidden Way of The Supreme Being." Tao philosophy was also the first known teaching outside of Egypt which held as the main idea that all creation is composed of two opposite but complementary forces. In Ancient Egypt this teaching was called *"Heru - Set."* In China it was called *"Ying and Yang."* It stresses the understanding of the interplay between the two major forces that comprise the universe (male and female, or pairs of opposites), the way to be in harmony with them (virtue), and the experience that lies beyond the pairs of opposites of Creation: unity with all that exists or the "way" of things. The following passage from the Gnostic Christian text, *Gospel of Philip*, examines the nature of opposites in order to uncover their illusoriness.

Light and darkness, life and death, right and left, are mutually dependent; it is impossible for them to separate. Accordingly, the good are not good, the bad are not bad, life is not life, death is not death. So each will be dispersed to its original source. But things that are superior to the world are indissoluble: they are eternal. [101]

Chi is the Chinese name for the single Life Force which exists all throughout the universe. The first writings in reference to Chi begins with Sage Huang Di in c. 2,690 B.C.E.-2,590 B.C.E. Knowledge about the human energy centers existed in Ancient Egypt at the inception of the Dynastic Period (5,500 B.C.E.) In China it took the form of snakes which are coiled three and one half times. This is the well-known symbol which gained popularity through the Indian Kundalini Yoga System in modern times. Like Indian Hatha Yoga, Chi Kung is a system of meditation and physical exercises for the development, sublimation and channeling of the Life Force energy, Chi (Sekhem, Prana, Kundalini), in order to promote spiritual transformation.

According to the Shaolin Temple system, where the disciplines Chi Kung and Kung Fu were developed, there must first be "internal purification" before there can be Chi Kung or Kung Fu training; that is, before the exercises can be performed effectively, the initiate or aspirant must follow a rigorous system of virtue and self control almost identical to the Ancient Egyptian system of Maat Philosophy. The same restrictions and detriments can be found in the Ancient Egyptian Books of Coming Forth By Day and the Wisdom Texts as well as the teachings given by Jesus in the New Testament.

The student must prepare himself for five restrictions:[1]

> *1. He must not be Frivolous.*
> *2. He must not be Conceited.*
> *3. He must not be Impatient.*

---

[1] From *Kung Fu History and Philosophy* by David Chow.

4. He must not be Negligent.
5 He must not be Lascivious.

and seven detriments:

1. Fornication depletes the energy.
2. Anger harms the breathing (CHI, Life Force Energy flow).
3. Worry numbs the mind.
4. Over-trustfulness hurts the heart.
5. Overdrinking (alcoholic beverages) *dilutes the blood.*
6. Laziness softens the muscles.
7. Tenseness weakens the bones.

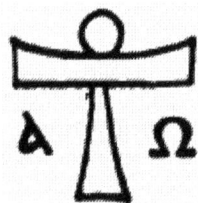

Above: Coptic cross from Stele of Abraham British Museum. #1257, showing Alpha and Omega.

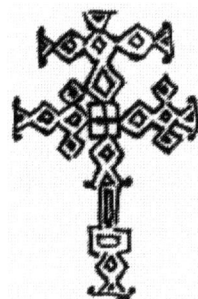

Above: Ethiopian cross from the Ethiopian Book of the Dead.

CHAPTER VI: THE DEVELOPMENT OF THE CHRISTIAN CHURCH

PROBLEMS IN THE EARLY CHRISTIAN CHURCH

Many people believe that the Christian doctrine, which has been handed down to them, is the same as Jesus Christ originally gave it to their forefathers. An in depth look at the history of Christian philosophy reveals that, from its inception, the followers of Christianity have been working out the meaning of the Christian teachings. The following chart shows several important beliefs of the early church and how they changed over time.

Doctrine	Early church doctrine	Later church doctrine
Who is Jesus Christ?	Savior	Son of God
When is Christ returning?	any day now	nobody knows for certain
What is the Christian church?	group of those who are preparing for Christs return	those receiving the message of Christianity
Who can be part of the church?	only Jews	Gentiles as well as Jews
What is the proper way of Christian worship?	in Synagogues and Jewish temple services	the Christian church and the Christian rituals

The notion of a phantasmal human existence is one of the central themes of mystical philosophy. However, this must not be seen as an unnatural state or something otherworldly. Rather, it can be better understood when we reflect upon the Dream State of consciousness and take a deeper look at what modern science has proven about "physical reality." In a dream you experience many situations. You have a body, and there are objects and other characters (perhaps animals or humans) with which you interact. While you are dreaming everything seems very real and tangible. If you are in a dangerous situation, you really feel as if it is truly happening. However, when you wake up the entire situation simply vanishes into thin air. Similarly, modern science has proven that this reality which is considered by most people to be so real and tangible is not really what it appears to the human senses to be. The mystics hold that when the ordinary human consciousness is freed of ignorance and attains "Gnosis," or intuitional experience of its true nature, it realizes this physical reality (the world) along with the physical body to be only a reflection of the true Self. This idea of the illusoriness of the world of time and space will be developed throughout this work since it is the most important element of mystical philosophy and also of modern physics. For now it is important to realize that this illusory projection of physical reality is what the Gospel of Thomas refers to when it says, "The Kingdom of the Father is spread upon the earth and men do not see it!" Thus, the terms "phantasmal" and "illusion," used by the Docetists to describe the appearance of Jesus, apply in the mystical sense outlined above.

Another idea that emerges about the relationship between Gnostic Christianity and Orthodox Christianity is that the Orthodox view is the elementary or preparatory teaching which should lead to the more advanced teachings of Gnosticism. In other mystery systems, the wisdom teachings were given according to the level of understanding of the aspirant. Some initiations such as those of the Essenes lasted for two to three years, a period in which increasing levels of teaching were given. Likewise, Gnosticism was meant for aspirants who were considered advanced in their understanding of the ritualistic aspects of the religion. These were students who were not given to holding on to symbols as realities, but who were ready to listen to the metaphorical and symbolic meanings.

Religions can be thought of as being composed of basically two aspects: one which is ritualistic and superficial *("exoteric"),* and the other which is secret and for the elect *("esoteric").* In religious systems, such as the Egyptian, Vedantic and Hindu, the higher teachings would be reserved for the "elect," those who had demonstrated sufficient maturity and strength of will to understand the subtlety of the philosophy and practice the rituals with the new mystical understanding. The masters or highly spiritually evolved leaders of religion would take care to lead the aspirant onward, beyond myth and ritual, with increasing wisdom according to her/his level of understanding in order to provide a steady movement on the spiritual path. If the movement is too fast, and the aspirant is given more than he/she is ready to understand, the movement may become stunted and may even become negative. Similarly, if the movement stagnates due to lack of guidance from an authentic spiritual preceptor or other spiritually advanced personality, the aspirant may quit due to disappointment and frustration, or become involved in negative activities which will lead her/him away from spiritual enlightenment, even without their being aware of it.

One of the problems encountered by early Christianity was the fanaticism with which the early Christian martyrs (most of whom were Orthodox) faced death at the hands of the magistrates and other Roman authorities. This fanaticism created such an interest among the Roman citizens that eventually more and more converts from the powerful segments of society were drawn until the orthodox groups finally gained control of the Roman government and its military forces. It then became possible for them to call all those who did not agree with them "heretics" and to persecute and destroy their churches and scriptures through the use of the Roman armies.

Matthew 16
18 And I say also to thee, That thou art Peter, and upon this rock I will build my church; and the gates of hell shall not prevail against it.

On the basis of the Biblical scripture above, the Pope in Rome and the Bishops of Rome claimed primacy as the center of the Christian church since they reasoned that Peter,[1] the disciple of Jesus, was said to be buried in Rome. This among other differences caused a split between the Catholic Christians of the West who were based in Rome, and those Christians of the East who followed the church at Constantinople, later called the Byzantine Empire. The Byzantine Empire was known also as the Eastern Roman Empire or Medieval Greek Empire since the two (Western and Eastern empires) were originally united under the authority of the Roman Emperors and the early Christian Popes. The history of the Byzantine Empire extended from A.C.E. 330 when the capital city of Constantinople was established by the Roman Emperor Constantine the Great, to the year 1453 A.C.E., when Constantinople was captured by the Ottoman Turks.

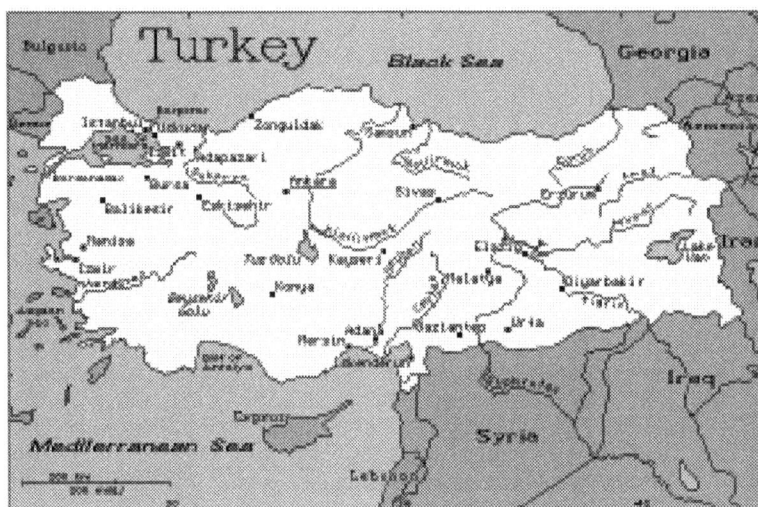

Above: Constantinople and the Eastern Roman Catholic Empire (modern day Turkey)

NOTE: Antakya, formerly Antioch; city in S Turkey, approx. 20mi (32km) E of Mediterranean coast, on Orontes River. It was an important Roman commercial and cultural center and early Christian center during the formation of the early church and the New Testament.

Constantinople was an important city because it was a well-fortified city on the Bosporus River and commanded one of the most important trade routes between Asia and Europe. The Byzantine Empire generally comprised parts of Asia Minor, the Balkans, Ravenna, Syria, Egypt, Greece, portions of Spain, the North African coast as well as South Italy during the expansion times.

THE COPTIC CHURCH

The Coptic Church is the major Christian church in modern day Egypt. The name, Copt, was derived from the Greek word for "Egyptian" and the Arabic "qubt" which was westernized as "Copt." The origins of Egyptian Christianity can be found in the Gnostic mystery schools, which developed the Hermetic teachings (teachings of the Egyptian God Djehuti), in the period immediately proceeding the Christian era. These schools were engendered by the early Greek philosophers who studied Egyptian philosophy and Alexander the Great who conquered Egypt and sought to establish a city of Enlightenment which would bridge the East and the West and spread the wisdom of Egypt to the world. Alexander knew, from his early instruction by Aristotle, that Egypt was the source of the most

---

[1] Peter: the name signifies a rock.

ancient knowledge and the repository of the world's greatest scholars and mystical philosophers. Thus, the Greeks under Alexander sought to appropriate and adopt the Ancient Egyptian traditions which they had been learning for the previous five centuries since the time of Thales, the first recognized Greek Philosopher (circa 700 B.C.E.), in order to carry on the mystical tradition of Egypt along with its highest technological advances. These Gnostic Hellenists intermixed with the Jews living in Alexandria in northwest Lower Egypt. Three centuries after Alexander's conquest of Egypt, notable Christian philosophers would emerge out of Alexandria who would exert a strong influence on early Christianity and later cause the separation of the Egyptian Christians (Copts) from the Roman and Byzantine Christians. Some of the important Christian theologians who emerged from Alexandria included Clement of Alexandria, Origen and Arius.

The debates in the church over the true understanding of Christ (Christology) led to a separation between the Church in Egypt (Coptic Church) and the churches of Rome and Constantinople (Western Empire and Eastern Empire). The majority of Egyptian Christians refused to go along with the decrees of the Council of Chalcedon in 451, that defined the person of Jesus the Christ as being "one in two natures." This doctrine of "two natures" seemed to imply the existence of two Christs, one being divine and the other human. These Egyptian Christians who refused the Council of Chalcedon faced charges of monophysitism. Monophysitism is the belief that Christ has only one nature rather than two. It is notable that the Council of Chalcedon was accepted both in Constantinople and in Rome, but not in Egypt. Thus, we see that the dualistic view of Christ was developed and promoted in Europe under the Roman church and in the Middle East under the church of Constantinople. It was Egypt, which sought to uphold the non-dualistic view of Christ, which viewed him as an all-encompassing Divine being. This was due to the tradition of non-dualism, which it assimilated from the Ancient Egyptian mystery schools. The Coptic Church of Egypt separated from Rome and Constantinople and set up its own Pope who, to this day, is nominated by an Electoral College of clergy and laity. The Coptic Church has survived up to the present in Egypt. There are over seven million Coptic Christians there today and 22 million in total.

The sacred music of Ancient Egypt lives on in the Christian Coptic tradition of the Coptic Church mass. Anthropologists believe that the primary characteristics of modern Coptic music were adopted from the music of the Ancient Egyptians. These characteristics include the use of triangles and cymbals, and a strong vocal tradition. The Copts are regarded as the genetically purest direct descendents of the Ancient Egyptians due to their lack of intermarrying with the other Egyptians who are of Arab descent. The whole of the Coptic service is to be sung. The singing is alternated between the master chanter, the priest, and a choir of deacons. A technique of chanting and singing was also used in Ancient Egypt during the processions and recitals of the mystery rituals.

THE IMPACT OF ANCIENT GREEK PHILOSOPHY ON CHRISTIAN PHILOSOPHY

Greek Philosophy has been equated with the origin of Western civilization. Ancient Greek philosophers such as Thales (c. 634-546 B.C.E.) and Pythagoras (582? -500? B.C.E.) are thought to have originated and innovated the sciences of mathematics, medicine, astronomy, philosophy of metaphysics, etc. These disciplines of the early Greek philosophers had a major impact on the development of Christianity since the version of Christianity which was practiced in the Western and Eastern empires was developed in Greece and alongside Greek culture, the Greek language and the philosophy which the Greeks learned from Ancient Egypt. However, upon closer review, the ancient writings of contemporary historians (early Christianity) point to different sources of Greek Philosophy and hence we are led to discover similarities in philosophy by tracing their origins to a common source.

> Solon, Thales, Plato, Eudoxus and Pythagoras went to Egypt and consorted with the priests. Eudoxus they say, received instruction from Chonuphis of Memphis, * Solon from Sonchis of Sais, * and Pythagoras from Oeniphis of Heliopolis. *
>
> –Plutarch (Greek historian c. 46-120 A.C.E.)
> *(Cities in Ancient Egypt)

Thales is the first Greek philosopher of whom there is any knowledge, and therefore, he is sometimes called the "Father of Greek philosophy." After studying in Egypt with the Sages of the Ancient Egyptian temples, he founded the Ionian[1] school of natural philosophy, which held that a single elementary matter, water, is the basis of all the transformations of nature. The similarity to the Ancient Egyptian Primeval Waters and the creation story in Genesis may be noted here. The ancient writings state that Thales visited Egypt and was initiated by the Egyptian priests into the Egyptian Mystery System, and that during his time in Egypt, he learned astronomy, surveying, engineering, mensuration and Egyptian Theology which would have certainly included the teachings related to Asar, Amun and

---

[1] The Ionians are one of the three important ethnic divisions of the ancient Greeks, the others are the Dorians and the Aeolians. Ionia itself is an ancient district which is located in the area which is now called Turkey. The area received the name from the Ionians or Greeks who emigrated there from the mainland of Greece.

Ptah. [107] Pythagoras was a native of Samos[I] who traveled to Egypt often on the advice of Thales and received education there. He was introduced to each of the Egyptian priests of the major theologies which comprised the whole of the Egyptian religious system based on the Trinity principle (*Amen-Ra-Ptah*). Each of these legs of the Trinity was based in three Egyptian cities. These were Heliopolis (Priesthood of Ra), Memphis (Priesthood of Ptah) and in Thebes (Priesthood of Amen {Amun}) in Egypt. [108]

> "If one were not determined to make haste, one might cite many admirable instances of the piety of the Egyptians, that piety which I am neither the first nor the only one to have observed; on the contrary, many contemporaries and predecessors have remarked it, of whom Pythagoras of Samos is one. On a visit to Egypt he became a student of the religion of the people, and was first to bring to the Greeks all philosophy, and more conspicuously than others he seriously interested himself in sacrifices and in ceremonial purity, since he believed that even if one should gain thereby no greater reward from the gods, among men, at any rate, his reputation would be greatly enhanced.
>
> –Isocrates, Busiris 27-30

Due to the immense impact, which Pythagoras had on the whole of Greek religion and philosophy, it is important to examine the writings about him. *Iamblichus* in the *Life of Pythagoras* writes "Pythagoras met all the priests (Egyptian), learning from each what they knew ...and it is in these conditions that he passed twenty-two years in the temples of Egypt. [112] He returned to Greece to teach in a way perfectly similar to the documents by which he had been instructed in Egypt." Plutarch confirms this by saying: *"Most of the precepts he taught he copied from the Egyptian hieroglyphic texts."* Plutarch also reports that not only did Thales and Pythagoras study under the Egyptian philosophers, but that Plato, Eudoxus, and Lycurgus did as well. [109]

The Ancient Egyptian Supreme Being in the form of Amun was identified with Zeus in Greek mythology and later with Jupiter by the Romans in Roman Mythology. The Greek philosophers acknowledged that the High God of Greek mythology, Zeus, along with the entire pantheon of Greek gods and goddesses, which originated with him, came from Ethiopia. One of the main titles of Zeus was *"Ethiops."* Ethiops means "Black" and also the name of the country, which is directly south of Egypt: Ethiopia. It is important to note here that the Ancient Egyptians also acknowledged their own origins in Ethiopia and that Kamit, the ancient name for the land of Egypt, also means "Black land or land of the Blacks."

The main difference in the Greek and Roman interpretation of Amun was in the emphasis on the anthropomorphic personality and gender aspects of the God as well as the reduction in importance of the principles of immanence and panentheistic features of the theology. The female aspect of Amun was not equally expressed in the European interpretations. Consequently, the high god of the Greeks, while being a copy of the Ancient Egyptian Supreme Being, lacks the transcendental quality, that beyond the human characteristics of the physical personality. Therefore, a more "male" oriented feeling was developed around the highest form of divinity, which reflected the view of male superiority within Western society. While it is true that early Greek mythology incorporated female deities, they were relegated to lower positions of importance. In the Ancient Egyptian and Indian systems, it is understood, not only that the female deities are equal in importance as the male, being complementary opposites to each other, but that the Supreme Being is the unification of those opposite elements. This means that the Supreme Being is both male and female and not just male. This emphasis on the male aspect is a factor, which has steered the course of developments in both secular and non-secular issues of western culture. The most negative effects of this idea of the maleness of the Supreme Divinity translates into the idea of male superiority in household life, business, politics and religion. Of course this ultimately also leads to sexism and the abuse of women and males who exhibit to much of their female natures. In Ancient Egypt, the equality of the gods and goddesses translated into social equality for men and women. This kind of society has not been seen in over two thousand years. Thus, in order to promote justice and peace in society there must be religious, i.e. spiritual equality, first. This can be accomplished first by establishing the truth about religion and its universality and then implementing the correct practice of true religious principles in the area of ordinary human activities.

The idea of the transcendental aspect of Amun, which goes beyond the name, and form of the symbols was thus misunderstood. This misunderstanding gave rise to a personal god, which was believed to really exist separate from humanity instead of to the understanding that it is a symbol for the divinity, which is the essence of all things. The Greeks did not look to a "Hidden" divinity within themselves, but to a tangible personality, whom they could call upon, seek out, converse with and pray to. This interpretation of divinity played an important role in the development of early Christianity since it was in the midst of Greek and Roman culture that Orthodox Christianity took form once it moved from Egypt to Palestine, Turkey, Greece and finally Rome.

[I] Samos is an island in southeastern Greece, in the Aegean Sea, near the coast of Turkey.

Pythogora's' theories of *Metempsychosis* or reincarnation and transmigration, the theory of communal living and poverty, the ideas of vegetarianism, his Ausarian style funerary customs and his medical knowledge all point to his education in Ancient Egypt. These ideas and teachings were passed on into early Christianity through the Pythagorean cults, which persisted into the Christian era as Neo-Pythagoreanism. Neo-Pythagoreanism was a philosophical movement begun in the 1st century B.C.E. which continued until it was diluted by the rise of Neo-Platonism in the 3rd century A.C.E. Neo-Pythagoreanism developed at the start of the Christian era and combined Hellenistic and Jewish elements with the more mystical and religious aspects of Pythagorean philosophy. It was an influence on Neo-Platonism and the Jewish cult of the Essenes.

Neo-Platonism

Neo-Platonism was a school of philosophy that came to prominence between the years 250 and 550 A.C.E. "Neo" means new, however this school of philosophy included more than just a new version of Platonic thought. It combined Stoic, Pythagorean, Aristotelian and Platonic ideas steeped in Egyptian philosophy, with portions from Jewish, Christian and Oriental religions. Thus, the newness does not refer to the introduction of new teachings, but rather to the consolidation of teachings and the revival of earlier teachings. Neo-Platonism tended to be mystical and poetic rather than philosophical. The formative leaders of the movement included two third century philosophers, Plotinus and Porphyry. When the Emperor Justinian closed the Neo-Platonic academies in 529 A.C.E. along with other cult systems such as that of the Egyptian Aset, Orthodox Christianity was closing its doors on the last links to the mystical traditions. Still, their influences on Christianity persisted through medieval times into the present because in order to be accepted, the Orthodox Church had to adopt many customs and symbols of other religions. They had to do this in order to convince the followers of the other religions that Christianity had those symbols and customs previous to their "pagan" religion and therefore, that they should come to Christianity which is, according to the orthodox, the "true" and "original" religion.

Hellenism

The term 'Hellenism' refers to the culture of classical Greece. It is most particularly associated with Athens during the 5th century B.C.E. Thucydides and Herodotus exemplified the writing of history and Socrates (469-399 B.C.E.), followed by Plato (427-347 B.C.E.), his disciple, established standards for philosophy.

Greek philosophy and mythology were inspired and carried on by Greek philosophers who had studied in Egypt and wished to enlighten their native country, as many others who had also come to Egypt from elsewhere. In West Africa, the Dogons[I] and the Yorubas[II] carried on the Ancient Egyptian teachings. In East Asia, the Vedantins[III] and later the Buddhists and Taoists carried on the tradition. Therefore, it is no surprise that reincarnation, transmigration, rebirth, or metempsychosis, the passage of the soul through successive bodies in a cycle of birth and death in order to gain varied experiences in order to grow spiritually, was a tenet of early Christianity. In the 6th century B.C.E. reincarnation was taught as a religious-philosophical doctrine in Ancient Egypt, Greece and India. This belief also appears in Hinduism, Buddhism, Jainism, and Sikhism. Herodotus informs us that reincarnation and the immortality of the soul was understood and taught by the Egyptians before any other peoples. [64]

Alexander the Great emerged as a student of philosophy and world conqueror. When he took control of the Greek Empire he tried to unite the entire civilized world under a single banner. He instinctively sought to conquer the major territories, which were the sources of religious and philosophical strength of the ancient world, which the Egyptian civilization had once covered.[IV] Having achieved control over Greece itself by putting down all dissenting factions, he stretched forth southward and eastward into Egypt, Mesopotamia and India, thereby controlling these three centers of Art, Philosophy and religion of the then known world.

Alexander The Great

Socrates (470? -399? B.C.E.) was regarded as one of the most important philosophers of ancient Greece. He ended up spending most of his life in Athens, however, he was known to have studied under the Ionian philosophers. This establishes a direct link between Socrates and his teaching with Ancient Egypt. Socrates had a tremendous influence on many disciples. One of the most popular of these was Plato. Plato in turn taught others including

---

[I] Dogon, people whose traditional ancestral dwellings are in remote cave-villages in the Hombori Mountains of the Mali Republic after they migrated from Egypt in Ancient times. Their religion is notable for its abstract concepts and a powerful creation myth and its similarities to Ancient Egyptian Religion. Dogon religion- religion-see Egyptian Yoga Volume I: The Philosophy of Enlightenment.

[II] Yoruba, Sudanic-speaking African people inhabiting southwest Nigeria. Yoruba religion-see Egyptian Yoga Volume I: The Philosophy of Enlightenment.

[III] Followers of Hindu-Vedanta philosophy from India.

[IV] Ancient writings tell of the Ancient Egyptian civilization encompassing southern Europe and East to as far as India in the time of Osiris and later during the rule of Pharaoh (king) Ramses II of Egypt.

Aristotle (384-322 B.C.E.) who was Plato's disciple for 19 years. After Plato's death, Aristotle opened a school of philosophy in Asia Minor. Aristotle educated Philip of Macedon's son, Alexander (Alexander the Great), between the years 343 and 334 B.C.E. Aristotle then returned to Athens and opened a school in the Lyceum (the school near Athens where Aristotle lectured to his students). He urged Alexander onto his conquests since in the process, he, Aristotle, was able to gain in knowledge from the ancient writings of the conquered countries. After Alexander's conquest of Egypt, Aristotle became the author of over 1,000 books on philosophy. Building on Plato's *Theory of the Forms*, Aristotle developed the theory of *The Unmoved Mover*, which is a direct teaching from Memphite Theology in Ancient Egypt. Among his works are De Anima, Nicomachean Ethics and Metaphysics.

Alexander the Great represented a great military force, which propelled Europeans for the first time out into the world. With the goal of uniting the known world under his realm, Alexander conquered Greece, Egypt, and reached as far as India, where he and other Greek philosophers recognized that the Greek gods and goddesses corresponded to the Indian pantheon of gods and goddesses of Hinduism and the gods and goddesses of Ancient Egypt. This *synchretic* view of religion was not held by the Jews. They would never say that Yahweh is equal to Shiva, Zeus or Asar. Trade between the Mediterranean countries and the Far East was flourishing during the time following the conquests of Alexander the Great. Alexandria, his capital city in Egypt, became the center of the sciences, philosophy and Enlightenment in the ancient world. At the height of the Roman Empire, which had by that time succeeded the Greeks, European conquests encompassed North Africa, Europe, the Near East and Britain. Throughout this time the Roman Empire used Persian soldiers and others who carried with them the varying religious beliefs throughout all parts of the empire. The opportunity to study at Alexandria with its great library[1] was the ambition of all who wished to attain the heights of excellence in every field. Thus, along with Buddhist monks sent to Egypt and the rest of the Mediterranean by the Indian emperor *Ashoka*, Indian yogis also traveled along the trade routs espousing the teachings of Yoga and Vedanta. From Hippolitus (c.225 A.C.E.), a Christian writer speaking out on the "heresies" of the time, we find Indian Brahmins included as one of the "pagan religions."

> There is...among the Indians, a heresy of those who philosophize among the Brahmins, who live a self-sufficient life, abstaining from {eating} living creatures and all cooked food... They say that God is light, not like the light one sees, nor like the sun nor fire, but to them God is discourse, not that which finds expression in articulate sounds, but that of knowledge (gnosis) through which the secret mysteries of nature are perceived by the wise.[39]

In the statement above we have Gnostic principles being compared with the mysteries of India and condemned by an Orthodox Christian as being equally heretical. One of the main goals of Indian philosophy is to lead the aspirant through philosophical as well as physical disciplines to understand his/her union with creation, the illusoriness of worldly objects and to understand the cause of misery as originating in the endless wellspring of desires which flow from the mind that suffers from ignorance of it's true nature. Therefore, by discovering the peace which lies beyond craving for objects and by developing a self-sufficient lifestyle free of worldly entanglements, spiritual enlightenment emerges. The understanding of the Divinity as light, Ra, was present in Ancient Egyptian religion from the earliest times and consequently, it was transferred into Egyptian and Christian Gnosticism (see Gospel of Thomas, verse 11). The light was also seen as the source of enlightenment. The abstention from eating flesh foods and cooked foods is a major tenet of the Ancient Egyptian Mysteries, Jainism, Buddhism and Indian Yoga disciplines.

From The Gospel of Thomas
>24
>His (Jesus') disciples said to Him, "Show us the place where You are, since it is necessary for us to seek it." He said to them, "Whoever has ears, let him hear. There is light within a man of light, and he (or "it") lights up the whole world. If he (or "it") does not shine, he (or "it") is darkness."

---

[1] *Alexandria, Library of,* The world's first state-funded scientific institution, founded 330 BC in Alexandria, Egypt, by Ptolemy I and further expanded by Ptolemy II. It comprised a museum, teaching facilities, and a library that contained 700,000 scrolls, including much ancient Greek literature. It sustained significant damage AD 391, when Theodosius I ordered its destruction.[126]

DRUIDISM, CELTIC CHRISTIANITY AND THE ARTHURIAN LEGENDS

The Celts[I] were a people who controlled a large quantity of central and Western Europe in the 1st millennium B.C.E. So their language, customs, and religion were passed on to the other peoples of that area.

The earliest archaeological evidence related to the Celts identifies them in the region that is now known as France and western Germany, around 1200 B.C.E. They are believed to have begun to settle in the British Isles during this time. Their influence extended from the area now known as Spain to the shores of the Black Sea between the 5th and 1st centuries B.C.E. The word Celt is derived from Keltoi. Keltoi or the Kelts was the name given to them by the Greek historian Herodotus and some other Greek writers. The continental Celts were known as Galli or the Gauls, and the Celts in Britain were called Britanni by the Romans.

The Celts invaded the Greco-Roman world (southern Europe) in the 4th century B.C.E. They conquered parts of the Roman empire, but as time passed, the Romans subdued them and finally Transalpine Gaul (the land known today as modern France and the Rhineland) was captured by Julius Caesar in the 1st century B.C.E. Most of Britain came under Roman control in the 1st century A.C.E. During the same time, the Germanic peoples dominated the Celts of central Europe.

Each Celtic tribe was headed by a king and was generally divided into three classes. These were the Druids (priests), warrior nobles, and commoners. Celtic mythology included various woodland spirits, earth gods, sun deities, elfin demons and tutelary[II] deities. These beings still exist in the lore of the followers of Celtic mythology or who have Celtic ancestry. Druidism is the religious faith of the ancient Celtic inhabitants of the British Isles and Gaul. In the areas of Britain that the Romans did not control, the practice of Druidism survived for many centuries until it was superseded and displaced by Christianity. The Druids believed in the immortality of the soul, and that at the time of death or shortly after the soul was believed to go into the body of a newborn child and thus reincarnate. The Druids also believed that they originated and descended from a Supreme Being.

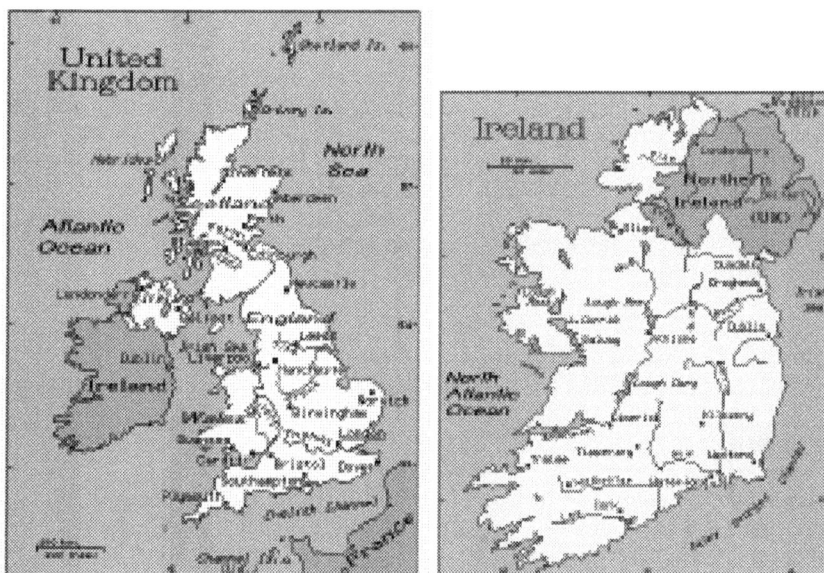

Above: the United Kingdom and Ireland.

The ancient accounts related to the Druids from 200 B.C.E. to 200 A.C.E. resemble the social order in Ancient Egypt during the same period, at the end of the Dynastic Egypt. Although there were no castes as such in Ancient Egypt, there were groups of professionals, priests politicians, nobles and the common folk. The priests were the most powerful group in Ancient Egyptian civilization. They guided every aspect of life in ancient times. The Druid priests were assisted by female sorcerers or prophets. They did not have the same privileges and powers of 5the Druids priests however. In earlier times, Ancient Egyptian priestesses were important in the Ancient Egyptian

---

[I] **Celt** (kĕlt, sĕlt) also **Kelt** (kĕlt) --*n.* **1.** One of an Indo-European people originally of central Europe and spreading to western Europe, the British Isles, and southeast to Galatia during pre-Roman times, especially a Briton or Gaul.[115]
[II] Being or serving as a guardian or protector.

143

temples. There were several high priestesses especially related to the temples of goddesses such as Aset and Hathor. However, as Ancient Egyptian society and culture declined and the Greeks and Romans gained permanent control over Egypt, the social order and the equality of women fell to the status of singers, chanters and assistants to the priests. The Druids also used the pyramid (triangle) symbol. When it is considered that in ancient times the Egyptian civilization extended into Europe, the similarities between the Druids and the Ancient Egyptian priesthood is understandable.

Celtic Christianity

In the 4th century A.C.E., the Christian faith was established in Celtic Britain. However, in the 5th century, the Saxons[I] invaded the country with the Angles[II] and Jutes.[III] The Christians Celts (Britons) were driven westward into Cornwall and Wales. During this time, St. Patrick and other British missionaries founded a new church in Ireland. This church became the center of Celtic Christianity. The monks from Ireland were devoted to religion and learning. They preserved the knowledge of the ancient Roman literature in Europe during the early medieval period. Then between the late 6th and the early 8th centuries, Irish missionaries were Christianizing the Germanic peoples who had conquered the Western Roman Empire. They founded many monasteries in the lands presently known as Switzerland, France, Germany, and Italy. Celtic Christianity was weakened in Ireland by the Viking[IV] invasions, which occurred in the 9th and 10th centuries A.C.E. The strong Roman church superceded the Celtic Christian tradition by the 12th century. Thus, the traces of Celtic mysticism were supplanted until recent times when many adherents to New Age spirituality sought to revive some of the Celtic (Druid) teachings.

Celtic cross

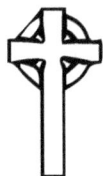

In modern times, the island of Ireland, which lies across the Irish Sea from Great Britain is divided into two governments. About five-sixths of the island is occupied by the Republic of Ireland. The northern part of the island, known as Northern Ireland, is known as Ulster because, in ancient times, six of the counties which had made up the Celtic Kingdom were located there in earlier times. In modern times, the people of Northern Ireland have cultural ties to England and Scotland. However, most of them settled there in the 17th century and most of them were Protestants. Southern Ireland is held to the Catholic-Celtic background. In the late 20th century, the Celtic influence has waned and most inhabitants remain as Roman Catholics.

In ancient times, the Celts had begun to move to Ireland around 300 A.C.E. It was then that Christianity influenced them. In 1169, England began to conquer Ireland, and from then on the Irish and the English-Irish were seen as enemies of England. The British controlled Northern Ireland for 750 years. In 1921 the British made South Ireland into a dominion, meaning a self-governing member of the British Commonwealth of Nations. In 1949 the association with Great Britain broke when Southern Ireland became a republic. However, Northern Ireland remained politically related to the United Kingdom. Great Britain or the United Kingdom is officially called United Kingdom of Great Britain and Northern Ireland. It consists of England, Scotland, Wales, the Channel Islands, Northern Ireland (Ulster), and the Isle of Man.

The issue of union or separation with the Republic of Ireland or United Kingdom has long dominated politics in Northern Ireland. This split has followed religious lines. The majority of the people have voted in favor of Northern Ireland remaining in the United Kingdom. Elections on the issue must be held at not less than ten-year intervals.[117]

The Arthurian Legends

The Arthurian Legends were important in the formation of European Christianity, and British Christianity in particular. The Arthurian Legends surround a group of tales written in several languages that developed in the Middle Ages concerning Arthur, a mythical king of the Britons, and his knights. The legend is a combination of Ancient Celtic mythology with later Christian traditions surrounding a possible historical personality.

The first references to Arthur appear in Welsh, the Celtic language of Wales circa 600 A.C.E. In later tales Arthur is identified as the son of the British king Uther Pendragon, and his counselor Merlin (Sage, Spiritual preceptor, Guru to Arthur) is introduced. Merlin is a personification of the Druid mystical wisdom teacher. The Arthurian Legends surrounded the life of the mythic king Arthur and the Knights of the Round Table who strove to establish truth and righteousness in the land after the fall of the Roman Empire. He was a protector and quasi-savior

---

[I] A member of a Germanic tribal group that inhabited northern Germany.
[II] A Germanic tribe who together with the Jutes and Saxons formed the Anglo-Saxon peoples.
[III] Early Germanic tribe of Denmark or northern Germany.
[IV] One of a seafaring Scandinavian people (Nordic people—Danes, Swedes, Norwegians) who plundered the coasts of Europe from the 9th to the 11th century. This period was known as the Viking Age.

who united the Britons against foreign attackers and who promoted truth and justice. The stories tell of the isle of Avalon, a magical place where Arthur went to recover from wounds received in his last battle. The stories also introduce characters such as Guinevere (Arthur's queen) and tell of her infidelity and the rebellion instigated by Arthur's nephew Mordred.

The first English Arthurian story appears in 1205 A.C.E. with the poet Layamon's Roman de Brut. Arthur is depicted as an epic warrior. The story of his magic sword Excalibur, which only he could extract from a rock, is included for the first time here. This parallels the Hindu epic *Ramayana* where the main character, Rama, an Avatar of the God Vishnu, extracts a bow which no one but he can remove from where it was, embedded in a rock.

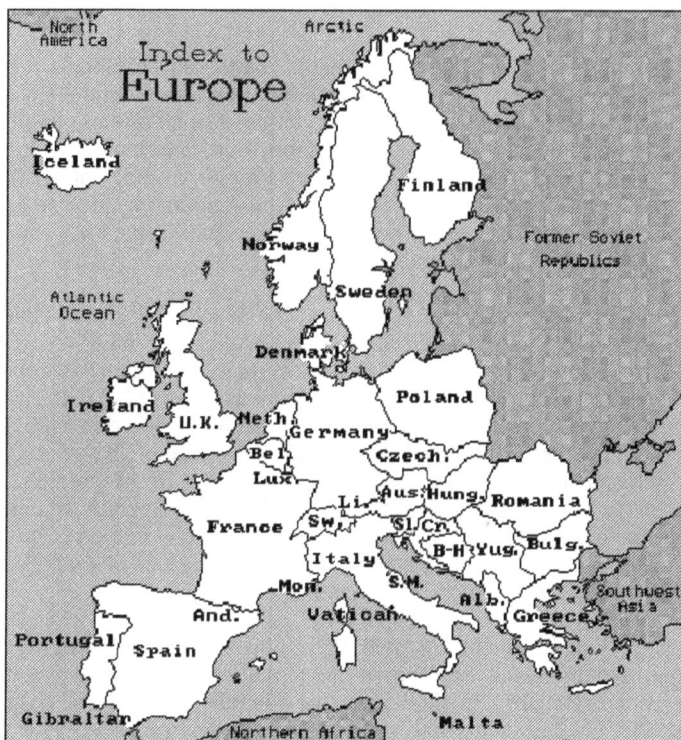

Left: Europe and the Western Roman Empire Below: A European Knight.

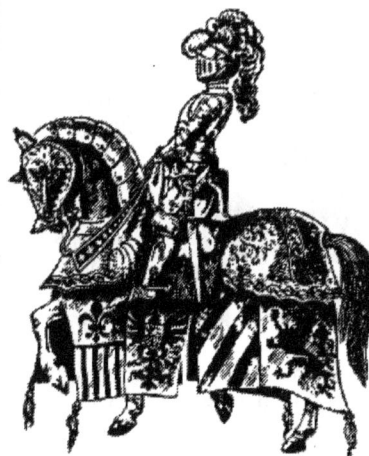

The possible historicity of the story in Britain emerges from the legend of a Roman soldier named Arthur, a native of Britain that was trained by the Romans in the art of war. The writers of the time, Nennius (c. 800 A.C.E.) and Gildas (d. 570) described him as a *dux bellorum* or "a leader in war."[58] He remained behind in Britain after the Romans withdrew and the Roman Empire fell. He was said to have rallied various groups and trained them in the art of warfare which he had learned from the Roman army, and led the British people to protect themselves from outside invasions.

An Arthurian tradition was developed in Europe as well. It most likely was based on stories, which were handed down from the Celts who had immigrated to Brittany in the 5th and 6th centuries A.C.E. The earliest French Arthurian romances are a series of poems by Chrétien de Troyes in the 12th-century. One of these introduced Sir Lancelot and Percival (Parzival). This is the earliest recorded 5story related to the search for the Holy Grail.

The Holy Grail ("bowl") is a medieval myth related to the sacred cup, which was used by Jesus Christ at the Last Supper. It was supposed to have been later piously sought after by the knights of the legendary round table of King Arthur. Tradition holds that the Grail was preserved by Joseph of Arimathea, who was, according to all four Gospels of the New Testament, a rich and pious Jew. After the crucifixion of Jesus Christ he requested the body of Jesus from the Roman procurator, Pontius Pilate, and placed the body in his own tomb. According to some ancient writers he was said to be the founder of Christianity in Britain, but most scholars however, reject these claims. In the writings of the Arthurian legends and in late medieval legend, he is said to have brought the Holy Grail into Britain. According to the tradition, Joseph of Arimathea collected the blood from the body of the crucified Christ in the Grail. The vessel was then taken to Britain where it was handed down within Joseph's descendants. The Grail was supposed to possess many miraculous properties. It had the power of providing food for those who were without sin, blinding those who were impure of heart, or striking dumb those who were irreverent. Many important facets of the

Grail story are now seen by scholars as having as arisen from a Celtic myth that was Christianized. The myth involves a hero and a magic vessel.

The deeper mystical meaning of the search for the Grail is the search for one's own connection to the Divine. In this case, the myth was intertwined with the personality of Jesus, but it relates to discovering one's own Christhood, which is the wellspring of all power and all glory because therein lies our own divinity in God. This search is most effectively exemplified in the Arthurian writings surrounding the knight known as Percival, whose purity and righteousness allowed him to discover it.

The Fall of Rome and the Breakup of the Church

After the fall of Rome in c. 476, the Western Roman Empire divided into unstable "barbarian" kingdoms. There was much strife and chaos in Europe at this time and the inhabitants of Europe suffered invasions from the Vikings as well as from northern hoards of barbarians such as the Vandals[I] and others. This period is often referred to as the Dark Ages.[II] Many of Europeans adopted Roman institutions and attempted to establish order in their own locals while at the same time fighting off outside invasions. During this time the Byzantine Empire became cut off from the West and the church in Rome. In the West Christianity became a powerful political tool among the barbarian kingdoms in the late Middle Ages.[III] Many students of history note that Christianity was almost wiped out and the kingdoms of the dark ages were almost destroyed by the invasions from outside.

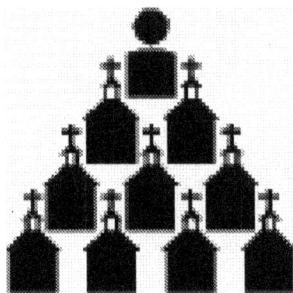

One figure was instrumental in the survival of the Western Christian church. Charlemagne (742-814 A.C.E.), was the king of the Franks,[IV] (768-814 A.C.E.) and the Roman emperor from 800-814 A.C.E. He captured the Lombard throne in Italy (773 A.C.E.). Due to the Saxon raids, he waged war from 772 A.C.E. to 785 A.C.E. and conquered Saxony, thereby securing Christianity. Charlemagne also captured Bavaria and defeated the Avars of the middle Danube in 791-96 A.C.E., 804 A.C.E., which added new lands to his empire. In 811 A.C.E. he strengthened Christianity in parts of northern Spain by establishing the Spanish March, a Christian refuge there. Pope Leo III in 800 A.C.E crowned him emperor. He had united the Germanic peoples for the first time, but his empire lacked strength and broke up after his death. Charlemagne was canonized[V] in 1165 A.C.E.

The challenge to the church hierarchy.

As time passed, various European kingdoms consolidated their power and used religion for political purposes. Christianity was used by Christian religious and political leaders as a weapon against rivals and foreigners who opposed them. In this sense the church assumed the right to persecute those who would not convert to Christianity and to suppress any dissenting religious and political views which it labeled as heresy. Thus, being in control of the government, the church was able to use religion as a way to accomplish political and economic goals as it wished.

The Byzantines considered themselves as Romans and therefore as heirs of the Roman Empire even though their society was a mixture of many social and cultural elements due to the cosmopolitan nature of the city. The Byzantines modeled their government after the Roman Empire while adopting Greek language and cultural customs in general. However, Orthodox Christianity determined their religious direction.

After the fall of Rome, the Byzantine State attempted to continue the Roman Empire. When the Roman Empire in the West had fallen into decline due to the Germanic invasions, imperial traditions were kept alive in the East. Emperor Justinian I (r.527-65) re-conquered the territory which had been held by the old Roman Empire, and codified the Roman law between the years 610 A.C.E. to 717 A.C.E. The empire defeated its Persian enemies under the Heraclian emperors. The Macedonian epoch of 867 A.C.E. to 1081 A.C.E. is referred to as the Golden Age of the Byzantine Empire. This was the time of cultural renaissance and territorial consolidation. The West was slowly emerging from the interminable wars and social crisis of the Dark and Middle ages. As the first millennium A.C.E. drew to a close, the West began to reconstruct Europe. Then the attention turned towards foreign conquests and on asserting control over all Christian churches, property and authority, which Constantinople had assumed after the fall of the Roman Empire. A struggle ensued between the Church leaders of Rome (Western Roman Empire) and

---

[I] A member of a Germanic people that overran Gaul, Spain, and northern Africa in the fourth and fifth centuries A.C.E. and sacked Rome in c. 455.

[II] The early part of the Middle Ages from about A.C.E. 500 to about A.C.E. 1000.

[III] The period in European history between antiquity and the Renaissance, regarded as dating from A.C.E. 476 to 1453.

[IV] Germanic peoples who settled along the Rhine river in the 3rd century A.C.E.

[V] When the church declares a deceased person a saint.

Constantinople (Eastern Roman empire) due to disagreements as to the canon of the Christian doctrine and the authority of the Christian church.

The Church of Rome claimed not only the primacy of Rome, but also the doctrine of papal infallibility, which held that the Roman Pope was the final authority on Church matters. Having regained military power after defeating the barbarian groups of Europe, the Western empire promoted the crusades which would effectively expand the Western Christian Church Empire and at the same time gain control over the domain of the Eastern Empire. The crusaders gained control over Byzantium during the dominion of the Latin Empire of Constantinople (1204-61). In 1261, Michael VIII, restored the Greek Empire (Eastern Church), and founded the Palaeologan dynasty (1261-1453). In 1453, Constantinople fell to the Turkish forces of Sultan Muhammad II and the Byzantine Empire came to a final end, never to rise again. Nevertheless, the Eastern Church subsequently broke up into two major sects, the Eastern Orthodox Church and the Coptic Church in Egypt which had, up to that time, remained in association with Constantinople. The following is a brief look at the modern history of the Christian churches.

Protestantism - Martin Luther (c. 1517 A.C.E.)

During the Dark and Middle ages, the Catholic Church had engaged in acts of political and religious repression. In addition, many other aspects of church conduct led to discontent, not only among the general populace, but also within the ranks of the nobility as well as the honest clergy. These included sexual misconduct by the priests, the perpetuation of sexists social rules which subjugated women, economic injustices that favored nobles and merchants, the religious wars of conquest (including the crusades). Later on in history, this contributed to the sanctioning of the African slave trade and the destruction of Native American civilizations. In response to the perceived corruption and straying from the original doctrines, Martin Luther and others developed new major Christian groups in an attempt to go back to the original teachings of the church. Luther believed that the church should go back to the original teachings of the Bible and that the Bible itself should be the highest authority in church matters instead of the theologians, bishops and popes. Protestantism became a popular religion for political reasons as well. In much the same way as the Roman Catholic Church used religion as a pretext to conquer other countries and capture the lands and economic resources of those who would not convert, many of those who followed the new religious sect did so in order to have a legitimate reason to separate themselves from the authority of Rome.

Matthew 16
18 And I say also to thee, That thou art Peter, and upon this rock I will build my church; and the gates of hell shall not prevail against it. {Peter: this name signifies a rock}

After this period there were several Roman Catholic Church Councils which met to reform the church in light of the new Protestant movements. Some of the most important ones were the Lateran Councils, and later the Council of Trent. Various denominations of Christian Churches developed between 1550 to the present. Currently there are over 600 different Christian Church denominations, all claiming to be the true Church. The question of what or where is the true church has puzzled all Christian groups since the time of Jesus. The passage above from Matthew 16:18 in the traditional New Testament is the theme upon which the Roman Catholic church has based its authority to create and build its organization. Certainly, Jesus never intended the church to become a monolithic organization, which controls vast resources and material wealth. The examples of saints such as St. Francis of Assisi and Mother Teresa, who gave their lives and wealth in the service of humanity, more closely follow the ideal of Jesus' own life and works.

Matthew 19
24 And again I say to you, It is easier for a camel to go through the eye of a needle, than for a rich man to enter into the Kingdom of God.

In any case, the way in which the church has used its authority has effectively alienated sufficient peoples around the world to cause a permanent rift, which will prevent a total reunification of the church under one ruling authority.

Among the most popular sects of the Protestants are the Baptists. Baptists are members of an evangelical Protestant church of congregational organization. They follow the reformed tradition in worship, and believe in individual freedom, the separation of church and state, and in the baptism of voluntary, conscious believers.

As stated earlier, Biblical scholarship proves that the scriptures of the Bible were not all created at the same time nor by the same person or persons. They were created, edited and revised over a period of more than 1,000 years until a final version was compiled and canonized in the first four hundred years of the first millennia A. D. As discussed, there are some differences between the Bible of the Christians and Jews. To elaborate on this point further, the Jewish Bible is made up of the Hebrew Scriptures consisting of 39 books, which were originally written, in Hebrew, except for some sections written in Aramaic. The Christian Bible is divided into two parts. These are the Old Testament with 39 books and the 27 books of the New Testament in the King James Version. The two main divisions of Christendom (Roman, Eastern) have structured the Old Testament into two slightly different formats. The Old Testament which is used by the Roman Catholics is the same as the Bible of Judaism along with seven other books and additions to the 39 books of the Jewish Bible. Some of the additional books along with the New Testament were originally written in Greek. The Protestants' version of the Old Testament is confined to the 39 books of the Jewish Bible.

The Apocrypha are certain writings of the Old Testament which are not considered canonical by Jews and Protestants, but which are generally included in the Roman Catholic canon. *Canon* in Christian terminology refers to a standard or rule. The word began to refer to the doctrines recognized as orthodox by the Christian Church in the middle of the third century. As time passed, the term was used to indicate collectively the list of books, which were accepted as, authorized scriptures or "canonized," by the "official church." The Apocrypha consists of the following books: *Second Esdras, First Esdras, Tobit, Wisdom, Judith, Ecclesiasticus, The Prayer of Manasses, Baruch, First Maccabees* and *Second Maccabees*. Also included are the following parts of these books: Esther 10.4 to 16.24 and Daniel 3.24-90, 13, and 14. The term "apocryphal" is sometimes also used to identify New Testament writings, which are considered by the church authorities to be inauthentic or not having originated from the true teachings, related to Jesus.

The Church of England, The King James Bible and the Struggle for Power between the Protestants and The Pope in Rome

The Church of England or the Anglican Church is the Christian church in England. It dates back to the first years of the third century A.C.E. and records referring to it can be found in the writings of the early church fathers. The early ritual and discipline of the early English church were largely introduced by the Celtic and Gaelic missionaries and monks. After the arrival of St. Augustine from Rome in 597 A.C.E., the fusion of Celtic and Roman influences occurred. After the Norman Conquest (1066 A.C.E.), the continental influence in the Church of England strengthened the connections between the English church and Rome. This promoted obedience to the papacy. The power of the church extended to secular affairs; the nobles and royalty of England opposed this. Several of them tried to limit the power of Rome in England but it was not until the reign of Henry VIII that the royalty took some power away from the Church of Rome.

The acts of the English Parliament between 1529 A.C.E. and 1536 A.C.E. marked the beginning of the establishment of the Anglican church as a national church, independent of papal jurisdiction. Henry VIII was upset because of the pope's refusal to annul his marriage to Catherine of Aragón. Henry VIII induced Parliament to enact a series of statutes denying the pope any power or jurisdiction over the Church of England. Henry VIII received the support of the overwhelming majority of clerical and lay Englishmen.

In 1549 A.C.E., the first Anglican Book of Common Prayer was published, and its use required of the English clergy by an Act of Uniformity. The second prayer book reflected the influence of continental Protestantism more strongly. It was issued in 1552 and was followed shortly by the Forty-two Articles, a doctrinal statement similar in tone.

The events outlined above led to the creation of the King James Bible. The King James Bible is a translation of the Bible ordered by King James I of England in 1604 A.C.E. It was completed in 1611, and is also called the Authorized Version. The King James Version became the standard Bible in Anglican Communion. There have been several revisions of the King James text. Some of these are the Revised Version in the late 19th century and the Revised Standard Version (1946-57). Thus, the King James Bible is a product of the Anglican vision of separation from Rome.

For a short period, the *Puritans* and other Protestants gained control of the government and ousted the monarchy of England. The Puritans were an advanced group (one of the first to arrive) of the Protestants in England in the days of the Reformation.[1] The division began among the religious exiles from England who sought refuge on the Continent during the Roman Catholic persecutions. In general, the Puritans were inclined to follow the lead of John Knox, Dr. Richard Cox, and the Swiss reformers, who rejected the Roman church because they could not find its authority in the Scriptures. They therefore reduced the worship in their churches to a bare simplicity. Their

---

[1] conflict separated the Christians of Western Europe into Protestants and Catholics.

opposition to written prayers, religious images and pictures in churches, instrumental music at services, etc., marked their form of worship.

Some of the Puritans wanted more than just to purify the church services. They also wanted to change the whole government of the church. The *Presbyterians* wanted to completely do away with the government system of bishops in the church, but would retain a system of state churches. Others sects, called *Independents* or *Separatists* wanted the state and church to be completely separated and they also wanted each congregation to manage its own affairs church. This sect was later called *Congregationalists*. More radical reformers called *Anabaptists* believed that baptism by immersion should be reserved only for adults. They also held other similarly unconventional views as to church and state. The government of most western countries has been so strongly influenced by the separatist tradition that this philosophy is now seen as a virtue. Yet, it developed as a backlash from the corruption of the catholic church's rule during the late Roman, Dark and Middle Ages, the Crusade period and afterwards leading up to the creation of Protestantism. In reality, those government officials who would like to do illegal or immoral acts use this argument because it frees them from having to deal with issues of righteousness. This philosophy has opened the door to the culture of greed and self-gratification. When business concerns override the public good there is bound to be injustice and degradation in the morals of society. Since this form of thinking is in opposition to caring and ethics, there is necessarily a large disparity between the rich and poor and the other manners of discrimination which are also easily practiced. Since God is the essence of Creation, spirituality has to be an integral part of every area of society. But the leaders of religion must be Enlightened Sages and not merely philosophers or theologians. In Ancient Egypt this teaching was understood well. The Pharaoh was not merely a political leader, but the head of the Church. The religious leaders who were lawyers, architects, business people, etc ran the government. In this manner they applied the strict rules of righteousness (Precepts of Maat) in every area of society. This is what allowed them to carry on a civilization, which flourished for over ***five thousand years.*** By contrast, the modern civilizations of the western world cannot be considered civilized because they have not reached a level of peace, stability and government based on righteousness and ethics. People consider the capitalist economic system and the democratic or parliamentary government system as signs of civilization but these, as practiced in modern western countries, produce economic imbalances and situations where some people get rich by taking advantage of others. Then they use their economic power to control public information, ideas and opinion. This is not freedom and it is not democracy. Thus, it is against Christianity. This called *Oligarchy* or Government by a few, especially by a small faction of persons or families.

Psalm 82

> 3 Defend the poor and fatherless: do justice to the afflicted and needy. {Defend: Heb. Judge}
> 4 Deliver the poor and needy: deliver [them] from the hand of the wicked.

In the Bible book of Psalms it says that the strong and powerful should defend the weak and abused. Jesus himself ministered and healed the spiritually and physically infirm. However, modern civilization has been constructed by subjugating poor peoples and exploiting them through slavery or creating economic conditions so that they remain in debt with no hope for improvement. This is un-Christian and must be remedied. It can only be remedied when Christians rise up to the true heritage of Christ Consciousness wherein one sees others in need as oneself, and one does not rest until everyone is healed, fed, educated, loved and provided for with every opportunity to enjoy and discover the meaning of life. In this area Mother Teresa led an exemplary life. Anything less than this lofty but attainable goal is un-Christian, it is worldly selfishness and sinful exploitation of others.

It was a group of the Separatists who migrated first to Holland in 1608 A.C.E., and then also to America in 1620. They founded Plymouth Colony (Plymouth, Mass.). Thus, it is clear to see from where the ideas of "separation of church and state" in the politics of the United States of America as well as the separation of Christians in America from the Church of Rome come. Since America was strongly influenced by these groups, the developing Christian churches have carried on these philosophies ever since. It is therefore important to realize that while the Anglican Christian tradition contains many of the same scriptures as does the church in Rome, they did away with those elements which lead to mystical or spiritual discovery and concentrate on those doctrines that promote political freedom of expression. This is a doctrine that was native to England and Europe due to the political upheavals, which they were experiencing at the time in the struggle for power between the Church of Rome and the royalty of Europe. These issues were not inherent in Africa or elsewhere, and the Anglican Church did not share the positive gains in the struggle against domination and exploitation with all peoples. Otherwise, they would not have condoned the slave trade and the stealing of America from the Native Americans. As a group, the Christian Churches that developed out of England were responsible for condoning slavery and murder. The church in Rome is also guilty because it did not do enough to denounce and stop the injustices.

The foundation of an independent Protestant Episcopal church in the United States dates from the time of the American Revolution, when members of the Anglican church in the former colonies could no longer give their allegiance to the mother church overseas. There followed the establishment of a number of other churches, centering upon the Church of England that became known as the Anglican Communion. In addition to the churches of England, Ireland, Wales and the Episcopal church in Scotland, separate and independent Anglican churches exist in Canada, the United States, Australia, New Zealand, western Africa, central Africa, the Republic of South Africa, India, China, Japan, and the West Indies. These churches and their numerous missions are located in nearly every area of the world, many of them among peoples of diverse origin who have become naturalized to the Anglo-Saxon culture. Thus, the influence of Anglo-Saxon culture has been felt around the world, and with it, the confusion over church doctrine, the rivalry between different sects, the church of Rome, and the political values of the Separatists and other Protestants.

The Church of England differs from the Roman Catholic Church mainly in that it denies the claims of the papacy to jurisdiction over the church and to infallibility as promulgator of Christian doctrinal and moral truth, and in rejecting the distinctively Roman doctrines and discipline. Also, unlike the Roman Catholic Church, the Church of England allows women to become priests. In 1975 the General Synod of the Anglican Church found the ordination of women to be theologically unobjectionable, although it was almost 20 years later before the first women were ordained in 1994.

The Church of England differs from the Eastern Orthodox Church to a lesser degree. The Anglican Church and its sister churches in the Anglican Communion differ from most Protestant churches in requiring Episcopal ordination for all their clergy. They also differ in the structure and tone of their liturgical services, which are translations and revised versions of the pre-Reformation services of the church. Other differences can be found in a spiritual orientation in which a Catholic sacramental heritage is combined with the biblical and evangelical emphasis that came through the Reformation. [75]

So if a person is looking for the original teachings of Christianity, there is much complicated history and dogma to sift through if they are searching through the church system and the various denominations. It is necessary to know the various political and social impetuses, which pushed people to promote certain doctrines over others. For these reasons, in the end, the church may not be the best source for those who want to go beyond the divisions caused by arguments over authority and jurisdiction. This problem has caused many to search elsewhere for answers. This of course is the path of those who are truly serious about discovering the important spiritual truths of life. The Christian church of Rome is an exponent of Western (European) culture, while the Church of England and its development in the form of the various churches in the Americas are exponents of Anglo-Saxon culture.

So, as we have seen, in tracing the roots of western religion Africa must be seen as not only the cradle of civilization, but also as the mother of the Christian church. In addition, any true reformation of the church must first include a repudiation of social injustice and must include the higher ideal of a mystical goal, rather than simply following some scriptures as the main practice and concern of the religion. How can the church promote peace on earth and good will to all when these virtues are lacking within the church itself?

Racism in the Christian Church and The Heroism of the Quaker Movement

The subject of racism in the Christian Church has been touched on throughout this text. However, this brief section will be devoted to acknowledging the movement within Christianity against racial injustices. Also, the point should be made here that not all Europeans believed in or supported the African slave trade or the mistreatment of Native Americans. Some fought hard and even died for the cause of freedom and universal fellowship among all peoples. They upheld the highest principle of humanity and civilization, the Golden Rule, a saying of Jesus, "Therefore all things whatsoever ye would that men should do to you, do ye even so to them: for this is the law and the prophets" (Bible, Matthew 7:12); also similarly stated Luke 6:31. These were the true Christians. We have seen how the church has been used by many people throughout history to promote the destruction and enslavement of others. Even though there have been some strides in curtailing the outward expressions of racism and discrimination, especially in western countries and the United States of America in particular, the ethnic groups remain divided and injustices continue to be perpetrated by so called Christians and others against peoples of non-European descent. At present (1998), the Christian services every week point up the factor of racial division, especially in the United States, as a majority of European Americans go to churches with predominantly all-white congregations and African Americans go to churches with predominantly black congregations. The stark reality is that many African Americans (blacks) feel resentment towards peoples of European decent, especially those who are descendants of the slave owners in the United States and those who promoted the African slave trade. On the other hand, European Americans (whites) feel a range of emotions from guilt, denial, and fear to bigotry and racism. Some feel guilt over what their ancestors did. Some deny responsibility, even though they enjoy the benefits of slavery. Many rich families owe their wealth to the institution of slavery. Others fear African Americans as a result of the portrayal of African Americans by racists government leaders and scholars as inferior and hostile, and erroneously or maliciously use the Bible teachings, such as those related to Ham (Genesis 9:25), to support their racist philosophy. Actually, the Bible does not support any separation of peoples with respect to their ethnicity, otherwise Abraham would not have married Hagar, an Egyptian woman (Genesis 16:1-3), and Moses would not have married an Ethiopian woman (Numbers 12:1). In both cases God blessed the union. Therefore, why do some people have a problem with something that God blesses? These ignorant and racist statements have caused a rift, which can only be repaired when the evil and erroneous nature of these teachings is addressed, and when the churches make an attempt to reconcile and affirm the true teachings of Christianity which support unity, regardless of ethnicity.

One problem in this area is that many people refuse to admit that the problem exists. Others want to forget about it and see it as a problem of the past, yet, to this day, there is more segregation than ever in the churches and there is more and more racial unrest in society. In recent years, the bombing of African American and other churches points to the failure of the church establishment, as a whole, to reconcile the sins of racism. It is unfortunate that no significant progress towards reconciliation has been made in the last thirty years after the civil rights movement of the sixties. As in other areas, people often remain complacent until there is some riot or other situation, which causes a major disturbance in society. Then the reaction is to focus attention on the problems of unfair economic opportunities and segregation, but not to implement laws that will redress the sins of the past and correct the problem at its roots. As long as the church does not denounce racism, sexism and economic unfairness of its own members, the society will stay the same since most of the people in the society are adherents to the Christian faith. If they are not shown the evil they are doing from a spiritual perspective, they will continue to lead lives of sin while feeling the church is supporting them.

The movement within the church against slavery did not come from the traditional church. Thus, it was not strong enough to overcome the scourge of racism. There are few fundamental problems in life that can be corrected without a righteous spiritual basis. Racism and sexism are two examples of these because people will always mistreat or be unfair to others if they see themselves as separate. They will rarely hurt those with whom they feel a kinship. Yoga and mystical religion are the only ways to engender a feeling of unity with others. Thus, Yoga is to be promoted not just for one's individual spiritual enlightenment, but to promote social harmony between ordinary people of all ethnic groups as well as between countries.

Slavery began in America around the year 1,619 A.C.E. Abolitionism was a 19th-century movement to end slavery in the United States. However, the antislavery sentiment went back as far as the 1,690s, when the Quakers began speaking out against it. The Quakers are a Christian religious group also known as members of the Society of Friends. George Fox in England started the religious movement in 1,647. Although it is puritan in spirit, they suffered persecutions in England and encountered difficulties when they moved to the American colonies. The Quakers established religious communities in Rhode Island after arriving in America in 1,656. In 1,682, William Penn settled a religious colony in Pennsylvania. The Quakers are known for their simple style of living and pacifist ideals. In the last one hundred years, splinter groups have developed within the sect, with an increasing movement towards organization. Worldwide membership is about 200,000 (1,990 A.C.E.). The yearly meetings in Africa, with about 39,000 members, and in Great Britain and Ireland, with about 21,000 members, are the next largest groups of Quaker congregations. Traditionally in the United States, members of certain religious sects (e.g. Quakers, Jehovah's Witnesses) have been excused from combat duty although they have generally been expected to serve in non-combat roles.

In the privileges and administration of the Quaker society, no distinction is made between the sexes. Membership is based on religious and moral grounds. The Friends interpreted the words of Christ in the Scriptures literally, particularly, "Do not swear at all" (Matthew 5:34), and "Do not resist one who is evil" (Matthew 5:39). Thus, they were persecuted from the time of their inception as a group. They refused, therefore, to take oaths. They preached openly against war and violence, and even about resisting attack. Since the general church and government sanctioned violence, wars and racism, they often found it necessary to oppose the authority of church or state. They refused to pay tithes[1] to the Church of England since they rejected any organized church. Moreover, they met publicly for worship, a violation of the Conventicle Act of 1664 A.C.E., which forbade meetings for worship other than that of the Church of England. Regardless of the trouble, many thousands of people in Europe and England adhered to the group's teachings.

Their teaching is that through voluntary suffering, they bear witness to God. They believe that the purpose of life is to worship God and to discover God within. The fellowship of spirit is the group form of worship. The Quakers approach God directly, with no need to distinguish a clergy. They believe in the independent and inward, individual nature and practice of religion, and therefore object to established ministries and churches. Their fundamental belief is that divine revelation is immediate and individual. Thus, any and all persons may perceive the word of God in their soul directly. Thus, they use terms such as revelation of the "inward light," the "Christ within," or the "inner light." Quakerism believes in peacefulness and goodness to all since God exists within every human being. [75/117]

It is remarkable to realize that the very teachings that impelled the Quakers to speak out against racism, violence, and the mistreatment of women (sexism) did not come from their adherence to the established church, but from a desire to emulate Jesus. However, where did their teachings related to the inner and inward view of spirituality come from? The Bible of course includes some verses alluding to this, such as in the New Testament *Gospel of Luke*: 17:21: ...the Kingdom of God is in the midst of you (within thee). However, the association of that inward view with the "light" is very Gnostic in character and expression. The following passages from the Gnostic *Gospel of Thomas* reveal the correspondence. Also, the very idea of direct, inner spiritual realization is perhaps the most important and defining principle of Gnosticism.

> 24 His disciples said to Him (Jesus), "Show us the place where you are, since it is necessary for us to seek it."

> He (Jesus) said to them, "Whoever has ears, let him hear. There is *light within* a man of light, and he (or "it") lights up the whole world. If he (or "it") does not shine, he or "it") is darkness."

> 55. If they ask you, "Whence have you come from?" tell them "We have come from the *Light*, from the place whence the *Light* is produced of itself." If someone says to you: "What are you?" say, "We are the sons and we are the elect of the living Father."

The writings of Hippolitus (c.225 A.C.E.), a Christian writer speaking out on the "heresies" of the time were introduced earlier. They are repeated here because they give insight into the teaching of light from the Indian spiritual perspective.

> There is...among the Indians, a heresy of those who philosophize among the Brahmins, who live a self-sufficient life, abstaining from {eating} living creatures and all cooked food... They say that *God is light*, not like the light one sees, nor like the sun nor fire, but to them God is discourse, not that which finds expression in articulate sounds, but that of knowledge (gnosis) through which the secret mysteries of nature are perceived by the wise.[39]

The heresy being denounced above is from Indian Vedanta philosophy based on the Upanishadic Tradition. The Bhagavad Gita is part of that tradition and a verse is presented below which shows an original text related to the inner wisdom which any human being can access.

Bhagavad Gita: Chapter 5

> 24. One who finds bliss within, rejoices within, and finds the *light of wisdom within himself* -- such a Yogi becomes Brahman, and attains absolute freedom (Nirvana).

---

[1] A tenth part of one's annual income contributed voluntarily or due as a tax, especially for the support of the clergy or church.

The teaching of the "inner light" is also a major tenet of Sufism. They believe that the *inner light (one's own soul-spirit)* is a sufficient source of religious guidance. The orthodox followers of Islam persecuted the Sufis just as the Orthodox Christian Church persecuted the Gnostics. Finally, Ancient Egyptian Religion also saw the *god of light*, Ra-Heru, as the *"God within the common folk"* (everyone).

Thus it is clear that the theology of inward reflection as opposed to the practice of orthodox, organized religions, produces a special insight into the nature of the inner self and the relationship with humanity. The inward view (Gnostic) sees all alike and worthy of respect and toleration. Respect and toleration lead to peace, sharing, universal love and compassion and spiritual enlightenment. The outward, externalized view, promoted by orthodox organized religion sees differences between peoples, separation between the sexes and intensifies the egoistic desires (greed, lust, power, etc.) of the human heart. This in turn leads to ideologies and policies based on greed and fear. Greed and fear lead to stealing, violence, hatred, segregation, delusions of superiority and inferiority of one group in relation to others, conflict and religious (spiritual) stagnation.

The Methodist and African Methodist Episcopal Churches

The Methodist Church was not originally planned as a new sect of Christianity. It started in England as a trend within Protestantism, which emphasized life rather than creed. The Anglican theology was continued. Anglican refers to all groups having to do with the Church of England or any of the churches related to it in origin and communion, such as the Protestant Episcopal Church. John Wesley, an Anglican priest, was the founder of Methodism. Methodism stressed God's mercy. In 1784, the Methodist Episcopal Church in America was founded. In Methodism, the Bible is studied as a continuing form of inspired revelation.

The African Methodist Episcopal (A.M.E.) Church is the second largest Methodist group in the United States. Objecting to the church's racial discriminatory policy, a group withdrew from the Methodist Episcopal Church in 1787. The first AME church was dedicated in 1793 in Philadelphia. Richard Allen was the first bishop and formal organization followed in 1816. Its doctrines are those of traditional Methodist churches. There are approximately 1.1 million members in African Methodist Episcopal Church.

African Methodist Episcopal Zion Church was formed in 1796 by a group of black members of the John Street Church (Methodist Episcopal) in New York City who protested racial discrimination. The name was approved in 1848, and James Varick was the first bishop. The church spread rapidly throughout the northern states, and some churches developed in the South. Missionary activity and education are stressed. There are approximately 900,000 members.

The Revival Movement

The understanding of the roots of the Methodist churches, and indeed other American churches as well, cannot be complete without an understanding of the *Revival Movement.* A revival is a meeting or series of meetings for the purpose of reawakening religious faith, often characterized by impassioned preaching and public testimony.

The term Revival, when used in religion refers mostly to the Protestants. The term has been used since the early 18th century to denote periods of marked religious attention. It is characterized by periods of prayer meetings and evangelistic preaching. These are frequently accompanied by intense emotionalism. These periods are intended to renew the faith of church members and to bring others to profess their faith openly for the first time.

In the Middle Ages, revivals occurred in connection with the Crusades. These were sometimes under the sponsorship of the monastic orders. At some revivals, fanatical practices were performed. Sometimes people would hit themselves with flagellas (whips) and practice a dancing mania. The Reformation of the 16th century was also accompanied by revivals of religion.

Some scholars feel that it is more accurate to limit the application of the term revival to the history of modern Protestantism, especially as it developed in Great Britain and the United States where such movements have flourished with unusual vigor. The Methodist churches originated from a widespread evangelical movement in the first half of the 18th century. This was later referred to as the Wesleyan movement or Wesleyan revival.

Churches soon came to depend upon revivals for their growth and even for their existence, and, as time went on, itinerant preachers, also called "circuit riders" also took up the work. The early years of the 19th century were marked by great missionary zeal, extending even to foreign lands. In Tennessee and Kentucky about 1,800, camp meetings and great open-air assemblies began to play an important part in the evangelical work of the Methodist Church, now the United Methodist Church. Organized evangelistic campaigns have sometimes had great success under the leadership of professional evangelists, among them Billy Sunday, Aimee Semple McPherson, and Billy Graham. The Salvation Army carries on its work largely by revivalistic methods.[75]

This brief look at the revivalist movement shows the origins of the Methodist Church. Many people believe that the traditions of modern day churches were in the original teachings when in reality they are new developments. The addition of emotionality, wild dancing and other fanatical type movements to the church which seem to stir up spirituality, most often only stirs up mental agitation and emotional exuberance. In this sense the original meaning of the term "filled with the spirit" becomes equated with uncontrollable shaking, shouting, etc. Many people also believe that the predominantly African American Churches practice a form of traditional service with singing and dancing originating in the indigenous African traditions. When Africans were brought to Europe and America as slaves, they were almost completely stripped of their identity as native Africans and forced to adopt the religion of the slavemasters. At the time when Europeans in America engaged in the business of slavery, the revivalist movement came into popularity and this aspect of European worship was readily adopted. Many critics point to the fact that since the African American churches developed during the period of slavery, they serve only to excite the masses without leading them to real spiritual or social upliftment. During the slavery years, the Black Churches were supervised by the white slave owners who made sure that no disruptive elements were allowed. Consequently, many of the African American churches became an instrument of the slavemasters where they could diffuse tension within the slave ranks and deflect the energy which would have otherwise been employed towards the struggle for liberation. Also, the churches became a reinforcement of the institution of slavery because the slavemasters introduced the idea that the Bible supported slavery, the separation of the races, the supremacy of the white race and the inferiority of the black race. Of course, as we have discussed, the Bible does not support these ideas. There is not a single scripture that does. Actually, as we have seen in the earlier sections of this book, the Bible actually speaks against racism and towards promoting the unity of all peoples.

When west Africans were abducted and made slaves, the traditional African religions which had come from northeast Africa (Egypt and Ethiopia) were not only being supplanted by Christian Zealots who desecrated the traditional religious practices, but they were also denigrated by the growing Islamic movement, whose followers conquered the areas from northwest Africa to Spain and all the way to India spreading the Islamic religion by force and imposing it on whomever they could conquer. It is these events which have led to the conflicts between the Indians and the Pakistanis as well as the conflicts of Bosnia-Herzegovina, Israel and Egypt, and internal conflicts within many African countries. Consequently, a mixing of traditions and often a confusing form of worship has emerged, where some of the old traditions are mixed with the new. Santeria is an example of the mixture of Yoruba religion and Christianity. In Santeria, the gods and goddesses of Yoruba religion are mixed in with the saints of Christianity.

While ancient traditional African religions incorporate music, dancing and singing, they were not created as a means to indulge in the pleasures of the senses or to engender emotional exuberance or egoistic passion. In their original form they were created as a means to promote spiritual knowledge and mystical experience. Modern traditions such as Gospel Music, Pentecostal revivals, etc., are of much more recent development than people realize.

Gospel Music is a genre of popular American music that emerged at about the year 1,870. At first it was a predominantly European American style of music. It later became prominent in the urban religious revivals led by the evangelist Dwight Moody, along with the musician Ira Sankey. Its roots were in Sunday school hymns, camp meeting spirituals, and the melodies and harmonies of popular music. In Gospel music, the bass voice often echoes the other parts. An early example is "I Love to Tell the Story" (1869) by William Fischer. The texts, notably those of the poet Fanny Crosby, often deal with salvation and conversion. Black gospel music, which became distinctive by 1930, is especially associated with Pentecostal[I] churches. It developed out of the combination of the earlier hymns, black performance styles, and elements from black spirituals. Singing, which may merge into ecstatic dance, is usually accompanied by piano or organ, often with handclapping, tambourines and electric guitars. In modern times, a fusion of R & B and Rap music has been accomplished with Gospel. Texts such as "Precious Lord" (1932) by Thomas Dorsey stress themes of consolation. Noted singers include Rosetta Tharpe and Mahalia Jackson. Although the black and white varieties of gospel music have remained distinctive, repertoire has been shared, and they have freely influenced each other stylistically. [75]

Much of the modern revivalist movement is directed towards large ministries and mass meetings, and deeper spiritual practice eventually requires introspectiveness, silence, reflection and meditation. If religion only promotes faith, without wisdom, exuberance and not reflectiveness, insight and meditation, the practice will be limited. This is why the church has lost so many followers to other religions. It is also the reason why the revival movement began in the first place, to make up for the vast numbers of people who were disillusioned with the promises of the British Empire since the 18th century. The British Empire (England) at one time controlled one quarter of the earth, but the wealth never reached the common people. Therefore they became disillusioned with the government and with the religion as well.

Modern Developments in the Christian Churches

In the last seventy-five years there has been a marked increase in the development of the form of Christian churches referred to as Charismatic and Evangelical. In theology, charismatic relates to a type of Christianity that emphasizes personal religious experience and divinely inspired powers such as healing, prophecy, and the gift of tongues.

The evangelical movement relates to, or is in accordance with, the Christian gospel, especially one of the four gospel books of the New Testament. It also relates to a Protestant church, which founds its teaching on the gospel. Other beliefs of the evangelical Christian church include the belief in the sole authority and infallibility of the Bible, in salvation only through regeneration, and in a spiritually transformed personal life. It also relates to the Lutheran and Protestant churches in Germany and Switzerland, as well as to a group in the Church of England that stresses personal conversion and salvation by faith. It is also characterized by ardent or crusading enthusiasm and zealousness in preaching and in services.

Fundamentalism and the Second Birth

Fundamentalism refers to a movement within the Protestant churches in the United States of America. It attempts to maintain what its believers consider to be traditional interpretations of the Christian faith. Fundamentalism arose in reaction to what was seen as modernist or liberal trends within Protestantism, which began in the later 19th century. The conservatives began to create conferences and schools, which emphasize literal interpretations of the Bible as opposed to mythological, metaphorical and mystical interpretations. The Fundamentalist movement received the name from "The Fundamentals," a series of small books produced by conservative scholars that were widely distributed in 1910-12. The doctrines most emphasized by fundamentalists are:

1- The divinely inspired and infallible nature of the Bible.
2- The Trinity.
3- The immediate creation by the command of God.
4- Man's fall into depravity.
5- The necessity for salvation of being "Born Again" by faith in Christ.
6- Christ's deity, virgin birth, miracle-working power and substitutionary atonement for man, and his physical resurrection, ascension, and imminent pre-millennial Second Coming
7- The physical resurrection of man for Heaven or Hell.
8- Fundamentalism also stresses domestic and foreign evangelism and is strongly opposed to evolution, Communism, and ecumenism.[117]

[I] Of, relating to, or being any of various Christian religious congregations whose members seek to be filled with the Holy Spirit, in emulation of the Apostles at Pentecost.

Born Again in the Bible and in the Christian Church

The teaching of being "Born Again" appears three times in the New Testament of the Bible. It is an exhortation that unless one turns away from worldliness and hearkens to the teachings of spirituality, one cannot aspire to discover higher aspects of spirituality. This is, of course, in keeping with every other spiritual tradition we have discussed in this volume. It is an absolute necessity to turn towards the Divine in order to discover the Divine. This means instituting, for oneself, a spiritual discipline of life, which allows the practice of an integrated program that includes prayer, chanting, good works, meditation, etc. Spiritual evolution is not an event, which occurs by someone praying over another in Jesus' name and declaring that the person has been "Born Again" or "saved" by the power of the Holy Spirit, etc. This is a simplistic and immature understanding. Their view is that anyone can be Born Again by simply saying that they want to be even if they have lived a life of intense worldliness. There have been many people who have turned to fundamentalism and become Born Again and then slipped back into their old patterns of sinful behavior. This is because in reality, the emotional exuberance of a revival meeting or a fundamentalist service is more like an initiation of sorts. It can encourage people to move in a new direction in their lives, but this is only a beginning which needs to be reinforced with additional practices of the spiritual program, and most importantly, with the correct understanding of the higher goals and objectives of spirituality, i.e. to become Christlike. Initiation into a religion or spiritual philosophy is the beginning of a journey, which, if completed, will lead a person to the Kingdom of God, the goal of all spiritual practices. This discovery of the Kingdom is the true second birth. The human mind is so filled with complexes, which have been gathered over the present lifetime, and from previous lifetimes, that there is much spiritual work to be done in order to be truly Born Again.

> John 3:3
> 3 Jesus answered and said to him, Verily, verily, I say to thee, Except a man be Born Again, he cannot see the Kingdom of God. {Again: or, from above}

> John 3:7
> 7 Marvel not that I said to thee, Ye must be Born Again. {Again: or, from above}

> 1 Peter 1:23
> 23 Being Born Again, not of corruptible seed, but of incorruptible, by the word of God, which liveth and abideth for ever.

Being Born Again in the higher sense of Biblical as well as Gnostic Christian mystical philosophy means having attained Christ Consciousness, to become an Enlightened human being, for there is no other way to "see the Kingdom of God" (John 3:3). Therefore, the form in which the Born Again teaching is used by Fundamentalists and Revivalist preachers is divergent from this original idea.

The Difficult Nature of True Christian Living

Many people feel that thy can essentially "have their cake and eat it too" as it were. In Christianity this translates to those who believe they can be Christians and still remain involved with the world and all of its distractions. In order for spiritual life to be successful it must be uncontaminated with worldliness. Jesus himself was celibate and practiced poverty, meditation, vegetarianism and non-violence. He shared everything he had, and cared for all regardless of their race, creed or religion. He promoted equal rights for women and made one of them his highest disciple. Why do the churches not advocate these ideals beyond simple rhetoric and preaching in the church? If you say you believe something but do not act in accordance with that belief, your belief is bogus. It is hypocrisy and hypocrisy will not enable a person to discover true inner peace or the discipline to discover their inner virtue. They will always lead themselves to sinful behavior again and again. How many Christians steal, commit murder, commit racial crimes, eat meat, believe in capitalism, sexism, etc.? If they believe in these things it is because their family and/or church also advocates them. How many pastors or preachers smoke, enjoy fame, fortune, indulgence in sexual pleasures, promote hatred of other people because of their sect, religion, race, etc.? The inability of most pastors to deal with Christianity honestly manifests as the selective study of certain passages of the Bible with the exclusion of others, which are considered "hard teachings" as well as the complete exclusion of two books in the Bible, Daniel and Revelations. Most times preachers stay with the Gospels and when asked about those books of the Bible which deal with dreams and prophesy, they shy away or say:

"These are only dreams. You need not read those books. They are very hard and nobody understands those books. It is better to read the Gospel."[128]

Another wanting aspect of modern Evangelism is the adherence to the idea that the Bible is the absolute word of God and therefore cannot be questioned. This point is held almost universally across Christian denominations including the Orthodox, Anglicans, Evangelists, Fundamentalists and Revivalists. As such they put forth the idea that true believers are those who take everything the Bible says on faith, even if it is not understood. This idea was not a dominant view of pre-Roman Catholic Christianity, and especially not of Gnostic Christianity and neither was exuberant preaching. The whole notion of the absoluteness, exactness and perfection of the Bible is destroyed within the Christian Churches themselves because, if the Bible has one single and correct interpretation, how can there be hundreds of different denominations, each saying essentially that they have the true teaching and they are the real church? Yet, the emotional fervor that the Evangelists, Fundamentalists and Revivalists drum up through forceful, exuberant and constant repetition of this idea acts to cloud their own intellects and that of their followers to the inner need of every human being to "Know" God. Therefore, they too are also prevented from discovering the means to accomplish that discovery through the disciplines of Yoga contained in the teachings of Jesus due to their own egoism.

Most Christian preachers acknowledge that the Bible was written by human beings, but they always overstep the question of the inconsistencies of the Bible such as those in the Gospels. Most importantly, they overstep the question of the versions of the Bible. Initially, The Old Testament was "The Word of God." The question arises, if the Old Testament was the absolute word then why was there a need to create a New Testament? Secondly, why was it necessary to edit the Christian scriptures, canonize particular ones and omit others in order to compile a Bible? If the Christian faith is the true faith, that truth should stand on its own. Why was it necessary for the early Roman Emperors who adopted Christianity to outlaw all other religions?

Some problems related to the translations or versions of the Bible were discussed earlier, but it is important to relate this issue to the preachers and church leaders who preach teachings from them because this dogma is so powerful in giving them authority. The American Heritage Dictionary defines the word "version" as *1. A description or an account from one point of view, especially as opposed to another. 2.a. A translation from another language. b. Often Version. A translation of the entire Bible or a part of it. 3. A particular form or variation of an earlier or original type.* A version is not an original. This is why the neither the Bible nor any other book can be read and understood without proper guidance. Since it is a compilation of writings selected by certain people for political reasons, it cannot be accepted as the single source of Christian teaching. Other scriptures need to be consulted (Nag Hammadi Library, Dead Sea Scrolls, Apocrypha, etc.). If this is not done there will be an incomplete understanding of the teachings, and one's faith will be based on misinterpretation. The only absolute truth or word that can be received from God is through direct intuitional revelation. Teachings based on books are indirect teachings. Books and scriptures lead a person to live life in such a way that the revelation becomes possible for them, but the writings themselves are not absolute truths. This is why they need updating from time to time by Sages who have purified themselves sufficiently to receive the revelations.

If you want to receive the absolute opinion of a person, it is necessary to go to them directly and not through intermediaries. This is the basis, which the Bible scriptures themselves point out. Otherwise the Jewish prophets and seers would have been looked down upon. This point was the main issue of contention between the Pharisee and the Sadducee sects of the Jews. They debated whether or not the scriptures should be the only authority, and whether the oral tradition should also be included?

The higher aspects of any religion are difficult for those who are worldly minded to grasp. Religions have instituted disciplines for the masses which are different (less stringent) from those of the monastic order. Otherwise, the churches would loose their entire congregation because people, beset with worldly-mindedness, would quickly realize that they cannot aspire to the higher disciplines of advanced religious practice. However, this system could work as follows. When the church leadership notices that a member of the congregation is ready for higher spiritual practice, the appropriate teaching could be given to that person at that time. The problem here comes in if the teachings are distorted and incomplete. Most preachers, as well as the masses of people, have come to believe that their lower practices of spirituality, which allow them to be involved in the world, marry, indulge in worldly pleasures, smoking, drinking, etc., are in line the goal of religion. Many people even become comfortable at this level, especially when things are going well with their job or business. They participate in the church services, and

157

then go home feeling that they have taken care of their spiritual responsibilities for the week. Others turn to the church as a source of support and may even attend services daily because they feel happy around others of like mind that share the same values. They come to depend on the emotional fulfillment and egoistic enjoyment they receive from the church and stagnate in their inner spiritual growth. It must be clearly understood that being content in a church is not the goal of religion. As with all things, a human being must grow up and out of the church, so to speak, in the same manner as one grows up and out of school. How would it look for a healthy, sane, fifty five-year-old man to continue attending elementary school? A true spiritual seeker should not delude himself or herself with the illusions of worldly life, either in the world or in the church. Did not Jesus say that one cannot have two masters?

Sages of Yoga give spiritual teaching in accordance with the level of understanding of the seeker. Worldly people are given what they can receive, but advanced aspirants are given more. This is why Buddhism and Islam split into two major divisions, one for the monks and nuns and the other for the masses. In Christianity, Mother Teresa is a modern example of the higher attainments of Christian Mystical Philosophy. When asked how she could bear to serve so many people in such wretched conditions she replied "I only see Jesus in their faces, I serve God." This is a profound example of "seeing" the Kingdom of God on earth. It is a great mistake for any person who calls himself or herself a Christian to believe that they cannot aspire to such heights. The only obstacle to discovering the Kingdom of Heaven is if a person does not act as a true Christian should act. If one does not act with righteousness, meekness, compassion, selflessness, etc., and aspire to the higher virtues (practice of celibacy, detachment, meditation, etc.) one is only fooling oneself and remaining involved with the world (maintaining one's ego-separation from God). Merely praising God and proclaiming oneself as a Christian is not enough to be a Christian. This point is made clearly in Matthew 7:21.

Matthew 7:21

> 21. Not every one that saith to me, Lord, Lord, shall enter into the kingdom of heaven; but he that doeth the will of my Father who is in heaven.

The same point is further elaborated in Luke 11 34:35

> 34 The lamp of the body is the eye: therefore when thy eye is sound, thy whole body also is full of light; but when [thy eye] is evil, thy body also [is] full of darkness.
> 35 Take heed therefore that the light, which is in thee, be not darkness.

The lamp or light of awareness being referred to above in a human being is the mind (consciousness). If the mind is contaminated with sinful thoughts such as anger, hatred, greed, jealousy, depression and even thoughts like elation, infatuation and desire, the light of the spirit, which illumines the mind and operates through the mind like a prism will be clouded. When the mind is contaminated in this way, it is as if a person sees everything as being contaminated, just as a person with blue sunglasses sees everything in blue. The blueness becomes their reality because that is all they can see. In the same manner, when there is lust in the mind, a person cannot have a platonic relationship. When there is greed in the mind, a person cannot look at the objects of other people and feel content with what they already have. Concepts and beliefs are like colors in the mind. As long as a person has closed concepts and beliefs, they will not be able to grow beyond these to discover the deeper aspects of their own religion and accept other people who espouse other philosophies, because these are not accepted by their closed concepts.

A person can experience a great deal of inner peace and harmony in their worldly life if they just live in accordance with the basic Christian values (Ten commandments, Beatitudes, etc.), however, their spiritual evolution is still limited because the worldliness will always distract them from the higher divine vision of the Kingdom. At this stage, all the shouting, dancing, praising the Lord and other emotionally exuberant experiences in or out of the church are in reality only experiences of the mind's imagination. They are illusions based on one's misconceptions about spirituality and one's deep-rooted egoistic desires for remaining in the world while still trying to be spiritual at the same time. Music, chanting, and praising God are all parts of devotional worship, but they are not ends in themselves. They are not the goal of spiritual life. At some point a serious spiritual aspirant must reach a quiet state, which will allow them to go beyond the noise of the world as well as the sounds of the church, regardless of how harmonious or heavenly the sounds may be. In order to discover God one has to go beyond the mind and senses.

This can only be accomplished by means of quiet meditation. This point is confirmed in Psalm 46, Verse 10: "Be still[I] and know that I am God!"

Therefore, if a person wants to continue a life involved with worldly pleasures (family, sexuality, fame, fortune, power, etc.), they may do so but they should not think that they will attain the higher vision of spirituality as well, at least not in the present lifetime, and perhaps not even in the subsequent ones. This can only come when a person turns away from the world through inner realization of one's Christhood. Jesus made this clear in his teachings related to turning away from worldliness (Mt. 6. 24), family entanglements (Mt.12 46:50) and sexuality (Mt. 19:12 and 22:30). Many preachers[II] are comfortable with the idea of preaching the Gospels while living a married life, which affords them the opportunity to engage in sexual relations and relationships. However, it must be clearly understood that the writers of the Bible scriptures were essentially monks who practiced celibacy and meditation.

Matthew 6:24 No man can serve two masters: for either he will hate the one, and love the other; or else he will hold to the one, and despise the other. Ye cannot serve God and money.

Matthew 12:46. While he was yet speaking to the people, behold [his] mother and his brethren stood outside, desiring to speak with him.
47 Then one said to him, Behold, thy mother and thy brethren stand outside, desiring to speak with thee.
48 But he answered and said to him that told him, Who is my mother? And who are my brethren?
49 And he stretched forth his hand toward his disciples, and said, Behold my mother and my brethren!
50 For whoever shall do the will of my Father whom is in heaven, the same is my brother, and sister, and mother.

Matthew 19:12 For there are some eunuchs, who were so born from [their] mother's womb: and there are some eunuchs, who were made eunuchs by men: and there are eunuchs, who have made themselves eunuchs for the kingdom of heaven's sake. He that is able to receive [it] let him receive [it].

Matthew 22:30 For in the resurrection they neither marry, nor are given in marriage, but are as the angels of God in heaven.

It must be clearly understood that being Born Again in the true, higher sense and being in the world is possible if one has the complete teaching (all three stages of religious practice) and authentic spiritual preceptorship (advanced teacher). However, if one's philosophy is limited in its scope and if one's leadership is ignorant, worldly minded or unwilling to accept the higher aspects of the teaching even for themselves, one's own spiritual evolution will also be limited as well. Sadly, most pastors, preachers, etc. are limited in their own knowledge of Christian spirituality and follow the doctrines that they have been handed down from others who were equally ignorant. They follow these doctrines blindly and have come to accept the literal interpretation of the Bible as the absolute word of God, and since their minds are unable to cope with anything other than this narrow understanding, change is difficult or impossible. This predicament is remindful of Matthew 23:13-16 where the scribes and Pharisees who minister to the Jewish people in Jesus' time are chastised for their worldliness and hypocrisy based on their limited understanding and practice of Judaism and their egoistic values which limits them as well as the masses of people practicing the religion.

Matthew 23
13. But woe to you, scribes and Pharisees, hypocrites! For ye shut up the kingdom of heaven against men: for ye neither go in [yourselves], neither permit ye them that are entering to go in.

[I] Strong's Bible Concordance defines the Hebrew word raphah {raw-faw'} 07503 as 1a3) to sink, relax, abate 1a4) to relax, withdraw1b) (Niphal) idle (participle) 1c) (Piel) to let drop 1d) (Hiphil) 1d1) to let drop, abandon, relax, refrain, forsake 1d2) to let go1d 3) to refrain, let alone 1d4) to be quiet. Thus, this word is most accurately rendered in modern Yoga discipline as "Meditation."
[II] One who preaches, especially one who publicly proclaims the gospel for an occupation.

14 Woe to you, scribes and Pharisees, hypocrites! For ye devour widows' houses, and for a pretence make long prayer: therefore ye shall receive the greater damnation.
15 Woe to you, scribes and Pharisees, hypocrites! For ye travel sea and land to make one proselyte, and when he is made, ye make him twofold more the child of hell than yourselves.
16 Woe to you, [ye] blind guides, who say, Whoever shall swear by the temple, it is nothing; but whoever shall swear by the gold of the temple, he is a debtor!

Remember that religion has three steps, stages or levels. These are Myth, Ritual and Mystical. Therefore, practices of the non-mystical Christian churches, i.e. churches that do not follow the threefold process of religion, are only related to the lower levels of spiritual practice (myth and ritual). This is the level of practice promoted by almost all Christian churches. This is because, in most cases, the understanding of the Christian myth is deficient. This in turn causes people to practice the religion (ritual stage) in a wrong or limited way. In Christianity, the problem is that the main doctrine of Christianity, since the time that the Roman Catholic Church, emphasized the literal interpretation of the life and teachings of Jesus. They hold that he existed as the one and only savior, a real human being who died and was bodily resurrected (literal interpretation). The mystical interpretation is that every human being's soul is Jesus, who has incarnated and been crucified by the world and its desires and distractions, turning it away from the divine vision of its own nature. The resurrection of Christ within the human heart is when the Christ Consciousness or vision of the Kingdom of God is regained. Further, the church doctrine holds that salvation, i.e. seeing the Kingdom of God, must occur through faith in Jesus and by Jesus' returning to the world and digging people out of the grave in order to resurrect them (literal interpretation). The mystical interpretation is that human beings are to grow into Christ Consciousness itself and resurrect themselves by discovering their ability to grow beyond the limiting weight of ignorance and worldly desire.

The belief in the literal interpretation of the scriptures closes the door to understanding Jesus Christ as a metaphor of our own life. With this understanding, or rather, misunderstanding, our own self-effort and responsibility for our own resurrection is negated, being dependent on Jesus alone. Thus, the last stage of religion, mysticism, is not even part of the spiritual plan of ordinary Christianity as it is understood and presented by most Christians in the world. The reason why people need constant revivals and emotional exuberance to keep them exited and interested is that the limited vision of the church will never satisfy the true yearning of the soul. This is because the worldly philosophy of the church is too limited. The soul, being Divine and infinite, will only find true peace and contentment through a mystical realization of its true nature, which is Divine and infinite. This is the higher message given by Jesus in the Bible book of John 10:34: *Jesus answered them, Is it not written in your law, I said, Ye are gods?*

When a human being becomes truly enlightened, there is no turning back. Why are there so many Christian priests and ministers who are exposed every year for suffering depression, engaging in drinking, wrong use of church funds, illicit sexuality with parishioners, prostitutes or children, etc.? Why are there so many preachers who confess their inability to keep the faith in the doctrine of the church? They question their calling and often times bury their own doubts under a mountain of memorized scriptures and impassioned proselytizing that distracts them from their own deeper spiritual needs. The limited vision of Christianity is not sufficient for them, so how can it be adequate for the masses who are even more removed from serious spiritual practice? Authentic teachers of the scriptures are those who are established in the teaching and who have had advanced spiritual experiences. They may not yet be Enlightened Sages, but they should be advanced students of those who are. Further, they should be monks and nuns who have engaged in serious spiritual practice involving all three stages of religion (especially mysticism) as opposed to seminarians[1] who are well versed in the academics of religion (myths, rituals and traditions) or preachers and others who are trying to live in two worlds (secular and non-secular) at the same time. Mysticism is the level of religion which enables a person to find true peace and fulfillment in life, to be in the world, but not of the world. Lacking this experience a person will remain vulnerable to the lower nature of the personality along with its desires, cravings and faults. They will therefore be limited in their ability to discover the deeper riches of spiritual life and lead others to discover them as well. It must be clearly understood that a truly advanced practitioner of Christianity in its three levels (myth, ritual, metaphysical) could go to a monastery or nunnery as easily as living in the world of human activity. The key is in the practice of the teachings and not in the location where they are practiced. Sages often remain in the world for the sake of leading others to blessedness and not due to personal desire for worldly enjoyments. If people were to practice the teachings given by Jesus, in their daily lives, they would automatically lead themselves towards a process wherein they would gradually begin to live the life of monks

---

[1] Students at a Seminary. A seminary is a school, especially a theological school for the training of priests, ministers, or rabbis.

and nuns, even while living in the world and being amongst others. Once again, what is necessary is to have the correct teaching to follow and an authentic teacher who can lead the process.

Overview of Christianity in Africa and The Missionary Movements

This vast subject cannot be fully treated in this volume of *Christian Yoga*, but it is a subject of paramount importance for understanding the history of Christianity in Africa as well as the future of Christianity in the world. Why? Because Africa is fast becoming the most Christianized part of the world.

> While every day in the West,[I] roughly 7,500 people in effect stop being Christians every day in Africa roughly double that number become Christians...[129]

Along with the statistics above, population growth in the world has changed dramatically in the last century. While population growth has slowed to .8% in North America and 0% growth for Europe (The West) as an average, or even negative growth for some parts of Europe, it is well over 3% in Africa.

> For the less-developed world as a whole, the 1990 growth rate of 2.0 percent per year is projected to be cut in half by 2025. Africa will remain the region with the highest growth rate. In 1990 this rate was 3.1 percent; in 2025 it is projected to be about 2.2 percent. Africa's population would almost triple, from 682 million in 1990 to 1.58 billion in 2025, and then continue growing at a rate that would almost double the population size in another 35 years.[75]

If the projections above hold it is possible that Africa will at some point in the future have one of, if not, the largest population of Christians in the world. How did this come to be? As we saw earlier, Christianity originated in Ancient Egypt (which included India). From there its adherents carried the Christian teachings to Canaan/Palestine, Turkey, Greece and the rest of Europe. Rome and Byzantium became the strongholds of Christianity, which enforced it by means of military power as they set out to spread the empire abroad including North Africa and Ethiopia. When the Roman Empire adopted Christianity, it banned all other forms of religion. At the same time as it subjugated its colonies around the Empire (200-450 A.C.E.) and forced people to pay heavy taxes to support Rome, the honest followers of Christianity practiced Christian charity and developed a great reputation as a religion of the masses. This reputation drew many adherents to the Christian faith in all parts of the Roman Empire. Thus, the negative economic situations that many people found themselves in provided a fertile soil for the propagation of Christian doctrines since Jesus' teachings on promoting justice and equality are the hallmark of Christian life in society. Jesus' teachings extol the virtue of sharing and helping others regardless of their race, religion or creed. The famous story of the Good Samaritan (Luke 10:33) is an example of this. Along with helping those in distress, Christianity emphasizes the virtues of loving one's enemies (Luke 6:27) and not developing resentment towards them, but instead showing them, through love and restraint, the blessedness of peace (Matthew 5:9), and the fellowship of all human beings in Christ (Galatians 3:28) and thereby, the error of their negative actions.

Galatians 3

28 There is neither Jew nor Greek, there is neither bond nor free, there is neither male nor female: for ye are all one in Christ Jesus.

Thus, the first Christian missionaries, such as the Apostle Paul, were very welcome for many reasons. However, in modern times the Christian missionary movement has come under fire for its denigration of native cultures and its hypocrisy for not dealing with its own issues of faith. For example, the Christian churches of North America have organized several movements to end hunger or to convert peoples of foreign countries, but there are people in North America who go hungry every day. Further, the pervasive problem of racism continues in a subtle form unopposed in the churches as well as the general society. Along with these problems there are several issues of Christian doctrine, which remain unresolved.

In modern times, the missionaries sent to the Americas and to Africa by the European nations sought to convert the native populations and at the same time convince them that the religion they were following up to that time was nothing more than idol or devil worship. The church carried out the missionary role while at the same time condoning the process of neocolonization.[II] Over the past 1,700 years since the adoption of Christianity by the Roman Empire, Christianity has experienced many low points throughout history. Some of these were the Crusades,

---

[I] **West**. The western part of the earth, especially Europe and the Western Hemisphere, controlled economically, politically and culturally by the European nations.

[II] A policy whereby a major power uses military force, coercion, illegal economic and political means to perpetuate or extend its influence over underdeveloped nations or areas.

the Inquisitions,[I] the Atlantic Slave Trade, and the Genocide of Native Americans. Consequently, many people became disillusioned with Christianity and it became an incidental part of life for many Western Christians. It was not until the emergence of the Revivalist movement that Christianity was revitalized. This was the primary force, which spurred the missionaries of the last hundred years. However, even today, the Earl of Spencer, the brother of Princess Diana of England, said publicly in an interview[II] that the death of his famous sister brought out some unexpected aspects of British life. He said that even though there is not much of an organized religion any more in the country, the outpouring of emotion took on an almost a spiritual quality as if they were expressing some "latent" feeling that had not found expression.

So, while Christianity emerged out of Africa and spread to Europe and America, it did not maintain its original form or its impact on people as an honest movement towards human fellowship and spiritual enlightenment. Thus, it is regarded by many as an inconsequential part of life even though they call themselves Christian by birth. Some people in Western countries even regard Christianity and religion in general, as a nuisance. They do not allow Christian principles to be considered in their government or business activities even though they claim that they are Christians, America is a Christian country and their motto is "in God we trust." In the eyes of many people who live in the European colonies, or who suffered slavery or military conquest at the hands of European Christians, Christianity became a symbol of European Imperialism and social injustice. Nevertheless, ironically, the missionaries that came into Africa before the independence movements[III] of the twentieth century were largely members of the revivalist Christian sects. The Reformation Movement[IV] was not as interested in missionary activities as the formation of a new church doctrine in Europe. The important influence came from the followers of the Evangelical Revival Movements. In the late eighteenth century, Protestant missionary societies increased, and after that the Catholics also sent some missionaries to Africa as well. Thus, using the map of "Africa and the West," we can trace the movement of Christianity through history.

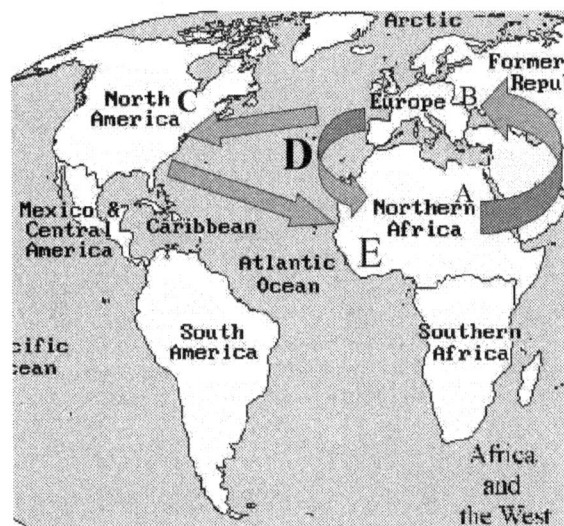

The missionary movement and the origin and return of Christianity to Africa.

A- Christianity emerges in Africa (Egypt) based on the Ausarian Resurrection Religion.
B- Christianity is adopted by some of the Jews who transfer it to Europe along with some of the previous Jewish teachings (Old Testament).
C- Missionaries come to Africa from Europe trying to convert Africans to the Christianity as it was practiced in Europe based on European culture and traditions which included images of Jesus and all of the characters of the Bible as Europeans (except for those images of the Black Madonnas). Christianity adopted the Jewish traditions and folklore (not found in the Bible) related to Egypt and Ethiopia as being heathens or pagans who were cursed for their blackness, thus denigrating the role of Africans in the Bible and promoting the enslavement and exploitation of African peoples during the slave trade.
D- The forms of Christianity practiced in the Britain, Anglican, Protestant, Separatist and Puritan churches, etc. were transferred to North America and were instrumental in sanctioning the colonization process which

---

[I] A tribunal formerly held in the Roman Catholic Church and directed at the suppression of heresy but became a means to murder and eradicate any person who disagreed with the church or its wealthy followers.

[II] Interview from 1998.

[III] Independence from European colonialism.

[IV] Reformation. A 16th-century movement in Western Europe that aimed at reforming some doctrines and practices of the Roman Catholic Church and resulted in the establishment of the Protestant churches.

included the stealing of land from Native Americans and murdering them, the enslavement of Africans through the slave trade, as well as the Jews, the Irish and others through indentured servitude.[I]

E- Missionaries from North America come to Africa to spread the revivalist movement.

CONCLUSION

It is extremely important to understand the dynamics of the spread of Christianity in its different forms. The propagation of ignorance and distorted teachings must be understood and corrected. Like Europeans and all those who have been touched by Western missionaries, Africans need to receive the knowledge about the origins and Gnostic teachings of Christianity, which come from Africa itself, and not just the doctrines of Protestants, Orthodox Catholics or Evangelicals from Europe. For the most part, wherever Western Christian missionaries have carried Christianity, they have attempted to eradicate the preexisting religion by labeling it as a pagan cult and not a "real" religion. Then they adopt some of the symbols or traditions of that cult and call them Christian. In modern times, with the power of Tele-evangelism it is even more important to promote the message of Christian Yoga, the mystical and universal Christian philosophy which affirms the Divine in all forms of religion as well as the equality of all human beings and the necessity to love all alike. Westernized Christianity resists attempts by some Africans to Africanize Christianity just as they themselves Europeanized it. As we have seen, in Europe Christianity adopted many rituals and symbols of Ancient Egyptian religion and later the Celtic religion, as well as from others. In Africa, the move is to identify God, the Father of Christianity, with for example, the "High God" of traditional African religions such as Chukwu of Igboland or Mwari of the Shona, etc. This understanding should be encouraged and the adoption of Christianity should be seen as an advanced African expression of the universal philosophy which is already being followed instead of a new, real religion which needs to be adopted while discarding the old, ignorant, pagan, false religions. When this occurs, African peoples as well as all Christians around the world will move into a new age of real Christian faith. Christian religion cannot be practiced in a church that is contaminated with economic, political or social doctrines, which are patently unjust. Also, it cannot be correctly practiced when the traditions and doctrines are based on the ignorance of Deism, corruption and dishonesty. The Church needs to acknowledge its role in promoting economic, social and religious injustices throughout history and then reaffirm the true Christian teachings, which have yet to be practiced. The church could begin with the teachings given by Jesus at the Sermon on the Mount. While these teachings have been advocated as propaganda or doctrinal principles by the church, they have never been implemented and upheld universally in the church.

A HISTORY OF MODERN CHRISTIAN AND NON-CHRISTIAN MYSTICISM

The Crusades were a period of crisis in western culture. The struggle for survival through the Dark and Middle Ages led to a low point in western culture, art and society in general. In much the same way that wars throughout history have stimulated economies and social interaction, the Crusades stimulated European countries by forcing the movement of thousands of people within Europe and between Europe and the Middle East. The Crusades were the military expeditions undertaken by European Christians in the 11th, 12th, and 13th centuries to recover the Holy Land from the Muslims from 1,095-1,272. The idea of the crusades began as a desire of the Catholic Church to control the Holy Land, but it turned into a means to destroy the Eastern Catholic Church (Byzantine Empire) after they had separated and began to have differences of opinion in reference to church doctrines and authority. Constantinople was sacked in 1,204, overthrowing the Byzantine Empire and establishing the Latin Empire of Constantinople. There were nine attempted crusades of which only one had any degree of success[II]. However, the success was short lived. The other crusades were ineffectual.

The cause of the crusades (recapturing the Holy Land-Palestine) soon deteriorated into a lust for plundering and pillaging any of the lands where the armies may have found themselves. For instance, on the way from Europe (France, Germany, Italy, etc) the armies had to pass through Greece and Turkey. On the way to the Holy Land they sacked many towns, raping women and destroying entire villages. Later, the attention of the West (Christians) turned to the conquest of the New World (Western Hemisphere - Americas).[75] With the religious mandate to conquer nature as well as all non-believers, the Muslims and Christians set out to acquire new lands, mineral resources and converts by force of arms without considering that all human beings are created by the same Supreme Being, and that all faiths have an equal right to exist. Some of the armies reached the Near East but were defeated.

[I] Indentured servitude and slavery were the economic factors which enabled the creation of the united States of America and its subsequent emergence as a Superpower in the mid twentieth century. A Superpower is defined in the American Heritage Dictionary as: **su·per·pow·er** (sōō′pər-pou′ər) *n.* A powerful and influential nation, especially a nuclear power that dominates its allies or client states in an international power bloc.

[II] The First Crusade captured Jerusalem in 1096-99.

Others never made it or their efforts simply turned into misguided attempts by lords and kings to gain power, land and wealth. Peasants searching for a better life conducted some of the crusades, or others who just engaged in the indiscriminate looting, murder, raping and pillaging of any city. In short, the crusades turned out to be a frustrating search for a better life. The last Latin Kingdom (city-state) in the Near East, Acre, fell to the Muslims in 1,291. However, the Crusades caused a mass movement of people and resources, which stimulated the arts, literature and commerce between the European nations as well as between Europe and foreign countries. This stimulation caused an interaction with the Near Eastern and with the Far Eastern cultures which led to the influential development of new literary forms in the 11th and 12th centuries such as the Arthurian romance tradition and the lyrical vernacular poetry of the troubadours. This was extremely important in the development of Western Christianity. They helped to develop a disdain for the church and engendered a love of individualism and self-expression.

After the period of the crusades, the Christian Church and Europe in general were in a state of stagnation. Then in the fourteenth century A.C.E. there came a revival of European spiritual culture. This period was known as the *Renaissance*. Historians refer to the period we currently live in today as "Modern Times." These Modern Times began with the period of Renaissance. The Renaissance began in Italy during the 14th century, reaching its height of expression in the 15th century. It spread to the rest of Europe in the 16th and 17th centuries. Renaissance means "rebirth." It refers to the rediscovery of the writings of the ancient Greeks and Romans by European scholars who were referred to as humanists. Humanism is a philosophical viewpoint that strives for human good in the present world and stresses human reason as a source of authority. The Renaissance period saw the discovery of new scientific laws, literature and new forms of art, new political and religious ideas, and new lands, such as America.

This period is critical to our understanding of modern Christianity and European thought because the very catalyst of the great renaissance in Europe was a rediscovery and not the creation of something. It was a rediscovery of the ancient mystical philosophy from Egypt, which fueled the movement towards progress in every field. How was this possible? Marsilio Ficino (1433-99) was an Italian philosopher and theologian. His translations and commentary on the works of Plato contributed to the Platonic revival during the Renaissance period. He studied philosophy, medicine and learned Greek as he prepared for priesthood. He was supported and encouraged by the Italian statesman and banker Cosimo de' Medici. Ficino made the first complete translation of Plato's writings into Latin (1463-69) and set up the Platonic Academy. He later translated works by Neoplatonic writers and the Roman philosopher Plotinus. Most importantly, he translated the Greek text of the Hermetic writings, which were brought from Byzantium into Latin, and thus the Corpus Hermeticum was brought to modern Europe.[58\75]

During the time prior to the creation of Orthodox Roman Catholic Christianity, Gnostic Christianity flourished alongside other mystical traditions. One of these was Hermeticism. The Hermetic Books were known as a collection of metaphysical and mystical writings and dialogues which dated from the middle of the 1st century A.C.E. to the 4th century A.C.E., that were the revelations of Djehuti, the Ancient Egyptian god of reason and spiritual knowledge. Hermeticism gets its name from Hermes. Hermes is the Greek name given to the Ancient Egyptian god Djehuti when the writings were translated from the Ancient Egyptian into Greek. The Corpus Hermeticum (body of Hermetic texts) deals with theological and philosophical questions. The central theme of the seventeen tracts of the Corpus Hermeticum is the deification and regeneration of humankind through knowledge of the one transcendent God.[58\75\117] Thus, Ancient Egyptian mystical philosophy is in great part responsible for the resurgence of European art, mystical philosophy and spiritual culture.

Traditional Christian literature and scholarship have recognized St. Paul as the first great Christian mystic. The New Testament writings best known for their deeply mystical emphasis are Paul's letters and the Gospel of John (John 10:30-34). Christian mysticism, as a philosophical system, is derived from Neo-Platonism through the writings of Dionysius the Areopagite, or Pseudo-Dionysius. The original Dionysius the Areopagite lived in the 1st century A.C.E. and became first bishop of Athens. Dionysius was martyred about 95 A.C.E. He is often confused with the Pseudo-Dionysius (c. 500) who created mystical writings using the name of Dionysius the Areopagite. He was later canonized as a Catholic Saint. Dionysius was converted to Christianity when he heard Paul preach the sermon concerning the nature of "the unknown God" on the Hill of Mars or Areopagus in Athens, as described in Acts 17:15-34.

These mystical writings provided a system of the cosmos and emphasized a union between God and the soul and the progressive deification of man. These were central elements of the Mysteries of Aset, which were still practiced up to that time. These writings had a very important influence on both the Eastern and Western Churches until their authenticity was contested in the 16th century. These Pseudo-Dionysiac writings, having originated in Egypt or Syria, were first cited at the Second Council of Constantinople in 553.

In the 9th-century, John Scotus Erigena, a scholastic philosopher, translated the works of Pseudo-Dionysius into Latin from Greek and thus the mystical theology of Eastern Christianity was introduced into Western Europe. Here it was then combined with the mysticism of the early Christian high-ranking clergyman and theologian, St. Augustine.

In the Middle Ages, mysticism often came to be associated with monasticism rather than the religious practice of the masses. Therefore, many of the most celebrated mystics are to be found among the monks of both the Western and the Eastern Church. A strong mystical influence developed particularly in the teachings and writings of the 14th-century, and it is evident in the following Christian theologians: Hesychasts of Mount Athos, Saint Francis of Assisi, Saint Bernard of Clairvaux, and John of the Cross.

Other important Christian mystical centers and prominent mystics included the French monastery of Saint Victor in the 12th century, St. Bonaventure who was a disciple of the monks of St. Victor, St. Francis, Jan van Ruysbroeck, Gerhard Groote of Holland who was a founder and religious reformer of the monastic order known as the *Brothers of the Common Life*, Johannes Eckhart, referred to as Meister Eckhart of Germany, Johannes Tauler and Heinrich Suso who were followers of Eckhart and became members of a group called the *Friends of God*. The writings of this group on German Theology later influenced Martin Luther. The *Cloud of Unknowing*, an influential discourse on mystic prayer, has been an influential mystical anonymous document.

There have been many distinguished female Christian mystics, notably St. Hildegard, St. Catherine of Siena, St. Teresa of Ávila, and Jeanne Marie Bouvier de la Motte Guyon who introduced the mystical doctrine of Quietism[1] into France.

The mystical undercurrent in Christianity, implying a need for a deeper, more effective means of religious experience, influenced the Christian reformation, a movement to eradicate abuse, malpractice and irresponsible and immoral practices in the church. This movement was a major change within Western Christianity between the 14th and 17th centuries, wherein a large segment of Christianity separated from the Roman Catholic Church under the leadership of several intellectuals such as Martin Luther and Ulrich Zwinglis. The papacy and the question of apostolic succession, church corruption and the straying from the "original teachings of the Bible" were the central issues of the reformers. Two of the most notable German Protestant mystics were Kaspar Schwenkfeld and Jakob Boehme, the latter being the author of *Mysterium Magnum* or "The Great Mystery."

The 20th century has seen a revival of interest in both non-Christian and Christian mysticism. An important commentator was the North American philosopher and psychologist, William James who wrote "The Varieties of Religious Experience" in 1902. In Zen Buddhism, the Japanese Daisetz Suzuki had become the leading commentator, in Hinduism, the Indian philosophers Swami Vivekananda and Savepalli Radhakrishnan, and on Islam, the British scholar R. A. Nicholson. The last half of the 20th century has experienced an increased interest in Eastern mysticism. Some of the most important commentators on Eastern Philosophy and mysticism in the West include Carl Jung, Joseph Campbell and Swami Jyotirmayananda. Their writings and discourses using the modern media (audio and video) have served to advance the understanding of Eastern mysticism to great heights.

In Judaism, the writings of the Cabalists of the Middle Ages and in the movement of the Hasidim of the 18th century were again emphasized by the modern Austrian philosopher and scholar, Martin Buber. Hasidim or Chasidim (Hebrew for "the pious ones") is the tradition in ancient Jewish history associated with especially pious persons who upheld Jewish traditions in the face of foreign conquerors. Their stories are related in the books of Maccabees and the Talmud. The term specifically refers to those who have distinguished themselves by charitable deeds and by loyalty to Jewish law.

Modern Hasidim surrounds a mystical sect that was established at about the mid-18th century by a charismatic leader named Baal Shem Tov. The name Hasidim also is applied to this group. Tov objected to the rigid formality and ritualism of Jewish religious practice and also the rule of the Jewish community by the masters of rabbinical scholarship, as well as the wealthy. He advocated joyous worship and stressed trust in God as a means to a closer relationship with God. Thus, it is possible to see that from time to time religion requires reform and the reaffirmation of religious principles. Often people begin to feel comfortable in the traditions of the past and loose sight of the meaning behind the rituals. This is when modern Sages must come forth to reaffirm the deeper values so as to permit their followers to have true spiritual movement. In this sense, Jesus, Buddha, Krishna, Asar, Muhammad, etc., were reformers and reaffirmers in their own time, of traditions, which were much older than they were.

---

[1] Quietism, type of mysticism that regards the most perfect communion with God as coming only when the soul is in a state of quiet. It is practiced in all forms of mysticism including Sufism.

NEW AGE SPIRITUALITY

The New Age Movement is regarded as a broad-based mixture of diverse spiritual, political, and social elements. The common aim is to transform society and individuals through inner spiritual awareness. It came into the mainstream of society in the 1980's A.C.E. Sometimes the New Age Movement is viewed as a resurgence of Paganism or Gnosticism of ancient times. The modern New Age Movement began in the 19th-century spiritualism movements, which were spawned by archeological discoveries in Egypt with the deciphering of the Ancient Egyptian hieroglyphic system in the early 19th century. In the late 19th century people also began to look towards Indian and Chinese spiritual philosophies as alternatives to traditional Christianity, western science and philosophy. Theosophy is the name that was given to one of the important early New Age movements. Theosophy (the name comes from the Greek theos, "god," sophos, "wise"), refers to any religio-philosophical system that attempts to provide knowledge of God, as well as the universe in relation to God, through direct philosophical inquiry, direct mystical intuition, or both. Its early proponents derived much of their teachings from the Indian Upanishads, Gnosticism, the Cabala and Ancient Egyptian mythology. Helena Petrovna Blavatsky became a popular exponent of theosophy 1875. She said that the teachings she espoused were based on the teachings of Oriental spiritual masters. The New Age Movement gained strength during the 1960's with the counterculture movement that rejected materialism in favor of Eastern forms of mysticism such as Yoga, Buddhism, Hermeticism and Taoism. People began to seek a direct spiritual experience rather than organized religion. The new Age Movement adheres to the Gnostic and Yogic idea that the individual is responsible for his or her own fate and that they are also capable of discovering their own spiritual reality.

The New Age Movement involves holistic thinking. This has influenced attitudes about medicine, family, the environment, regional planning, the work environment, cultural relations and world peace. Some of the ideas associated with the New Age movement include teachings related to inner transformation, reincarnation, biofeedback, extraterrestrial life, chanting, yoga, alchemy, transpersonal psychology, martial arts, the occult, shamanism, astrology, extrasensory perception, psychic healing, divination, acupuncture, astral travel, massage, Zen, tarot, mythology, and creative visualization.

In recent years Christians within the New Age movement have fostered the creation of new texts which the authors claim were channeled (dictates psychically) by higher beings through human beings acting as mediums. Two of the more famous texts are The Aquarian Gospel of Jesus and The Course in Miracles. These new texts present much of the Gnostic view of Christianity and are comparable, in some respects, to the Yogic (Mystical) texts of Ancient Egypt and India.

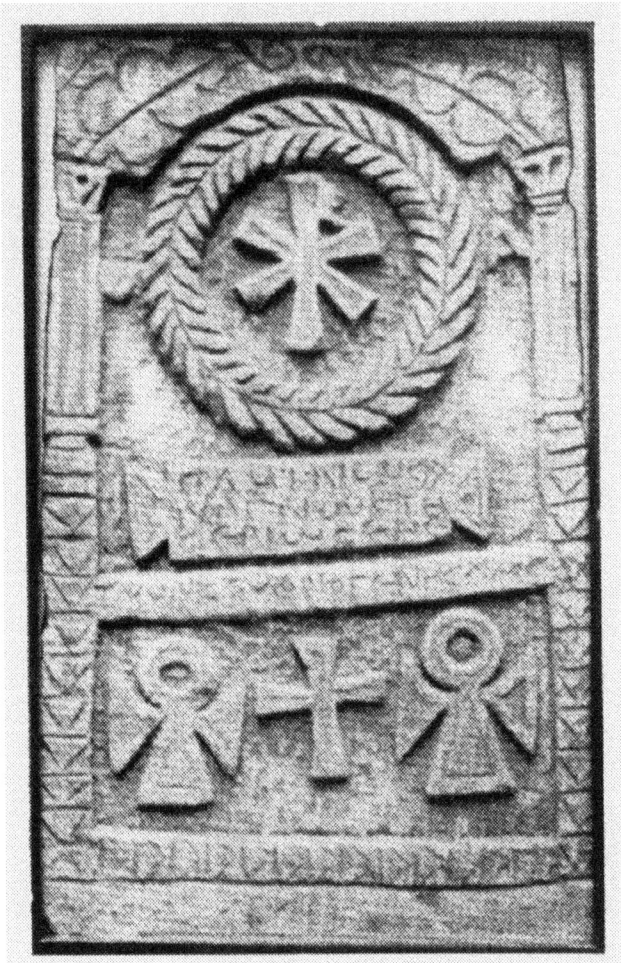

Above: Sepulchral Stele of Plêïnôs, a "reader."
Sculptured with Alpha and Omega, the
Christian Cross and Ancient Egyptian Ankhs
from 8th or 9th century.

CHAPTER VII: INITIATION INTO CHRISTIANITY YOGA

Christianity as a Spiritual Discipline
For Spiritual Transformation

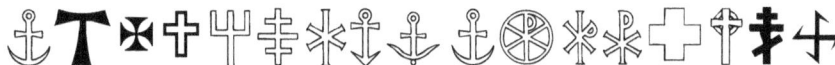

From the Upanishads:

"As a river flows to the Ocean and becomes one with it, so too is the individual soul."

From the Tao Te Ching:

"Tao in the world is like a river flowing home to the sea."

A DEEPER LOOK AT YOGA PHILOSOPHY

Introduction

In this chapter we will explore in depth the teachings of Yoga and we will see how they were taught in early Christianity. We have already introduced many concepts and wisdom teachings from Ancient Egypt, which were instrumental in the creation of Christian Mysticism. Now we will take a closer look at yoga philosophy as it developed in India and then we will see how the Christian scriptures themselves reflect the same yogic wisdom which is designed to lead a person to attain a spiritual union with God. Yoga philosophy has four major aspects of practice, the Yoga of Wisdom, the Yoga of Action, the Yoga of Devotion and the Yoga of Meditation. This final section of the book will introduce the Yoga of Wisdom and the teachings of Christian Yoga Wisdom. In Christian Yoga, Volume II we will present the teachings of the remaining forms of Yoga. (See the Preview of Christian Yoga, Volume II at the end of this book.

VEDANTA AND YOGA IN INDIA

Vedanta philosophy originated from the ancient spiritual scriptures of India called the *Vedas,* meaning "knowledge," and later developed with the creation of the Upanishads. The Vedas are related to a specific kind of knowledge, more specifically, knowledge which is heard. The ancient Sages who recorded the Vedic hymns were said to have heard them, inspired by the transcendental realms of consciousness. Therefore, they wrote out of their own inspiration.

Vedanta refers to the end of the Vedas or the scriptures commonly referred to as *the Upanishads,* which constitute a revision as well as a summary or distillation of the highest philosophy of the Vedas. The term Upanishad means "wisdom achieved by sitting close to a spiritual master." The following segment from the *Mundaka Upanishad* details the view of the two sets of scriptures in relation to each other and the two forms of knowledge.

> *Those who know Brahman (God)... say that there are two kinds of knowledge, the higher and the lower. The lower is knowledge of the Vedas (the Rik, the Sama, the Yajur, and the Atharva), and also of phonetics, grammar, etymology, meter, and astronomy. The higher is the knowledge of that by which one knows the changeless reality.*

Vedanta philosophy, as it exists in the present, is a combination of Buddhist psychology, Hindu mythology relating to the gods and goddesses of India, the ancient metaphysical philosophy from the Upanishads and the mental and physical disciplines from Yoga practice. Having its original roots in the philosophy of the oneness of God who manifests in a myriad of ways, Vedanta achieves a balanced blend of all the philosophies and has been adapted by the present day Sages to teach modern day society the ancient philosophy of spiritual evolution and spiritual practice. Modern Vedanta includes the 16 Yogas (8 major, 8 minor) from the classical yoga of Sage

Patanjali, adapted from the Buddhist *Wheel of Life* which had been developed as an alternative to the Brahmanic ritual religious system.

BASIC YOGA PHILOSOPHY

The True Essence of Humankind: Divine, not mortal - Omnipotent, not weak.

The Problem with Humanity*:* Identification with one's body, sensual pleasures, desire, imaginations, passions as abiding realities due to a mind overcome by mental fetters which originate in *IGNORANCE.*

The Solution to the Problem: KNOW THYSELF- Self Realization (Salvation, YOGA).

The Process of YOGA:

The process of Yoga is usually understood as consisting of three steps:

1- **Listening** to Wisdom teachings.

2- **Reflection** on those teachings and living according to the disciplines enjoined by the teachings until the wisdom is fully understood.

3- **Meditation** leading to expansion of consciousness culminating in identification with the Absolute Self: Brahman (God).

Yoga Stage 1: Listening to the Wisdom Teachings

> By association with the exalted, who would not become uplifted?
> The thread which strings the flowers becomes a garland for the head.

Nagarjuna (c 100-200 A.C.E.)

Satsanga is the practice of keeping company with the wise (Saints and Sages) who can direct the aspirant on the path of wisdom. Satsanga is one of the main directives of all Yoga philosophy texts, beginning with the Egyptian hieroglyphic texts to the Vedas and Upanishads of India. Satsanga literally means: *Sat* or "that which is real," the truth, the only reality and *sanga* means "attachment to." Thus one should learn the highest teachings by practicing attachment to the truth given through discourses from a qualified teacher. Such discourses are based on the wisdom of yoga and mystical religion instead of the illusoriness of the world and worldly-minded people. Through *satsanga*, the aspirant is able to achieve wisdom and understanding of the teachings and their main goal, learning *how to get close to God.* This process has also been called *the Guru - disciple relationship.* The disciples of Jesus employed this very same principle when they left their families and previous life endeavors in order to follow the teachings of Jesus and to *"find rest with their own people."*

The Gnostic *Book of Thomas* Chapter 4:14-15:

> Thomas answered Jesus and said: "Is it good for us, Lord, to find rest among our own people?"
> The Savior said, "Yes, it does help. It is good for you, since what is visible in human existence will pass away."

Spending time among one's own people has several implications. If you do not practice Yoga, your people are ordinary members of society, the masses of un-enlightened people who seek after the pleasures of the world. If you live in this manner you will soon lead yourself to experience pain and sorrow, because all things in human existence pass away. Your search to fulfill your worldly desires will never succeed. This will turn you towards Yoga. If you are a practitioner of Yoga, your people are other practitioners of Yoga. If you spend time with them you will discover deeper and deeper wisdom about life until you eventually outgrow your worldly desires and begin to seek after a higher truth, enlightenment, the Kingdom of Heaven, which brings inner peace, joy and supreme contentment. Therefore, both roads lead to the same ultimate goal, but the first is full of pain, sorrow and frustration, while the second may be painful in the beginning, but the pain gives way to understanding and great rapture.

Vedanta philosophy has been called *The Heart of Hinduism* since it represents the central teachings upon which Hindu philosophy is based. Just as Christianity has many denominations, there are many traditions in India which

168

follow different gods or goddesses. However, like the gods and goddesses of Ancient Egypt, the deities of India all emanate from the same Supreme Being and this is acknowledged in all of the different systems, thus leading people to the same goal, although sometimes under different names. This is why Vedanta is referred to as the end of the Vedas, "end" implying distillation or an extraction of the purest essence of the Vedas, the raw mystical philosophy which underlies all of the systems. Therefore, the Upanishads are the principal *Vedantic* texts.

Vedanta Philosophy is summed up in four *Mahavakya*s or *Great Utterances* to be found in the Upanishads: 1- *Brahman, the Absolute, is Consciousness beyond all mental concepts.* 2- *Thou Art That* (referring to the fact that everyone is essentially this Consciousness). 3- *I Am Brahman, the Absolute* (I am God); to be affirmed by people, referring to their own essential nature). 4- *The Self is Brahman* (the Self is the essence of all things).	Compare to the Bible: On the essence of God: *"God is everywhere and in all things."* (Deuteronomy 4:7) On the name of God: *"I Am That I Am."* (Exodus 3:14) Jesus speaks of his own origin and identity: *"I and the Father (God) are ONE."* (John 10:30)	Compare the preceding statements in the Indian Upanishads and the Christian Bible to the following Ancient Egyptian scriptures (*Metu Neter, Sacred Speech*) taken from the *Egyptian Book of Coming Forth By Day* and other hieroglyphic texts: *Nuk Pu Nuk.* ("*I Am That I Am.*") In reference to the relationship between God and humankind: *Ntef änuk, änuk Ntef.* *("He is I and I am He.")*[I]

Yoga Stage 2: Reflecting on the Teachings and Practicing them in Everyday Life

The following passages below from the *Secret Book of John* are of particular importance because they contain a description of God which is characteristic of those found in Egypt, India and China in reference to Amun, Brahman and the Tao, respectively. There are many such passages in the Gnostic text, *Thunder, Perfect Mind,* as well. The idea of God as Absolute Existence is usually expressed in the form of contradictory statements because the Ultimate Existence is considered to be beyond the mental concepts of a God or deity with name, form and other attributes. When the Sages who wrote the scriptures experienced the Absolute, they tried to express their understanding but found that it is not possible to do so in rational terms because the Absolute is beyond mental concepts.

The mind considers things by using a frame of reference. It understands new information by making comparisons to other information which it has gathered in the past. Popular religion (exoteric, myth and ritual level) is designed for the rational mind through teachings that appeal to reason. To this end, characters that ordinary people (novices on the spiritual path) can relate to are developed. These characters, if properly understood, are symbols which can lead aspirants to the reality which lies beyond them. This is the reality which the Sages and Saints experience.

Mystical experience, however, transcends all ordinary human conceptualization. Is and is not, being and not being, existence and non-existence, these are only concepts of the mind which are all transcended in the mystical experience. Therefore, seemingly contradictory and paradoxical statements like, *"God is neither corporeal nor incorporeal"* are used in the attempt to lead the mind of a spiritual seeker to eventually be able to transcend the meaning of the words and their rational interpretations, attaining understanding which transcends mentation and culminates in intuitive understanding. In this manner, Christ leads us to the *Kingdom of Heaven*, Heru of Egypt leads us to *Manu, The Beautiful West*, and Krishna leads us to *Brahman*. The following Hermetic text elaborates on the teaching.

3. It is the invisible Spirit, One should not think of it as a God, for it is greater than a god, because it has nothing over it and no lord above it.

11. It is neither corporeal nor incorporeal.
   It is neither large nor small.
   It is impossible to say, How much is it? or What kind is it?
   for no one can understand it.

13. It is not one among the many things that are in existence: it is much greater.[63]

[I] From the Ancient Egyptian Book of Coming Forth By Day (Book of the Dead).

The next passages are from the *Upanishads* and *The Tao Te Ching*. They convey the same paradoxical nature of the Absolute, called *Brahman*, which is beyond ordinary mental capacity. In the same way that Jesus cautioned about false Christs and prophets, the Upanishads caution against mistakenly thinking that one has progressed spiritually when in reality one has indulged the ego and become more involved with its illusions. The Upanishads caution against asserting that one has found Brahman (God) since this may be merely the product of mental imagination. Rather, they continuously assert that those who have discovered Brahman, the seers, report it as being beyond mental comprehension. Despite this apparent confluence of ignorance and knowledge, the seer knows without any doubt that she/he has found Brahman when the true discovery is made.

Kena Upanishad

> If you think you know well the truth of Brahman, know that you know little. What you think to be Brahman in yourself, or what you think to be Brahman in the gods — that is not Brahman. What is indeed the truth of Brahman you must therefore learn.
>
> I cannot say that I know Brahman fully. Nor can I say that I know him not. He among us knows him best who understands the spirit of the words: "Nor do I know that I know him not."

Tao Te Ching 32

> The Tao is forever undefined.
> Small though it is in the unformed state, it cannot be grasped.

Gospel of Thomas saying 17 (Gnostic)

Jesus said, "I shall give you what no eye has seen and what no ear has
heard and what no hand has touched and what has never occurred to the
human mind."

Matthew 24:24

> For false Christs will arise, and false prophets, and shall show great signs and wonders; so that, if [it were] possible, they would deceive the very elect.

Mark 13:22

> For false Christs and false prophets shall rise, and shall show signs and wonders, to seduce, if [it were] possible, even the elect.

From the Ancient Egyptian Hymns of Amun

> 10. The One, *Amun*, who hideth himself from men, who shroudeth himself from the gods, His color and appearance is not known.
> 11. The gods cannot pray to him because his name is unknown to them.

Yoga-Vedanta Philosophy Continued: Human Desire as the Cause of Pain and Suffering

According to Vedanta philosophy: Desires cannot be fulfilled through the world of time and space because:

1- There is no object or person in the realm of time and space that can satisfy the desires of any person's ego-personality because the desires of the mind, like all things in creation, are illusions. This process whereby the mind becomes deluded by its ignorance about nature is referred to as *MAYA.*

2- The pursuit of objects and relationships causes mental agitation so that the active mind cannot see beyond its immediate reality: *VIKSHEPA*. The analogy to explain Vikshepa is of a person holding a mirror to see his face but the hand is shaking. The shaking (mental agitation) of the mind due to ego-based desires which cause the image of the deeper Self to be blurred is referred to as Vikshepa.

3- At the most elementary level, the human being is in reality composed of three bodies which are supported by the Absolute Self, God: A- Causal Body, B- Astral Body, C- Physical Body.

4- The desire for objects and their pursuit through various lifetimes causes subtle impressions in the causal body which lead the jiva (individual soul) to reincarnate endlessly in an attempt to fulfill those desires: *KARMA.*

5- All objects that exist in time and space are in reality Brahman: one absolute reality, The Self. By reflecting on the teachings we can discern the real from the illusion: *VIVEKA.*

6- By following the various disciplines (spiritual disciplines), the subconscious is cleansed of illusions and desires: *DHARMA.*

7- Inner dispassion and detachment from worldly objects and human associations, *VAIRAGYA,* and renouncing the world as an illusion, *SANYASA,* lead to equanimity and peace of mind.

8- By following the wisdom teachings the mind is calmed: *SHAMA.*

9- All paths of Yoga and Yogic meditation lead to greater and greater concentration of the mind, gradually calming the mental thought waves: *DHARANA.*

10- Prolonged concentration leads to meditation and succeeding levels of greater and greater peace. Concentration is maintained without effort, *DHYANA,* and the subconscious impressions cannot arise unnoticed. The true will, *SAT SAMKALPA,* develops, allowing the divine qualities to emerge: Universal love.

11- Increased practice of meditation leads to expansion in consciousness reaching to the level of cosmic consciousness. This is called *SAMADHI.*

12- At this point the true reason for existence is realized. Knowing that one is immortal and separate from the body and that creation is a projection of one's own consciousness, one is free from MAYA. Therefore, the pain and sorrow of life is no longer experienced and there is no more reincarnation. One is supremely fulfilled in one's essential nature: BRAHMAN. All things are intuitively understood to be BRAHMAN. This is the state of *JIVAN MUKTI*: "Liberated while still alive."

13- Now there is no reason for worry. All situations can be experienced in the spirit of play or sport. This is the concept of Divine Sport: *LILA.*

14- Existence is experienced without any perception of duality. The individual merges into the ocean of existence. There is only the experience of absolute oneness, beyond all mental concepts - even those of YOGA philosophy: *KAIVALYA* (LIBERATION*).*

At this point it would be useful to examine more in-depth features of yoga philosophy. With this understanding it will be possible to discover those features in early Christian texts as well as in two of the most prominent versions of the Christian Bible.

The practice of Yoga, as developed by Sage Patanjali in India (c. 200 B.C.E.), is classified as a science with eight steps:

1- Self control (yama): Non- violence, truthfulness, chastity, avoidance of greed.

2- Practice of virtues (niyama, nyama): Actions to avoid in order to maintain yama.

3- Postures (asanas): To condition the body and prepare the mind and body for meditation.

4- Breath control (pranayama): Controlling the breath is controlling the Life Force; controlling the Life Force is controlling the mind.

5- Restraint (pratyahara): Disciplining the sense organs to avoid overindulgence and physical temptation of the body: food, sex, drugs, etc.

6- Steadying the mind (dharana): Focusing the mind. Concentrating the mental rays on one subject over a short period of time.

7- Meditation (dhyana): When the object of concentration engulfs the entire mind, concentration continues spontaneously.

8- Deep meditation (samadhi): Personality dissolves temporarily into the object of meditation, experience of super-consciousness.

Yoga Stage 3: Meditation on the Teachings

This stage is dedicated to Self-discovery through the *DIRECT INNER EXPERIENCE* of one's own true nature, leading to complete Enlightenment (salvation-liberation) by the transformation of one's consciousness. Meditation means transcendence of ordinary mortal consciousness and the achievement of the mental state of cosmic consciousness (knowledge of true Divine Self) by cleansing the subconscious mind (heart) when it is *"stilled"* (state of peace - meditation). This stage does not imply that thoughts cease forever. Meditation means the practice of stopping the thoughts and allowing the mind to become free of vibration. When this occurs the soul is able to see through it, as through a clear piece of glass. Otherwise the movements of the mind are like a reflection in the water, which is constantly moving due to waves. Consider a lake. If you are trying to see the bottom of the lake the view will be difficult if the water is agitated. The agitation caused by waves obstructs the vision of the bottom of the floor because it stirs up the silt. When the clarity which comes from the practice of stopping the vibrations (agitation) of the mind is achieved, the soul is able to see through the mind (lake) in an unobstructed way. It is at this point that it is said that the mind is nonexistent in such a person, meaning that it is transcended. The *"world has come to an end"* for that person. The world here refers to the world of illusions and misconceptions (egoism, ignorance) about the Self and about the nature of Creation.

In the Yoga Sutras of Sage Patanjali, the following instruction is given for the practitioner of yoga:

योगश्चित्तवृत्तिनिरोधः

YOGASH CHITTA VRITTI NIRODHAH.
Sutra 2: Yoga is the intentional stopping of the mind-stuff (thought waves).

This is desirable because:

वृत्तिसारूप्यमितरत्र

VRITTI SARUPYAM ITARATRA.
Sutra 4: "At times when the mind-stuff flows indiscriminately, "the seer" becomes "identified" with the thought-waves."

Patanjali goes on to say that due to the identification of the seer (our true Self) with the thoughts, we believe ourselves to be mortal and limited instead of immortal and immutable. He further says that there is no need to worry because through the steady practice (repeated effort) of yoga (dispassion, devotion, mind control exercises of meditation), even the most unruly mind can be controlled. Thus, the individual will discover their true Self when the *"Chitta"* (thought waves) are controlled. It is as if one looks at oneself through colored sunglasses and believes oneself to be that color. In the same way, Yoga is the process of uncovering the eyes from the illusion of the mind's thought waves.

The goal of all yoga disciplines is to destroy all *KARMA*. Karma is not destiny, as most people believe. Karma may be defined as worldly actions which leave impressions in the unconscious mind that lead a person to have desires or entanglements during life and at the time of death impel a person to reincarnate again. Some people erroneously try to stop the process of karma by retreating from the world so as to not have to perform actions which will lead to karma. However, this does not work since merely stopping actions does not stop the underlying cause of karma which is ignorance: *AVIDYA*. Ignorance may be defined as "absence of the knowledge of the Higher Self." Therefore, upon experiencing the Self through the various practices of yoga which lead to the mystical meditative practice of Samadhi, ignorance itself is rendered void and the light of wisdom of the Self becomes the shining reality. This is why the state of liberation from ignorance is often referred to as "Enlightenment." Attaining wisdom is like shining a light on darkness.

INTRODUCTION TO YOGA IN CHRISTIANITY

In an earlier section it was stated that Yoga philosophy has five major disciplines: The Yoga of Wisdom, The Yoga of Devotional Love, The Yoga of Righteous Action, The Yoga of Tantrism and The Yoga of Meditation. This chapter will explore the wisdom aspects of the teachings presented in Christianity. However, we will not deal with ordinary knowledge, but with mystical teachings which lead a human being from ignorance to light and from death to immortality. In order to learn the teachings properly we need to be initiated into the philosophy and practice of mysticism. Otherwise it would be like going to a library and just picking up any book and reading without a deeper understanding as to the higher purpose of the information being presented. The teachings will be ineffective if a person is not properly prepared to listen to them. This would be like sitting down to eat dinner and using the same plates from yesterday without having washed them. Therefore, we must begin by understanding the initiatic way of education and the meaning of initiation into the teachings as well as the journey of enlightenment.

What is necessary to allow a person to grow spiritually? First it is necessary for a spiritual aspirant to come under the influence of an authentic spiritual teachers. This is known as good association or *Satsanga* in India and *Sheti* in Ancient Egypt. This is the kind of relationship that Jesus had with his disciples. This is a study group led by an authentic spiritual master for the purpose of delving deeply into the meaning of the teachings for the purpose of learning how to apply them in one's daily life. This form of study must relentlessly go over the teachings again and again so the mind becomes brighter and understanding deepens. Eventually an understanding dawns in the mind that one is more than just a mortal human being, that one has an immortal spiritual heritage. All of this falls under the heading of the Yoga of Wisdom.

It is also necessary to adjust your life-style. You need to live the teachings, to make every part of your life permeated by them. Your occupation in life should be something that is good for humanity. This discipline is known as the Yoga of Righteous Action. Also it is necessary to practice prayer, chanting and channeling the emotions within you. You must learn to control your feelings and not allow the negative feelings to control you. You should develop the attitude that you are serving God in humanity and that your actions are worship of the Divine in the same way that you may light incense or bring flowers to an altar. Then you can direct your feelings towards discovering the divine essence within you which is the source of your true desires. Through the development of devotion towards the teachings and towards the deity of the Christian myth (Jesus), it is possible to discover boundless Divine Love, bliss and joy within your own heart. This is known as the Yoga of Devotional Love. When all of these teachings come together, a mystic movement allows an aspirant to transcend the thinking mind through meditation. This meditative movement leads to the experience of oneness with the Divine. This is known as The Yoga of Meditation.

Christian Yoga concentrates primarily on three forms of yogic spiritual practice, wisdom, devotion, and righteous action, however the other forms are closely related to them. The most important form of yoga in Christianity is the Yoga of Devotional Love. When Jesus speaks of taking refuge in him, when he says that he is the way to salvation and when he tells everyone to love others as they love themselves, he is expressing the practice of the Yoga of Devotional Love. Along with the Yoga of Devotional or Divine Love, the Yoga of Righteous action is also emphasized. When Jesus admonished his followers to keep the commandments and to follow the beatitudes with a new insight, to take up the cross and follow him, etc., he is expressing the practice of the Yoga of Righteous Action. When Jesus gives the special inner teachings and parables to his disciples and says that he is one with the father, that the Kingdom is spread upon the earth but people do not see it, and that a person has to develop vigilance, detachment and dispassion, this is the Yoga of Wisdom. In this Yoga the mystical teachings which relate the soul to the Divine are imparted. The Yoga of Meditation and the Yoga of Tantrism are closely related to the Yoga of Devotion in Christian practice, and these will be explored further in great detail in Christian Yoga, Volume Two.

THE MYSTICAL JOURNEY FROM JESUS TO CHRIST

THE GENERAL PLAN OF CHRISTIAN YOGA

The mystical plan of life as conceptualized by the Gnostic Christian philosophy may be conceptualized as follows:

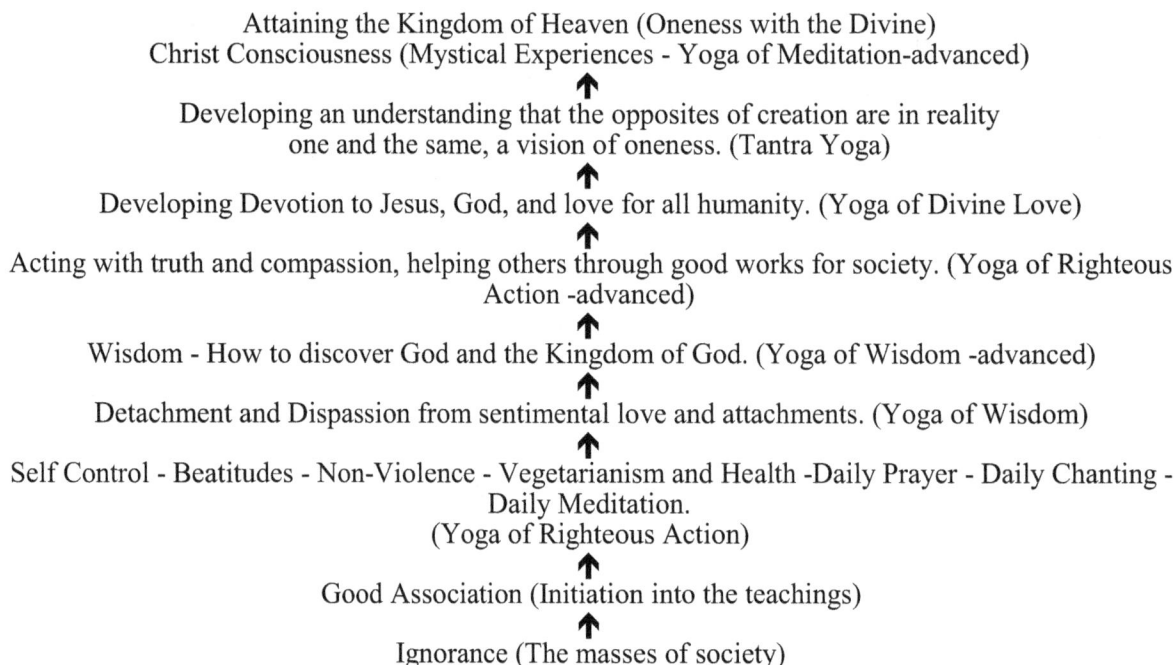

Attaining the Kingdom of Heaven (Oneness with the Divine)
Christ Consciousness (Mystical Experiences - Yoga of Meditation-advanced)
↑
Developing an understanding that the opposites of creation are in reality
one and the same, a vision of oneness. (Tantra Yoga)
↑
Developing Devotion to Jesus, God, and love for all humanity. (Yoga of Divine Love)
↑
Acting with truth and compassion, helping others through good works for society. (Yoga of Righteous
Action -advanced)
↑
Wisdom - How to discover God and the Kingdom of God. (Yoga of Wisdom -advanced)
↑
Detachment and Dispassion from sentimental love and attachments. (Yoga of Wisdom)
↑
Self Control - Beatitudes - Non-Violence - Vegetarianism and Health -Daily Prayer - Daily Chanting -
Daily Meditation.
(Yoga of Righteous Action)
↑
Good Association (Initiation into the teachings)
↑
Ignorance (The masses of society)

THE INITIATIC WAY OF EDUCATION

As discussed earlier, the loss of an authentic link to traditional mysticism allowed a situation of confusion and debate over the original Christian teachings to ensue amongst the early Christian Fathers and Bishops. This situation has been the cause of continued misunderstanding throughout the history of Roman Catholicism. In contrast, Western religions are regarded even by Westerners as inexact exercises in faith.

Every true mystical tradition, be it religious or non-religious, requires a traditional mystical link. Initiatic teachings, or the teachings given to those who become initiated into a tradition, need the benefit of a teacher who has actually experienced the mystical state of consciousness and who can explain the meaning of the texts and how to apply their teachings. When aspirants try to understand mystic teachings without the guidance of such a master, it is, as an Eastern parable explains, like blind people trying to learn from another blind person what the world looks like by simply using imagination and wit.

Intellectuals who come to believe that they have attained "Enlightenment" merely by reading the scriptures often experience a rude awakening when they are tested by natural human situations of adversity. At such challenging times they realize that they cannot control their emotions or find mental peace. Others study the teachings with earnestness and great seriousness, yet find that they cannot realize the subtlety of the teachings in order to achieve their Enlightenment. They find that they cannot control their minds, emotions or desires, and thus are unable to discover the deeper meaning of the teaching due to their inability to calm the mind. One example of this personality type is someone who needs constant activity so as not to feel lonely or bored. Such a person is constantly searching for action by turning on the television, calling someone, gossiping or having some other interaction or activity. In its extreme, such a personality type seeks to agitate themselves constantly by finding something to be upset or argumentative about. Unless there is a fight or other intense emotion present, such a person feels lost. Even if there is no trouble they will create trouble so as to agitate their minds and feel "alive."

An example of one who is unable to control the mind is the cigarette smoker. He or she "knows" that smoking is poisonous and yet they are unable to stop. Why? Because their intellect is overpowered by the need to satisfy their dependency on the cigarettes. They have not discovered the wellspring of will and inner fulfillment which is within them, so they continue to search outside of themselves through objects which seem to satisfy the needs but which are in reality leading to greater pain and disappointment. They live on a superficial level, concerned with a life based on the body, physical senses and the fulfillment of worldly desires.

A sage does not live a life based on the sense perceptions nor on the desires of the mind and body. He or she has discovered the illusoriness of the senses, the emptiness of desires and the futility of trying to fulfill them in the realm of time and space. Those who are advancing on the spiritual path have discovered that they do not need to lean on sense perceptions or on emotional or physical dependencies to feel alive. They have discovered that sustenance and happiness comes from within. It is there that all desires are truly fulfilled. For this reason, proper initiation into a teaching and learning under the instruction of an enlightened master or her/his direct disciple is a necessary process in order to develop the correct understanding and practice of the teachings. While the teachings may seem explicit to the highly intellectual mind, there are nuances of misunderstanding which will occur. This is why association with an authentic teacher is essential on the spiritual path for those who are serious about their spiritual development. Any other learning process is subject to error and confusion which will lead to disappointment and frustration.

The initiatic teachings exist as an alternative to ordinary worldly life, and Christianity, having originally been an initiatic mystery religion, was no different in its approach to the transference of the teachings from teacher to student. Long before the establishment of Christianity as a religion, water was used in initiation ceremonies to initiate new followers of the philosophy. Prior to entering a temple people would bathe as a symbol of inner purification. Christianity adopted this ritual and it was used at the initiation of Jesus by John the Baptist. This ritual act served to join Jesus to a tradition into which he would initiate his own future disciples. But what was this initiatic relationship all about? What was its purpose and how was this purpose to be accomplished. How could it be possible for Jesus or any other teacher to impart the most profound teachings of spirituality to others? These are very important questions for anyone considering treading the spiritual path in a serious way. Therefore, it is appropriate here to discuss what aspiration really means and what an authentic teacher is.

THE ASPIRANT

When a person begins to wonder about the origin of the universe, about the purpose of life, the cruelty of life, the inability to be truly happy in the world and the transitoriness of all things, such a person may be ready to inquire about the deeper truths of her/his own existence and to seek after answers which have plagued them for perhaps many lifetimes. Sometimes people say that they are serious about spirituality, but when they begin to learn about what it entails they develop a fear or distaste for spiritual practice because they begin to realize that they need to make dramatic and fundamental changes in their life to stop the negative patterns of behavior and control the mind and its endless desires.

The reason that most people accept the injustices, cruelties, and sorrows of the world is that they tend to overlook the obvious illusoriness of relationships and the fleeting nature of sensory pleasure. There is a lack of thoughtfulness about the nature of pain, so people go on believing that they will find happiness in the world. They almost never entertain questions about the unreality of the world and life in general, or the fact of eventual death. When they do so, they often turn to others who are intensely involved in the world and, by so doing, become once again distracted with the burdens of life, hoping to get some happiness and pleasure out of life's experiences. Sometimes people delude themselves into ignoring a serious question because they feel they cannot reach an answer, or the answer is perceived as being too painful.

The Qualities of a Spiritual Aspirant

In the Indian scripture, the *Shiva-Samhita* (III.16-19), an *adhikarini* or "qualified person" to learn Yoga is said to need the quality of *vishvasa* or "positive frame of mind" as the most important quality. This is followed by moderate diet, sense restraint, impartiality, and veneration of the teacher.

For those who come to a Yoga counselor or a Yogic Spiritual Preceptor (Guru), the benefits are a step beyond those of ordinary psychology which seeks to help a person cope with ordinary life problems by accepting them. In the beginning, the Yogic counselor must help the individual to somehow turn the anguish and pain experienced from the world into a desire to rise above it, not to go along with it and live with it, but to understand it and transcend it. The Yoga counselor helps the seeker to channel those disappointed energies into healthy dispassion towards the world and its entanglements, towards spiritual aspiration and self-effort directed at sustaining a viable spiritual discipline or program. Gnostic Christianity has incorporated these universal techniques for spiritual transformation.

In Ancient Egypt, a devotee of the goddess Aset is: *One who ponders over sacred matters and seeks therein for hidden truth.* It is not enough to just hear the ancient myths or to understand them at an intellectual level. The aspirant must go deep within him/herself to discover the subtle ideas being conveyed. *Plutarch* describes the character of an initiate of Aset as:

> *He alone is a true servant or follower of this Goddess who, after has heard, and has been made acquainted in a proper manner (initiated into the philosophy) with the history of the actions of these gods, searches into the hidden truths which lie concealed under them, and examines the whole by the dictates of reason and philosophy. Nor indeed, ought such an examination to be looked on as unnecessary whilst there are so many ignorant of the true reason even of the most ordinary rites observed by the Egyptian priests, such as their shavings[1] and wearing linen garments. Some, indeed, there are, who never trouble themselves to think at all about these matters, whilst others rest satisfied with the most superficial accounts of them: They pay a peculiar veneration to the sheep,(sacred to Amun) therefore they think it their duty not only to abstain from eating flesh, but likewise from wearing its wool. They are continually mourning for their gods, therefore they shave themselves.*

One particular statement in reference to the teachings, *...the hidden truths which lie concealed under them....,* begs the question: What are these "hidden truths" which are "concealed" within the "history of the actions of the gods?" The following statement from the *Yoga Vasistha* (Indian Vedantic text) sheds light on this question, introducing us to the esoteric or metaphysical level of religion as opposed to the ritualistic-mythological level.

> "O Rama, gods and goddesses and other deities with name and form are representations created by Sages for those whose intellect is weak as a child's..."

Yoga Vasistha Nirvana Prakarana Section 30

The elaborate system of gods and goddesses as well as the symbols representing a Supreme Being are merely metaphors created by the Sages of ancient times for those who are not spiritually mature (possessing a highly developed sense of intellectual subtlety) to understand that God transcends all thoughts, symbols and concepts of the mind. Until the intellect *(Saa)* is developed, the symbols are used, but when spiritual sensitivity dawns, the hidden or esoteric meaning of the symbols is revealed, leading the initiate to greater and greater levels of inner awareness or Enlightenment. While religion is expressed as a system of gods and goddesses or angels and saints, in reality these refer to symbols and metaphors whose understanding will lead to insight into the nature of existence and the innermost Self. Thus, polytheistic systems are, in reality, an intricate code system which holds the wisdom of life.

> Isis says: "I Isis, am all that has been, all that is, or shall be; and no mortal man hath ever unveiled me."

Aset (Isis) represents the preceptor of the mysteries, the high goddess. Having attained spiritual knowledge by listening to the teachings of Aset, the task of the initiate is to continuously reflect upon them until the veil of ignorance (egoism) is lifted. Through the process of continued intellectual refinement (reflection on the teachings), the veil is gradually torn away. Thus, the mortal consciousness (symbolized by the veil) is transcended and Aset is realized in her unveiled form. In order to behold her unveiled form, ordinary human perception cannot be used. This is why *no mortal man* has unveiled her. Only those who have become like Aset (divine in consciousness) can see her. Through gradual intellectual refinement attained through the process of reflection and meditation, the mind of the initiate becomes transformed. Thus, the initiate sees with Divine eyes and not with mortal ones. He or she is now beyond birth and death (mortality).

Unveiling Aset is unveiling your true Self. One must go beyond the "mortal" waking, dream-sleep and dreamless-deep-sleep states of consciousness to discover (unveil) one's true nature. Over five thousand years before the rise in prominence of the cult of Aset and Asar in Greece and Rome, the Egyptian *Pyramid Texts* described the process of spiritual transformation through the mythology surrounding the *Eye* of Heru and its return to the initiate following its theft by Set.[II] In later times, the struggle against Set was carried on in the mysteries of Aset which

---

[1] *In the *Papyrus of Nes-Menu*, there is an order to the priestesses of Isis and Nephthys to have "the hair of their bodies shaved off". They are also ordered to wear fillets of rams wool on their heads ▯ ⌐ ⌐ as a form of ritual identification with the hidden (Amun) mystery. Wool was also used by the Sufis, followers of esoteric Islam. The name *"Sufi"* comes from "Suf" which means "wool." The name Sufi was adopted since the ascetic‡ followers of this doctrine wore coarse woolen garments (sufu). ‡ An *ascetic* is one who practices severe and austere methods of spiritual practice.
[II] See the book *Egyptian Yoga: The Philosophy of Enlightenment*.

lasted until the year 394 A.C.E. when the Temple of Aset at *Philae* was closed by Christian Zealots who had taken over Egypt and Ethiopia. The process of initiation and spiritual awakening may be further defined as follows.

In the Indian system of classification of spiritual aspirants, the categories are further classified by the characteristics that are favorable and unfavorable for spiritual disciplines. The serious aspirant should study these well, in order to understand what is required for the successful practice of spirituality and to promote them within him/herself.

The *Yoga Sutra* (III.7), the textbook of classical Yoga, lists the following impediments on the yogic path: illness, languor, doubt, heedlessness, sloth, dissipation, false vision, non-attainment of the higher levels of the spiritual path, and instability in a given level of attainment. These are also called distractions (*vikshepa*) of consciousness, and the *Yoga Sutra* (I.29) prescribes the practice of mantra[1] recitation (*japa*) and contemplation (*bhavana*) of the sacred syllable *OM* for their swift removal. The *Linga Purana* includes: lack of faith, suffering, and depression. This work states that such obstacles can be removed through constant practice and devotion to one's teacher. The *Bhagavata-Purana* includes *siddhis* (paranormal psychic powers) as mental distractions.

The *hatha yoga* work, *Shiva-Samhita* (V.10 ff.), states that the weak aspirant *(mridu)* is unenthusiastic, foolish, fickle, timid, ill, dependent, rude, ill-mannered, and un-energetic. He is considered fit only for *mantra yoga* or the recitation of empowered sounds (*mantra*).

The mediocre aspirant (*madhya*) is endowed with even-mindedness, patience, a desire for virtue, kind speech, and the tendency to practice moderation in all things. He/she is considered capable of practicing *laya yoga,* or dissolution of the mind through meditative absorption.

The exceptional aspirant (*adhimatra*) is someone who shows such qualities as firm understanding, aptitude for meditative absorption (*laya*), self-reliance, liberal-mindedness, bravery, vigor, faithfulness, willingness to worship the "lotus feet" of the teacher, and delight in the practice of Yoga. This reference to the lotus feet of the teacher refers to the understanding that the teacher, having attained God-consciousness or Self-realization, is indeed God incarnate and, therefore, his/her feet should be venerated as God's feet.

The extraordinary aspirant (*adhimatratama*), who may practice any type of yoga, demonstrates the following virtues: great energy, enthusiasm, charm, heroism, scriptural knowledge, the inclination to practice, freedom from delusion, orderliness, youthfulness, moderate eating habits, control over the senses, fearlessness, purity, skillfulness, liberality, the ability to be a refuge for all people, capability, stability, thoughtfulness, the willingness to do whatever is desired by the teacher, patience, good manners, observance of the moral and spiritual law, the ability to keep his struggle to him/herself, kind speech, faith in the scriptures, the readiness of the divine, knowledge of the vows in his/her particular level of practice, and the active pursuit of all forms of Yoga.

THE TEACHER

How do you know when you are growing spiritually? When the troubles of life are no longer insurmountable, when you become slowed to anger, when you begin to discover a higher vision of yourself which goes beyond any mental conception, that is when you are moving towards self-discovery. That is the art and practice of Yoga in life.

When you are practicing Yoga and you are living in the world, you are continually being challenged. Have you controlled your anger? your fears? your lusts? etc. This is how you know when you are progressing. When you face life with the teachings of Yoga, then you are as if equipped with a suit of armor which insults, annoyances, and egoistic values cannot penetrate. You begin to discover an inner peace which surpasses both outer pleasures and pains as well as internal desires of the ego. This occurs in degrees, so be patient. When you are sincere and repeatedly practice the teachings, even though you may fail many times before succeeding, you will achieve progress.

> *When the Student is ready the Master will appear!*
>
> *-Ancient Egyptian Proverb*

When you are growing spiritually you will recognize those who are spiritually advanced. You will be led to them in a mystical way and you will receive the teaching which you need at that time. First, you need to begin to purify yourself and make yourself into a good student because only then will you be able to recognize a good teacher. Only

---

[1] Hekau in Ancient Egyptian Terminology.

then will you be fit to receive teachings and to understand them and put them into practice. Spiritual development does not occur in a flash or through a magical touch. It occurs with incremental practice of the teachings as you gradually integrate them into your life. Once you learn the correct methods of spiritual discipline you can then choose those forms (meditation, selfless service, study of scriptures, etc.) which suit your personality. Then gradually you can increase the intensity of your practice even while you carry on the normal duties of life. This process leads to peace and enjoyment of life and to spiritual Enlightenment in an integrated and balanced way.

The need for a true teacher of spirituality cannot be overemphasized in the course of spiritual practice. An aspirant (anyone seriously seeking spiritual development) is like an athlete. He or she needs coaching and practice in order to attain the mastery over the lower self. True spiritual Enlightenment cannot be achieved through magic or through unnatural means. It is achieved through understanding and hard work, not ordinary work, but that activity which leads to purification of the heart (eradication of anger, hatred, greed, jealousy, etc.). Books can only go so far in explaining the true practice of spirituality because the mind tends to develop many misconceptions and illusions about what is read. Therefore, a guide or coach who is advanced in the practice should be sought out and approached. This is the process of spiritual teaching called initiation. The aspirant is initiated into a philosophy and way of life which he or she needs to learn and practice by studying, reflecting, practicing and meditating on the teachings. Initiation is a conscious choice to adopt a teaching and to embark on the task of basing your life on it in order to purify your mind and body and become a conduit of the Divine.

The wisdom texts and scriptures are like a painting of fire. They provide information about wisdom just as a picture gives an idea of what something looks like. However, in order to understand the subtlety of the scriptures, something more is needed. A true teacher is one who lives the teaching. Such a one can breathe life into the scriptures and myths to make them understood in the language of today. This is the fire of knowledge which burns away ignorance and illusions, which are the causes of human suffering and misery.

There is no nobler occupation than teaching Yoga philosophy because there is no greater endeavor than relieving the burden of those who are beset by ignorance and mental suffering. Also, there is no greater force to dispel the mental anguish of society than Yogic mystical philosophy. Therefore, meeting an authentic teacher of Yoga philosophy is a highly coveted event by those who have begun to recognize the deeper levels of their own being.

One of the main problems of society is the relative lack of interest in the scriptures and another is the relatively small number of authentic spiritual preceptors available to teach them. Many people do not find spirituality attractive because they feel they would "lose out" on life if they became seriously involved. They do not realize that their attempts to experience joy from the world are doomed to failure. Further, they do not understand that they already have all they need to be truly happy without continuing to search outside of themselves. Their problems arise from the intensification of their ego-body identification, erroneous concepts about religion and Yoga, as well as misconceptions about life and the possibility of fulfilling desires.

A *Guru* is not only someone who is advanced on the spiritual path or even just someone who has reached the fully enlightened state. A Guru, in the Upanishadic (teachings of the Indian Upanishads) sense of the word, is someone who is spiritually enlightened and who also is well-versed in the scriptural teachings and methods of training aspirants according to their level of understanding. Therefore, a counselor of Yoga must first achieve a high degree of understanding and personal - spiritual emancipation since the subtleties of the mind must be well understood. The teacher must be able to be a refuge for all people, have the ability to succeed in his/her struggle, have complete knowledge of the teachings pertaining to her/his level of attainment, and enthusiastically pursue all forms of Yoga. The *Guru*, is referred to as the "weighty one" or "enlightener of the cave," is so called because his/her judgment and counsel are "weighty" and that person shines the light of wisdom on the darkness of ignorance in the "cave" of the heart. The *Advaya-Taraka- Upanishad* speaks of the guru in the following way:

The (true) teacher is well versed in the Veda (wisdom teachings), a devotee of Vishnu (God, The Self), free from envy, pure, a knower of Yoga and intent on Yoga, and always having the nature of Yoga.

THE HISTORY AND PHILOSOPHY OF MYSTICAL CHRISTIANITY

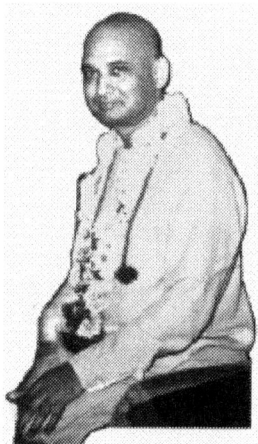

Left: Swami Jyotirmayananda lecturing on the wisdom of Yoga.
(Swami Jyotirmayananda, the Spiritual Preceptor of Dr. Muata Ashby)

"Yoga is a universal religion. It gives insight into every religion...Yoga embraces all religions of the world. It does not see the need of contradicting them. Its interest lies in giving a wider meaning to one's love for God. What is contradicted is limitation in understanding God, and a mental obstruction in developing love of God. All great mystics, saints and seers in all parts of the world proclaim the same reality, but, in different expressions, in different languages. Yogic principles are verified through all great personalities. Some thinkers and seers have especially named Yoga as the basis of their inspiration. Many practiced universal Yoga without giving it a Sanskrit name. The philosopher Schopenhauer was inspired by the Upanishads. The teachings of Jesus were inspired by the Yogic teachings that prevailed in antiquity through Buddhism. Socrates was inspired by Yogic wisdom. Directly or indirectly, all great personalities drink deep from the universal stream of wisdom which is Yoga...therefore Christianity is nothing but Yoga."

—Swami Jyotirmayananda

Sri Swami Jyotirmayananda now lives in the United States, where he conducts weekly classes on Integral Yoga from his Ashram in Miami, Florida. Swami Jyotirmayananda is a living Saint who is dedicated to the enlightenment of all peoples of every faith and ethnic background.

Many scriptures admonish the aspirant to submit to and serve the Guru in all things since the guru's contact with the Absolute (*Brahman*) gives him/her a unique insight and unfailing understanding of the teachings and the human mind. The relative scarcity of Self-realized[1] gurus has led many seekers to disappointing experiences. In modern times many self-proclaimed gurus who required absolute obedience have exploited many seekers, prompting a mistrust in gurus. Western television evangelists and local preachers have also tarnished the view of spirituality in the minds of many. *Guru-yoga* or the practice of submission to the guru's will in all matters is still practiced around the world.

A personality who is perfect in his/her identification with the transcendental Self has been seen as an embodiment of the teaching itself and is, therefore, deserving of full veneration as an incarnation of the Divine. However, the relatively few numbers of truly realized personalities has given rise to many self-styled spiritual personalities, not only in modern times, but in ancient times as well. The *Kula-Arnava-Tantra* (XIII.106ff) from around 500 A.C.E. speaks on this issue:

O Devi (Goddess), there are many *guru*s on the earth who give what is other than the Self, but hard to find in all the worlds is the *guru* who reveals the Self.

Many are the *guru*s who rob the disciple of his wealth, but rare is the *guru* who removes the disciple's afflictions.

He is the (true) *guru* by whose very contact (association) there flows the supreme Bliss *(ananda)*. The intelligent person should choose such a one as his *guru* and none other.

---

[1] Those who have "realized" their union with the transcendental Self.

Many teachers (psychologists, psychiatrists, yoga instructors) are deluded as to their understanding of the scriptures and of their own attainment. This ignorance results in their failure to cope with their own afflictions as well as the afflictions of others and their inability to help others in a permanent way. Due to their ineffectiveness in their own professional and personal life, the erring teacher is unable to provide treatment to others which is viable and, therefore, lasting.

The teaching is often understood differently at different levels. Just as there are increasing levels of religious practice (Myth - Ritual - Mystical) there are varying levels of aspirants. Only one who has experienced and matured to greater levels of attainment through *personality integration* can assist others in understanding those higher levels. Here, personality integration refers to the extent that the individual has realized his/her own ego-lessness and identification with the transcendental Self. One on the spiritual path who intends to help others needs to understand this well by first helping him/herself, by profoundly practicing the teachings.

An authentic teacher of yoga philosophy is someone who is advanced on the path of self-control, indifferent to both positive or negative situations, unaffected by praise or censure. Such a teacher is not desirous of any object in the phenomenal world and thus able to utilize various objects and manage various situations in a detached manner for the welfare of humanity. He or she has discovered inner fulfillment and is a wellspring of joy and peace to all they meet.

They are not interested in developing relationships with students based on emotionality or other egoistic sensibilities. They do not keep disciples as servants for their own amusement or to inflate their own egos, because they have transcended all of these human frailties. They are fulfilled through their realization of their own divinity and help others out of the compassion and universal love which flow through them directly from the divine source.

In this manner, Sages carry out the work of enlightening others and relieving the pain of life. The actions of a Sage affect incalculable numbers of people because their actions ripple through the world as a wave ripples across a calm lake when a stone is thrown into it. By their writings, expositions, subtle spiritual influence, and their example as living embodiments of wisdom, they have an effect on the course of the world and on all with whom they come into contact, whether directly or indirectly.

Enlightenment occurs in degrees like the sun rising at dawn. The light of wisdom grows; this light grows to infinity. As a person grows in inner peace and inner awareness, they are moving towards Enlightenment. Therefore, there are different degrees of teachers. This idea was reflected in the original Christian Church hierarchy. The Holy Orders in the Eastern Orthodox, Roman Catholic and Anglican churches is the sacrament through which a person becomes a minister of the Gospel. The orders of bishops, priests, and deacons were said to have been set up by Christ. The authority of the bishops is thought to extend in succession from Jesus' Apostles. Only bishops are allowed to ordain new ministers in this system. There are some churches which ordain ministers but do not believe in the Apostolic Succession. Religions other than the Judeo-Christian tradition had priesthoods and/or priestesshoods. A class of clergy was recognized by the ancient civilizations of Egypt, Greece, Rome, Britain, the Celtic tribes of Ireland, and Gaul. In modern-day Shintoism, Buddhism and Hinduism, the priestly function is still held to be important.

It is acceptable to have advanced Yoga instructors (disciples) provide initial Yoga instruction including the introduction of exoteric and esoteric knowledge and providing support and encouragement to aspirants, but as a rule, the lower level priests or priestesses do not initiate the disciple into the subtle mysteries of advanced spirituality. This role is reserved for the fully enlightened Guru or spiritual master.

In Ancient Egypt the spiritual teacher was known as *Sehu*. A preceptor is a teacher who may or may not have the function of a *Sehu* or *Guru*, or spiritual guide proper. It should be noted here that enlightened personalities are not necessarily nor exclusively to be known as Gurus. They may reside in any part of the world and may be engaged in various activities or occupations. They may not write voluminous works of philosophy or preach, yet they are Sages nonetheless. What denotes them is their way of working, the manner in which they deal with life and how they serve humanity through their work. Also they may be either male or female. Thus, in order to be effective, preceptorship needs to be given by those who are part of a lineage of true spiritual practitioners. So the leader as well as the lowest order of clergy can provide adequate spiritual support to society. This will occur if their teaching is authentic, if they teach at the level of their individual attainment and individual personal practice, and if they receive proper guidance from the level of priesthood above their own. If one of these areas is deficient, the church system will be inadequate to meet the spiritual needs of the community as well as the clergy itself.

When the priest determines that the aspirant is ready to receive more advanced spiritual instruction, he/she may consult with the more advanced enlightened personality (Sage, Saint, Guru, etc.) or refer the aspirant directly for advanced teaching while continuing the counseling-teacher relationship. Therefore, the lower order of the priesthood or priesteshood and the higher order can complement each other, though not necessarily working together. The *Yoga Vasistha* text states the importance of teaching the wisdom of the Self as a way of raising one's spiritual consciousness. This is because, by keeping the teachings foremost in the mind through the teaching process, it (mind) does not stray to sense objects or to other distractions. The mind, therefore, flows to the Absolute in a continuous manner.

Sage Vasistha continued: One who is ceaselessly devoted to *Brahman* (God), who exists for the sake of the Self, who rejoices in talking about *Brahman*, and who is engaged in enlightening others about their essential nature, he attains Liberation even in this life. III. 9:1

Since all human problems are understood as proceeding from the original cause of ignorance of one's true nature, all efforts are directed to dispelling the mental illusions which lead to misunderstanding of spiritual truth.

To this effect the program of Yoga is imparted in three stages:

1-Listening to the wisdom teachings. The nature of reality (creation) and the nature of the Self.
2-Reflecting on those teachings and incorporating them into daily life.
3-Meditating on the meaning of the teachings.

Note: It is important to note here that the same teaching which was practiced in Ancient Egypt of **Listening** to, **Reflecting** upon, and **Meditating** upon the teachings is the same process used in Vedanta-Jnana Yoga of India of today: **Jnana Yoga.** "The Yoga of Wisdom" is a form of Yoga based on insight into the nature of worldly existence and the transcendental Self, thereby transforming one's consciousness through development of the wisdom faculty. The three steps in the process of Jnana Yoga are equal to the teachings of the Temple of Aset of Ancient Egypt. In Sanskrit these steps are known as:

1- *Shravana*: Listening.
2- *Manana:* Reflection.
3- *Niddidhyasana:* Meditation.

Lastly, it would be an exceedingly great error for someone to claim to be a realized spiritual master if they are not. This is because the psychic illusion that would be created within their own mind would hamper their own spiritual movement. However, the imitation of spiritual personalities and their behavior is permitted and even promoted to the extent that it is grounded in reality and honesty. The idea is that we are what we feel, act, believe and think. Therefore, as we feel, act, believe and think in a particular way, we become like onto that. Therefore, it is all right to emulate the qualities of a Sage because this process helps to control the ego and promote the process of becoming sagely.

CHAPTER VIII: THE FEMALE ASPECT OF CHRISTIANITY

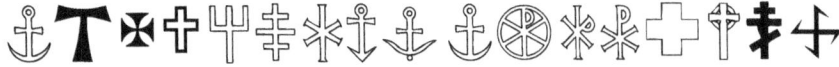

What good is it to me if Mary gave birth to the son of God fourteen hundred years ago and I do not also give birth to the son of God in my time and in my culture?

—Meister Eckhart (1260?-1328?)

We are the mother of Christ when we carry him in our heart and body by love and a pure and sincere conscience. And we give birth to him through our holy works which ought to shine on others by our example.

—Francis of Assisi (1182-1226)

GOD AS MOTHER

While the male aspect of God in Christianity has been expressed and affirmed throughout the history of Roman Catholicism following the early Orthodox Church councils, the theme of the Supreme Being as a female personality in Christian religion existed in previous times. Traces of this majestic ideal survive in the present day versions of the Bible. The female essence of Divinity was implied to be present in all "High God" male deities of the ancient religions which predated Judaism. Most prominent in ancient times were Aset (Isis) from Egypt and Durga (Kali) from India, but there were many others. Thus, God could be equally worshipped as Father or as Mother without any contradiction. In a deeper sense, the ancient religions correctly sought to express the idea that God is in reality both male and female to those who were ready to understand this transcendental reality. Therefore, the presence of the goddess is to be expected in Christianity as well, having originated in the land of Egypt where the cult of Aset was the strongest mystery religion during the time of the early development of Christianity. In the beginning stages of Christianity, Mary, the mother of Jesus, received many of the attributes of the female goddesses which preceded her. The following lines from Bible illustrate the idea of God, not as an aging man sitting on a throne in heaven, but of a mother who tenderly nurtures her child and compassionately watches over the fruit of her own being.

I [Yahweh] groan like a woman in labor, I suffocate, I stifle.

Isa. 42:14

14 But Zion said, the Lord hath forsaken me, and my Lord hath forgotten me.
15 Can a woman forget her nursing child, that she should not have compassion on the son of her womb? Yea, they may forget, yet I will not forget thee.

Isa. 49:14,15

9 Shall I bring to the birth, and not cause to bring forth? saith the LORD: shall I cause to bring forth, and shut [the womb]? saith thy God.
13 As one whom his mother comforteth, so will I comfort you; and ye shall be comforted in Jerusalem.

Isa 66:9,13

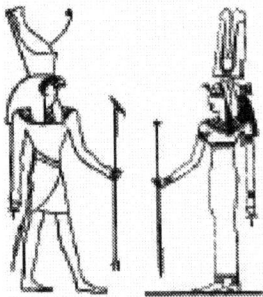

Left: Above: the divine couple from Ancient Egypt, Horus and Hathor.

In order to experience the divinity within yourself, you must begin to discover the complementary nature of your being. If you possess a male body, you must realize that half of your genetic structure, indeed, half of your physical being, is female. If you possess a female body the opposite is true. The difference in the genes which causes the difference in physical appearance is illusory, as a mental thought is illusory. In your dream you may take any form, but when you wake up you realize that no matter how real the experience felt, it was not true. Likewise, this physical reality is not the absolute truth of your existence. The human body is not an abiding reality. It is a transient vehicle which you have created according to your past feelings and the current needs of your soul. It is not a truth to be held onto. However, even if you were to examine the body, thinking that it is an abiding reality, you will realize that it is never stable. Blood is constantly flowing and cells are constantly changing. If you were to compare the male and female physiology you would see that both men and women have the same organs, but these are developed in slightly different ways to suit the task of the gender. So maleness and femaleness are illusory concepts which are supported by spiritual ignorance. When the body is seen as the utmost reality and your identification with the body is intense, the desires, pleasures, and discomforts of the body take precedence and your intellect and willpower are reduced. The inability to control your desires leaves you prey to the animal feelings and base emotions of the mind. These lead the ignorant on an endless search for bodily comforts which are always illusory. At this level people convince themselves that they are happy when they attain some physical comfort, but this never lasts. Therefore, use your intelligence to see through the mist of ignorance by using the light of reason and wisdom. Open up to the greater reality which is what you truly are. You are more than an aggregate of elements and chemicals arranged into the form of flesh and bones. You are the transcendental Self, the Christ.

> "Souls, Horus, son, are of the self-same nature, since they came from the same place where the Creator modeled them; nor male nor female are they. Sex is a thing of bodies not of Souls."

Ancient Egyptian Proverb from
The teachings of Isis to Horus

Jesus and Mary Magdalene

In Ancient Egypt, there were several prototypes for the ideal spiritual couple who exemplify the highest qualities of spiritual aspiration in a male-female relationship. One of these was Asar and Aset (Osiris and Isis). Their relationship formed the basis of the Ausarian Resurrection myth, which we reviewed earlier, and also became the basis for the resurrection teachings of Christianity as well as the final judgement of the soul. Another important couple is Heru and Het-heru (Horus and Hathor). Their part of the Ausarian Resurrection myth is also integral to the teaching and in their own right they convey powerful mystical principles as well.[1] In fact, all of the major gods and goddesses of Ancient Egypt had their male or female counterparts, and it is therefore expected that we might see the same teachings reflected in Christianity, given that it was in Ancient Egypt where Christian philosophy originated.

Below: Jesus and Mary Magdalene. Drawing by Hamsa Yogi (Lou Lochard)

In Indian mythology, the characters of Krishna, an incarnation of Vishnu (God), and Radha, his consort, are prime examples of the male-female elements and their relation to spiritual development. Like Heru and Het-heru of Ancient Egypt, their relationship is complementary. It closely resembles the relationship of Jesus and Mary Magdalene with respect to the message of intense devotion. The character of Krishna, as a devotional representation of God, developed out of a need for a relationship between a personal God and the human self (ego). Prior to the emergence of the teachings related to the characters of Krishna and Rama in India, the spiritual tradition focused on ritualism and on intellectual studies. The Sages saw the need to provide a vehicle whereby the devotional aspect of personality could be developed in order to foster an integral spiritual movement. In India, the devotional idea developed out of the *Svetasvatara Upanishad* and the *Bhagavad Gita*. Through increasing levels of devotion, which has the effect of consuming one's attention and concentration, one is gradually able to see the object of devotion in all things, regardless of the activities in which one is engaged. Thus, the Christian image of supreme devotion took form as the personality of Jesus, and the example of devotion towards the Divine was portrayed as the greatest devotee, Mary.

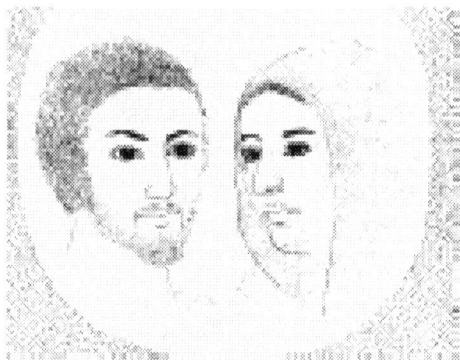

In the Indian text, *Bhagavata Purana*, also known as the *Shrimad-Bhagavata*, written in the tenth century A.C.E., Krishna is portrayed as a God-man who is husband to 16,108 women (Gopis). However, the point of this story is not to advocate polygamy. It is a metaphorical teaching given to describe, in tantric terminology, the nature of the Divine Self, God, who as if makes love with all human beings who seek after him with love and devotion their heart. While human beings see God as one, in reality God is one for all. Therefore, while there may be many religions in the world, they all refer, with equal validity, to the same Divinity. Through the passionate stories of the devotion of the *Gopis* (shepherdesses), the Purana illustrates the levels of devotion necessary for the individual human souls, symbolized by the Gopis, to achieve union with God, symbolized by one God, Krishna, manifesting for all as an individual, giving all his attention to each of them as an individual. So taken are they with their fascination for Krishna that the Gopis drop all other interest including their

---

[1] See the Ausarian Resurrection: The Ancient Egyptian Bible by Dr. Muata Ashby.

husbands and families. At times, Krishna appears to become many in order to satisfy each individual Gopi, each one of whom thinks she is making love with the one Krishna. In this manner, the one absolute God is understood as being all pervading, ever present and available to each soul because the individual soul is essentially one with the Absolute Self. So when you are loving your spouse, a friend, a relative or an object, you are in reality loving God, who has assumed that particular shape and form, just as the Gopis have become enamored with Krishna. The error in the human mind is in believing that the shape and form is real and separate from God instead of understanding that it is an expression (illusory modification) of the Divine.

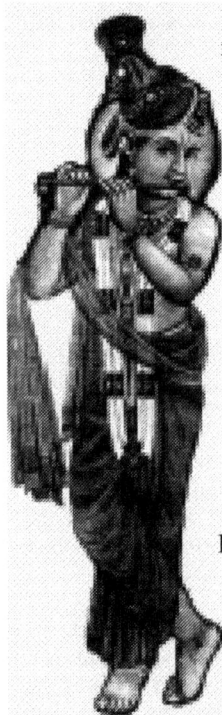

In section VII.1.30 of the text, it is established that any emotion, even anger, may be used as a means to attain yoga if the intensity is strong enough. All that exists gradually comes to be known as being permeated and sustained by the object of intense Divine love, God. Therefore, due to the power of attention and concentration that unfolds on the path of devotion, that devotional path is affirmed as a means to spiritual movement in much the same way as the other practices of yoga which seek to control the mind through concentration and meditation practices, through wisdom or through righteous action.

Everywhere I behold you {you who are} of endless Form, with many arms, bellies, mouths, and eyes. I can see no end, middle, or beginning in you, O All-Lord, All-Form! (XI.16)

In the *Gita Govinda* or *"Song of Govinda,* a twelfth century Indian text, the story of Krishna and his favorite shepherdess (Gopi), *Radha,* is to be found. Radha exemplifies the height of the devotional feeling in a human being, which transcends physical love. She is in many respects the Hindu counterpart of Mary Magdalene in Christianity. One of Krishna's names, Govinda, means, "cow finder," referring to his occupation of cowherd. The Sanskrit word "go" (meaning "wisdom") leads to the esoteric understanding of Krishna as the finder or shepherd of wisdom. Thus, we note here that the title or appellation of *"shepherd "* is the same as that of Jesus, Djehuti-Hermes and Asar, who all share the title *The good shepherd.*

Above: Krishna, the eight Avatar of God (Lord Vishnu) in Indian religion.

Lord Krishna is usually depicted as a child or adult man playing the flute. The flute on which he is playing symbolizes hollowing one's personality from ego consciousness and thereby allowing God to use one as an instrument to bring good to the world.

Radha represents the female spiritual ideal. Her love is so strong that it includes and transcends its gross aspects (physical sex) and touches the very heart of the beloved, becoming one with him. The *Gita Govinda* reflects a passionate style of Tantrism, using sexual metaphors to illustrate the passionate desire (*Rati*) which the devotee feels. In the following segment, Radha describes her feelings for Krishna to a friend.

He laid me down on a bed of shoots. For a long time he rested on my breast, while I caressed and kissed him. Embracing me, he drank from my lower lip. (III.13)

This is similar to the relationship of Jesus and Mary where Jesus is said to have *"kissed often on her mouth.*[14\93] Krishna and Radha were also said to have kissed but their relationship was also not sexual. While the Tantric traditions practice various techniques which include physical and non-physical exchanges between a male and female partner, there were also equivalent mystery traditions in Ancient Egypt which later transferred to Rome and also became part of Gnostic Christianity. Among the cults which practiced Tantrism in ancient Rome prior to the development of Christianity were those of *Aset* (Isis) and *Vesta.* The *Vestal Virgins* were the priestesses of the cult of Vesta. They tended the sacred fire and officiated at ceremonies in the goddess' honor. The Vestals serviced the temple under vows of absolute chastity. An esoteric tradition holds that their purity was necessary for tantric rituals in which they would dance and gesture (without physical contact) in light veils before male initiates in order to excite the sexual energies in them.[98] The male initiates, in turn, through sublimation of their gross passion, would develop advanced spiritual capabilities. Thus, through the exchange of subtle energies, male and female aspirants can increase their spiritual development. This tantric understanding sheds light on why the male God cannot exist without his "female" manifesting power.

In ancient times some ceremonies could not be performed by *Brahmin* priests without wives.[100] In the same way, early Judaism contained similar ideas as those expressed in the Indian *Mahanirvanatantra*, in which the male God figures, *Shiva, Vishnu and Brahma*, were said to be powerless without their Shaktis (female aspect) *"without whom they avail nothing."* Similarly, the early Jewish tradition believed that the incantations and spells of Rabbis would be useless if they were unmarried.[99]

While it is not necessary to have a physical family with a particular spouse and children etc., in order to mature spiritually, it is important that the natural energies, which exist in the body, are channeled in a spiritual direction. Thus, when sexual energy is indiscriminately expended in a gross (physical) way through sexual intercourse and other sensual means such as anger, hate, greed, passion for worldly attainments, etc., spiritual movement is slowed or blocked. This blockage occurs because the object of attention and the expenditure of energy are not spiritual, but material, and the psychic energy, which could have been used for mental discipline, has been lost.

It must be clearly understood that using sexuality and sense pleasures as a part of spiritual practice does not mean engaging in physical intercourse. It means that when sexual desire arises in the mind, it, and the energy which those thoughts engender, should be harnessed and sublimated, channeled and directed towards the higher spiritual centers of consciousness, through higher devotional feeling towards God, in order to more effectively explore the inner reaches of the Self. Then it is possible to create in the plane of spiritual thoughts instead of physical offspring. It is then possible to create wisdom, understanding, spiritual strength and endurance, qualities that are needed for success on the spiritual path.

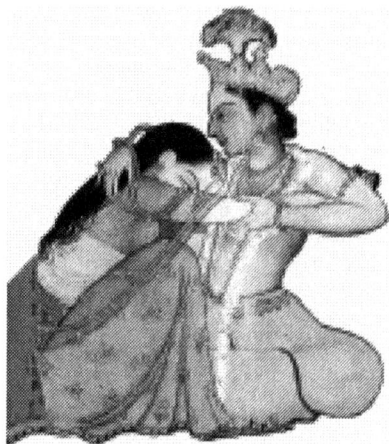

The relationships between Krishna and the Gopis in the Indian Puranas are reminiscent of the parable of Jesus, which likens the Kingdom of Heaven to *brides* and the *bridegroom.* The brides are his disciples, symbolizing the human soul, and he himself is the bridegroom, the God-man.

Left: *The Divine couple, Krishna and Radha of India.*

Matthew 9
14. Then came to him the disciples of John, saying, Why do we and the Pharisees fast often, but thy disciples fast not?
15 And Jesus said to them, Can the children of the bride chamber mourn, as long as the bridegroom is with them? But the days will come, when the bridegroom shall be taken from them, and then they shall fast.

Matthew 25
1. Then shall the Kingdom of Heaven be likened to ten virgins, who took their lamps, and went forth to meet the bridegroom.
2 And five of them were wise, and five [were] foolish.
3 They that [were] foolish took their lamps, and took no oil with them:
4 But the wise took oil in their vessels with their lamps.
5 While the bridegroom tarried; they all slumbered and slept.
6 And at midnight there was a cry made: Behold, the bridegroom cometh; go ye out to meet him.
7 Then all those virgins arose, and trimmed their lamps.
8 And the foolish said to the wise, Give us of your oil, for our lamps are gone out. {gone out: or, going out}
9 But the wise answered, saying, [Not so], lest there be not enough for us and you: but go ye rather to them that sell, and buy for yourselves.
10 And while they were going to buy, the bridegroom came; and they that were ready went in with him to the marriage: and the door was shut.
11 Afterward came also the other virgins, saying, Lord, Lord, open to us.
12 But he answered and said Verily I say to you, I know you not.
13 Watch therefore, for ye know neither the day nor the hour in which the Son of man cometh.

Mary, the Mother of Jesus, and Aset, the Mother of Heru and the Black Madonna

The prominence and importance of women in the Gnostic texts is evident in texts such as *The Gospel of Thomas, The Gospel of Philip, The Gospel of Mary, Pistis Sophia* (Faith Wisdom), and *Thunder, Perfect Mind.* In most cases the female element of creation and humanity is exalted alongside the male aspect, indicating the importance of the female element for spiritual development in Gnostic Christianity. Further, there is an underlying idea of androgyny and sexual sublimation, wherein the disciple is directed to balance her/his male and female halves in order to become "ONE" or androgynous. Therefore, we are thus directed towards a transpersonal understanding of Gnostic Christianity as it relates to each individual aspirant or disciple rather than to the historical personality of Jesus.

THE MYSTICAL JOURNEY FROM JESUS TO CHRIST

The Ancient Egyptian Cult *of Auset* (Isis) which was part of the Ausarian Myth that flourished until c. 394 A.C.E. was so strong that it was one of the last to be overcome by the Roman Catholic religious persecutions. In giving birth to Heru as a virgin, Aset provided the prototype for Mary, who gave birth to Jesus. This virgin birth is a symbol of the "second birth," the birth of the inner spiritual life that can occur in all humans. Out of a mind, which is concerned with materialism and pleasures of the body, comes a new consciousness. Aset suckling Heru is a common symbol in art and mythology throughout Africa. It represents the importance of the mothering, nurturing principle in the making of a human being, as well as the nurturing that must take place in order for one to give birth to one's own spirit. This is the true meaning of the "virgin birth." Out of one's animal (lower self) existence one brings forth a higher vision and aspiration in life beyond the sensual pleasures of the physical body. This is the idealized symbolic form of the Madonna and baby Jesus.

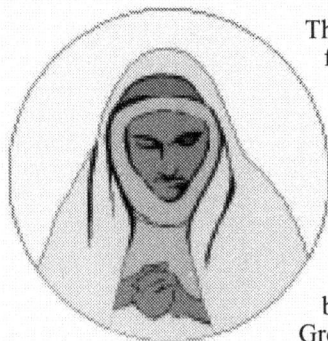

The *Immaculate Conception* teaching is a Roman Catholic dogma, which holds that from the very beginning of its creation, the soul of the Virgin Mary was completely free from any original sin. This idea developed as a way to explain how Jesus, the son of God, could have been born from a mortal woman who was susceptible to human sin. This doctrine must not to be confused with the doctrine of the *Virgin Birth*. The virgin birth holds that Jesus Christ was born of a virgin mother through the spirit of God and not the seed of a mortal man. The dogma of the immaculate conception is damaging to the original concepts of Christianity because it confuses the true meaning of the idea behind original sin as it sets Mary and Jesus apart from the rest of humanity as "perfect" or "untainted" human beings. It places them on a divine level while leaving humanity on the sinful earth. Grounded in an egoistic and left brain thinking rather than a mystical, egoless and right brain oriented understanding, this idea of the immaculate conception makes it more difficult for the ordinary Christian to identify with the possibilities of Jesus because he or she will see him as superhuman and unreachable. The original teaching, as we have discussed, is that Jesus was as human as any other human being. His mother and father were humans, and he had siblings. What made him different was his spiritual attainment. He achieved it through hard work and self-effort during his childhood and adolescent years in Egypt, his initiation from John the Baptist, his subsequent meditations and spiritual practices in the wilderness and his successful struggle over the inner temptations (anger, hatred, greed, jealousy, fear, etc.). All of this should lead a Christian aspirant to understand that Jesus' attainment of the highest spiritual realization is possible for anyone.

Above: Mary, the Mother of Jesus. Her ancestry can be traced to Ethiopia.

From the Gospel of Thomas

112. Jesus says: "He who drinks from my mouth *will become like me*. As for me, I will become what he is, and what is hidden will be revealed to him."

Shortly after the creation of the Christian church, the position of Mary was challenged. Was she a Saint or just a woman? If she gave birth to the son of God then is she a mere mortal woman or is she a goddess? Should she be revered or worshipped? These questions, along with the position of women in general, have caused confusion and disunity in the church for over 1,500 years. As stated earlier, the need for translation along with the inexactness of some of the writings of the early Christian era lends the scriptures of the Bible to wide interpretation and therefore, controversy as well. For example, even though the Bible clearly states that Mary, the mother of Jesus, was a virgin prior to her marriage to Joseph and that later she had sex relations with him (Matthew 1:25) and later the New Testament tells us about Jesus' brothers and sisters, some religious scholars have held that this does not mean that Jesus really had "brothers" (Mat. 12:46-50) and "sisters" (cf. Mk 6:3). Their reasoning is that the ancient Hebrew language had no special words for different degrees of relationships, such as are found in more modern languages. In general, all those belonging to the same family, clan and even tribe were sometimes referred to as "brethren." This controversy is in reality caused by an attempt to prove that Mary remained a virgin after she had given birth to Jesus and did not ever "soil" herself with sexual intercourse or worldly desires. The argument stems from the doctrines of the Immaculate Conception and the Virgin Birth. It is thought that since Jesus was Divine he could not incarnate through a vessel (Mary) that was not pure. Therefore, the church theologians set out to prove their point long after the New Testament scriptures were canonized. The Christian Gnostics refuted this doctrine as soon as the orthodox theologians advanced it. The Gnostics hold that Jesus was born of a human mother and father but that his spirit was Divine, just as every other human being's. This idea was rejected by the orthodox due to their misunderstanding of the Christian philosophy, which they themselves were espousing. Due to the destruction of the mystical traditions, Christianity has not maintained a direct line from the founders of Christianity, who originally intended these teachings to be understood in a metaphorical and mystical sense. Consequently, a struggle to determine the meaning of the New Testament scriptures emerged between year 0 and the year 200 of the Christian era and continues to the present.

Right: *The Ancient Egyptian Goddess Aset (Isis) with Heru.*

From very early times, Indian religion contained the statements and teachings of female Saints and Sages. One of the oldest Indian texts, the *Rig-Veda*, explains the perennial philosophy of the innate unity between creator and the created, between God and the human soul in a passage called *Devi Sukta*.

> I am Queen, source of thought, knowledge itself!
> You do not know me, yet you dwell in me.
> I announce myself in words both gods and humans welcome.
> From the summit of the world, I give birth to the sky!
> The tempest is my breath; all living creatures are my life!
> Beyond the wide earth, beyond the vast heaven,
> My grandeur extends forever!

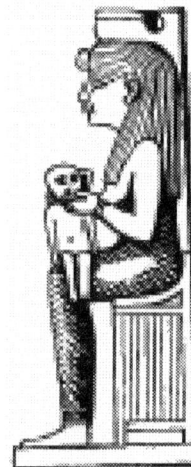

The preceding passage uses the traditional self-proclamation style (I am...) in the first person. As a revelation discourse, it is equal to those, which are found in other Indian texts, the only difference being that it is a female revealer of the spiritual mysteries, the Goddess. The following passages from the *Nag Hammadi*, come from a Gnostic text called *Thunder, Perfect Mind*. In style and format it is equivalent to the revealer style in the first person. At the same time, it makes use of the scriptural technique of paradoxical or antithetical statements, which are meant to express the absolute transcendence of the revealer, who is beyond comprehension through ordinary rational thought processes. Further, paradoxes are used to describe the absolute in an attempt to emphasize the idea that the absolute transcends the pairs of opposites: good-evil, light-dark, here-there, you-me, etc. Roman Catholicism, which is based on Zoroastrian and Aristotelian rationalism (left brained thinking), objected to this form of mystical reasoning.

> I was sent forth from the power, and I have come to those who reflect upon me, and I have been found among those who seek after me...
>
> For I am the first and the last.
> I am the honored one and the scorned one.
> I am the whore and the holy one.
> I am the wife and the virgin...
>
> You, who know me, are ignorant of me, and those who have not known me, let them know me.
> For I am knowledge and ignorance...
> Why then have you hated me, you Greeks?
> Because I am a barbarian among the barbarians?
> For I am the wisdom among the Greeks and the knowledge of the barbarians.
> I am the judgment of the Greeks and of the barbarians.
> I am the one whose image is great in Egypt and the one who has no image among the barbarians.
>
> I am the knowledge of my inquiry, and the finding of those who seek after me, and the command of those who ask for me, and the power of the powers in my knowledge of the angels, who have been sent at my word, and of gods in their seasons by my counsel, and of spirits of every man who exists with me, and of women who dwell within me.
>
> Hear me, you hearers, and learn from my words, you who know me.
> I am the hearing that is attainable to everything; I am the speech that cannot be grasped.[14]

The female revealer was also a prominent part of Ancient Egyptian religion in the form of *Arati*, the divine Goddess, her most prominent form of course being Aset.

THE MYSTICAL JOURNEY FROM JESUS TO CHRIST

ASET (Isis): The Egyptian Goddess - Prototype of Mother Mary

Aset speaks:

> "Moved by your prayer I come to you - I, the natural mother of all life, mistress of the elements, first child of time, Supreme Divinity, Queen of those in Hell, First of those in Heaven.... I, who's single Godhead is venerated over all the Earth under manifold forms, varying and changing names. Only remember me, fast in your heart's deep core, if you are found to merit My love by your dedicated obedience, religious devotion, and constant chastity, you will discover that it is within My power to prolong your life beyond the limits set to it by Fate; and after death live on praising Me in the Fields of Reeds.[63]

During the Ancient Egyptian pre-dynastic period (>10000 B.C.E.-5000 B.C.E.) in which the *Realm of Light* mythology was prominent, God was conceived as being the cause of all existence, but not as having any particular form. In later predynastic times, God in the female form reigned supreme in Egypt as well as in the rest of Africa (especially in Ethiopia), her power of fertility being identified with creation itself. God as the "Great Mother" (Hathor), who gave birth to the elements, cosmic forces and life itself, was depicted in various zoomorphic (non-human) forms such as a hippopotamus, a cow, a cobra, a crocodile, and a lioness to emphasize specific female oriented forces in nature and her life-giving qualities. In early dynastic times, the Divine Cow (Hathor), the Cobra Goddess (Buto), Nekhebet the Vulture, and Sekhmet the Lioness were major forms representing the Goddess. In later times, the Goddess in the anthropomorphic forms of Aset, Nut and Nephthys became prominent, although never supplanting the previous zoomorphic depictions or mythologies[64]

A striking example of the integration of the female principle into Ancient Egyptian mythology is to be found in Chapter 78, Line 47 of the Egyptian *Book of Coming Forth By Day*, where it is stated to the initiate:

> "To the son (initiate), the gods have given the crown of millions of years, and for millions of years it allows him to live in the Eye (Eye of Heru), which is the single eye of God who is called Neberdjer, the queen of the Gods."

The previous passage is of paramount significance since it states that the primary Trinity, *Nebertcher (Neberdjer),* the High God of Egypt, which is elsewhere primarily associated with male names, *Amun-Ra-Ptah,* is also *"the queen of the Gods."* Therefore, the primary *"Godhead"* or Supreme Being is both male and female. The concept of the Godhead as being female in nature translated to the original Jewish theology which eventually gave birth to Christianity. The Hebrew term *Elohim* means *"the goddesses and the gods."* Elohim is also a general term which is used frequently in the Old Testament referring to any divine being, however it is more commonly used in reference to the God (the Father) of the Israelites. Elohim is the plural of the Hebrew word Eloah which means "God." However, even though this teaching is part of the scriptural writings, both the Jewish and Christian Churches emphasize the male aspect almost exclusively. This is a stark example of machismo (an exaggerated sense of masculinity), spiritual ignorance and immaturity (egoism).

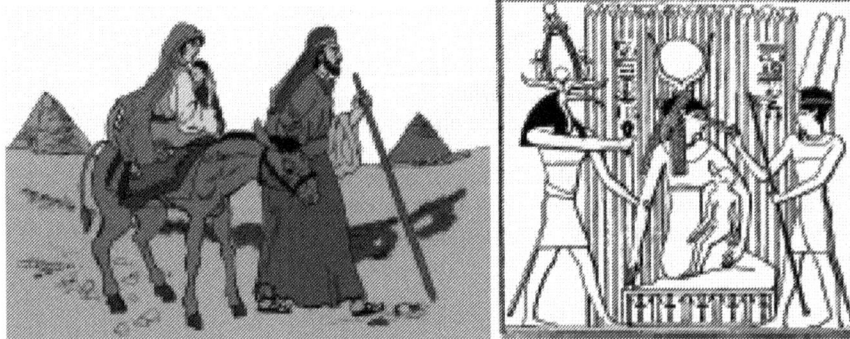

Above left: Mary and Joseph flee to Egypt for safety in order to save Jesus.
Above right: The goddess Aset (Isis) flees into the papyrus swamps of Egypt to save Heru.

This understanding of the Supreme Divinity as being androgynous, and being one entity expressing as many entities including both sexes, parallels the Ancient Egyptian and Hindu understanding. As societies have changed to a male dominant structure, the translation in the Bible is usually simply "God." In the original manuscripts of the book of Genesis, Yahweh was only one of the *Elohim*. This understanding is more accurately reflected in Cabalism, the esoteric form of Judaism.[I]

In the New Testament Book of Matthew 1:20-23, the story of the Annunciation, Conception, Birth and Adoration of the Child Jesus is presented. The "angel of the Lord" appeared to tell Joseph that his wife Mary is pregnant by the Holy Spirit of God. Once again, the transcendental themes of Christianity reach far into Ancient Egyptian antiquity. In the Holy of Holies or *Mesken* in the Temple of Luxor (1,700 B.C.E.) there is a special image which parallels the Christian teaching of the annunciation and birth of the savior, complete with three kings or wise men. In the first scene at left, the god Djehuti or the transmitter of the *word* (logos), is depicted in the act of announcing to queen Mut-em-Ua (who has assumed the role of Aset) that she will give birth to the child who will be the righteous, divine heir (Heru). In the next scene Knum (Kneph), the ram headed god (also associated with Amun), along with Hathor, provide her with the Life Force Energy (spirit of God). In this scene the virgin is pictured as pregnant through that spirit. In the following scene, the mother is being attended to while nurses are supporting the child. The next scene is the Adoration wherein the child is enthroned and adored by Amun, the hidden Holy Spirit behind all creation. Also, there are three men behind Amun who offer boons or gifts with the right hand (open facing up) and life with the left (holding the Ankh).

This scene and its usage attests to the deeper significance of the virgin birth mystery. Every mother is a Goddess and every child is a product or mixture of the earth or physical nature and the spirit of God. Through this metaphor we are to understand that each human being has a divine origin, heritage and birthright. Therefore, it is clear to see the meaning of the Christian statements: *I and [my] Father are one. Jesus answered them, Is it not written in your law, I said, Ye are gods?* From John 10:30 and 34, respectively.

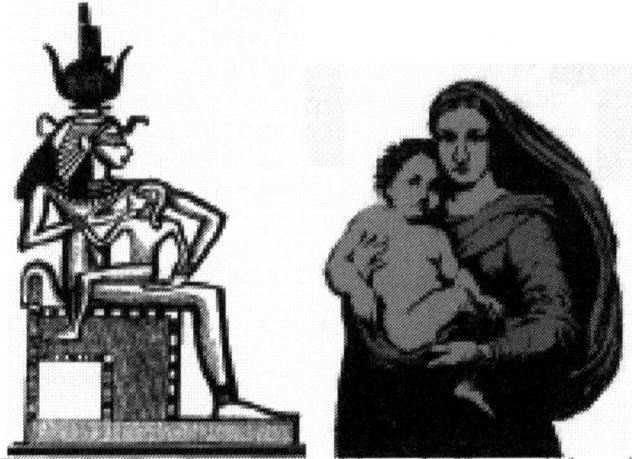

Above right: The Ancient Egyptian prototype of the savior Heru, and his mother, Aset (Isis).
Above left: The Christian image of Jesus and his mother Mary.

The Black Madonna

As an adjunct to European Christianity there is an unofficial cult which reveres the images of Mary, the mother of Jesus as a Black woman. There are literally hundreds of images located in shrines and churches in Europe, some of which have been painted over or defaced in the last one hundred years. When the priests of churches or curators at museums are asked about the reason why she is depicted as a black woman several incongruous answers are usually given. For example, a priest in the church at Lucera gave the following reason in 1944: "My son, she is black because she is black." In 1980, the proprietress of a souvenir shop across the Orcival church, which displays an image of the Black Madonna, told a questioner: "Because she is."

The Encyclopedia Britannica once reported that "Isis" was worshipped in Egypt, Greece, Rome, Gaul and almost all of the remainder of Europe and England. This was true before and during the emergence of Christianity. Thus, it is well established and accepted by most scholars that the image of the Ancient Egyptian goddess Isis (Aset) sitting with the child Horus (Heru) is the source of the Madonna and child paintings and sculptures.[130] The noted Egyptologist A. Wallis Budge considered the mythology and iconography of Aset to be "identical with those of Mary."[23] The world-renowned psychiatrist Carl Jung also said she is Isis. The Ancient Egyptian tradition clearly

---

[I] See section entitled "Kabbalism, the Mysticism of the Tree of Life."

states that the divine family of Asar, Aset and Heru were black skinned. Asar (Osiris), Heru's father and husband to Aset (Isis) was known as the "Lord of the Perfect Black" and is often depicted as being black or green of hue. Aset, the daughter of Nut (the black night sky).

In the temple of Denderah (Egypt), it is inscribed that Nut gave birth to Aset there and that upon her birth, Nut exclaimed "Ås" behold, *I have become thy mother"*. This was the origin of the name "Åst," later known as Isis to the Greeks and others. The inscription further states that she was a dark-skinned child and was called *"Khnemet-ankhet"* or the *lady of life and love.*[I] Thus, Aset also symbolizes the "blackness" of the vast un-manifest regions of existence, Asar.

The images of the Black Madonna, also known as the Black Virgin, can be found in many shrines and churches throughout Europe including Germany, Poland, Italy, Russia and especially in France. France has more than 300 sites displaying the Black Virgin, with over 150 images of Black Virgins still in existence. In France they are called "Vierge Noires" or Black Virgins; in other countries they are called Black Madonnas.

The evidence given by the Christian tradition and its documents suggests that these images of the Black Mary were taken as is, renamed (rededicated as it were) and used in Christian worship. This practice was compatible with the customs on *inculturation*, also known as co-optation,[II] the process of adopting symbols and rituals from other religions and calling them Christian, which were officially confirmed and endorsed as church policy by Pope St Gregory the Great in a letter given to priests written in 601 A.C.E.:

> "It is said that the men of this nation are accustomed to sacrificing oxen. It is necessary that this custom be converted into a Christian rite. On the day of the dedication of the [pagan] temples thus changed into churches, and similarly for the festivals of the saints, whose relics will be placed there, you should allow them, as in the past, to build structures of foliage around these same churches. They shall bring to the churches their animals, and kill them, no longer as offerings to the devil, but for Christian banquets in name and honor of God, to whom after satiating themselves, they will give thanks. Only thus, by preserving for men some of the worldly joys, will you lead them thus more easily to relish the joys of the spirit."

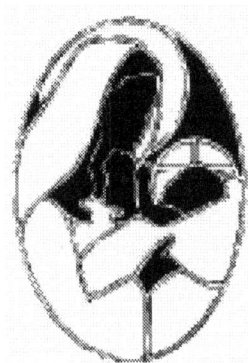

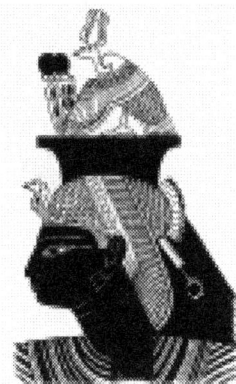

Far left: The Black Madonna within the Mandorla (vertical-oval).

Right: The Black goddess Aset (Isis) of Ancient Egypt.

Aset is the mother of Heru. She is known as the "beautiful Black one" as are her mother, Nut and sister Nebethet.

[I] From an inscription in the temple of Denderah, Egypt.

[II] To neutralize or win over (an independent minority, for example) through assimilation into an established group or culture.

The Female Savior of Humankind

The idea of a "savior" is not to be considered a high philosophical concept, but it is useful in a symbolic way to help us understand early on in our spiritual quest that there is a higher power which we can call upon to assist and guide us through our lives. Thus, from a more advanced perspective, the main gods and goddesses of Ancient Egyptian mythology such as Heru and Hathor should be viewed as guides or teachers, rather than as "saviors" in the Western religious sense of the word. The western concept of a savior leads to the idea that it is through the efforts of someone "outside of ourselves" (i.e. Jesus Christ, Gods, Angels, Saints, etc.) that we will be liberated. However, the Gnostic understanding is just the opposite. It is we who must do the work of saving ourselves through the application of the teachings. Thus, when discussing the idea of a savior we must consider that it is our own Higher Self who is being described. Therefore, we must strive to acquire those "saving" qualities in our personality, which will lead to our own liberation.

In modern day society, a Sage is usually defined as *a venerable, wise person*. In terms of mystical philosophy, a Sage is not only a wise person but also someone who is highly spiritual and capable of teaching others on the spiritual path. *Agastya* is a Sage who is reputed to be one of the composers of the Rig-Veda of India. He was known to receive teachings from his wife, who was a female Sage. Two important stories from the Vedas illustrate their relationship. One of these relates the story of how Agastya leaves his family and home to seek out a master (guru) who can teach him the wisdom, which leads to Enlightenment. The teacher directs him to the master from whom he himself learned the teachings. When he realizes that this master lives in his (Agastya's) own home, Agastya exclaims: "But that's my wife!"

These stories illustrate the Tantric philosophy, which existed since the time of the Vedas. Lopamudra taught Agastya that self-mortification and extreme asceticism were not the only ways to achieve God-realization. If worldly activities are performed with an attitude of wisdom, by offering them to God as one would offer flowers or incense in the spirit of inner renunciation as in *Bhoga Tyaga* (renunciation of worldly enjoyments), those very activities will lead to spiritual realization. Further, when using this tantric wisdom one realizes that Divinity is in all things and that what society considers good or evil is neither good nor evil from the perspective of spiritual realization. This is because the view from the perspective of society and the individual is conditioned by mental ignorance, while the view from a spiritually realized perspective is free from mental conditioning. Actions and objects are nothing but the Self (God); therefore, all activities and all interactions with objects are Divine encounters if they are understood from the highest perspective.

In Ancient Egypt one of the most important annual festivals was the festival of lights. It symbolized the goddess in all her forms as the sustainer, enlightener and bringer of good fortune to all people. The most important site for this worship was in the city of Sais, but the celebration was nationwide. Everyone would light lamps on the special evening.

In like manner, the early Christians adopted the practice and instituted a Festival of Lights. Also, the Hindus instituted a Festival of lights as well. The Hindu ritual is called *Divali.* The light symbolizes the Divine Consciousness which illumines the mind and which operates throughout the universe to sustain all life.

The festival is a celebration as well as an affirmation of divine reality. This process leads to reflection and meditation upon the most profound truths of spirituality.

Mary Magdalene, the Female Sage and Apostle of Christianity and Partner of Jesus

Mary Magdalene has been canonized by the Catholic Church as a Saint. A Saint is usually described as: "A person considered holy and worthy of public veneration, or a very virtuous person." In the capacity as Saint, Mary's position in Christianity has been only half-expressed. In the Gnostic Christian texts her position emerges as a teacher to common people and to the Apostles as well. In a sense she is an Apostle to the Apostles. The term Apostle means, "to preach the Gospel," the teachings of Christ or any of the first four books of the New Testament. In the following text from the *Gospel of Philip*, we see a new interpretation of the New Testament relationship between Jesus and Mary Magdalene. It may be compared in one aspect to the relationship between Krishna and Radha of India or that of Heru and Hathor in Egypt, in that it implies a complementation of each other, a completeness that is above and beyond the ordinary conjugal experience. In this sense, the sum of the two is greater than the parts.

Three women always used to walk with the lord: Mary his mother, his sister, and the Magdalene, who is called his companion, and it is the name of his partner.

.... The companion of the {Savior is} Mary Magdalene. {But Christ loved} her more than {all} the disciples, and used to kiss her {often} on her {mouth}. The rest of {the disciples were offended}...They said to him, "Why do you love her more than all of us?" the Savior answered and said to them: If a blind person and one with sight are both in the darkness, they are not different from one another. When the light comes, then the person with sight will see the light, and the blind person will remain in the darkness.

In the canonical Gospels, Mary Magdalene or "Mary from the village of Magdala" (city on the west bank of the Sea of Galilee) is known to be a fervent follower of Jesus. She believed in his message so strongly that she left her home, her possessions and her family and devoted herself to follow Jesus' teaching. According to the New Testament Gospels, she accompanied Christ on his preaching in Galilee and witnessed the Crucifixion and burial of Jesus. Her belief in the teaching of Jesus was so great that it made her worthy of being absolved of seven demons.

Mark 16
9. Now when [Jesus] was risen early the first [day] of the week, he appeared first to Mary Magdalene, out of whom he had cast seven demons.

The *seven demon*s which were cast out of Mary are not specifically mentioned here, however, other writings give reference to *seven deadly sins* as the characteristics that prevent spiritual development. These seven sins are known as *anger, covetousness, envy, gluttony, lust, pride* and *sloth*. These sins are "fatal" to human spiritual progress. These are the sins or demons being referred to here. In the section on *"the seven demons of Mary"* and the *"temptations"* of Jesus and Buddha, these sins and the philosophy behind them will be discussed further. These seven sins correspond to the teaching of *Mala* or gross impurity of the heart in Vedantic philosophy or the *Fetters of the soul* in Ancient Egyptian mythology. This teaching holds that ordinary human consciousness is beset with gross impurities, which must be overcome before advanced spiritual disciplines can be practiced successfully. These impurities are known as ignorance, anger, hate, greed, jealousy, passion, etc. Until the gross impurities are controlled, it will not be possible to progress on the path of advanced yoga instruction. Control of the gross impurities is accomplished through the practice of what Indian Yoga and Buddhism calls *Dharma* or what Ancient Egyptian Yoga calls *Maat*. Both of these terms signify the practice of righteous living, which is of course the same goal of the Christian Beatitudes, the teachings that Jesus gave in the Sermon on the Mount. Righteousness purifies a person because when a person practices living in accordance with truth they cannot also act in egoistic ways. Therefore, the ego becomes less and less important and the mind, unburdened by the desires of the ego, becomes clearer and sensitive to the spiritual wisdom. Other important yoga aspects of spiritual practice are *abhyasa* (repeated effort in spiritual practice), and *satsanga* (company of sages-good association). These help a person to overcome obstacles in the practice of the teachings and to understand the deeper meaning of the teachings.

Mary Magdalene was the first to witness the resurrection of Jesus and to report it to the Apostles, who, in almost all versions of the story from the New Testament Gospels, refused to believe that the Master (Jesus) would reveal himself to a "woman." In accepting women into his cult, Jesus was seen as a radical since women were thought of more as possessions than as free thinking individuals equal to men. A woman who was not legally attached to a man was considered an impure woman, a harlot, etc. In so far as these customs persisted, it required great courage for women to seek the company of a man who was not their husband, father, owner, etc. Also it required great courage to accept them into the cult since this drew controversy to the movement and further inflamed the animosity towards Jesus from the Jewish leaders.

A similar situation existed in the east under the social organization in India, which was based on patriarchal values and the caste system. Buddhism and early Vaishnavism (worship of God as Vishnu) developed during a time of extreme social unrest and perceived inequity. Buddha's acceptance of women caused a similar stir of emotion in India, since under the Aryan-influenced Brahmanic system women were considered subordinate to men and not to be taught the mysteries of religion. However, both Buddhism and Vaishnavism were preceded in the fair treatment of women by the Upanishads and the Tantric tradition. In the *Brihadaranyaka Upanishad,* instruction of the mysteries of *Brahman* is given to a woman. In addition, Tantric traditions, which went under ground as it were due to the surge of the Vedic Aryans who imposed a caste system which asserted male dominance over women, kept alive a tradition which included women as central figures of religion and the worship of God as Mother. Thus, there have been and continue to be women priestesses and enlightened masters even to this day outside of Western countries. They are venerated alongside their male counterparts. The following statement from Chapter 9 of the *Bhagavad Gita* shows how, as a reformist text, the *Gita* refutes the caste system and sexism in much the same way as Jesus did hundreds of years later.

32. O Arjuna, those who take refuge in Me, whether men born in a lowly class, or women, or Vaishyas, or Shudras, even they are sure to attain the highest goal.

In *The Acts of Paul*, a Christian Apocrypha, there is a story of *Thecla*, a saintly personality who was worshipped in *Seleucia*, a new city capital built by the Seleucid dynasty in 275 B.C.E. after Babylon was abandoned. The following passage tells of how she practiced ascetic living and meditation. Later in the story she undergoes trials and tortures by the Romans, but survived due to the miraculous intercession of God in response to her devotion and piety. Thecla then traveled the land preaching until she *"sleeps a noble sleep."*

Indeed, for three days and three nights Thecla has not risen from the window either to eat or to drink, but gazing steadily as if on some joyful spectacle she so devotes herself to a strange man...[14]

In the same text, the following passage appears. Once again the idea arises that resurrection refers to a change in consciousness and not to the physical body. It brings up the idea of a resurrection that has already occurred but which needs to be realized as fact.

"And we shall teach you concerning the resurrection which he says is to come, that it has already taken place in the children whom we have, and that we are risen again in that we have come to know the true God."

The fact that Mary Magdalene was the first to witness Christ and to report this to the Apostles endows her figure with great importance. Later, during the Dark Ages of Europe, she was confused with Mary of Bethany (sister of Lazarus). It was not until Pope Gregory combined her image with that of a repentant prostitute who anointed Christ's feet that she came to be known as "Mary the repentant prostitute." While some believe that this combination was an intentional effort to denigrate the position of women in the Bible, it also gave impetus to the idea that even a person who committed the "worst sins" could be absolved and hope to achieve sainthood. Even today, long after the Vatican has issued edicts (1969) correcting the error, the image of Mary Magdalene as a reformed prostitute or her portrayals as a "sexual saint" persist among misguided individuals and among certain feminist groups.

While the openness of modern society is allowing the expression of many points of view with respect to the image of women, there are some significant psychological aspects to the continued development of the image of Mary Magdalene as a sexual saint. The continued use of an avowed erroneous interpretation may signify a need by some to validate their status as legitimate sexual outsiders[I] while still identifying with the religious aspect within themselves. In exploring these aspects of themselves, some women view themselves as holy temptresses, as a combination of the whore and the saint, while others may simply seek to honor the two impulses (sexual desire and spiritual devotion) within themselves in an effort to find a balance or resolution of these important human feelings.

However, when we turn to the Gnostic Gospels and other Gnostic Christian texts, a deeper mythology surrounding the relationship of Jesus and Mary Magdalene emerges. In the following comparison of the *Gospel of Luke* from the Bible and the *Gospel of Mary* from Egypt, there is a prime example of the complementary and esoteric function, which the Gnostic texts serve to the Bible texts.

Luke 24
10 It was Mary Magdalene, and Joanna, and Mary [the mother] of James, and other [women that were] with them, who told these things to the apostles.
11 And their words seemed to them as idle tales, and they believed them not.
In the following segment from the *Gospel of Mary*, the feelings, emotions and issues associated with a female as a spiritual master are explored. It seems to take up where the traditional gospel ends.

Peter asks:
"Did he really speak privately with a woman, not openly with us? Are we to turn about and all listen to her? Did he prefer her to us?"
Mary replies:
"My brother Peter, what do you think? Do you think that I thought this up myself in my heart, or that I am lying about the savior?"
Levi interrupts the argument:
"Peter, you have always been hot-tempered. Now I see you contending against the woman like the adversaries. But if the Savior made her worthy, who are you, indeed, to reject her? Surely the Lord knew her very well. That is why he loved her more than us."[39]

[I] Legitimizing their preferred sexual behavior before the general masses.

THE MYSTICAL JOURNEY FROM JESUS TO CHRIST

In the *Pistis Sophia* text, Mary complains to Jesus about Peter's disapproval of her. In this passage Mary symbolically verbalizes the plight of women in general, while Peter symbolizes the male dominance and ignorance which subjugates women to subservient roles.

"Peter makes me hesitate; I am afraid of him, because he hates the female race." [36/71]

When Peter asks Jesus to silence her he quickly reproves Peter's attitude and admonishes him to understand that women and men are equal in matters of divinity, and that anyone who is inspired by the spirit to speak has an equal right to do so. In the *Dialogue of the Savior* text, Jesus includes Mary as one of the three disciples who would receive special teaching and also praises her above Matthew and Thomas:

"She spoke as a woman who knew The All."

This reference to **The All** is of special significance since, as we have already seen, in Gnostic Mysticism it relates to the all-encompassing supreme divinity, God, in the transcendental way of understanding. Thus, Mary is being hailed as an Enlightened Sage. This places her on the level of the other enlightened personalities we have already mentioned so far, Buddha, Krishna, Jesus, Asar, Aset, etc. Such is the wonderful heritage of Mystical Christianity, which acknowledges and affirms the equal status and power of female human beings. This is one of the most important aspects of Christianity, which the church needs to regain because as women are elevated to their proper status, society as a whole will be elevated. For where there is ignorance such as sexism there can be no true peace, harmony or enlightenment, but only strife, violence and degradation such as that which society is currently experiencing. Women need to be allowed to preach as legitimate priestesses of Christ as they did in the early years of the church.

At the end of the second century, the orthodox Christians retaliated against the prominence of women through the *Apostolic Letters*. The Apostolic Letters were treatises written by Catholic bishops many years after the compilation of the Bible, but later attributed to the Apostles. Seeking to establish a hierarchy and male superiority in the church, the letters declare that the bishop is the father of the congregation, and that the bishop must be a man whose wife and children are to be *"submissive in all ways to him."* Prior to this time women had served as bishops in Gnostic and Catholic sects. The following excerpt from the *Apostolic Tradition* depicts Mary as an unworthy aspirant, and it is on this tradition that the Orthodox Church bases its decision to bar women from preaching in the church.

When the master blessed the bread and the cup and signed them with the words, "This is my body and blood, he did not offer it to the women who are with us." Martha said, "He did not offer it to Mary, because he saw her laugh."

The alleged immaturity and disrespect of Mary never happened. It was a fictional event composed for the purpose of denigrating women and justifying their placement in a lower state. This movement against women would have severe consequences, not only for women, but also for the whole of society in the next 1,700 years.

CHAPTER IX: CHRISTIAN YOGA WISDOM

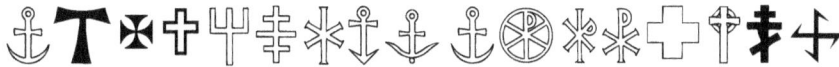

⚓ ✝ ✚ ✝ ☥ ✝ ✡ ⚓ ⚓ ☸ ✳ ✚ ✝ ☥ ✝

WHAT IS KNOWLEDGE?

The main goal of Christian Yoga, or any Yoga system, is to discover God, but how can this discovery be accomplished? What are the tools that will be needed and how will those tools be used? Philosophy is the main tool. The practice of philosophy is the means to reach the goal and the mind is the instrument, which will allow a person to use philosophy. However, first an aspirant must understand what knowledge is. Then it will be possible to understand the mind, how it works and how it will be affected through the process of following the teachings, and its ultimate transformation.

Gnostic Christianity, Jnana Yoga from India as well as the wisdom teachings of Ancient Egypt all emphasize that knowledge must be gained in order to transcend the mortal form of existence. But what this is knowledge and how is it to be found?

In the *Bhagavad Gita* Chapter 5, Line 16, Lord Krishna says:

"For those whose ignorance has been destroyed by the knowledge of the Self (Yoga of Wisdom), wisdom shines forth like the sun, revealing the Reality of the Transcendental Self."

When a person thinks of knowledge and information, they usually think about the things that they have heard, seen, felt, tasted, etc. The cognitive abilities and psychic structure of a human being (how a person sees themselves and the world) are based on the information they have gathered from their life experiences, which are based on their intellectual limitations and the limitations of their senses. The ordinary human being's concept of self is bound by the categories of thought (rules by which they have learned to judge, know and accept reality). Thus, in examining themselves they begin to think that they cannot know anything that does not fall into the parameters of their categories of thought or cannot be perceived and proven with the senses. These categories of thought are based on the mode of thinking, which they have learned to accept throughout their present and previous lifetimes. Thus, in collecting information about the world they are bound by the ignorant concepts of the mind and the limited instruments for information gathering, which they have, available to them.

As discussed earlier, the information gathered through our senses is limited to the parameters of the information sensing abilities. For example, if we had the ability to smell as a dog or hear as a bat, we would experience a particular way of life based on that heightened sense of information gathering ability. We would experience the world with sensitivity. Therefore, we need to examine the possibility that there is more to the world beyond our ordinary abilities of perception. This has been one of the most important themes of mystical philosophy. Modern physicists have come to realize that creation is not what it appears through their experiments in quantum physics. Scientist-writers such as Albert Einstein, Frijot Capra and Stephen Hawking have revolutionized the world of modern physics and the view of time, space and existence by showing how the phenomenal universe is not solid or real as people believe it to be. However, this very message has been the theme of ancient mythology for many millennia. In the myths from all over the world, there are metaphorical stories, which have been trying to lead us to the transcendental understanding of reality. These refer to a reality which is understood not through the ordinary senses, but through an intuitional state of mind—a new sense of reality which surpasses intellectual understanding and sense perception, but is nevertheless more real than ordinary life experience.

Maya or *Cosmic Illusion* is a term used in Hindu mythology to describe the process by which the human mind is deluded due to the triad effect of the mind. *Maya* is further understood as the perception by our senses of objects, when, in reality, they are illusory modifications of a transcendent, absolute existence (Pure Consciousness) and not real "objects" at all. This means that when you perceive a chair composed of wood or metal, you are perceiving an illusory modification of what is really there. In reality, there is only the Self, which has been modified by your limited, conditioned consciousness to appear as something, which it is not (an object composed of matter). In the Hindu Upanishads there is a teaching which explains this point. Suppose there is a rope on the floor in a dark room. If you go into that dark room and step on the coiled object, you may think it is a snake and become afraid though in reality it is only the rope. You superimposed the idea of the snake onto the rope and on the basis of this illusion (the existence of the snake) you have developed fear and anxiety. However, once you turn on the light and see the rope, the ignorance about the nature of what you stepped on and consequently your fear, disappeared. In the same way, due to the darkness of ignorance in the mind, a person believes that what they are experiencing is the world of different objects. If, however, they were to turn on the light of yoga wisdom, they would clearly perceive the true nature of what they are experiencing not as a world of objects (snake), but in fact the Kingdom of God (rope).

Thus, from the point of view of mystical philosophy, human consciousness is understood as a limited expression of Absolute Consciousness, just as a wave is a limited expression of the ocean or a patch of blue created by clouds covering the sky is a limited manifestation of the vast expanse of the sky. It is Absolute Consciousness (God) which takes the form of individual consciousness in all living things, and assumes the role of inert objects in creation for the individual consciousness to perceive and through which it can interact. Within the Christian context this can be understood by reflecting on the teaching that since God is divine, God's creation too must be an expression of divinity. Therefore, creation must be divine as well. If all Christians could develop this attitude in dealing with other human beings, animals, plants and all Creation, and if this understanding became the basis of all personal and business dealings, then there would be no racism, sexism or any other type of "ism" in human interaction. The earth would not be polluted because nature would be recognized as God himself. The mind and the mental process are, therefore, intricately related to *maya* as the following quotation from Yoga Vasistha Vol. II, sec.45p220, elucidates:

> ...though apparently real, this world is illusory. Just as objects reflected in a mirror do not exist in reality, in the same way this world, being of the nature of reflection, has no real existence.

> The body, the numerous worlds, and the expansion of time and space are all projections of the mind. They are experienced through the mind, and without the mind have no reality.

> There is no object that has not been created or projected by the mind. There is no object in the world that the mind cannot acquire and realize. There is nothing impossible for the mind to achieve because all objects are nothing but projections of the mind.

WHAT IS THE MIND FROM THE GNOSTIC PHILOSOPHICAL POINT OF VIEW?

According to mystical philosophy, the mind is both the cause of bondage to and the source of release from the world of time and space (Maya). The mind is that which allows a human being to be aware of the varied experiences faced at every moment. In a world created out of a combination of dense and subtle energy and various states of consciousness, it is necessary to have an instrument that will discern and discriminate between the opposites of creation (good and evil, hot and cold, here and there, etc.), in order to carry on the affairs of life. This process of discernment is what causes the appearance of distinct and different objects and situations in nature. Therefore, the process of mental discrimination is a dualizing mode of consciousness, due to which there seems to be "many realities" rather than the one reality, the Self—Pure Consciousness (God). When the mind is only aware of the apparent duality, the idea arises that we are "thinking" individuals, separate from other individuals, and that we are also separate from the objects of the world and from the universe. In this state of ignorance, we interact with the world in an action-reaction mentality, following our lower nature (anger, greed, hate, etc.), based on instinctive desires, instead of our higher nature (feeling of oneness), which will lead to the experience of universal love, sharing and peace.

The experience of oneness is likened to the experience of peace because there are no desires to create unrest. There is no duality to cause partiality or repulsion in the mind, but only equanimity and tranquility. This is the nature of the Kingdom of Heaven. Therefore, the experience of oneness is considered to be the state in which all apparent realities cease to exist. This is the original primordial state of consciousness. The experience of duality is the state in which opposites exist and therefore, the struggle between those opposites exists as well. In the mental state of duality, there is always a desire to acquire something to feel complete or whole and to get rid of something undesirable in order to get rid of pain or discomfort. When this state is transcended, there is no longer a need to acquire or efface objects, because there are no more objects, only the Kingdom, the Self. When intuitional wisdom dawns, what appeared in the state of ignorance to be objects to be acquired is discovered to be what is already in one's possession—universal oneness underlying multiplicity and duality. Also the subject, whom you thought you were, the individual mortal human being, is discovered to be that same Pure Consciousness beyond individuality, just like a wave discovering its true essence to be the entire ocean, encompassing all waves. Thus, there is no more need to pursue or acquire that, which is already possessed. All the objects are within you because you are the source of them. You are the ocean-like Self, not a wave-like personality. This is the state of Enlightenment.

Spiritual movement is the development of the higher mind, which leads one's consciousness to the discovery of truth rather than illusion. Thus, as we change the patterns of conditioned thoughts, we break away from our cyclical pattern of ignorant thoughts, feelings and desires and enter into an upward spiral of growth and transformation.

Since the mind is essentially energy emanating from the Self, which is the innermost reality of your being, that energy of the mind can be trained to act or perceive in particular ways. According to the texts, most people are incapable of controlling their emotions, moods and feelings because they do not realize that their real Self is separate from these. They cannot separate themselves from their thoughts or mental complexes or conditioning. This is the process known as identification, wherein a person sees him/herself as the emotions, feelings and thoughts—as the body itself.

The teaching of Adam and Eve must be clear to the Christian aspirant. This phenomenal world which seems to be composed of a mixture of misery, pleasure, happiness, pain, etc., is nothing but the Garden of Eden. According to the book of Genesis in the Bible, in the beginning, God is said to have created Adam and Eve, who lived happily in the Garden of Eden, without worries or cares. They did not feel desire or pain. They felt one with nature. Once they ate of the forbidden fruit (from the Tree of Knowledge of Good and Evil) they represent human consciousness having fallen prey to ignorance of their true nature and the egoistic desires which ensue from this forgetfulness. The Garden of Eden and the Kingdom of Heaven are synonymous with human consciousness when it is devoid of desires and ignorance. Desire and ignorance are overcome through the practice of Yoga.

Most worldly-minded people believe that desires are to be satisfied whenever possible and that this is the sole purpose of life. They believe deep down that if this is not possible then life is not worth living. They come to accept the notion, reinforced by the society at large, that happiness means acquiring wealth and enjoying sensual pleasures. Further, it is believed that the more of these possessions and pleasures that can be acquired, the more happiness there will be and the more successful a person is. This is an extremely dull state of mind, which leads to constant mental agitation as well as untold suffering and frustration. A person who operates under this philosophy will be disturbed if they cannot get what they want and elated if they seem to get it. However, when there is an opportunity to briefly fulfill a desire, there emerges the need to satisfy it again and again, much like a drug addict who seeks a more potent dose each time to feel the same high. If the desires are not fulfilled, there is misery and anger, and if there is a favorable situation, there is a feeling of gain. Then a longing develops to seek more opportunities to reproduce the pleasurable situation. This leads to craving and greed, which leads to stress and anxiety. This is why Buddhist philosophy emphasizes that both pleasure and pain are painful, because worldly pleasure merely creates an ongoing desire to acquire the situation or object which is perceived as being the source of pleasure, again leading the soul into greater and greater delusion.

In this condition there are uncontrollable urges to do things which you think will cause others to act in your favor to give you what you want, but you are disappointed when you discover that they have their own desires, feeling, and goals, which do not necessarily match your plans, or that life does not always provide what the ego desires. You acted in a certain way expecting others to act reciprocally, but were disappointed when they did not give you what you wanted, after all of your trouble. Therefore, there is never any peace, rest, fulfillment or contentment, without which the heart cannot fathom the depths wherein mystical experience is enjoyed. This predicament has gone on for many life times, and there is no way that the endless desires will ever be fulfilled. So a wise person will turn away from the ignorance and egoism which makes life miserable and enter into the intensive practice of Yoga.

When you realize that all occurrences in the world, good or bad, are transitory and stressful, you will turn away from the world of egoistic human activity to discover the true wellspring of bliss. You will break the bonds, which compelled you to act unrighteously, to act with exaggerated expectations of gaining something, to suffer bitter disappointments. You can seek to advance in worldly life, but that advancement should not be seen as the source of happiness. Your inner spiritual attainment is the only true source of abiding happiness. All outer forms of pleasure are in reality a manifestation of your inner feeling. Therefore, as you grow spiritually you will discover greater peace and happiness with the world.

WHO IS GOD? THE ANCIENT EGYPTIAN ORIGINS OF MONOTHEISM AND THE CONCEPTS OF GOD IN THE WORLD RELIGIONS AND THE CHRISTIAN GOSPELS

Akhenaton, Moses and the Concept of One God in Ancient Egyptian Mythology

Many people have come to believe that religions such as Judaism, Christianity and Islam were the first to put forth the teaching of monotheism. Upon closer review, however, we see that the monotheism of the western religions is related to a personalized idea of God. This form of monotheism holds that there is a personality who has a particular form, a particular location of residence and a particular religion. The mysticism of Ancient Egypt and of all other mystical philosophies shows that there is a Supreme Being who manifests as all forms, gods and goddesses, animals, human beings, etc. This goes a step beyond monotheism, thereby accepting God as the reality behind all things. This form of thinking may be classified as "monism," "panentheism" or "non-dualist Divinity." This understanding is a departure from the ordinary way of thinking and it is the cornerstone of mystical philosophy, differentiating it from orthodox, logical and dualistic thinking.

> "God is the father of beings. God is the eternal One... and infinite and endures forever. God is hidden and no man knows God's form. No man has been able to seek out God's likeness. God is hidden to Gods and men... God's name remains hidden... It is a mystery to his children, men, women and Gods. God's names are innumerable, manifold and no one knows their number... though God can be seen in form and observation of God can be made at God's appearance, God cannot be understood... God cannot be seen with mortal eyes... God is invisible and inscrutable to Gods as well as men."

Portions from the Egyptian *Book of Coming forth by Day* and the papyrus of Nesi-Khensu

The statements above give the idea that God is the unfathomable mystery behind all phenomena, which cannot be discerned "even by the gods." However, God is the unfathomable mystery as well as the innermost essence of his children. This means that God is transcendental, the unmanifest, but also what is manifest as well. In order to perceive this reality it is necessary to transcend ordinary human vision. When this transcendental Self is spoken about through different names and metaphors, the idea often emerges that there are many faces to the ultimate deity or Supreme Being. Nevertheless, as has been previously discussed, it must be clear that all spiritual traditions are in reality referring to the same Supreme Being, the transcendental reality.

The many Egyptian cosmogonies and ritual systems are in reality leading toward the realization of the same Supreme Being. However, during the period of the 18th dynasty, Egyptian religion went through a short-lived phase in which only one god symbol was worshiped. This occurred under the reign of Akhenaton, r.c.1379-1362 B.C.E. He suppressed the older god symbols, including Amun-Re, and instituted Aton, represented by the solar disk, as the only God. Renouncing the old gods, he introduced worship of the sun God, Aton or Aten, and established a new capital at Akhenaton. Aton symbolized the underlying essence of reality.

Many researchers of Egyptian religion have considered Akhenaton to be the first monotheist; however, he only wanted to return to the original idea of the Supreme Deity which had existed prior to the development of the various companies of gods and goddesses. This point is proved by the following passages from the Ancient Egyptian texts concerning Amun, Ra and Ptah and the creation myths, which existed prior to the reign of Akhenaton. In essence he was trying to reform the worship of God and of society in general, just as Jesus was trying to reform Judaism, Krishna and Buddha Indian religion, and Lao Tzu Chinese religion.

UA ⸻ or "One,"
UA NETER ⸻ or "One God,"
"Only One" ⸻,
"Only One Without a second" ⸻
"One One" ⸻

The following passages come from the Egyptian *Book of Coming Forth By Day* (Chapter. clxxiii):

"I praise thee, Lord of the Gods, God One, living in truth."

The following passage is taken from a hymn where princess Nesi-Khensu glorifies Amen-Ra:

198

"August Soul which came into being in primeval time, the great god living in truth, the first Nine Gods who gave birth to the other two Nine Gods,[I] the being in whom every God existeth One One, ⟨hieroglyphs⟩, the creator of the kings who appeared when the earth took form in the beginning, whose birth is hidden, whose forms are manifold, whose germination cannot be known."

Sometimes religious practice becomes ritualistic and traditional, and the meaning is lost over a period of time. A similar situation occurred in Christianity during the time of the creation and rise of Islam. This is when a highly developed personality comes to reform the religion and once again emphasize the mystical aspects of it in order to promote its proper function in society. The ideas of monotheism, monism, pantheism and panentheism exited in Egypt and Ethiopia prior to their emergence anywhere else in the world. Akhenaton wanted to encourage a more naturalistic style of Egyptian royal portraiture and life in general, as well as a deeper relationship with the Divine as opposed to the increasingly ritualistic development in religion, which was taking place. He saw Aten (Aton) as the benefactor of all religions and sought to establish a new order of social justice wherein all citizens would partake in the riches of society.

The corruption of some of the Egyptian priesthoods and dissatisfaction with the level of spiritual experience prompted a call for reforms. The high philosophy, which spawned the creation of the Temples and Pyramids, had degenerated to where many scribes and priests were selling religious texts to the highest bidder without imparting the true meaning of the teachings. Thus, Akhenaton attempted to make reforms in the spiritual character of Egypt. He confiscated much of the wealth of the priests of Amen and redistributed it among the people. He tried to foster an atmosphere of brotherhood among the neighboring countries by reducing appropriations for the military and thus reducing the belligerent stance of the Egyptian civilization. The priests of Amen and many people who had practiced the cults of various Egyptian deities for thousands of years rejected his efforts. Foreign countries used this opportunity to encroach upon Egyptian territories and, after Akhenaton's death; Egypt reverted to the system of gods and goddesses, which it had before.

It would be correct to note that the Jews who entered Egypt at various times throughout its history were strongly influenced by the theology of Egypt. However, they did not carry on the ideal of universality which Akhenaton sought to foster. He viewed Aton as the supreme deity who is revered everywhere under different names. It must be understood that he never saw the sun itself as Aton, but as a dynamic aspect of Aton which sustains the world and all life. This is actually the same teaching, which was inherent in the teachings related to the Ancient Egyptian god Ra. Thus, he was merely transferring the same attributes, which were previously held to the form of Aton. The Jewish idea that the Jewish God is the only true god, and he belongs to them alone, is a factor of Zoroastrian influence coupled with the occidental tendency of the Jewish religion to concretize images and to exclude and segregate themselves. Nevertheless, the instruction, which the early Jews received in Egypt about the oneness of Divinity, which they transferred to the personality of *Yahweh*, cannot be overlooked.

Akhenaton was at the same time a king and mystical philosopher. He introduced not a new religion, but a form of worship, which was highly philosophical, and abstract, thus less suited for the masses and more appropriate for the monastic order. The tenets of his hymns can be found in hymns to other Ancient Egyptian gods such as Amun (Amen), Asar (Osiris), and Ra, which preceded those to Aton. However, the form of their exposition brings forth a new dimension of Ancient Egyptian philosophy, which is unsurpassed in some ways even by the Hymns of Amun[II]. However, he was not able to reconcile the worship of Aton with the pre-existing forms of worship in Ancient Egypt. Also, he was not able to balance the duties of kingship with those of his position as High Priest. While he was not able reconcile these issues, he did bring forth the most advanced exposition of Ancient Egyptian philosophy. Scholars of religious studies have classified him as the first monotheist, before Moses, but his contributions to religion go much deeper than that.

Upon closer study, the philosophy, which Akhenaton espoused, is comparable to the most advanced spiritual philosophies developed in India, known as Vedanta philosophy. In Vedanta two important forms of spiritual philosophy developed. They are expressions of non-dualist philosophy known as Absolute Monism. The Hymns to Aton, which also espouse Absolute Monism, were recorded at least 579 years before its exposition in India through the Hindu Upanishads which are considered to be the highest expression of Hindu mystical philosophy. Akhenaton's teachings were given less than 200 years before the supposed date for the existence of Moses. However, Moses' teaching was not understood as Absolute Monism, but rather as monotheism. Therefore, whether the Jewish Pentateuch was written by a person named Moses or by Jewish scribes much later, as most modern biblical scholars

---

[I] Ancient Egyptian mythology conceives of creation as an expression of God in which there are nine primordial cosmic principles or forces in the universe. These first nine may be seen as the cause from which all other qualities of nature *(the other two Nine Gods)* or creative forces in nature arise.

[II] See the book "Egyptian Yoga Volume II" by Dr. Muata Ashby.

now agree, the influence of Akhenaton's teachings would have been foremost in the instruction of Moses. Remember that the Bible says Moses learned the wisdom of the Egyptians (Acts 7:22). While all of the attributes of Yahweh, the Hebrew God, are contained in the teachings related to Aton, the Hymns to Aton go farther in espousing the nature of God and God's relationship to Creation and humanity. They are based on Monism. Absolute Monism means that there is a recognition that there is only one reality that exists: God. All else is imagination. This means that everything that is perceived with the senses, thoughts, etc., is a manifestation of God. Modified Monism views God as the soul of nature, just as the human body also has a soul, which sustains it.

The next form of philosophy present in Akhenaton's hymns is pantheism. There are two forms of Pantheism, Absolute and Modified. Absolute Pantheism views God as being everything there is. In other words, God and Creation are one. Modified Pantheism is the view that God is the reality or principle behind nature. Panentheism is the doctrine that God is immanent in all things but also transcendent, so that every part of the universe has its existence in God, but God is more than the sum total of the parts. God transcends physical existence. Aten or Aton was represented not as a human being, but as the sun, from which extended rays that terminated with hands which bestowed Ankhs (Life Force), to all Creation. This image was used exclusively and constituted a non-personalized form of Divine iconography pointing towards the abstract and transcendental nature of the Divine as principle as opposed to personality. This was not a departure from Ancient Egyptian philosophy but an attempt to reinforce elements, which were already present in the very early forms of worship, related to the formless, nameless *God of Light* teaching. The following exerted verses from the Hymns to Aten approved by Pharaoh Akhenaton exhibit the most direct exposition of the philosophies mentioned above.

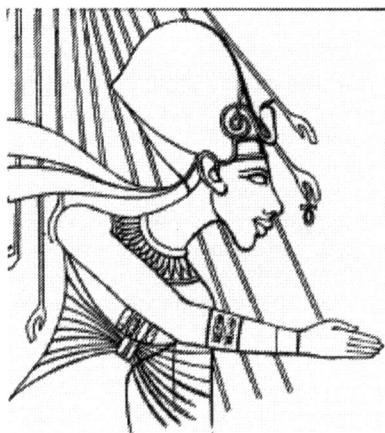

The Ancient Egyptian Pharaoh and High Priest Akhenaton.

Hymns to Aten	Philosophical Principle
A- The fish in the river swim towards thy face, thy beams are in the depths of the Great Green *(i.e.,* the Mediterranean and Red Seas). The earth becometh light, thou shootest up in the horizon, shining in the Aten in the day, thou scatterest the darkness.	A-From time immemorial God was worshipped as the Sun in Ancient Egypt. This has prompted many scholars in ancient and modern times, ignorant of the metaphorical symbolism, to refer to their worship as idolatry. This verse shows that God is seen as the principle <u>operating through</u> the sun and not the sun itself.
B- Thou makest offspring to take form in women, creating seed in men. Thou makest the son to live in the womb of his mother, making him to be quiet that he crieth not, thou art a nurse in the womb, giving breath to vivify that which he hath made.	B- God is not only the Creator of human life but also the very Life Force that sustains it. Worldly people would see the mother as sustaining the baby in the womb. Akhenaton affirms the higher source of sustenance i.e. God. The exact word used is "vivify." God is therefore not remote but intimately involved with Creation.
C- [When] he droppeth from the womb on the day of his birth [he] openeth his mouth in the [ordinary] manner, thou providest his sustenance...The young bird in the egg speaketh in the shell, thou givest breath to him inside it to make him to live. Thou makest for him his mature form so that he can crack the shell [being] inside the egg. He cometh forth from the egg, he chirpeth with all his might, when he hath come forth from it (the egg), he walketh on his two feet.	C- The philosophy of "breath" or breath of life has a very important teaching behind it. Breath relates to the Life Force energy, which vivifies everything. The force is subtle and thus interpenetrates all creation, thereby enlivening and sustaining it from within, much like the later Holy Spirit of the Bible. There is a recognition here that it is this same force, which causes vegetation and human life to grow and thrive.
D- One God, like whom there is no other. Thou didst create the earth by thy heart (or will), thou alone existing, men and women, cattle, beasts of every kind that are upon the earth, and that move upon feet (or legs), all the creatures that are in the sky and that fly with their wings, [and] the deserts of Syria and Kush (Nubia), and the Land of Egypt.	D- This important verse brings forth the understanding that there is a Supreme Being above the gods and goddesses. God caused all to come into being by his will and is not just the Creator of what exists (nature, living beings etc.) but that God and Creation are indeed one and the same, "alone existing" in the form of or manifesting as animals, people of all lands, etc.
E- Thou settest every person in his place. Thou providest their daily food, every man having the portion allotted to him; [thou] dost compute the duration of his life. Their tongues are different in speech, their characteristics (or forms), and likewise their skins (in color), giving distinguishing marks to the dwellers in foreign lands... Thou makest the life of all remote lands.	E- God has Created all peoples, all nations and countries and has appointed each person's country of residence, language and even their ethnicity and physical appearance or features. So all people, including those of foreign lands, have the same Creator and owe their continued existence to the same Divine Being.
F- Oh thou Lord of every land, thou shinest upon them...	F- In no uncertain terms, there is one God (Lord) who is the Supreme Being of all countries.
G- Thou hast made millions of creations from thy One self (viz.) towns and cities, villages, fields, roads and river. Every eye (i.e., all men) beholdeth thee confronting it. Thou art the Aton of the day at its zenith.	G- God manifests as and in countless forms, indeed, everything that exists, including life forms but also inanimate objects as well. Thus, when a person uses their senses and perceives objects, they are in reality perceiving God who is manifesting as Creation. This realization indicates the attainment of the highest goals of spiritual realization. This attainment is also known as non-dual vision, seeing God everywhere without separation between Creation and Divinity or the soul from God. This is of course the same teaching given by Jesus in the Gnostic Gospel of Thomas from Egypt where he asserts that *"The Kingdom is spread upon the earth but people do not see it!"*

THE CONCEPTS OF GOD IN WORLD RELIGIONS AND MYSTICAL PHILOSOPHIES

The Concept of God in Vedanta and Yoga Philosophies from India

The Absolute Reality (God) is named **Brahman**. Brahman signifies that which is the underlying essence of all phenomena. The manifesting universe is an appearance of Brahman only, an illusory modification of Brahman. Therefore, Creation never had a beginning and will never have an end, because it is only an appearance. Brahman or the ultimate reality, God, Supreme Being, is ALL that exists. All the objects of the world and universe, even though appearing to be different, are really one entity, having the same essence. All physical reality is an illusory manifestation of Brahman, which Brahman sustains at all times, yet is detached from—just as the sun sustains life on earth and yet is detached from it. Brahman is pure consciousness devoid of thought vibrations. All that exists is essentially Brahman, or *"Sat-Chit-Ananda*—Existence - Knowledge - Bliss Absolute, or Pure Consciousness involved with thought vibrations.

The Concept of God in Confucianism

"What the undeveloped man seeks is outside; what the advanced man seeks is within himself."

The Concept of God in Buddhism

"If you think the Law is outside yourself, you are embracing not the absolute Law but some inferior teaching."

The Concept of God in Shintoism

"Do not search in distant skies for God. In man's own heart is He found."

The Concept of God in Taoism

"Being at one with the Tao is eternal...
the great Tao flows everywhere, both to the left and to the right..."

The Concept of God in Hinduism

"God abides hidden in the hearts of all."

The Concept of God in Sikhism

"Why wilt thou go into the jungles? What do you hope to find there? Even as the scent dwells within the flower, so God within thine own heart ever abides. Seek Him with earnestness and find Him there."

The Concept of God in Islam

7:65 Section 9. To the Ad people, (We sent) Hud, one of their (own) brethren: He said: "O my people! Worship Allah! Ye have no other god but him. Will ye not fear (Allah)?"

The Concept of God and Creation According to the New Testament and the Gnostic Gospels

In the New Testament, the triad of "Father, and of the Son, and of the Holy Spirit" is used to describe the idea of God (Matthew 28:19). The Trinity is the central teaching of Christianity. It holds that God is three personalities, the Father, the Son, and the Holy Spirit [or Holy Ghost]. The idea is that there is only one God, but that he exists as *"Three."* Christian theologians claim that the true nature of the Trinity is a mystery, which cannot be comprehended by the human mind, although they can grasp some of its meanings. The Trinity doctrine was stated in very early Christian creeds whose purpose was to counter other beliefs such as Gnosticism. However, as we saw earlier, later church authorities misunderstood it.

The Concept of God and Creation According to Ancient Egyptian Religion and Mystical Philosophy

The term *"Trinity"* was misunderstood by the Orthodox Catholic Christians and, because of this misunderstanding, some Gnostic groups even ridiculed them. However, the three in one metaphor was ancient by the time it was adopted by Catholicism. It was a term used to convey the idea of different aspects of the one reality. This same idea occurs in Egyptian as well as in Indian mythology. However, for deeper insights into the mystical meaning of the Trinity we must look to Ancient Egypt. In Egyptian mythology, the Trinity was represented as three *metaphysical neters* or gods. They represent the manifestation of the unseen principles, which support the universe, and the visible aspects of God. The main Egyptian Trinity is composed of Amun, Ra and Ptah. Amun means that which is hidden and unintelligible, the underlying reality which sustains all things. Ra represents the subtle matter of creation as well as the mind. Ptah represents the visible aspect of Divinity, the phenomenal universe. The Ancient Egyptian "Trinity" is also known as a manifestation of *Nebertcher* (Neberdjer*)*. Nebertcher means "all encompassing" Divinity. Thus, the term Nebertcher is equivalent to the Vedantic Brahman, the Buddhist Dharmakaya and the Taoist Tao. The Ancient Egyptian text reads as follows:

"Nebertcher: Everything is Amun-Ra-Ptah, three in one."

The following passage from the *Hymns to Amun* (papyrus at Leyden) sums up the Ancient Egyptian understanding of the Trinity concept in creation and that, which transcends it.

He whose name is hidden is *AMUN*. *RA* belongeth to him as his face, and his body is *PTAH*.

Thus, within the mysticism of the Ancient Egyptian Trinity, the teaching of the triad of human consciousness (seer-seen-sight) is also found. Amun, the hidden aspect, is called the "eternal witness." This witness is one of the most important discoveries in mystical philosophy because it points to the existence of a transcendental awareness, which lies beyond the conscious level of the mind. This "witness" is also to be found in Indian philosophy under the Yoga teaching of *Sakshin* and the Buddhist teaching of *Mindfulness*. Sakshin is the "fourth" state of consciousness beyond the waking, dream and dreamless sleep states. It is the goal of all mystics to achieve awareness with this state.

The visible "gods" and "goddesses" with a name, form and other attributes are considered to be emanations of the one God. One name used was the Neter of neters: *NETER NETERU* or "God of gods" also known as "Pa Neter," meaning "The God" and "Nebertcher," meaning that which is without name, form or attributes (absolute). In the same way the Indian Trinity (Brahma, Shiva, and Vishnu) arises out of Brahman, the Absolute. They are responsible for the direction (management) of creation at every moment. In Indian mythology, each male aspect of the Trinity of Brahma - Shiva - Vishnu had his accompanying female aspect or manifesting energy: Saraswati - Kali - Lakshmi. Similarly, in the Egyptian system of gods and goddesses we have:

Male		Female
Amun	-	Amenit
Ra	-	Rai
Ptah	-	Sekhmet

There is one important difference between Ancient Egyptian Mythology and Yoga and other mystical systems. The idea of God being the Father who begets the Son, who is His *Paraclete* (advocate or intercessor) and revealer, occurs first and with most primacy in Egypt in the mythology of Nebertcher and Asar. While Buddha and Krishna are *Avatars*, incarnations of God, Heru in Ancient Egypt was the reincarnation of Asar, his father, who was himself an incarnation of the High God Ra who was, in this particular mythology referred to as the Absolute Self. At the same time, Heru is the symbol of the human soul, the essential nature and the innate hero/heroine within every human being. In much the same way, Jesus is the revealer and Paraclete of the Father, the Lord, and the Holy Spirit. The original idea of Avatarism was that from time to time God manifests himself in order to restore virtue in the world, to reform religion in a sense. In Hindu tradition, the god Vishnu had ten important avatars. Avatars also appear in the Jain tradition.

The acceptance, adoption and transformation of religious teachings from Ancient Egypt, India and other traditions into the particular form of Christianity espoused by Rome and the Byzantine Empire fostered the development of new terms for previously existing concepts. The terms used in the New Testament and the Gnostic Gospels, *Kingdom of God* or *Kingdom of Heaven,* are new terms not found previously in Jewish texts. Most often the Kingdom is described in parable form, but if we look past the facts of the mythology itself, a mystical meaning directed towards the individual is discovered. As such these terms convey a concept which is in exact agreement with the Vedantic, Buddhist, Egyptian and Taoist understanding that the realm of God is not in some far distant location which we must aspire to reach, but that it is everywhere, all around us and within us. What we must strive to do is realize this fact through virtuous living as well as growth in knowledge and wisdom.

As previously discussed, the Ancient Egyptian gods and goddesses are called *neteru,* and they emanate from *Pa Neter* or the Supreme Divinity. A very important aspect of Ancient Egyptian Religion and ritual can be related to Christian myth and ritual. This aspect is the consumption of the gods and goddesses or *neters* as a means of *becoming like onto them* in Ancient Egyptian mythology and ritual. This idea of consuming spirits occurs in a limited fashion in certain elements of Hinduism, such as in the battles of Krishna where he defeats the demons and they become absorbed by him. However, it does not occur with the same intensity and emphasis as in the Ancient Egyptian ritual and religious thought which appear as early as the *Pyramid Texts* (5,500 B.C.E.) in the Ancient Egyptian religious scriptures. In Christianity this notion was transformed into the idea of the *Eucharist.*[1]

The use of the word *Amun* or *Amen* in the Ancient Egyptian religion and later in the Christian religion requires further exploration here. The word Amen in Ancient Egyptian mythology connotes the Absolute Reality or transcendental Deity (Supreme Being). In the Hebrew religion the word Amen is usually explained or defined as an interjection meaning *so be it.* It is used at the end of a prayer or to express approval. However, in Egyptian myth and symbolism, Amen signifies an extremely sophisticated and elaborate explanation of the absolute and transcendental mystery behind all physical phenomena, in much the same way that the term *Brahman* is used in Hindu mythology and religion.

The mystical concept of Amun or Amen is the central theme of not only Ancient Egyptian religion and mystical philosophy, but also of every world religion. Having been intertwined with religious iconography and ritualism, the idea of an "eternal witness" has been mythologized by the Sages of ancient times in such a fashion that it may be possible to discover ever-increasing layers of the mystery behind it. The name *Amun (Amen)* appears in the remotest times of Egyptian history and came to prominence in the ancient city of *Waset or "Thebes,"* Egypt. The mysteries of Amun represent a quintessence of Ancient Egyptian philosophy concerning the nature of the unmanifest aspect of all existence and the understanding of human consciousness. It contains within it the teachings, which predate all other similar teachings. These teachings speak of God as an unmanifest, nameless, formless Pure Consciousness, which supports Creation.

Thus, in Ancient Egypt, the concept of the ultimate and Absolute Reality behind all physical manifestations was called *Amn, Amun, Nebertcher, Pa Neter, Asar, Aset* and *Ptah.* In Hindu mythology it is *Brahman, Shiva, Krishna, Vishnu, Kali or Rama;* to the Taoists it is *The Tao;* in Judaism it is referred to as *Yahweh;* in Islam it is *Allah;* in Christianity it is *God* and the *Kingdom of Heaven;* and in modern physics it is *energy.* There are, however, deeper meanings to the symbolic names given to explain the Absolute. They hold formulas, which convey mystical teachings about human beings and the nature of existence. Nebertcher carries with it various additional attributes referring to the Supreme Divinity: "Utmost Limit," "All Being," "All Powerful," etc. Nebertcher, as a name for the Supreme Being, appears in the Coptic texts and the attributes associated with this name were transferred to the idea of God Almighty of Christianity.[109]

As stated earlier, when you, as the spiritual aspirant, remove your own egoistic mask (individualism, desire, ignorance, etc.), you will discover that your underlying essence is one and the same as that of the Trinity, for indeed the Trinity is a symbol of cosmic and human egoism. Like the Ancient Egyptian Trinity, the Christian Trinity incorporates deep psycho-mythological implications. God the Father is the hidden creator, while the Son (Jesus) is the incarnating spirit, the body of creation. The Holy spirit is the enlivening force, which vivifies the creation. Every human being is an aspect of this Trinity, and the universe is also an aspect of the Trinity. The human ego, mind and body are the Son who suffers and the Holy Spirit is the force by which the soul enlivens the ego and body. With this understanding, God the Father is the witnessing consciousness, which supports the existence of the Son and of the Life Force energy of Creation.

In the original understanding of the early Christian theologians, the three aspects of the Trinity (Father, Son, and the Holy Spirit) were seen as equal in power and importance and as being one in their underlying essence. However, due to the zealous destruction of competing theologies, the Orthodox Christians developed a distorted view of Divinity. Only the dualistic, male-oriented view of the Trinity was understood and promoted, although reformers such as *Arius* sought to establish the non-dualistic view.

If one were to strip from the mind the mental concepts of duality which have been engendered by an elementary understanding of religion, the non-dual reality will emerge. This means that the spiritual aspirant must leave behind the understanding of the outer form of the Trinity and discover the underlying essence. When this is accomplished, the essence of the Trinity is discovered to be the same as that of every human being. When Jesus says, *I and the Father are One,* he is not referring to two individual personalities (Father and Son) which are one in a spiritual sense. Although this is certainly true, he is referring to the fact that there is only one being in existence and this being transcends the personality of Jesus and the Father. So take away the "Father" image and take away the "Son" image and what is left in the mind is the underlying basis of these concepts. That underlying basis is the ground upon which all mental concepts exist. It is this ground which is "one" with all things. This is what is referred to as the transcendental Self or the Supreme Being, etc. This is what is eternal, while the father and Son are mere temporary manifestations of that. The mental concepts are only images of this ultimate ground, which has taken on a

---

[1] See the section entitled: The Eucharist of the Ancient Egyptian Mysteries.

particular name and form. The name and form are related to time and space, but everything in time and space is temporal and illusory. In this ultimate ground there are no opposites. The opposites only seem to exist at the superficial conscious level. Therefore, in reality all names and forms have the same underlying basis and are composed of the same material: thoughts. The Self underlies all thoughts and, therefore, the Self is the Goal of all spiritual movements.

If you go beyond your ego-self, your thoughts and your concepts, you discover that your underlying essence is also One and undifferentiated Consciousness. Ultimately, you will discover that this personality of yours, all of nature and all representative forms of religion (Jesus, Buddha, Krishna, Allah, etc.) are all masks which are covering the transcendental Self. This is the pure non-dualistic view of Divinity which is to be reached by an aspirant through the practice of the Yoga disciplines. Nature and the human ego are only reflections of Divinity and not abiding, individually existing entities. This non-dualistic experience of the Divine is what constitutes true sainthood and is therefore the most laudable goal of life. All other goals are illusory and transitory; this is the only absolute truth of existence. All other goals are perishable in time, but this truth transcends time. For this reason early Christianity incorporated the idea of reincarnation and the need to serve and love others as yourself. If you were to practice seeing everything before you, including your own body and your own thoughts, as an expression of God, you would discover that God is all that exists and that you are God, expressing as a triad of *seer, seen and sight*. You would discover that you are transcendental, immortal, infinite and non-dual. You have always existed, and you will always exist for all eternity. Your identification with your transient ego-personality, which is subject to birth and death, will be ended.

GOD AS THE ALL AND THE ABSOLUTE

Bible, Revelation 1:8
I am Alpha and Omega, the beginning and the ending, saith the Lord, who is, and who was, and who is to come, the Almighty.

Gospel of Thomas
81. Jesus says: "I am the All, and the All has gone out from me and the All has come back to me. Cleave the wood: I am there; lift the stone and thou shalt find me there!"

In Egyptian mythology, the God *Ra* represents Cosmic Consciousness, The All, which manifests as the *sight* aspect of consciousness within the system of Amun-Ra-Ptah. Asar is Ra in material form, and Heru represents *the way* to reach the father, Ra. As previously stated, the visual forms and ideas presented in each of the gods were created by the Sages of ancient times to help us understand the qualities and characteristics of God through the descriptions of the various neters or deities. Similarly, the Biblical statement from the book of Revelations and the Gnostic Christian quote above, attributed to Jesus in the Gospel of Thomas, describe the same idea, even calling it by the same name, "The All." In Hermeticism we encounter the same terminology. A comparison between the following Hermetic teachings and the Gnostic Christian teachings reveal the same meaning and mode of expression.

"There is only one Supreme Being, All is It; It manifests itself through infinite forms and many Gods."
"In its essence, The All is Unknowable."
"The Universe is Mental, held in the mind of The All. The All is Spirit."
"The infinite mind of The All is the womb of Universes."
"The All creates in its Infinite Mind, countless Universes, which exist for eons of time; to the All, the creation, development and death of a million Universes is as the time of the twinkling of an eye."
"While All is in The All, it is also true that The All is in All. To him who truly understands this truth hath come great knowledge."

The All refers to the whole of existence. We normally perceive reality as being composed of separate objects, people, planets, stars, etc., but the ancient mystical philosophy view is that there is an all-encompassing existence, which encompasses everything. Further, what we call time and space or the passage of time and the cause and effect experiences of the world are only expressions of or emanations from the Transcendental Being which is beyond time and space. It is from this being, The All, that time and space come, and it is into this same being that time and space as well as human life and consciousness dissolve after a certain period of time. This is the idea that Jesus is referring to in the Gospel of Thomas, line 81: *"The All has gone out from me and the All has come back to me."* It is also the mystical implication of the ocean metaphor. All transient phenomena—life, birth, death, animals, planets, stars, etc.—are like waves, which rise and subside continuously in the ocean of the Self.

This Great Being has a thousand {meaning countless} heads, a thousand eyes, and a thousand feet. He envelops the universe. Though transcendent, he is to be meditated upon as residing in the lotus of the heart, at the center of the body, ten fingers above the navel.

He alone is *all thi*s—what has been and what shall be. He has become the universe. Yet he remains forever changeless, and is the lord of immortality.

From the Svetasvatara Upanishad 47

The same idea is expressed in the *Bhagavad Gita* where Krishna, having identified himself with all creation, states that all creatures come from him {send forth} and merge in him again.

Bhagavad Gita, Chapter 9, Raja Vidya Raja Guhya Yogah— The Yoga of Royal Knowledge and Royal Secret

7. O Son of Kunti, all beings merge into My Prakriti at the end of the Kalpa, and with the commencement of the next Kalpa it is I who send them forth.
8. Keeping Prakriti under My control, I, again and again, send forth these beings which are helplessly under the control of Prakriti.

In other chapters of the *Gita*, Krishna also discusses the oneness of God and the one who aspires to realize God by using phrases such as: "attains Me," "attains Brahman," "realizes Me," "abides in Me," "enters into Me," etc.

The main idea of the All is that it is inconceivable by the ordinary human mind. It is beyond thoughts, transcendent while at the same time all-encompassing. It is transcendent of being or non-being, and even transcendent of being beyond the pairs of opposites or no opposites. The transcendent is exactly that— transcendent. Therefore, words, ideas, similes, metaphors, sacred scriptures, etc., which are grounded in images from time and space will always be deficient in describing that which is transcendent of them. Somehow, the mind must go beyond the normal thought-concept processes it is used to in order to realize the meaning of the scriptures. If this is not done, the mind becomes stuck in the mental world of time and space, causation, and there is no breakthrough to the source of consciousness and mental activity. Therefore, religion needs to allow a person to transcend the religious symbols, myths and rituals in order to attain the higher goal of religion.

Even when speaking of God as the male spirit and creation as being the female aspect which is enlivened by God (the spirit), dualism is still implied. In the end we must break through the duality to understand that, in reality, there is no male and female except in our thoughts. In essence, creation is one substance. That substance is not separate from God, and we are indeed one with all of that. To know this intellectually is the first step towards realizing it in actuality. This realization which goes beyond rationality and non-rationality is the Kingdom of Heaven, the fruit of the Tree of Life: Spiritual Enlightenment.

CHAPTER X: THE DEEPER MEANING OF SYMBOLS, RITUALS OF CHRISTIANITY

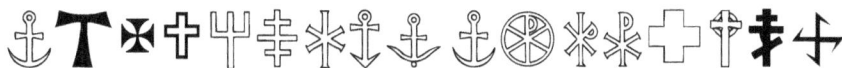

THE POWER OF SYMBOLISM

The unconscious can be reached and expressed only by symbols, which is the reason why the process of individuation can never do without the symbol. The symbol is the primitive expression of the unconscious, but at the same time it is also an idea corresponding to the highest intuition produced by consciousness.

C. G. Jung (1875-1961)

The understanding of symbolism is of primary importance prior to any study of ancient forms of religious or philosophical concepts because those very concepts are heavily mixed with and sometimes entirely described in symbolic forms. Often, we try to understand ideas and concepts of the past through the eyes and mind of a 20th century scholar rather than through those of a keen student of life thousands of years ago. Thus, it is appropriate to begin with a quotation from an ancient Greek philosopher on this very issue.

"If anyone suggests that it is disgraceful to fashion base images of the Divine and most Holy orders, it is sufficient to answer that the most holy Mysteries are set forth in two modes: one by means of similar and sacred representations akin to their nature, and the other to unlike forms designed with every possible discordance ... Discordant symbols are more appropriate representations of the Divine because the human mind tends to cling to the physical form of representation believing for example that the Divine are "golden beings or shining men flashing like lightning." But lest this error befall us, the wisdom of the venerable sages leads us through disharmonious dissimilitudes, not allowing our irrational nature to become attached to those unseemly images ... Divine things may not be easily accessible to the unworthy, nor may those who earnestly contemplate the Divine symbols dwell upon the forms themselves as final truth."

– Dionysius the Areopagite

The previous quotation by Dionysius provides us with insight on the nature, purpose and dangers of creating images of the Divine for the purpose of worshiping. Making images of God and the gods and goddesses in human likeness can be either helpful or dangerous for the follower. The mind is a wonderful tool but it easily indulges in emotion and illusion, developing attachment to that which it understands and fear towards that which it does not. The danger arises when the mind becomes fixed on the image rather than the essence of the symbolic meaning of the deity to be worshipped. Instead of worshipping those qualities and developing them in oneself, the worshipper might believe that those qualities belong to the statue or painting, or are for some special person who lived long ago, or belong to a special religious or philosophical system to the exclusion of others. They do not realize that the symbols such as "Heru," "Christ," and "Buddha" are representations of the qualities which lie deep within every individual, not somewhere "out there," but right in here inside each one of us. So very often the wise Sages of ancient times chose radical images, such as an animal head with a human body, that were so far from the norm that the attachment-oriented human mind would not get "hung up" on the picture or symbol and thereby concentrate on the *meaning* behind it. For example: the Hawk is the symbol of Heru, the God of light, vision and speed. The symbol may be the picture of a hawk or a human body with the head of a hawk. When looking at the hawk, we should be immediately drawn to those qualities (vision, tenacity and speed, freedom, Heru, etc.) instead of to the image itself.

Symbols have great psychological significance because without them there would be no possibility for the mind to exist, function and interact with creation. A deeper examination of symbols reveals that they are more than just representations of images or ideas. The human mind understands things by first making a mental picture of it and then associating that mental concept with other ideas and thoughts. When we think of a chair, a three-dimensional mental image appears in the mind of what a chair looks like. We do not think of the letters that make up the word C-H-A-I-R. Therefore, to most efficiently and quickly convey an idea or thought, symbols are far superior to written forms of communication. Then, just a glance at them will convey the ideas, thoughts and feeling associated with them, which were learned in this volume. When we understand that we are not the body, but spirits, it becomes obvious that all our mental notions are only elaborate symbols. In fact, all the objects in creation are really symbols or ideas, not absolute realities. They are representations of the thoughts in the mind of God, which have been projected through cosmic energy in much the same way as a human being projects the dream world during a dream. Therefore, symbols are a vital key to understanding the workings of the mind and the nature of existence.

In Ancient Egyptian mythology and philosophy, as well as in other mythological and philosophical systems, it is often necessary to learn about a symbol's meaning(s) by its relation to other symbols. In many cases, symbols from seemingly separate cultures may shed light on each other's meaning. Another important point to understand is that symbols do not have absolute meanings. Actually, nothing in the realm of time and space has absolute meaning because objects are illusory, transient and the human capacity to know an object is limited due to the restrictions of the human mind and senses. In addition, the symbolic meaning is subject to the frame of reference of the individual. For example, the symbol of a cow may be an image of food to one person, or a symbol of the goddess to another. Sometimes the meaning of symbols is lost in religions because the creator of the symbol passed on without having an opportunity to pass it on through the initiatic tradition, to a successor or disciple. In the absence of a spiritual preceptor, people may turn directly to the scriptures themselves as sources of guidance. Since the scriptures can always be misinterpreted, intentionally or unintentionally, the true intent of the founders of the religion may not be grasped, and thus, their practice of religion becomes something other than a viable method for spiritual evolution. The meaning of something discussed in mystical philosophy refers to a context, which leads to determining the transcendental nature of the object as opposed to the secular reference. This is accomplished by discovering its source and sustenance. For this reason, a Yogi or mystic strives to know the transcendental nature of an object by discovering its source and sustenance. Since God is the sustainer and true nature of all that exists, if God is discovered, then all objects are simultaneously discovered as well.

It was not until the emergence of Western religions in Mesopotamia that the religious symbols which had existed previously for thousands of years were thought of as realities in fact, rather than conveyers of wisdom about nature and its relation to the individual. Now, with this concretized vision and the self-appointed mandate to subdue nature and convert all peoples, man began to see himself as the conqueror of nature instead of as part of nature.[65] The ordinary human being identifies him/herself as being within his own ego-personality, and views him/herself as an individual rather than as one with the universe.

In modern times people often confuse their identity with their job roles and get so caught up in that false identification that they cannot find happiness without it. The executive dresses up in executive clothing, works in an executive office, drives an executive car, comes home to the executive neighborhood to the executive wife to be greeted by the executive children, and so on. If he/she is not treated in an executive manner, he/she will get upset. If others do not live up to his/her social standing, they are chastised. There are many forms of delusion, which can arise when a person begins to identify with their occupation, birthplace, ethnicity, gender, etc. A person may feel "I am an American and all other countries are primitive" or "I was born in the city and I am sophisticated and not like you country people" or "I am a man and I'm stronger, so you women are inferior." The soul, identified with the personality as a woman, may feel, "I cannot enjoy life unless I become a mother." As a result, she will proceed to get pregnant whether or not she is healthy, can financially take care of the child, or is at a stage in life where she can handle the responsibilities, etc. This happens because ignorance, lack of will, and desire have deluded the mind and the ability to reason has been impaired. Indoctrination with ideas like "life is for having babies and becoming a mother" or the pressure from society with ideas like "if you don't get pregnant you are not worth anything" hold sway in the weak and ignorant mind. When the soul is caught up in such mental delusion, one forgets that one's role (mother, father, boss, employee, etc.) in life is only a vehicle for spiritual discovery, not an end in itself. It is not who you are. What would you say about an actor who gets off the stage but continues to play the role when they go home, to the market, church, etc? You would call them insane! Yet people are constantly playing roles, in their ordinary lives, based on their erroneous notions of reality, and these ignorant notions are constantly being reinforced by society at large (government, media, misguided religious people).

Paganism and Idolatry in the Christian Church

The Christian Church has indoctrinated many Christians with the idea of paganism. The church leaders have the idea that anyone who deviates from the Christian faith is a "pagan."[1] Further, they have promoted the idea of paganism not only with divergent faiths or religions, but also with atheism. In effect, the underlying message of the Christian leaders is if you do not have the Christian faith, and more specifically, if you do not believe that Jesus Christ will come and save you, it is the same as if you have no faith at all. This is evidence of the self-righteous attitude and conceit of Christianity, which comes down in history from the Jewish tradition, which it developed out of, and the Zoroastrian tradition, which strongly influenced Judaism. This closed-minded view of the world has led to repudiation of other religions and the unwillingness of Christians to understand and accept other peoples. The

---

[1] pa·gan (p³"g...n) n. 1. One who is not a Christian, Moslem, or Jew; a heathen. 2. One who has no religion. 3. A non-Christian. 4. A hedonist. -- pa·gan adj. 1. Not Christian, Moslem, or Jewish. 2. Professing no religion; heathen.

passages below denote the ironic disdain of the Bible for the religion of other lands, including Egypt. We have seen so many correlations between Christianity, Judaism and Ancient Egyptian Religion, yet the biblical writings in many places seek to set themselves apart from these, referring to them as abominations.

Ezekiel 20:7

> 7 Then said I to them, Cast ye away every man the abominations[1] of his eyes, and defile not yourselves with the idols of Egypt: I [am] the LORD your God.
> 8 But they rebelled against me, and would not hearken to me: they did not every man cast away the abominations of their eyes, neither did they forsake the idols of Egypt: then I said, I will pour out my fury upon them, to accomplish my anger against them in the midst of the land of Egypt.

Along with this idea the Christian tradition also looks down upon those peoples who worship nature, animals and heavenly objects as part of their religion. As we will see, Christianity, in its attempt to separate itself from other religions, has itself committed the offence of idolatry. In turning away from so called pagan religions, Christianity has tried to turn away from its own roots. As far as the worship of animals and natural objects as part of the religious tradition, Christianity has, since its inception, incorporated these and still continues to do so, even while looking down on other religions, as well will see shortly.

Another prime example of this problem is the case of Christhood. The original meaning attached to the word Christ by early Christians is contrary to the later definitions and philosophical understanding. People identify the experience of Jesus Christ as being "His" experience instead of understanding that he is a symbol of the potential, which is within all people and must be achieved by all people via his example. While most Christians profess to not be idol worshipers, failure to understand the true meaning of Christ is an expression of extreme idolatry. Thus, idolatry and egoism are closely related.

If the definition of idolatry is *the worship of a physical object as a God,*[68] then concretizing religious symbolic images as facts and not as myths must, therefore, be considered idolatry. In this sense, religious traditions which view their specific philosophy as the only truth or their images of deities as entities that exist as revealed facts from which creative powers emerge are also to be considered as *idolatrous philosophies.* In concretizing the image into one religion or one personality or philosophy, they are in effect saying that God has been defined into a particular form and that form is separate from human beings.

Ancient mystical philosophy holds that God is transcendent. This means that any one concept, symbol or image cannot define God. Concepts, symbols and ideas can only be used to direct the mind towards the understanding, but the understanding itself is transcendent of thought. Human consciousness must go beyond the picture, idea or symbol in order to connect with the reality which *transcends* them. If this is not possible, spiritual development stops or becomes distorted due to contraction in consciousness. Contraction is the nature of egoism, while expansion is the nature of Enlightenment. Deep down the soul knows the transcendental truth, but at the conscious level of mind, a human being who is not in tune with the soul follows the path of egoism and ignorance, and these lead to mental conflicts which manifest as delusion, anger, hatred, frustration, desire, etc.

According to the *Raja Yoga* philosophy of India, when the soul ceases to expand in consciousness, the mind contracts into ever-increasing delusions, complexes and miseries. These are collectively called mental illness. They may also be seen as increasing levels of egoism or hardening of the ego. On a planetary scale, mental illness manifests as wars, denigration of whole populations and the destruction of nature.

> There is no greater intoxication than that of love when it transcends the human object and is directed towards the Divine Being.
>
> Pir Vilayat Inayat Khan (born 1916)
> Sufi Priest

---

[1] Strong's Concordance of the Bible defines Abomination as: 1) a disgusting thing, abomination, abominable 1a) in ritual sense (of unclean food, idols, mixed marriages)1b) in ethical sense (of wickedness etc)

Zoomorphic and Natural Symbols used in Christianity (0-1,600 A.C.E.)	Zoomorphic and Natural Symbols used in Ancient Egyptian Religion (6,000 B.C.E.– 400 A.C.E.)
St. Luke – the Bull	
The Bull symbol is used in relation to St. Sylvester. He performed the miracle of bringing a bull back to life. The bull is also a symbol of St. Eustace (top right). He was martyred with his family by being jailed on a bull, which had a fire burning under it	The Bull is especially related to the god Asar (Osiris). It is a symbol of his power to create the world.
St. Mark – the Lion. The lion is the symbol of strength and courage. It is related to the Resurrection as the symbol of Christ. It appears as one of the four animals in the prophecy of Ezekiel. Lions appear as attributes of St. Paul the Hermit, St. Mary of Egypt, St. Onuphrius and St. Euphemia.	The lion is the symbol of power, strength and courage. It is related to the god as well as the goddess (lioness) in Ancient Egyptian mythology.
In Christian iconography the Falcon represents the Holy man.	The falcon or hawk (left) is the symbol of Heru (Horus), the Ancient Egyptian savior and holiest of personalities. The falcon is also related to each individual in the form of the falcon body with the human head.

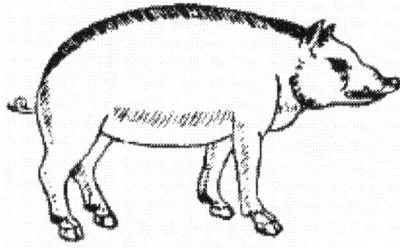

C-1

In Christian iconography the Hog represents the demon of sensuality and gluttony.

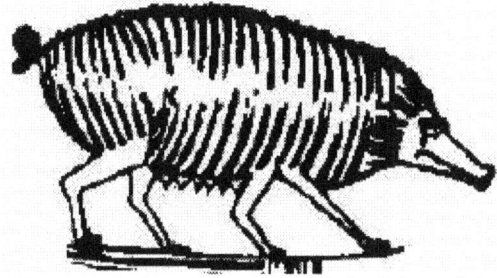

In Ancient Egypt the Hog was a symbol of the god Set, the personification of indiscriminate sexuality, gluttony, anger, hatred, greed, violence, etc.

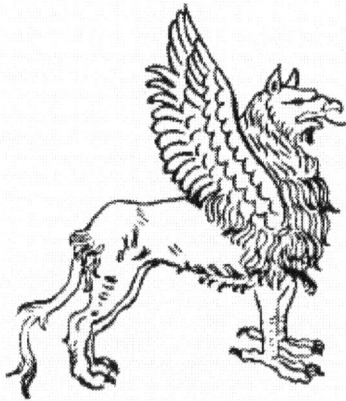

C-1

The Griffin is the symbol of the Savior and the supreme power.

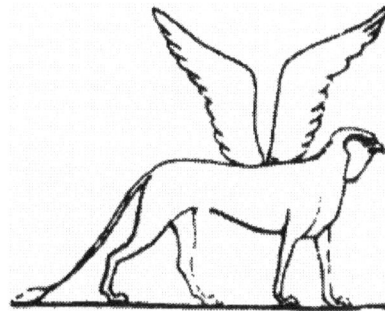

The Ancient Egyptian Sefer or Griffin is the symbol of the most powerful creature, which is above all creatures. It is the goddess in her form as the incarnating instrument of God, which he uses to punish those who are evil.

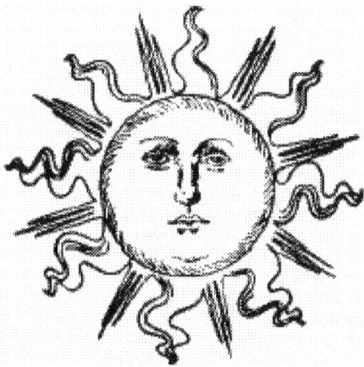

C-1

The Sun is the symbol of The Christ. This interpretation is based on the prophecy of Malachi 4:2 'But unto you that fear my name shall the sun of righteousness arise with healing in his wings.'

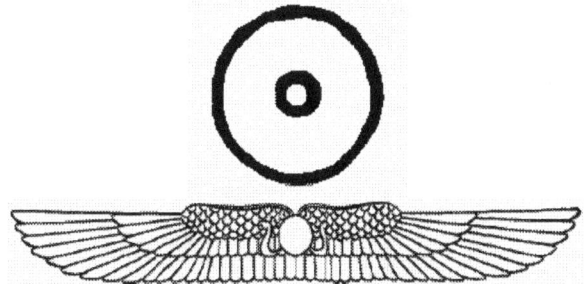

In Ancient Egyptian mythology the sun is the symbol of the dynamic aspect of the God, Ra, though which he engenders life on earth. Heru in the horizon is the aspect of the savior who is rising with the sun in the east. Below: The Ancient Egyptian Symbol of the Supreme Spirit – Heru (Egyptian Savior), the Winged Sun-disk.[64]

C-1

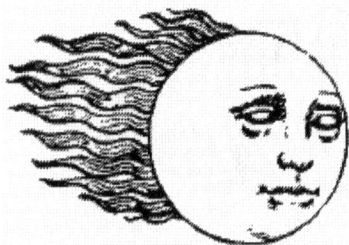

The Moon and the Sun are symbols of the Virgin Mary. She is referred to as the 'woman clothed with the sun, and the moon under her feet.' (Revelation 12:1)

The Sun and Moon are also frequently used in scenes of the crucifixion to symbolize the sorrow of creation at the death of Christ.

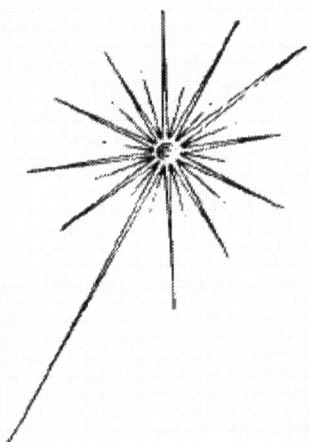

C-1

The Star symbolizes divine guidance. It guided the Magi to the place where Jesus was born. Twelve stars symbolize the twelve Apostles and the twelve tribes of Israel. The star is the symbol of the Virgin in her aspect as the Star of the Sea ('Stella Maris').

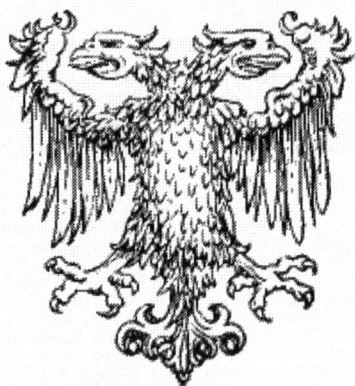

C-1

The Phoenix is an ancient symbol related to the sun. In Christianity it is related by St. Clement in his first Epistle to the Corinthians. It relates to the resurrection of the dead and the victory of eternal life over death. It is also a symbol of the resurrection of Christ and it appears many times in connection with the crucifixion.

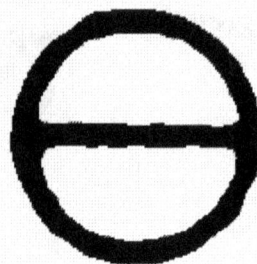

The Moon is the symbol of the goddess and of the mind. It is the reflection of the God or Spirit. As such, the moon as a symbol of the goddess represents creation itself. The moon is also a symbol of the god Djehuti, who is the minister of Ra. Djehuti represents mind. The human mind is the reflection of the Cosmic Mind, Ra, just as moonlight is a reflection of the sunlight. The goddess Hethor [Het-Hor or House of Hor (Heru, Horus)] is understood as creation itself, which is illuminated by Heru, the sun or spirit.

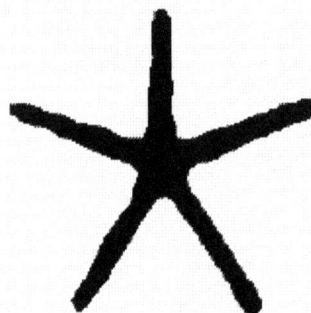

In Ancient Egyptian mythology the star (Sba) is the symbol of a journey across water. The term Sbau means the pilot who leads the ship and its crew skillfully. Sba also means star in the heavens. It is also a symbol of the netherworld (Astral Plane).

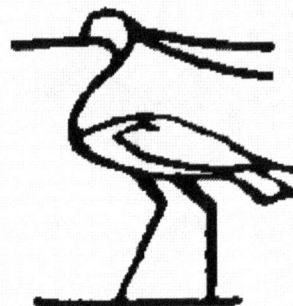

The Ancient Egyptian Bennu bird is the forerunner of the European and Middle Eastern Phoenix, which the Christians adopted. It is a symbol of Ra, God, who renews himself as if rising from death to new life. Thus it is a symbol of God, the sun and resurrection.

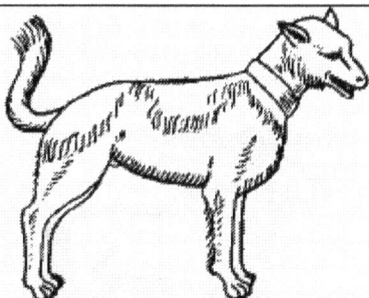

C-1

The Dog is a symbol of faithfulness, watchfulness and, fidelity and vigilance. It is related to the dog of Tobias and the dog of St. Roch. A dog with a flaming torch in his mouth is a symbol of St. Dominic. Black and White dogs are used as symbols of the Dominicans. They are known as the 'Dogs of the Lord.'

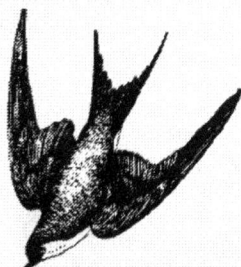

C-1

The Swallow is the symbol of the incarnation of Christ since it hibernates in the winter and appears in the spring hailing the new season.

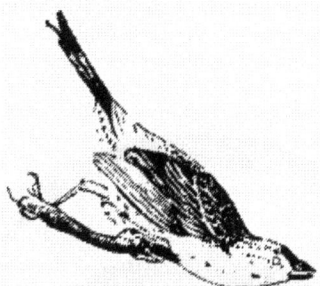

C-1

The Sparrow is the symbol of that which is lowly since it is seen as the lowliest of birds. Thus, it is seen as the lowest among people, who regardless of their lowliness are taken care of by God.

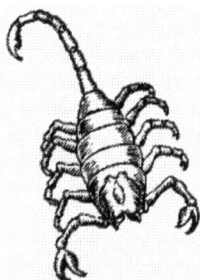

C-1

The Scorpion is the symbol of evil, pain and suffering due to its sting. In the Bible the following scripture appears. '... and their torment was the torment of a scorpion, when it

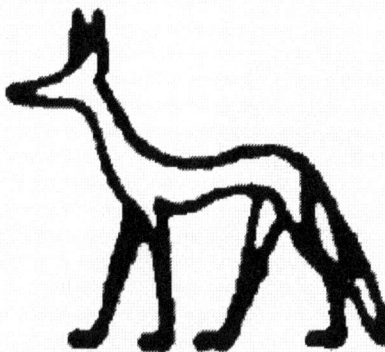

In Ancient Egyptian mythology the Jackal is a symbol of the dog god Anubis. Because of his intellect and quality of discernment between friend (right) and foe (wrong), he is the one who leads the spiritual aspirant to discover God. He is the knower of the ways and his vigilance prevents the aspirant from moving in the wrong direction.

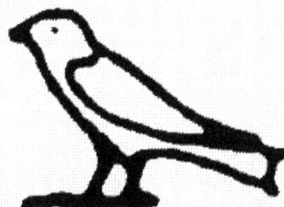

In Ancient Egyptian mythology, the swallow is the symbol of the goddess Aset (Isis) who will bring forth the salvation of the earth by giving birth to the Savior Heru, the Christ. Thus the swallow is also the symbol of greatness and of anointing (Christ). The tail expands in the swallow, denoting expansion in character, wealth, and spiritual enlightenment.

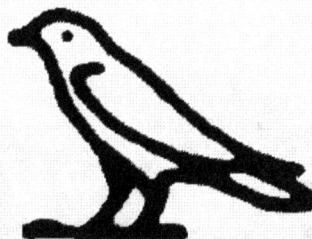

In Ancient Egyptian mythology the Sparrow is seen as the lowly man or woman and the retched conditions of life. It is also a symbol of that which is defective, small, bad, inadequate, small and insufficient. The rounded tail signifies constriction and contraction as well as self-centeredness and selfishness.

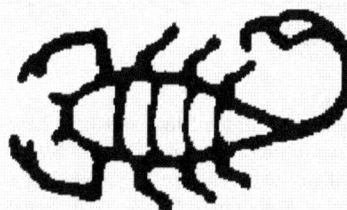

In Ancient Egypt, the Scorpion had two aspects. One of them was the evil and vicious Set, who transformed himself into the form of a scorpion and stung and killed Heru, the Ancient Egyptian Christ. Heru's mother Aset resurrected him and Heru then challenged and defeated Set and thereby established

'...and their torment was the torment of a scorpion, when it striketh a man' (Revelation 9:5). Due to its treachery it became a symbol of Judas.

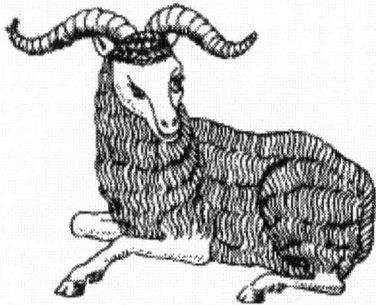
C-1

The Ram is the leader of the herd. It is used as a symbol of Christ. Since the ram fights with the wolf to keep him away and eventually defeats him, the symbol is related with Christ who fights with and defeats Satan. Also, since God gave Abraham a ram to sacrifice instead of his own son, Isaac, the ram is seen as a symbol of Christ, who led people to salvation. Also, the lamb is a symbol of Christ who sacrificed himself for humanity. (see below)

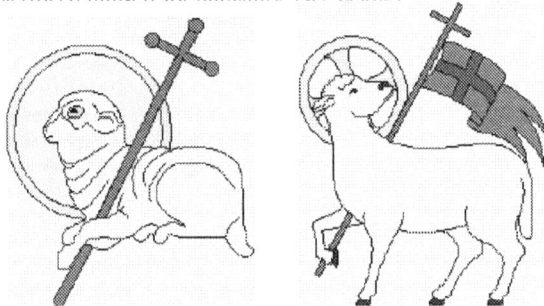
C-1

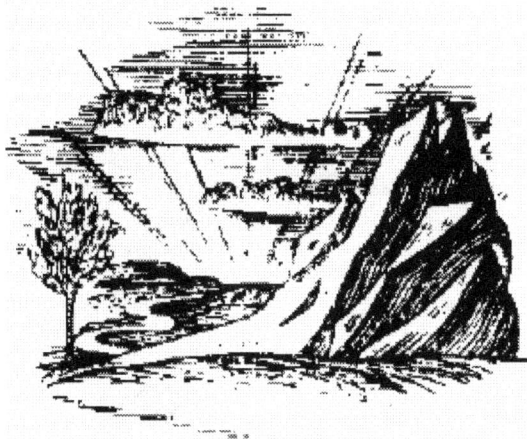
C-1

The Dawn is a symbol of the Blood of Christ because by the shedding of Christ's blood human kind is able to overcome the darkness of sin. Dawn is also the symbol of the coming birth of Christ. Sometimes Christ is depicted as being enveloped in the glow of the rose colored morning sunlight.

justice in the land and showed the way to blessedness and enlightenment again. The other aspect is the benevolent goddess, Serket, who helps Heru in his time of need.

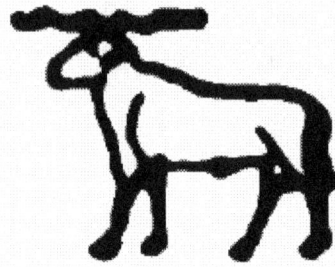

In Ancient Egyptian Mythology the Ram is the symbol of Amun. Amun is the hidden aspect of the god Ra and is therefore, the highest, innermost reality of Creation. In the aspect of Amsu-Min, Amun is also identified with Heru or the Ancient Egyptian Christ.

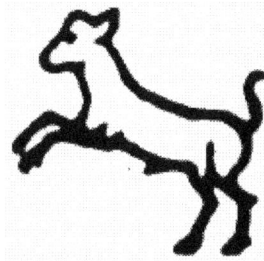

In Ancient Egyptian Mythology the young ram (lamb) is a symbol of the newborn child and is sometimes used to symbolize Heru, the Ancient Egyptian Christ.

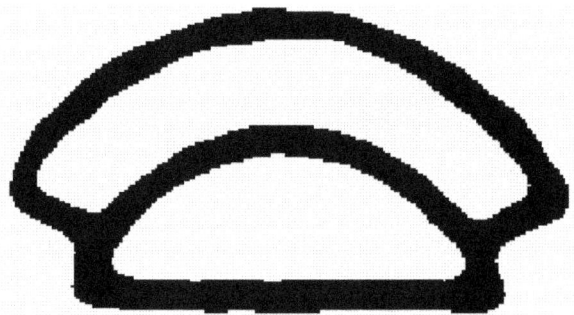

In Ancient Egyptian mythology, the symbol of sunrise refers to the coming of God over the horizon to enliven the earth. It also means resurrection and the birth of the new sun in the form of Heru (the Ancient Egyptian Christ), the sun child who will bring light and spiritual upliftment to the world.

214

The Origins of Angels

The biblical verse, Exodus 33, also speaks of another important feature of Judaism, Christianity and Islam, namely, the *angels*. Angels are thought of as messengers between the Divine and the world of human activity. However, they also point to some contradictions in the philosophy. While Orthodox Judaism[I], Christianity and Islam claim not to be polytheistic, their mythology as related to the angels and saints clearly shows that they have substituted the older notion of multiple gods and goddesses for the hierarchies of angels and numerous saints.

This point is very important to realize. Most followers of orthodox religion believe that since they follow one God, even though their system incorporates a host of saints and angels, they are still following a monotheistic system of religion. However, when other so called polytheistic religious systems, such as Shetaut Neter (Ancient Egyptian Religion) or Hinduism, which have been dubbed as pagan religions in the biblical texts are correctly evaluated and understood, the true character of the religious philosophy emerges. In reality these are systems which portray a single Supreme Being. The many deities (gods & goddesses) symbolize the many manifestations or aspects of this one God. The orthodox traditions have the same systems, only substituting the gods and goddesses with saints and angels.

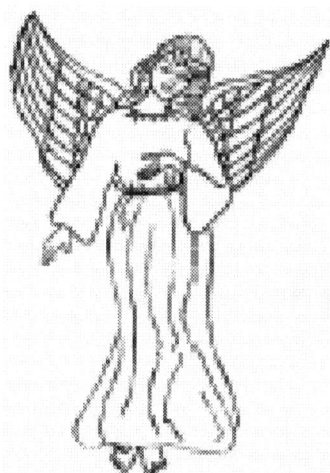

Left: Modern rendition of the Christian concept of an angel. In Christian mythology, angels are the doers of tasks. They perform the bidding of God. They help human beings, acting as conduits for God's message.

Right: Ancient Egyptian image of the Maati goddesses. They manage the orderly process of the universe. Note that they too are adorned with wings, like the angels.[II]

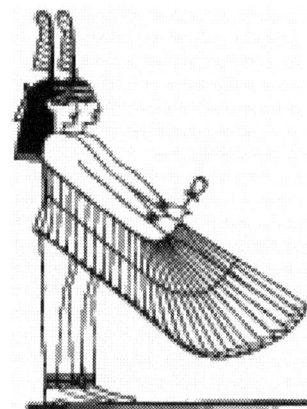

The Symbol of the Eyes and Trinity of God

Matthew 6
> 22 The light of the body is the eye: if therefore thy eye be single (good), thy whole body shall be full of light.
> 23 But if thy eye be evil, thy whole body shall be full of darkness. If therefore the light that is in thee is darkness, how great [is] that darkness!
> 24 No man can serve two masters: for either he will hate the one, and love the other; or else he will hold to the one, and despise the other. Ye cannot serve God and money.

Matthew 18
> 9 And if thy eye causeth thee to sin, pluck it out, and cast [it] from thee: it is better for thee to enter into life with one eye, rather than having two eyes to be cast into hell fire.

Mark 9
> 47 And if thy eye causeth thee to fall into sin pluck it out; it is better for thee to enter into the Kingdom of God with one eye, than having two eyes to be cast into hell fire.

The statements concerning the *eye* and *vision* certainly refer to the ordinary sense of vision, but also have a deeper esoteric symbolism as evinced in the Ausarian Resurrection mystery of Ancient Egypt which is the earliest

---

[I] **Orthodox Judaism** *n.* The branch of Judaism that is governed by adherence to the Torah as interpreted in the Talmud.

[II] Definitions: **an·gel** (ān'jəl) *n.*

1.a. *In Theology.* An immortal, spiritual being attendant upon God. In medieval angelology, there are nine orders of spiritual beings. From the highest to the lowest in rank, they are: seraphim, cherubim, thrones, dominations or diminions, virtues, powers, principalities, archangels, and angels.
b. The conventional representation of such a being in the image of a human figure with a halo and wings.
2. A guardian spirit or guiding influence.
3. *In Christian Science.* God's thoughts passing to man.

known usage of the symbol. Like other senses, the eyes see something of interest and immediately report that information to the mind. The eyes are also the symbol of consciousness, which at the ordinary human level perceives a subject, object, and the interaction between them. The interrelationship between these three factors is referred to as the triad of the human mind. The eye is the symbol of consciousness and awareness, which characterize the essence of life and existence. There can be no existence and hence no life, if there is no consciousness to be aware of it.

When the human mind is aware of a triad of consciousness (object-subject-relationship), this mental condition is said to be the state of spiritual ignorance because the underlying identity of all three characters in the *"Triad"* are in reality the *"Self,"* (Ra, Asar, Brahman, Krishna, Kingdom of Heaven, The Tao). In reality, there is no separation between these three aspects of consciousness except in our mistaken identification with them as our true being. This philosophical point can be better understood if you examine the waking, dream and dreamless states of human consciousness. In the dream there is also a subject, an object and a relationship between them, but upon waking they all vanish. In the dream state your consciousness has become modified (taken the form) and identified itself with the subject who is experiencing the dream. However, upon waking up the occurrences, which seemed so real were discovered to be nonexistent. Also, when you fell asleep, the waking world became nonexistent. This study leads to the understanding that neither the waking nor the dream states are absolutely real. Only that which supports them and makes it possible for them to exist is real because it is always there and unchanging. If you put on different glasses, which have different color tints, you will see things with a different tinge, but the consciousness, the looker (you) is always the same. When you are able to discover this underlying reality behind the multiplicity and transience of the waking and dream states, you will have discovered the truth of your real self. This is the objective of yoga mystical practice.

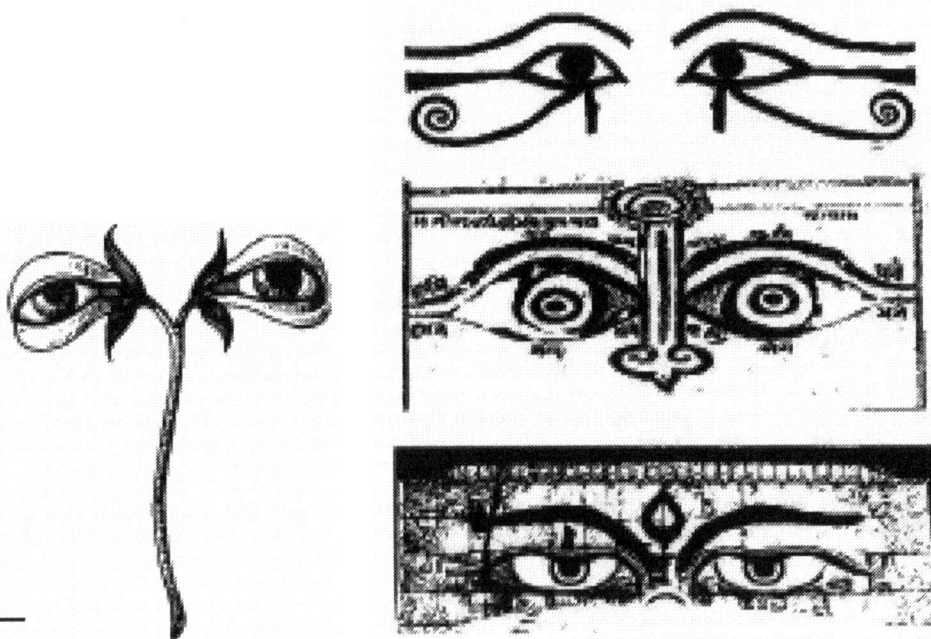

Left: The Eyes of God (Christian).
Top right: The Eyes of Heru (Egyptian).
Center right: The Eyes of Krishna (Indian).
Bottom right: The Eyes of Buddha (Indian).

Below left: A symbol of the Christian Trinity using the Fish.
Below center: The fish symbol used in Buddhism.
Below right: The Legendary fish symbol of the Ancient Egyptian tradition.

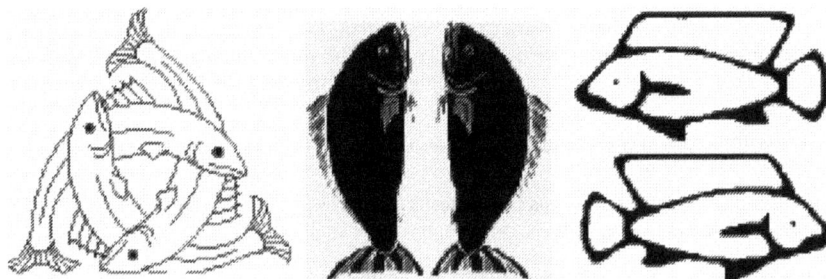

Secret Codes in the Bible?

Many followers of Jewish mysticism have advanced the idea that there is a special hidden code in the Bible, which if understood, contains prophecies about the future as well as special spiritual wisdom. To this end they say that each letter in the Bible corresponds to a number related to the Hebrew alphabet. These number combinations are said to provide the secret wisdom. Also, they promote the idea that hidden teachings can be discovered by looking for individual words throughout the text. Some people believe that by using a computer program to scan text blocks and pick out every 3rd, 7th, 10th letter, and so on a method called Equidistant Letter Sequences, ELS, they can discover phrases, words, and whole sentences from the Bible. Some of the words that can be found in the Bible seem to be amazing, like Princess Diana, Hitler, President Clinton, Holocaust, Auschwitz, etc. Other examples might be the words "tomorrow," "comes," "Armageddon." These words can certainly be found in this book (*Christian Yoga*) if it were to be scanned, but now the words are being taken out of context and any meaning can be applied. This process can also be done with the encyclopedia, a novel or a newspaper. What you find depends on how you adjust the letter count and what you're looking for. Using this system you can find just about anything you want! The proponents of this idea hold that this is a secret code which they can decipher and thereby lead people to spiritual enlightenment. In reality, they have created computer programs that they are selling and getting rich.

Using this method virtually any message can be derived from a large block of text. This kind of technique is baseless and should be abandoned at once. The most secure path to spiritual enlightenment is to study the teachings of an authentic spiritual preceptor and then to practice those teachings and thereby discover the supreme truth, which is hidden in your own heart.

THE MESSAGE OF RITUALS

A natural outgrowth of symbolism and mythology is ritual. In their original forms, early ritual systems, in relation to society, were directed to assisting the individual to learn about the specific group or culture in which he or she lived. These may be rites of passage rituals or rituals to mark the acceptance of a post in society. A modern day college graduation exercise is an example of a social ritual, but there are many others, which are used by society to manage or control individuals within society. An example of these might be mandatory retirement. More advanced rituals may serve the purpose of relating a person to society and to a tradition, such as patriotism and pride about one's country or one's group. This kind of feeling can be good for society in many ways, if it is based in righteousness. This means that people should care, not only for their own groups and communities, but for all people in the world. However, when this feeling is not based in truth and righteousness, it can be taken to extremes because people become so greedy or prejudiced about other groups and peoples that they develop animosity towards them, and feelings of hatred and violence emerge. Everything has a purpose and role, but if the purpose is not understood and managed by the wise, society will degenerate into the lower emotions, ignorance and negativity.

In their original forms, ancient religious rituals such as those from Ancient Egypt and India exhibit the advanced purpose of relating a human being not only to a spiritual tradition, but to the deepest mysteries of Creation as well. There are two forms of rituals. One seeks to promote psycho-spiritual transformation and the other seeks the fulfillment of worldly desires.

Throughout this volume we have introduced the idea that when Jesus said "I and the father are one" and "The Kingdom is within thee," he meant that God is within every human being and not just within himself alone. In the *Egyptian Book of Coming Forth By Day* and in the *Yoga Vasistha* from India, there are rituals directing the performer to feel, think and act like a particular deity, that deity being a symbol of the hidden, omnipresent, omniscient, transcendental power behind all things. The underlying theory of this form of spiritual practice is that in acting a certain way, one begins to feel that way as well, a concept, which is utilized in the field of psychotherapy for counseling patients. These rituals are directed to the transformation of the psychological makeup of the individual.

Then there are *Yajnas* or ritual sacrifices for the fulfillment of desire. These rituals are performed by those who want to achieve some end in the realm of time and space, the physical world. In any case, the *bhav*[50] or mental disposition or feeling is the most important factor in a ritual. Whenever you perform ordinary actions, you are creating mental impressions in your unconscious mind. If, for example, you went to a store for the first time and did not feel it was well stocked, you will hold that impression in your mind. When you think about that store, the impression will emerge to color your memory. These impressions are what determine a person's likes and dislikes as well as the circumstances a person leads themselves to experience. The negative impression about the store will push a person to avoid it in the future. This is just a simple example. The mind works in many more subtle ways, storing impressions over many lifetimes.

Many of your day-to-day activities are rituals. The feeling and purpose you attach to your actions determine the direction of the development of your consciousness either towards evolution or devolution, by causing an expansion (enlightenment) or contraction (karmic entanglement) of your consciousness. The feeling and purpose you attach to your actions also affects the new mental impressions (subconscious) you are gathering, which determine your waking reality and your future experiences. If you have to go someplace everyday as part of your job and you attach a positive feeling to it, you will be creating positive impressions related to your work. If society promotes rituals, which support negative feelings about something, those rituals will create negative impressions, which will have tremendous repercussions down the road. Therefore, it is clear that rituals are very important to every human being, but of particular importance to a spiritual aspirant because rituals can support positive ideals, spiritual principles, understanding and harmony. This is the highest purpose of rituals.

A popular ritual in ancient times referred to finding the *promised land* and/or *bathing in the sacred waters*. In Egypt, there was Kamit (Egypt) herself - the Black Land and the Nile River, in India, Benares and the Ganges River, in Biblical traditions there is Jerusalem and the Jordan River, in Persia, Damascus and the Euphrates River, etc. The crucial idea from each tradition is that there is a need to search for a new place where God has promised eternal peace, where people can feel that they belong. This feeling of belonging is not for the purpose of owning real estate, but for the purpose of having a viable place where spiritual practice may be performed without obstruction. The river represents the idea that it is necessary to cleanse oneself. Water, being a universal principal of inexhaustible life giving energy, is the cleanser of all things. It washes the land in the form of rain and allows plants to grow. In the form of a river it brings new sacred waters all the time so that people may bathe themselves and allow it to carry away their impurities. In modern times the household plumbing serves the purpose of the river, but people have seemingly forgotten where water comes from and their connection to it. The land and the river are two most important elements of spiritual practice. However, if the act of a ritual is to be performed physically, it must be accompanied with the meditation on the idea behind it. The Upanishads themselves speak about the negative consequence of performing rituals without correct understanding:

> Those who desire offspring and are devoted to alms giving and rituals, considering these the highest accomplishment, attain the world of the moon and are born again on earth.
>
> Prashna Upanishad

The world of the moon refers to that which is transient, a worldly goal. This is what most people pray for. An example of this is praying to win a lottery or a contest, to have a baby or to find a mate, etc. This kind of ritual leads to what is perishable and eventually a person who has gained all of the riches of the world has only gained perishable objects which must be given up at the time of death. However, the impressions gathered from chasing after objects and longing for them remain in the unconscious mind even after death, and cause a person to return again and again in the cycle of birth and death called reincarnation.

The *Yoga Vasistha* text makes the point clearer in the following passage:

> All virtuous deeds in the form of performance of sacrifices, visiting pilgrimage centers, austerities of various types, acts of charity and so forth, give rise to the pleasures of the senses alone. C.6: 24

The statement above alludes to the idea that external rituals benefit mostly the emotions and desires dictated by the ego. What is needed in the true practice of religious ritual is a desire to surpass the ego and to cleanse the mind of its desires in order that it may find peace and freedom, even from the pleasurable feelings generated by church-going. With higher philosophical insight, one learns that the true promised land, the true pilgrimage site, and the true sacred river are all to be found within oneself. Deeper mythical and mystical understanding enable us to make any location into a "sacred" place. A local river or even a small apartment can become our own "sacred river" and "promised land." At even a higher level of thought, the idea of the land can be understood as the "mental landscape" and the river as "the stream of thoughts" in our minds. We need not travel to Egypt, Jerusalem, Mecca or Benares to obtain the highest blessing of spiritual experience. In reality, this can only come from within.

Thus, for the advanced aspirant, taking a physical bath in a distant, sacred river or visiting historical sites or temples found in a specific geographic location on earth are not at all necessary. In fact, this concretization of the idea behind the ritual could be considered an idolatrous and dualistic interpretation of the ritual which could lead to further mental illusions and subconscious impressions of separation from God.[37/58] Out of the thousands of people who visit spiritual centers around the world, how many experience a profound enough transformation to attain Sainthood or Sagehood?

However, in the beginning stages of spiritual development, it is helpful to visit sites, temples or churches, which will help to direct the mind towards the Divine. Likewise, spiritual images, symbols and icons are useful in directing the mind towards spiritual teachings and in facilitating the remembrance of one's spiritual goals. This is the idea behind the atmosphere of the church or temple. When you walk inside you should feel that you have been transported away from the world of time and space and human situations into a meditative state of mind. Therefore, if possible your own environment should be as conducive as possible to lead you to have harmonious feelings, and it should put you in tune with the spiritual philosophy you have chosen.

YOGA, CHRISTIANITY, REINCARNATION AND TRANSPERSONAL PSYCHOLOGY

The essence of what is presently considered to be a new field of psychological thought, Transpersonal Psychology, has appeared throughout recorded history in the mystical writings of the philosophers of Ancient Egypt, Greece, and other countries as well. Nowhere, however, has it received more extensive literary exposition than in the religious and philosophical schools of the East. The spiritual practice of India in particular, having enjoyed an unbroken tradition for over 3,000 years, is yet an undiscovered treasure of psychological understanding and experience. Carl Jung, the eminent Western psychiatrist, remarked that the West is far behind the East in the understanding of the psyche. The advent of the "New Age" movement in modern society, coupled with the availability of foreign ideas due to modern technology and mass communications has allowed a renaissance, as it were, to occur in Western thinking about human psychology and the understanding of consciousness itself. Modern Western science is confirming many ancient mystical ideas, thereby expanding the understanding about the universe outside of us as well as within.

Modern practitioners of Western psychology have performed extensive research with respect to theories and therapies during the last one hundred years since the emergence of Western psychology as a scientific discipline with Sigmund Freud. In contrast, the psychology of the East has remained relatively unchanged for over 2,000 years in the form of Yoga disciplines which are essentially programs which promote the natural psychological transformation which every human being must undergo. But what is the nature of this transformation? What are we transforming into and for what purpose? According to Western Philosophy, psychology is for making the abnormal mind normal, again using society's standards of normalcy. This means that people, who are occasionally angry, elated, depressed, jealous, hateful, etc. are considered to be normal by society. Those who cannot function in a society, which is full of violence, greed and cruelty, are looked upon as too sensitive or as neurotic. However, the goal of Yoga is to make a "normal" mind supernormal by eradicating its negative aspects (anger, hatred, greed, depression, jealousy, etc.).

The term "Yoga," and the disciplines and practices related to it have been associated with various Eastern, African and Western religions throughout human history. Yoga is essentially a nondenominational, nonsectarian philosophy and psychological discipline for self-improvement. As stated earlier, the literal meaning of the word Yoga is to *"Yoke"* or to *"Link"* back. The term "Yoga" may be understood as the process which unifies individual and Cosmic Consciousness, God, but it should also be understood as the actual attainment of the transcendental state of union itself as well. The implication is: to link individual consciousness back to the original source, the original essence, that which transcends all mental and intellectual attempts at comprehension, but which is the essential nature of everything in Creation. Any practice, which assists a person in realizing her/his true Self, is known as Yoga.

Many disciplines have been evolved to affect a profound change in those who wish to discover the true nature of their being. While there are several systems of philosophy and several religions, it is also true that there are certain common spiritual principles to which they all adhere. These are the yogic disciplines. Most of these disciplines have been developed as physical, mental, and emotional exercises to turn the mind away from the illusion of the phenomenal world and allow it to discover the truth behind it. As previously discussed, there are four major forms of Yoga practice, and from these several minor forms branch off. The four main forms are the Yoga of Devotion, Yoga of Wisdom, Yoga of Meditation and Yoga of Action.

The predominant form of Yoga practiced in Orthodox Christianity is a limited form of Devotion, while the predominant form of Yoga practice in Gnostic Christianity is a combination of Gnosis or Intuitional Wisdom and Devotion. Orthodox Christianity is limited because it takes a person only part way in the realization of the objective of devotion in spiritual practice. Orthodoxy admonishes a person to love Jesus and God, and to follow their example. Gnostic Christianity not only admonishes a person to love Jesus and God and follow their example, but also leads a person to allow that devotion to reach full expression. This means that a true devotee unites with the beloved and thereby becomes one with the beloved. This is the true meaning of Jesus' statements "I and The Father are One" and "Know ye not that ye are gods." The Orthodox Church would consider it blasphemous for a Christian to say "I am God," but Yoga would consider any statement to the contrary as blasphemy and a reinforcement of spiritual ignorance.

The Science of Yoga constitutes the teachings required to achieve perfection in consciousness, which is the innate potential of every human being through conscious self-effort. However, there are two ways in which Yoga may occur. The first is the path of nature. Nature herself offers one path to perfection. This path requires learning through mistakes and suffering over countless incarnations in a seemingly endless cycle of births and deaths, first in the process of becoming a better human being (free from vices), then transcending one's egoistic human nature (spiritually). The path of nature is the process of trial and error, pain and elation, adversity and prosperity—like a never-ending roller coaster ride. It is arduous and requires many thousands and perhaps millions of reincarnations. Therefore, the path of nature is to be avoided if possible.

This path is likened to the *Passion* of Jesus and Asar as symbolized by their deaths. Few people are aware of the fact that early Christianity accepted the teaching of reincarnation fully, and even fewer people are aware of the fact that the Bible also accepted reincarnation up to the seventeenth century A.C.E., when it was edited out by the church authorities. The Bible still contains references to reincarnation. In Mark 8, Jesus is believed to be an incarnation of John the Baptist or of Elijah.

Mark 8
27. And Jesus went out, and his disciples, into the towns of Caesarea Philippi: and by the way he asked his disciples, saying to them, Who do men say that I am?
28 And they answered, John the Baptist: but some [say], Elijah; and others, One of the prophets.
29 And he saith to them, But who say ye that I am? And Peter answereth and saith to him, Thou art the Christ.
30 And he charged them that they should tell no man of him.

The passage above shows the remnants of the teachings of reincarnation in the modern Bible. The fact that Jesus' disciples asked him if he was one of the sages who had passed on (***John the Baptist: but some [say], Elijah; and others, One of the prophets***) shows that reincarnation was not only part of the culture of Christianity at the time, but that it was so strong as to make it into the Roman Catholic version. This is extremely important because the historical evidence shows that the Orthodox Catholics tried to excise all traces of Gnostic Christianity. It may also have been left in as a hint for those who are inclined to understand the concept of reincarnation, but since the church publicly repudiates this teaching, why did they allow it to remain in the cannon? The church leadership preferred the concept of a single life and a single death for its simplicity, but simple or not, the concept cannot be used if it is inconsistent with reality. Consequently, people in modern society have come to fear death. The modern field of parapsychology has discovered evidence to prove that reincarnation does occur. Therefore, we must take a new look at the Christian teachings from an expanded point of view, taking into account the vast span of time that the human soul experiences human existence.

THE PURPOSE OF MENTAL CONCEPTS IN SPIRITUAL STUDY

What does it mean when the mystical teachings speak of going *beyond all mental concepts* or *transcending the world and ordinary human consciousness?* These statements refer to the fact that everything that is "known" by the mind is a concept. Think about it. You do not really know anything about the world outside of the mind and senses, which bring you information about the world. This information is based on some frame of reference, which you have developed in your life. Nothing can be known without being compared to something you already previously knew, and therefore, you cannot know anything through your mind for which you do not already have a frame of reference. Modern society has learned to conceptualize the nature of matter based on the concept of atoms and electrons. However, if the masses of people would inquire further, as modern physicists have done, they would discover that atoms and electrons don't really exist. They are composed of smaller particles, and these in turn are composed of what modern physics calls "energy." But what is energy composed of? It is Consciousness, God, itself in the dynamic aspect, the divine creative *Word* that has come into being as matter with form, texture, volume, etc.

The concept of human individuality is also illusory because individuality means indivisible. While human beings seem to have one body, their minds are in constant duality, thinking divergent thoughts, trying to make decisions between two or more different things, etc. True individuality would mean being single and independent in all areas, a singularity of mind, body and spirit. However, the ordinary person has grown up to think of her/himself in a dualistic manner and therefore, considers him/herself to be a separate unit among many distinct human personalities and physical objects. As a result of this incorrect basis of understanding, one of the most powerful and erroneous concepts that have become engrained in people's minds is that the desires of the mind need to be satisfied by pursuing objects (including people) and situations in the world of human experience. Even though the satisfaction attained by acquiring objects and engaging in human relationships is fleeting, most people have become convinced that this is the best or the only way to find happiness in life.

This understanding is in complete contradiction with the teachings of Yoga as well as those of modern physics. While all things seem separate and unconnected, there is an underlying reality of the universe, which supports all of the apparent multiplicity. To discover this truth, one must re-train the mind to discard the concepts by which it has learned to label "things" in nature. This truth can only be discovered by studying, reflecting, practicing and meditating upon the teachings of Yoga.

When the mind is retrained so that erroneous concepts no longer distract it from the truth, then the truth is revealed as an ever-present reality. Happiness and true fulfillment CANNOT and DO NOT come from objects, relationships or any activity you can perform or any achievement you can reach. They can only reflect it in small quantities and for short periods of time, because they are not the true source. Physical objects, including the human body, are limited and temporary expressions of the Divine. Therefore, they have some potential to allow us to experience happiness. However, the experience is an internal one, based on our mental conditioning. Otherwise there would be some universal object, which could bring happiness to everyone, and there is no such object in existence. In addition, all worldly attainments are perishable in the end. Therefore, a wise person turns away from the folly of looking to the world for happiness and turns to the wise for help in ending the illusion or "disease" from which the mind is suffering: ignorance of one's essential Divine nature.

It must be understood that Enlightenment itself is not a concept. It is not an opinion or a view held about the world. Enlightenment is not dependent on a person's ability to debate or sustain good arguments to convince others of its existence. It cannot be attained by simply stopping the thoughts in the mind or by being extremely virtuous nor can it be achieved through any other kind of extreme, be it good or bad. It cannot be achieved by amassing voluminous works of wisdom or through intellectual prowess. A supreme sense of peace and a feeling of all-pervasiveness and unity with all things characterize it. Enlightenment is revealed as an ever present and transcendental reality, a fact, which becomes obvious once the mind is able to transcend the concepts, which agitate the mental substance and cloud it with misunderstanding.

All of the disciplines employed in the practice of Yoga are necessary to promote physical and mental health. There must be an atmosphere of peace, serenity and a profound understanding of the nature of the Self, within as well as without (in the outside world). Therefore, even the teachings of yoga must be transcended in order to attain the glorious experience of Gnosis (Enlightenment). Thus, Yoga, in its true practice, is not a philosophy in the strict sense of the word because a philosophy is a point of view, which is supported by argument. Yoga is a spiritual discipline which allows a human being to transcend ordinary human consciousness, the realm of concepts, and to attain the realm which is Absolute, beyond duality.

THE IDEA OF CHRISTHOOD

The word *"Christ"* is not a name but a title, like Vice-President. *"Christ"* means: *"He or she whose head is anointed with oil"* or simply *"The Anointed One."* In ancient times the holy oil used for anointing was called *Chrism* (Christos) in Greek. The Anointed One was a title of many Middle Eastern and African gods. Among these were Asar, Tammuz, Adonis and Attis. Heru, Sage, Saint, Buddha, Christ, Krishna, etc., are terms or names to describe the same thing. In some cults and tantric traditions, the sacrificial God's erect penis was anointed for easier penetration by his Goddess. In others the sacrificed hero was anointed for the marriage with the earth. Of course, this sexual union is metaphorical, referring to the coming together of individual consciousness and universal consciousness, even though it is acted out in rituals.

With this expanded understanding, the purpose of the anointing of Jesus becomes clearer. Jesus was anointed before his passion (Mark 14:8) as well as after (Mark 16). Both times he was anointed by women, first by a female follower and then by Mary Magdalene, his mother and his other female disciples. The anointing represents the ecstasy and glory of spiritual expansion.

Mark 14

8 She hath done what she could: she is come beforehand to anoint my body for the burial.

Mark 16

1. And when the Sabbath was past, Mary Magdalene, and Mary the [mother] of James, and Salome, had bought sweet spices, that they might come and anoint him.
2 And very early in the morning of the first [day] of the week, they came to the sepulchre at the rising of the sun.

The ritual of anointing was pictorially depicted in the Ancient Egyptian *Books of Coming Forth By Day* at the stage when the initiate would reach the inner shrine, which signified coming face to face with God. This anointing was symbolized by the change into gleaming vestments and the *"grease cone"* on his head ("A" below). In much the same way as the term Christ refers to anyone who has attained "Christhood," the term Buddha refers to any one who has attained the state of enlightenment. In this context there have been many male and female Christs and Buddhas throughout history.

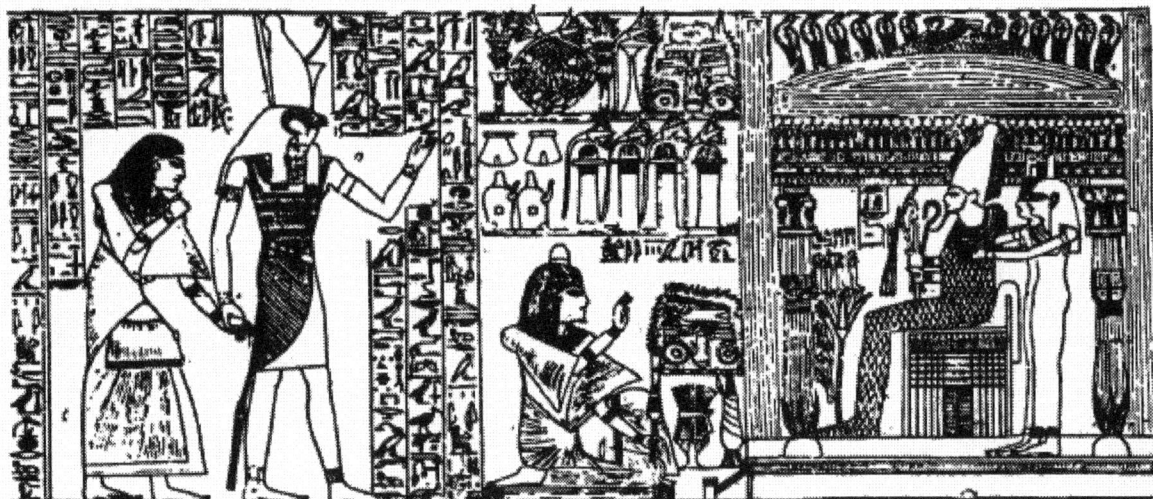

The Anointing of Asar Ani
From Ancient Egyptian *The Book of Coming Forth By Day* of Ani

Among the Essenes, the priest was also known as *Christos*, the Redeemer or Sin Bearer. Among such early Christian cults, women were known to lead worship services. Therefore, there also were female Christs. Names such as Heru or Christ refer to certain qualities exhibited by mythological or historical personalities as symbols representing the potential state of Enlightenment of every sentient being in the universe.

In psycho-mythological terms, Christs are those persons who have attained complete purification of their psychological personality. They experience Cosmic Consciousness, the experience of being one (identifying oneself) with everything in the cosmos. This is a state of supreme bliss that comes from becoming one with one's essential nature: God. This is a state which cannot be achieved through earthly pleasures or relationships, although earthly existence allows one the possibility of achieving Cosmic Consciousness by giving one the opportunity to evolve one's mind through experiences, challenges, suffering and struggle.

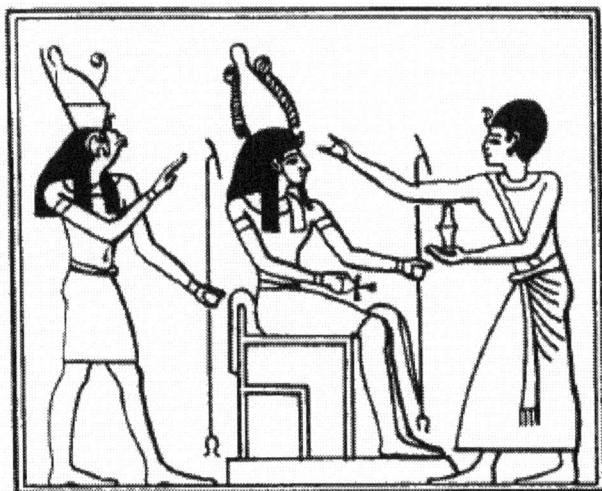

The anointing
of Asar in
Ancient
Egypt.

When Cosmic Consciousness is attained, an anointing occurs with an etheric oil, secreted from the energy centers (Chakras) into the brain and the body's circulatory system including the heart, the mystical seat of the soul. The body and mind are transcended and one experiences a higher level of existence beyond the joys and sorrows of the world. Christhood means to attain the beatific vision of oneself as God. One becomes consciously established in the realization that one IS God. This is in contrast to the masses of people who believe themselves to be only a perishable body of flesh and bones.

In psychological terms, the Son of man is the person on the path of spirituality, the seeker who knows of but has not yet realized the Kingdom in full consciousness. In terms of Yoga philosophy, the *wicked one* would be considered one's own negative mental qualities (karmas) which impede one from pursuing virtuous actions. We ourselves have sown these negative qualities through our indulgence in the world of sensual pleasures and desires. Our soul is driven by the constant pursuit of satisfaction through physical means, which in turn reinforces our belief that we are separate from the Kingdom. What is required is that we develop a discriminating intellect in order to separate that which is good (knowledge of the Kingdom), that which is real (virtue, peace, dispassion, detachment) from that which is unreal and leads to pain and suffering (illusions worry, hate, greed, anger, etc.).

In previous sections, we introduced the controversy over Jesus' humanity. You will recall that in the developing period of the Christian Church there were debates, which sought to determine the nature of Christ (Christology). Some claimed that he was human and Divine and others that he was a man, etc. The passage from Mark 14 gives us an idea why this debate ensued. Just before Jesus was to be taken prisoner and executed, he prayed to God and asked if this passion which he was fated to experience could be prevented, or if it was possible that he could be excused from going through it.

Mark 14
   35 And he went forward a little, and fell on the ground, and prayed that, if it were possible, the hour might pass from him.
   36 And he said, Abba, Father, all things [are] possible to thee, take away this cup from me: nevertheless not what I will, but what thou wilt.

Jesus asks what he wants but in the end surrenders his will to the Divine will. He did feel the fear of what was to come and he later felt the pain of the torture and suffering onto death. So he felt as a human being, but what made him Divine? The difference between Jesus Christ and an ordinary person is that he worked for the good of all and surrendered his will, his ego, to the Divine will. While feeling the sentiments of a human being he also experienced the glory of the Divine and this is what carried him through the ordeal.

If Jesus was supposed to be an enlightened being, beyond ordinary human egoism and experiencing Christ Consciousness, then why would he be feeling and suffering as a human being? A similar story occurs in Hinduism and sheds light on this question. In the myths related to the god Krishna, he was once battling a demon that possessed the power of illusion. This demon projected an image in Krishna's mind of Krishna's father dying. For a brief period Krishna became sorrowful until he realized that this was an illusion. Krishna is the Hindu exemplar of enlightened consciousness, so why was he also susceptible to human emotion?

The scriptures are giving an important simile to gain insight into the ideal state of enlightenment. While there is experience of the transcendental, there remains a level of contact with the phenomenal world of time and space. Otherwise, how would it be possible for Sages to interact with human beings? Enlightened beings interact and are aware of human emotions, but they experience these in a different way than ordinary human beings. They are detached from their emotions and therefore remain clear of inner delusion and grief. While a Sage may appear to be suffering on the outside, he or she is not really suffering deep down. Their ability to feel the human predicament allows them to sympathize and commiserate with others and serve humanity in a real way. They serve not just with instructions from afar, but by working with people and showing them by their own example how to live in happiness, sorrow, pain, birth and death.

SELF-KNOWLEDGE AND THE BAPTISM OF TRUTH

The Gnostic text, *Testimony of Truth*, makes patently clear to us the true source of authority on spiritual matters. It is the acquisition of *"self knowledge"* within the individual that leads to salvation. It is a transformation, which occurs within the psyche of the aspirant. A person cannot expect eternal life merely by being baptized or by studying wisdom texts. The author of the *Testimony of Truth* rejects all the marks of ecclesiastical[1] authority. He states that

---
[1] Of or pertaining to a church, especially as an organized institution

faith in the Catholic sacraments shows a naive and a magical form of thinking. He explains that Catholic Christians are practicing baptism as a kind of initiation rite which will guarantee them *"a hope of salvation,"* further, they believe that only those who are able to receive baptism are *"headed for life."*[18]

If the logic of the church with respect to the resurrection is examined, the point brought up by the *Testimony of Truth* becomes evident. The ecclesiastical doctrine of resurrection asserts that at the end of time, all faithful souls will be resurrected from their graves. This means that the decayed, worm-eaten flesh will be somehow miraculously reconstituted or that those whose bodies died so long ago and have turned back into dust will magically come back to life again. It is a wonder that modern Christians believe in this doctrine but refuse to consider the Gnostic teachings such as reincarnation. This doctrine also implies that people of other faiths are headed straight for hell. What does all this say about God? Does this mean that God plays favorites? Does this mean that God created a world of misery where some people can be saved and others are doomed to hell and damnation? This would mean that the world is imperfect and that God has no compassion. Further, it would mean that God is capricious and takes pleasure in human suffering.

The *Gospel of Truth* rejects the Catholic "lie" that baptism is a guarantee of salvation, asserting that the true testimony comes only when a man *knows himself* and God who is the truth. Only then will he be saved. One must experience Enlightenment as a new life and new consciousness. This is the real meaning of *"resurrection."* In much the same way as Advaita Vedanta and Buddhism proclaim that Enlightenment is an inner-psychological experience that cannot be accomplished through outward ritualism, the *Gospel of Truth* proclaims that physical rituals such as baptism, etc., are irrelevant since:

"The baptism of truth" is something else; it is by renunciation of the world that it is found."[96]

Below: Jesus being baptized (Initiated) by John the Baptist.

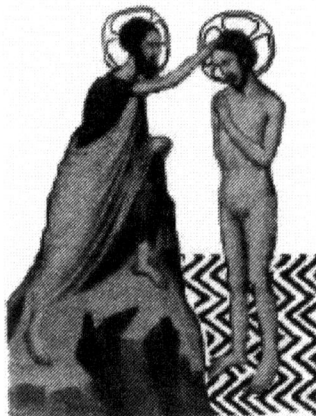

The previous text from the *Testimony of Truth* includes some very important themes which merit further elucidation and may be used as a basis to directly compare Gnostic Christianity to other philosophies. Specifically, these themes are (A)- *Knowing Oneself* and (B)- *Renunciation of the world.* These are paths to discover the ultimate truth of existence. Both of these themes are strong elements in Ancient Egyptian mythology, Hermeticism, which developed out of it, as well as in Vedanta philosophy in India where monks or renunciates are called *sanyasis.* It should be noted here that Christian monasticism, a discipline dedicated to profound introspection and renunciation, first began in Egypt and Asia Minor around 200-350 A.C.E.[75]

In the following statement from the *Gospel of Thomas* we also find an emphasis on the need for the practice of renunciation.

114. Jesus says: "He who has found the world and become rich, let him renounce the world!"

Many forms of renunciation emerged through the millennia of time. When understood as a purely physical discipline, aspirants strive to keep a physical distance from objects and people which can disturb their minds and distract them from their spiritual practice. At advanced levels, the practice of renunciation takes on completely new dimensions. Psychological resurrection is given more emphasis than physical resurrection. Buddhism was one of the first disciplines, in the Indian tradition, to emphasize that psychological renunciation is more important than physical renunciation. This idea gave rise to other theories in certain sects, which held that since *samsara* [1] *is equal to Nirvana* (Enlightenment), *bhoga* (worldly enjoyment) *is the same as Yoga.* The idea that the world process *(samsara)* is equal to Enlightenment *(Nirvana)* occurs in Christian philosophy where Jesus states that *"The Kingdom of the Father is spread upon the earth and men do not see it!"* Where some of the orthodox eastern theologians erred, was in equating worldly enjoyment and pleasure *(bhoga),* without the benefit of any form of spiritual discipline or philosophy, to a process of transcendence of the illusion of the world (Yoga). When *bhoga* is engaged in without the benefit of spiritual knowledge (gnosis), it has the effect of intensifying the illusions of the mind and the power of the personal ego. Further, even when a spiritual aspirant engages in enjoyments of the world, there is a danger. Enjoyments can become enslaving if he/she has fooled themselves into believing they are detached from the activity while, in reality, they are unknowingly reinforcing worldly mental impressions. This process is described in later forms of *Advaita Vedanta* (non-dualistic Vedanta philosophy) as espoused in the *Yoga Vasistha:*

---

[1] The transient, phenomenal world of time and space.

Yoga Vasistha 6:29

"When cravings increase, the disease of the world process (illusion) is intensified. When cravings are gradually destroyed, the disease of the world process begins to wane. Therefore, renounce all cravings of the mind and remain a detached witness to all of the functions of the mind and senses."

Yoga Vasistha 6:50:

"By thinking of the objects of the world and by entertaining desires for the pleasures of the senses, the mind becomes increasingly involved in the world-process. This is called fattening of the mind. By considering the body as the Self, and by developing attachment towards one's wife and children, and towards the objects of the world, the mind becomes fattened."

In order to correct the misunderstanding between enjoyment and renunciation, the concept of *bhoga tyaga* was introduced. *Tyaga* means renunciation, therefore, the discipline means to renounce enjoyment and pleasure. Renunciation is not to be understood as a discipline of deprivation and self-denial. The subtlety of engaging in worldly enjoyments must be well understood by an aspirant who wishes to practice Yoga at the same time as participating in the world. *Bhoga tyaga* requires that whenever one experiences worldly pleasure or enjoyment (happiness), they should be attributed to the Self within, rather than to worldly objects. Since the objects of the world do not hold happiness or pleasure in and of themselves, it must be understood that it is our deepest consciousness, which produces a feeling of enjoyment in the mind, and the source of this consciousness is the transcendental Self. Therefore, we should attribute any enjoyments we may perceive to that deeper Self which is within us. This philosophy is known as renunciation of worldly enjoyments. Once the art of renouncing worldly enjoyments is learned, a person will not be trapped by the illusory pleasures of human existence.

Some of the Gnostic sects of early Christianity practiced orgiastic rituals in much the same way as the Indian *Tantrists* do even today. They attributed the orgasmic flow of energy to God, the light within us, while considering excrement as that which is impure. Hence, they performed elaborate purification rituals and ate special diets as part of the discipline. This discipline is of a very advanced nature. It may be understood as an extension of the yogic discipline of seeing God (the Kingdom of Heaven) in all things. The key lies with the spiritual sensitivity of the disciple, his/her level of mental awareness and self-control. If misunderstood, this philosophy of *Tantrism* can be degraded into a gross form of debauchery, an egoistic excuse to satisfy the lower desires in the erroneous title as Sex Yoga, as it has come to be misunderstood in some New Age circles of modern times.

The entire text of Chapter 5 of the *Bhagavad Gita* is devoted to the practice of renunciation.

"ab"
Ancient Egyptian Hieroglyph meaning cleansed, purified, washed.

Before entering the temple the Ancient Egyptian priests would wash in the sacred pool of the temple.

10. He who performs actions by invoking *Brahman* (God) and by renouncing attachment to the fruit of action, is not touched by sin, even as a lotus leaf remains untouched by water.

11. A Yogi (practitioner of the Yoga of action) continues to perform actions merely with his body, mind, intellect and senses. He performs actions without attachment and out of the purity of his heart.

12. One who is devoted to Yoga (Karma Yoga) attains peace by renouncing the fruits of action. But one who is not united with Karma Yoga is impelled by desires, attached to the fruits of action, and therefore, goes to bondage.

Compare the previous statement with the following passages from Ancient Egyptian mythology:

"Know thyself as the pride of creation, the link uniting divinity and matter; behold a part of God Itself within thee; remember thine own dignity nor dare descend to evil or meanness.[63]

"To Know God, strive to grow in stature beyond all measure. Conceive that there is nothing beyond thy capability. Know thyself deathless and able to know all things, all arts, sciences, the way of every life. Become higher than the highest height and lower than the lowest depth. Amass in thyself all senses of animals, fire, water, dryness and moistness. Think of thyself in all places at the same time, earth, sea, sky, not yet born, in the womb, young, old, dead, and in the after death state.[63]

"I am the Mind - the Eternal Teacher. I am the begetter of the Word - the Redeemer of all humankind - and in the nature of the wise, the Word takes flesh. By means of the Word, the world is saved. I, Thought - the begetter of the Word, the Mind - come only unto they that are holy, good, pure and merciful, and that live piously and religiously, and my presence is an inspiration and a help to them, for when I come, they immediately know all things and adore the Universal Spirit. Before such wise and philosophic ones die, they learn to renounce their senses, knowing that these are the enemies of their immortal Souls.[63]

Those who have learned to know themselves, have reached that state which does transcend any abundance of physical existence; but they who through a love that leads astray, expend their love upon their body, they stay in darkness, wandering and suffering through their senses, things of anxiety, unrest and Death.[63]

"A soul, when from the body freed, if it has fought the fight of piety (between good and evil)-to Know God and to do wrong to no one, such a soul becomes entirely pure, whereas the impious soul remains as it is, a slave to its passions, chastised through death, by its own self.[63]

In Chapter 26, utterances 7-9 of the *Egyptian Book of Coming Forth by Day*, once the initiates know they have gained control (power) over their heart (mind), when they *"know their heart,"* then they will *"not lose consciousness"* as an ordinary person would at the time of the death of the physical body. Rather, they will retain the power to go in and out of the spirit world according to the desire of the spirit. Also, an initiate will not suffer through reincarnation, but will live on in the spirit form because he/she is well-established (enlightened) in the spirit rather than the body-consciousness:

"I know my Heart, I have achieved power over it, I have achieved the power to do what pleases my Ka (spirit), I will remain aware in my Ab (heart), my Ba (soul) will not be fettered or restrained at the entrance of the west, I will be able to come and go as I please."

The importance of purifying or *"washing the heart"* appears throughout the entire *Book of Coming Forth by Day*. Washing before entering a temple was a long-standing spiritual ritual, as previously discussed. It was a precursor to the Christian baptism. However, the washing of the heart has deeper implications. Washing the heart means that the heart is relieved of sentimental attachments and feelings, be they feelings of joy, happiness, anger or sorrow. Developing dispassion is also a classic tenet of Indian Vedanta and Buddhist philosophies. In Ancient Egyptian mythology and philosophy, the symbol for cleansing or purifying the heart (mind) is composed of a leg and/or human figure (sometimes beside the symbol for water) over which a jug of water is poured. Also, outside of all of the Ancient Egyptian temples there was a "sacred pool" that symbolized the primeval waters of creation. It was customary to bathe in the pool prior to entering the temple to perform the rituals of the faith. Some of the pools had sculptures of *Khepri* within them. Khepri is the Ancient Egyptian god Ra in the form of the morning sun, the Creator of the universe. So the cleansing also symbolizes the renewal of life, a new spiritual awakening, just as Khepri rises and creates a new day. Washing the heart is called *"ab."*

Chapter 1- utterance-24: *"I am the ab* (cleansed-washed one) *in Tettetu"* (stability, establishment in the Divine Self, see Djed pillar).
Chapter 81- utterance 1: The initiate states: *"I am the ab* (pure-washed one) *coming forth from the fields."*

The following quotes from the Bible, while somewhat cryptic in reference to the practice of curtailing one's worldly activities, may be better understood when compared to the Gnostic Christian, Indian and Ancient Egyptian texts below.

Matthew 5
29 And if thy right eye shall cause thee to sin, pluck it out, and cast [it] from thee: for it is profitable for thee that one of thy members should perish, and not [that] thy whole body should be cast into hell {offend... or, do cause thee to offend}.
30 And if thy right hand shall cause thee to sin, cut it off, and cast [it] from thee: for it is profitable for thee that one of thy members should perish, and not [that] thy whole body should be cast into hell.

Mark 9
45 And if thy foot causeth thee to fall into sin, cut it off: it is better for thee to enter lame into life, than having two feet to be cast into hell, into the fire that never shall be quenched. {offend... or, cause thee to offend}
46 Where their worm dieth not and the fire is not quenched.
47 And if thy eye causeth thee to fall into sin pluck it out; it is better for thee to enter into the Kingdom of God with one eye, than having two eyes to be cast into hell fire. {offend... or, cause thee to offend}.

The Gospel of Thomas:
32. If you do not fast from the world, you will not find the Kingdom. If you do not make the Sabbath the {true} Sabbath, you will not see the Father.

In Matthew 5:29-30 the aspirant is expected to cut out all activities which lead to indulgence in the senses and draw him or her away from the Divine. The reference in *The Gospel of Thomas* (32) above refers to engaging in a more profound spiritual practice during the Sabbath than simply taking time off from work or spending a few hours of the day praying or reading prescribed texts. Rather, this reference requires intense forms of what would today be called concentration and meditation upon God, while at the same time withdrawing one's attention from any concerns or worries about the world. This form of spiritual practice can be achieved through the control of the wandering senses by practicing concentration and meditation exercises. The *Gita* provides extensive instruction as to the necessity for and procedures to achieve control of the senses.

Bhagavad Gita Chapter 2

58. When he is able to withdraw his senses from the sense-objects, even like a tortoise that withdraws its limbs from all sides, he is then established in wisdom.

59. When the personality is not fed with sense objects, the objects turn away from him, but their taste continues to linger in his mind; but, even this taste turns away from him when the Supreme Self is realized.

60. O Son of Kunti, the turbulent senses carry away violently the mind of even a wise man who is striving to control them.

61. Having controlled his senses and having collected his mind with one-pointed devotion to Me, he should sit steadfast in the Self; for one whose senses are under control, his wisdom becomes steady.

62. By constantly dwelling upon objects, one develops attachment to them; from attachment there arises desire, from desire there is born anger.

64. But the self-controlled Sage, though moving among the sense-objects, with his senses restrained and free from attachment and hatred, goes to Peace.

65. In that peace of the mind all sorrows are brought to their cessation, because the intellect of the Sage, whose mind is full of bliss, becomes established in Brahman.

66. There is no intuitive intellect for one who is not united with the Higher Self, and there is no meditative movement in the unsteady mind; and to the un-meditative there is no peace. How can there be happiness to one who is without peace?

67. Whatever wandering sense the mind follows after, it (the sense) robs the mind of its intuitive vision, just as the wind carries away a boat on the waters.

68. Therefore, O Mighty Armed Arjuna, one whose senses are completely restrained from the sense-objects, his intuitive wisdom is firmly established.

70. Just as waters from different rivers enter into the ocean from all sides, and yet the ocean continues to be immutable, in the same way he in whom all desires enter without affecting him, he alone attains peace, not the desirer of sense-objects.

From the teachings of Hermes:

"To free the spirit, control the senses; the reward will be a clear insight."

"Something is added to thee unlike to what thou seest; something animates thy clay higher than all that is the object of thy senses. Behold, what is it? Thy body remaineth perfect matter after It is fled, therefore It is no part of it; It is immaterial, therefore It is accountable for its actions."

"Knowledge derived from the senses is illusionary, true knowledge can only come from the understanding of the union of opposites."

"The senses give the meaning from a worldly point of view; see with the Spirit and the true meaning will be revealed. This is the relationship between the object and its Creator, it's true meaning."

"Before such wise and philosophic ones die, they learn to renounce their senses, knowing that these are the enemies of their immortal Souls."

"To free the spirit, control the senses; the reward will be a clear insight."

WHAT IS CONSCIOUSNESS?

Consciousness is the primordial state of existence. In Ancient Egyptian and Indian mythology, as well as in Christian mythology, Pure Consciousness or the *Primeval Water*s are considered to be *Unformed Matter, The Self, God,* before creation took place. Pure Consciousness is the stuff of which everything, including thoughts, are composed. In the same way that modern physics has discovered the same basis behind all matter (energy), the Sages of ancient times discovered that there is one underlying substance which underlies all Creation. *Pure Consciousness* is behind all things, matter, thoughts, energy, etc. The "Primeval Waters" is a symbol of Pure Consciousness, unmodified or unconditioned into any particular form or another.

Think of clay for a moment. Clay has no particular form, but when the artist gives it shape and a name it is recognized as a pot or a bowl, etc. Through the process of thought, Consciousness is able to become whatever it desires, that is, to take on any form by the power of vibration. Vibration causes ripples in Consciousness and these ripples are what constitute movement, shape, color, dimension, sound, light, etc. This is the meaning of the teaching in Genesis, which speaks of God as hovering or blowing air on the waters in order to stir them up.

In the primordial state there is only the Self, Pure Consciousness, without even a thought about anything other than itself. Upon the emergence of the first thought, immediately there is something besides the Self, an objectified form, the experience of duality and of the triad: seer-seen-sight or subject-object-interacting media. However, it is only through illusion that the Self is able to see anything as if it is other than itself. It is the conditioned mind that allows the illusion of the triad to exist. However, this objectified form is composed of the same Self.

Think once again about your dream state of consciousness. When you dream you are creating an entire world which seems to be separate from yourself, but in reality it is all within you. The universe is all within the Self, God, in the same way. The material out of which dreams and waking consciousness arise is the same. Sages have discovered that Pure Consciousness is the underlying basis of the human mind, but when thoughts arise, Consciousness takes and identifies with the various forms.

From a mystical standpoint, when Creation occurs, God is said to have created him/herself in the form of that which is created, in the same way that the consciousness of a dreaming person takes on the forms of the dream. When Consciousness becomes something, anything, from the grossest form to the subtlest—a tree, a rock, a planet, a human body, air, radiation, etc.—then it is said to have created a physical object; creation is created. This process is described in the book of Genesis in the Bible.

Genesis 1:1-2

1 In the beginning, God created heaven and earth.
2 And the earth was without form, and void; and darkness [was] upon the face of the deep. And the Spirit of God moved upon the face of the waters.

Romans 8:9

9 But ye are not in the flesh, but in the Spirit, if the Spirit of God dwelleth in you. Now if any man hath not the Spirit of Christ, he is not his.

In the two verses above from the Bible we are to understand that the Spirit of God is the same Spirit who is responsible for Creation and at the same time also responsible for human existence. When a human being lives consciously in this awareness, the Spirit is of Christ. Thus, we are to understand also that God is the subtlest of all matter, who underlies all and is within all things. When the Spirit objectifies itself as gross matter, the Spirit no longer simply just exists in complete peace and stillness. When the Self enlivens a physical object such as an animal, a plant, or a human body with the soul (higher consciousness), then that object is said to be "living." When the Self becomes involved with the thoughts and forgets itself, thinking that it is the subject, then this process is called *identification,* and the Self, thinking itself to be limited to the form it has become involved with, identifies itself as the limited individual. This is the emergence the individual of a soul and the process of egoism. Therefore, the soul is in reality the Self which has forgotten its true, all-encompassing nature. The Self who was Pure Consciousness has become involved with the thoughts through a process of becoming ignorant of its real nature.

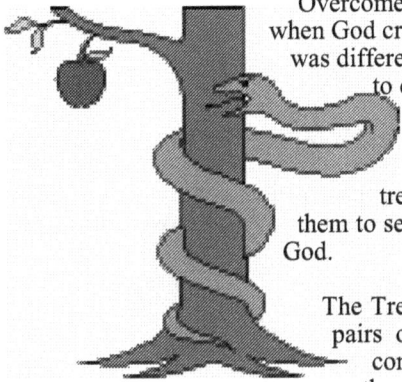

Overcome by desire for sensual experiences, the soul becomes blinded. In the Bible, when God created Adam and Eve (male and female), it was a way of saying that now there was differentiation (duality) in Consciousness. Adam and Eve were tempted by a serpent to eat a fruit, which had been forbidden to them. Prior to the eating from the tree of knowledge of good and evil, Adam and Eve did not have any special feeling of differentiation between themselves or with nature. Everything was the same, equal and united. However, desire led them to eat from the tree of knowledge of good and evil, and this knowledge immediately caused them to see differences between themselves, within nature and between themselves and God.

The Tree of Knowledge of Good and Evil is, therefore, a metaphor representing the pairs of opposites. Instead of there being just oneness, pure awareness of one consciousness, singularity, now there is awareness of multiplicity and duality, the pairs of opposites, you-me, here-there, up-down, male-female. Consciousness is now aware of individual parts of itself, as it were. Having eaten from the tree, everything became as if transformed by magic—from a place of joy and bliss into the world of time and space, i.e. the opposites.

Above: *The Tree of Knowledge of Good and Evil and the Serpent of Ignorance.*

However, there is also another tree in the Garden of Eden, the *Tree of Life*. It is in the center of the Garden of Eden and it represents regeneration and the return to the primordial state of being. This is the tree of knowledge *(gnosis)*, and when it is realized, humankind regains whole consciousness: consciousness of that which is mortal, changeable, and also of that which is immortal and changeless. This is the state of Enlightenment which Jesus expresses in the words: *"I am Alpha and Omega, the beginning and the ending..."* from Revelations 1:8. In the same way that Heru of Egypt as well as Buddha and Krishna of India are masters of *"Above and Below"* (mortal consciousness and divine consciousness), Jesus is also. Both trees are in the same place, human consciousness. Therefore, the Tree of Knowledge of Good and Evil has caused us to forget about the Tree of Life. As previously discussed, in the psycho-mythology of Ancient Egypt, there is also a Tree of Life which is propitiated for its sustaining food and drink which is given by the Goddess of creation. In the religion of Asar, the tree is known as the Tet or Djed Pillar, the body of Asar himself, which is in the center of Creation. In Egyptian mythology there is also a serpent. He is called *Apophis* and he represents the destructive, mischievous nature of the mind, which diverts the soul from its consciousness of oneness into the world of time and space duality. This is the same serpent which distracted Adam and Eve and which afflicts humankind today, every time one is distracted by emotions of anger, hate, greed, passion, desire, etc. Through these feelings and emotions, one's mind is driven away from the peace of pure, undifferentiated consciousness. However, if one learn the art of true Christian living (universal love and forgiveness), it is possible to eradicate stress and mental unrest and uncover the peace of the Self, which is always there patiently awaiting rediscovery.

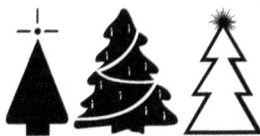

Left: The Modern Christmas Tree.   Right: The Ancient Egyptian Pyramid

In the development of early Christianity, there was a tradition, which held that Jesus was crucified on the Tree of Knowledge of, Good and Evil. Jesus, like Asar, represents the soul who is leaving the Garden of Eden in order to come into the field of human experience (duality, multiplicity, happiness and sorrow, etc.), the physical world. Therefore, the crucifixion of Jesus is a symbol for the soul being crucified by duality and multiplicity (separation from the oneness of God by the ego and the ignorance of the mind). This is the same idea as Asar's being dismembered by his evil brother, Set. Asar' dismemberment represents the scattering of the consciousness of the soul due to desires, egoism and ignorance. It was not until later that the tree symbol gave way to the cross symbol due to the numbers of Christian martyrs who were crucified by the Roman Empire. However, as mentioned earlier, the mystical symbolism of the Christian Cross is that it represents time and space (duality and multiplicity) consciousness, so there is no real contradiction in the use of the tree or the cross if the mystical symbolism is well understood. In a subtle way, this mystical symbolism may be seen in modern day Christmas Trees, since they are cut in such a way that they taper towards the top, ending in a point surmounted by a single star ornament. This is the same symbolism represented in the great pyramids of Egypt, wherein each side represents duality and opposing forces which unify at the top and are transcended in the *Capstone* or uppermost point.

Thus, the way to rediscover one's original essence is to find the Tree of Life. In the New Testament, John 11:25, Jesus says that "I am the resurrection, and the life: he that believes in me, though he were dead, yet shall he live." Like Jesus, Heru was the symbol of "the resurrection and the life" and he, as the Son of God (Asar), was also known to walk on water. Thus, by following the examples and teachings of Heru and Jesus, spiritual Enlightenment is achieved.

The project of Enlightenment from a Christian point of view is to regain the knowledge of your divine nature (Tree of Life) and thus achieve complete Consciousness within yourself. In this sense the Christian Tree of Life is equal to the *Caduceus* of Djehuti-Hermes or the Djed Pillar of Asar of Egypt, the *Chakras of Kundalini* in Indian Yoga and the *Sefirotic Tree of Life* in the Cabala. All of these symbols represent an onward movement leading towards self-discovery and enlightenment.

The Pillar of Asar

In the myth of Asar and Aset, after Asar was killed by Set, his body grew into a tree. The pillar of Asar was made from this tree. The tree had developed such beauty and fragrance that a king of Syria discovered it and cut it into the shape of a pillar for his palace. Aset discovered the whereabouts of her husband's dead body and revived him. This is the source of the Ancient Egyptian ritual of "Raising the Tet." The Pillar of Asar is a mystical symbol representing the four highest stages of spiritual experience. It also refers to the four higher psycho-spiritual energy centers of the subtle human (astral) anatomy known as Chakras, in the Indian system, which are developed through the various practices of mystical spirituality (Yoga) outlined here. Aset represents intuitional wisdom. Therefore, it is through the practice and discovery of the ultimate wisdom, your true Self, that you can return to, rediscover or resurrect your essential reality as an immortal, eternal being who is united with the source of all creation, the Divine Self.

The mind, which is weakened by ignorance and lacks, will and self-control will fall sway to the myriad visions and experiences of the *Duat* just as you fall prey to the experiences of a dream during sleep. The *Duat* is the Ancient Egyptian name for the Netherworld or Astral Plane. It is equivalent to Heaven in Christianity, but this heaven is not THE heaven to be sought after by a spiritual aspirant. The orthodox understanding of heaven is a place where you go after death, retaining your ego consciousness, to live for eternity alongside Jesus and God. The Kingdom of Heaven described in the Gnostic Christian texts is equivalent to the Transcendental Consciousness which Ancient Egyptian, Buddhist, Vedantic and Taoist texts speak of, recognizing all Creation as the Kingdom itself. The physical world, the mental world and that which transcends these is God. The objective of the mystic is to discover and become one with this kingdom and not become enamored with the idea of an everlasting heaven, and not to reside in this heaven as a tenant for all eternity. This is the higher understanding of heaven.

Through the practices of Yoga (control of senses, dispassion and detachment toward sense objects, meditation, etc.), a Yogi is able to gain control of the mind. As a result, he/she is no longer caught up in the illusions of the *Duat* or the physical world and is able to discover Asar within him/herself and become *sound and strong in the Netherworld,* i.e., he or she attains *Nehast,* Enlightenment, resurrection.

BODY CONSCIOUSNESS

The Gnostic *Book of Thomas,* Chapter 4:14-15:

Thomas answered Jesus and said: "Is it good for us, Lord, to find rest among our own people?"

The Savior said, "Yes, it does help. It is good for you, since what is visible in human existence will pass away. For the fleshy body of people will pass away, and when it disintegrates, it will find its place in what is visible and can be seen.

The idea expressed in the passage above is similar in tone and feeling to the following texts from Ancient Egyptian Religion, where it is explicitly stated that there are two parts to the human being. One part of the human being is divine and heavenly while the other is transitory, belonging to the earth.

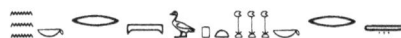

Thy essence is in heaven, thy body to earth. (VI dynasty, c. 5,000 B.C.E.)

𓂋𓏤𓆳𓏛𓆓𓅱𓆓𓆓𓏲𓆓𓅱
Heaven hath thy soul, earth hath thy body. (Ptolematic period, c. 300-100 B.C.E.)

Many Egyptologists have suggested that the Ancient Egyptians embalmed their dead with the idea that the dead person would attain immortality, and that the Ancient Egyptians believed that the physical body, which was mummified, would rise up again some day. This idea spurred many Hollywood[1] movies. The statements above, from the early and late periods of Ancient Egyptian culture, clearly show that the Ancient Egyptians never sought a bodily resurrection or eternal life in the physical body. They understood death as a passageway to the next existence, and just as the physical body needs nourishment, the spiritual body was also provided for by means of the subtle essence of the solid food that was buried with the mummy.

The problem of human existence is the forgetfulness of the Divine essence of the Self and the identification with the body as the Self. Through concern with the body and its needs and desires, the true Self becomes identified with worldly concerns and the fulfillment of desires of the body, mind and senses. This is the development of the ego and individual soul. This identification with the desires of the body is what leads the soul to further ignorance of its true Self. It is the pursuit of desires that keeps the mind occupied with worldly thoughts such as the fear of disease and death of the body, the pursuit of pleasure and happiness, and the eradication of things which cause displeasure.

Gnosticism, Hinduism, Buddhism, Taoism and Ancient Egyptian Religion all emphasize the need to practice detachment and dispassion toward the body. This discipline relieves the pressure of the lower desires, which impel a person to run after the illusions of life. These traditions hold that only through detachment is it possible to calm the mind enough for it to perceive the transcendental reality.

The constant preoccupation with the body is incessantly reinforced through many years of living with family and others in society. Such body consciousness leads to the conviction that the psychophysical complex (mind and body) is indeed the Self. It is this idea that is to be dispelled through the spiritual discipline of constantly turning towards the Divine (through the various disciplines of Yoga) instead of to the body and to the world of illusion.

This process becomes easier to understand through reflection on the fact that the body is composed of physical elements, which are themselves, transient. The body you have today is not the same as the one you had nine years ago. Every cell in your body has been regenerated. Even your bones are different. As surely as people are born, just as surely their body will some day cease to exist. Is it wise to hold onto something that you will definitely lose at some point in time? Impermanence is a given fact of life. Flowers grow, live and die. Insects grow, live and die. Yet people accept these changes. Why is it that people do not cry when the flower dies, or when a leaf falls from a tree and dies or for every creature in nature that has died? The fact is that it is not only death that causes fear, but attachment to that which died and has met the "unknown." So fear of death is due to ignorance of one's true nature.

Likewise, people hold on to life, no matter how miserable a situation they may be in, because they don't know any other way of thinking or acting, and also because they have the illusion that there is a chance they may find happiness someday or they may somehow come into some money. Wealth is a big illusion. You can read the papers and see how wealth destroys a person's peace of mind through the endless worries associated with acquiring, investing and protecting it.

Matthew 19
23. Then said Jesus to his disciples, Verily I say to you, That it is hard for a rich man to enter into the kingdom of heaven.
24 And again I say to you, It is easier for a camel to go through the eye of a needle, than for a rich man to enter into the Kingdom of God.

An even greater illusion comes into play when a person tries to figure out which part of the body contains the soul. There is no body part which contains the soul or which can be considered to be the "Self." No body part can be called "me," yet somehow the conglomerate of thoughts, memories, physical body and senses is understood to be "me." This error or misunderstanding is the cause of human misery and pain because it involves the soul in the mishaps and troubles of the mind-body complex and its attending desires. If the mind and senses were transcended, these problems along with individual identification with the body-mind would cease, and the true Self would be discovered to be infinite and eternal. This is the discovery of the Saints and Sages. For this reason they have

---

[1] Hollywood, Calif., area of greater Los Angeles known throughout the world as the home of the US movie industry.

proclaimed that the soul has been overtaken by ignorance of its true Self, and due to this ignorance, it is subject to experience the pain of human existence.

A simple philosophical study of the body reveals the error in thinking that the body is the Self. If the senses fail to perceive, or a limb or organ ceases to operate, consciousness is still there. The awareness of being alive remains even if the perceptions of the senses or nerves fail. The practice of spirituality involves discovering that which transcends the body, as well as learning how to become attached to that transcendent reality as the truth, rather than remaining attached to the physical body and its desires and impulses, as well as to one's emotions throughout the ups and downs of human existence.

The world of unenlightened human existence is likened to being out in the middle of the ocean when there is a raging storm. The desires of the mind and body are the waves thrashing the mind about. Spiritual practice is the boat, which allows a person to weather the storm of the world with its ever-changing situations. It gives the power to move forward in life and not be disturbed by the choices, desires and unpredictability of the world-process.

WHERE CAN TRUE HAPPINESS BE FOUND?

Romans 14:17
   17 For the Kingdom of God is not food and drink; but righteousness, and peace, and joy in the Holy Spirit.

Matthew 6
   21 For where your treasure is, there will your heart be also.

Yoga philosophy helps us to have no illusions about true happiness. It can be ours, but on the condition that we work to purify our minds as well as our bodies. When we are disillusioned by all that is temporary and transient in this world, we will be led by that same disappointment to search for stability and truth. Stability or steadfastness is the most important element of happiness, but it cannot be discovered if the mind is constantly buffeted by the stormy winds of egoistic desires and ignorance about how to live in harmony with nature.

Righteousness can be equated with happiness. If you learn how to act rightly, you will lead yourself to correct actions. Correct actions will lead to positive conditions. Positive conditions will lead to prosperity. Prosperity will lead to all that is good and true. The joy of acting righteously and being in control of your life itself will be a source of happiness even if you are not materially prosperous. Once true happiness is found, it will never be lost. Regardless of the situation—rich or poor, scorned or famous—you will be above human frailties. To be truly happy, you must have a stable point to hold onto permanently and this is your faith in the teaching. Once you are firm in this faith you will never lose your balance and it will lead you to discover the highest spiritual realization. That center of firmness is within your own heart and it can be discovered if you determine to do so. Once you discover it, you can always return to it at any time.

If, due to ignorance, you don't know how to think, act and feel about life, you will become uneasy, afraid, and at the mercy of every situation that arises. Happiness is a state of consciousness, a way of understanding, thinking, feeling and behaving. It is an attitude you can learn through study and knowledge of the science of Yoga. But this science does not become effective until you put it into practice right here and now. If you do, you will learn how to appreciate your existence every second, every hour, and every day on earth, and beyond.

Happiness cannot be found in the world of time and space. This is because the happiness derived from objects or sensual pleasures is transient. No person on earth can control life. It is unpredictable and traitorous. No sooner does a person become rich than they contract cancer and die. You can work hard for a job, only to see it lost due to the changing economy. Any happiness that you seem to experience in life is only a fragment of the boundless bliss of the Self. You may have noticed that a feeling of happiness occurs whenever there is a release of stress. Whenever you relieve some stress by acquiring something you wanted or by achieving some pleasurable circumstance that you desired, there is an immediate feeling of expansion and brief satisfaction. But this expansion or relief is short lived. Imagine what would happen if you could experience that relief in an infinite way, boundless and unobstructed, no matter where you were, what you were doing, or what was going on in your life. What would that be like? Many people like to think that if they were to become suddenly rich they would be able to make this happen; they fail to understand that the money would only intensify their ego as well as the pain and suffering that are inseparably linked to the ego. When people succeed in acquiring wealth, they immediately set out to pamper their desires with objects they always wanted. Soon, however, they become bored with those objects and enter into an endless search for other objects that they think will lead to greater happiness, ultimately to be disappointed. Look how many rich movie stars have died of drug overdoses, depression, and disputes over finances, etc.

In the New Testament *Gospel of Luke* we find the following statement:

> 17:21 Neither shall they say, Lo here! or, lo there! for, behold, the Kingdom of God is in the midst of you (within thee).

Ephesians 2
> 8 For by grace are ye saved through faith; and that not of
> yourselves: [it is] the gift of God:
> 9 <u>Not by works,</u> lest any man should boast.
> 10 For we are his workmanship, created in Christ Jesus to good works, which God hath before ordained that we should walk in them. {ordained: or, prepared}.

Many people feel that by doing good works alone they can attain the highest goal of spirituality. Good works means that a person has decided to make their life a conduit for divine inspiration and action, a medium for allowing God to transform the world. Faith is not just believing but also trusting that all events which transpire (good or bad) are divinely ordained for a higher purpose and therefore must be accepted willingly. How many people who profess to believe in God get upset when things don't go their way? How many people go to church every week but remain remorseful, envious, angry or frustrated with others, or with their own life? This is not real faith. It is a deluded movement in which people make themselves believe they are spiritual, but in reality they are spiritually stagnant, and this way of feeling will bring frustration and failure in life. Faith is that movement in life when you know something is true even though you cannot yet experience it, and so you move forward anyway. True faith brings solace, mental peace and fortitude. This movement of spiritualizing your actions and the adoption of an attitude towards life based on faith, allows your mind to expand and your spiritual sensitivity to grow. This is true Divine Grace, which leads to ever increasing awareness of the Divine.

The happiness and peace, which comes from the successful practice of Yoga, cannot be found anywhere in this world. True happiness can only come from following the spiritual path. The path of spiritual discovery is the only endeavor, which allows a human being to satisfy their true need to rediscover their true identity, which is the source of all sweetness, peace and love. Therefore, the practices on the path of Yoga should be thought of as a great treasure. Like a miser who is constantly thinking of his treasure, the disciple should keep the teachings in mind (the heart) at all times in order to discover the greatest treasure, God (the Absolute Reality). The mystical path allows you to discover that happiness does not come from any activity you can perform or cause to happen. It is something you discover within yourself, which expresses as the outer world in which you live.

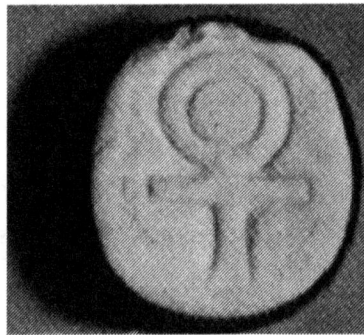

Above: A Gnostic Christian Amulet bearing the Ancient Egyptian Ankh Cross.

CHAPTER XI: THE PEARLS OF MYSTICAL CHRISTIAN WISDOM

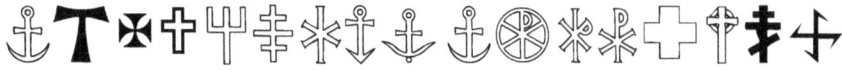

Matthew 7

6 Give not that which is holy to dogs, neither cast ye your
pearls before swine, lest they trample them under their feet, and
turn again and rend you.
7. Ask, and it shall be given you; seek, and ye shall find;
knock, and the door shall be opened to you:
8 For every one that asketh receiveth; and he that seeketh
findeth; and to him that knocketh the door shall be opened.

—Jesus

The Wisdom of the Sermon on the Mount and the Ten Commandments

The following tables show how Ancient Egyptian wisdom was adopted by the early Jews and incorporated into the teachings of the Bible. Beyond this however, it must also be understand that the objective is not just to show the origins of Judaism in Ancient Egypt, but to point to a deeper understanding of those same teachings so that our understanding of the Bible may be more profound and our spiritual practice of Christianity more intense and fruitful. The wisdom teachings provide us with guidelines for how to conduct our daily affairs. This is important because if we do not have harmony in our day to day life, our spiritual practice will be unbalanced. Therefore, the wisdom teachings and their proper practice are the first step in a viable spiritual program for life.

The most forceful expositions of the wisdom teachings contained in the Christian Bible are to be found in two primary locations. The first is the Sermon on the Mount, which presents the teachings of Jesus in a condensed form. Supporting these teachings are the Ten Commandments, the teachings given by Moses. The first chart below presents the Sermon on the Mount and relates each teaching to the virtuous qualities to which they refer. The succeeding charts will review the Ten Commandments in more detail as they relate to the Ancient Egyptian Wisdom teachings. The virtuous qualities that are extolled in the Sermon on the Mount are disciplines for Christian living. As such they form the disciplinary aspects for the practice of true Christianity. When these qualities are perfected in a human being, one is able to discover blessedness in their own lives and bring it forth to others in the world as well. Thus, they are the essence of Christian wisdom as it relates to human interaction and all aspects of Christian social life including politics, economics, family, etc. Therefore, a Christian businessperson, a Christian government official and even a Christian engineer must live their professional and social life in accordance with these principles, otherwise they are not really practicing Christianity in its most elementary level.

The following charts are a comparison of the teachings. They are presented here in this way for the sake of showing their origins in previous teachings as well as to give a greater depth in understanding them. Many Egyptologists now believe that the early Jews were well aquatinted with the Ancient Egyptian Wisdom Texts, especially the *Instructions of Amenemope*. The *Instructions of Amenemope* is strikingly similar in concept and the form of the literary expression with the Bible book of Proverbs.[61] In *Christian Yoga Volume II* we will present a more detailed study of the precepts and their application in daily life.

The Sermon on the Mount and Its Virtuous Qualities

SERMON ON THE MOUNT (THE BEATITUDES)[I]	VIRTUOUS QUALITIES
Matthew 5	
1. And seeing the multitudes, he ascended a mountain: and when he was seated, his disciples came to him: 2 And he opened his mouth, and taught them, saying, 3. Blessed [are] the poor in spirit: for theirs is the kingdom of heaven.	Virtue of Humility.
4. Blessed [are] they that mourn: for they shall be comforted.	Virtue of desiring spiritual life - aspiration to discover God instead of perishable worldly desires.
5 Blessed [are] the meek: for they shall inherit the earth.	Virtue of self-effacement.
6 Blessed [are] they who hunger and thirst for righteousness: for they shall be filled.	Virtue of seeking truth and justice.
7 Blessed [are] the merciful: for they shall obtain mercy.	Virtue of compassion, sharing and caring for others.
8 Blessed [are] the pure in heart: for they shall see God.	Virtue of right thinking – absence of anger, hatred, greed, jealousy and lust in the mind.
9 Blessed [are] the peacemakers: for they shall be called children of God.	Virtue of non-violence as opposed to aggressiveness and violent behavior.
10 Blessed [are] they who are persecuted for righteousness' sake: for theirs is the kingdom of heaven.	Virtue of speaking and doing right action as opposed to perpetrating injustices or allowing these to exist.
11 Blessed are ye, when [men] shall revile you, and persecute [you], and shall say all manner of evil against you falsely, for my sake. {falsely: Gr. lying}	Virtue of not being resentful.

[I] Beatitudes, group of blessings spoken by Jesus at the opening of the Sermon on the Mount, as recorded most fully in Matthew 5:3-12.

The Ten Commandments and Their Origins in Ancient Egyptian Wisdom

The Ten Commandments and the Teachings of Maat:

TEN COMMANDMENTS	TEACHINGS OF MAAT (Ancient Egypt)
Exodus 20 3:17 1. Thou shalt have no other Gods before me.	(30) "One should revere The God (Supreme Being)"*
2. Thou shalt not make to thee any graven image.	(42) "I have never thought evil or slighted the God in my native town." (64) There is no perfection before The God**
3 Thou shalt not take the name of the Lord thy God in vain.	(38) "I have not cursed the God."
4 Remember the Sabbath day, to keep it holy.	(21) "I have not violated sacred times and seasons. "
5. Honor thy father and thy mother.	Thou shalt never forget what thy mother has done for thee, she beareth thee and nourished thee in all manner of ways.***
6. Thou shalt not kill.	(5) "I have not murdered man or woman."'
7. Thou shalt not commit adultery.	(19) "I have not committed adultery."
8. Thou shalt not steal.	(4) "I have not committed theft."
9. Thou shalt not bear false witness against thy neighbor.	(17) "I have not spoken against anyone."
10. Thou shalt not covet thy neighbor's house, thou shalt not covet thy neighbors wife, or his male servant, or his female servant, or his ox., or his donkey, or any thing that is of thy neighbors.	(41) "I have never magnified my condition beyond what was fitting or increased my wealth, except with such things as are a justly mine own possessions." *The Instructions of Merikara (c. 2,135-2,040 B.C.E.) **The Instructions of Amenemope (c. 1,500-1,200 B.C.E) ***Egyptian Proverbs

The Teachings of the Bible and The Teachings of Sage Amenemope

THE TEACHINGS OF THE BIBLE	THE TEACHINGS OF AMENEMOPE (Ancient Egypt)
PROVERBS XXII. 17-XXIII. 14; The "teachings of King Solomon" 0 Israel 1. Incline thine ear, and hear my words, And apply thine heart to apprehend; For it is pleasant if thou keep them in thy belly,	1. Give thine ear and hear what I say, And apply thine heart to apprehend; It is good for thee to place them in thine heart,
1a. That they may be fixed like a peg upon thy lips.	1a. Let them rest in the casket of thy belly. That they rally act as a peg upon thy tongue.
2. Have I not written for thee thirty sayings of counsels and knowledge! That thou mayest make known truth to him that speaketh.	2. Consider these thirty chapters; they delight, they instruct. Know how to answer one who speaks, To reply to one who sends a message. So as to direct him on the paths of life…
3. Rob not the poor for he is poor, neither oppress the lowly in the gate.	3. Beware of robbing the poor, and of oppressing the afflicted.
4. Associate not with a passionate man, nor go with a wrathful man, lest thou learn his ways and get a snare to thy soul.	4. Associate not with a passionate man, nor approach him for conversations: Leap not to cleave to such a one, that the terror carry thee not away
5. A man who is skillful in his business shall stand before kings.	5. A scribe who is skillful in his business findeth himself worthy to be a courtier.

The Teachings of the Bible and The Teachings of Sage Ptahotep

The Teachings of the Bible	The Teachings of Ptahotep (Ancient Egypt c. 2,300-2,150 B.C.E.)
PROVERBS 3:7; " Be not wise in thy own eyes: fear the LORD, and depart from evil."	1) "Don't be proud of your knowledge"
PROVERBS: 27.1; "Boast not thyself of tomorrow; for thou knowest not what a day may bring forth."	2) "One plans the morrow but knows not what will be."
PROVERBS 25:9; "Debate thy cause with thy neighbor himself; and discover not a secret to another."	3) "If you probe the character of a friend, don't inquire, but approach him, deal with him alone....."
PROVERBS 25:13; "As the cold snow in the time of harvest, so is a faithful messenger to them that send him: for he refresheth the soul of his masters."	4) "If you are a man of trust, sent by one great man to another, adhere to the nature of him who sent you, give his message as he said it."
PROVERBS 9:9; "Give instruction to a wise man, and he will be yet wiser: teach a just man, and he will increase in learning."	5) "Teach the great what is useful to him."
PSALM 78:5; "For he established a testimony in Jacob, and appointed a law in Israel, which he commanded our fathers, that they should make them known to their children: 6; That the generation to come might know them, even the children which should be born; who should arise and declare them to their children:"	6) "If every word is carried on, they will not perish in the land."
ECCLESIASTES 6:2; "A man to whom God hath given riches, wealth, and honor, so that he wanteth nothing for his soul of all that he desireth, yet God giveth him not power to eat thereof, but a stranger eateth it: this is vanity, and it is an evil disease."	7) "Guard against the vice of greed: a grievous sickness without cure. There is no treatment for it."
ECCLESIASTES 9:17; "The words of wise men are heard in quiet more than the cry of him that ruleth among fools."	8) "If you are a man of worth who sits in his master's council, concentrate on excellence, your silence is better than chatter... gain respect through knowledge ... "
PROVERBS 18:21; "Death and life are in the power of the tongue: and they that love it shall eat the fruit thereof."	9) "The wise is known by his wisdom, the great by his good actions; his heart matches his tongue..."
PROVERBS 23:1; "When thou sittest to eat with a ruler, consider diligently what is before thee:"	10) "If you are one among guests at the table of one greater than you, take what he gives as it is set before you."

The Commandments of Jesus	Teachings of Ancient Egypt
Mark 12	† Ancient Egyptian Hymns of Amun. (c. 2,500-1,500 B.C.E.) ‡ Ancient Egyptian Teachings of Sage Amenemope.
28. And one of the scribes came, and having heard them reasoning together, and perceiving that he had answered them well, asked him, Which is the first commandment of all?	
29 And Jesus answered him, The first of all the commandments [is], Hear, O Israel; The Lord our God is one Lord:	4. His unity is Absolute. Amun (God) is One, One [without a second].†
30 And thou shalt love the Lord thy God with all thy heart, and with all thy soul, and with all thy mind, and with all thy strength: this [is] the first commandment.	46. Thy beauties take possession of and carry away all hearts [minds], and love for Thee make all arms to relax, Thy beautiful form make the hands to tremble, and all hearts [minds] melt at the sight of Thee. †
*In the First Letter of John in the Bible it is stated that God is love: 1 John 4:8 8 He that loveth not knoweth not God; for God is love. 1 John 4:16 16 And we have known and believed the love that God hath to us. God is love; and he that dwelleth in love dwelleth in God, and God in him.	In Ancient Egypt love of God was so important that God was referred to as: "Beloved one or love itself God- *Merr*"[132] **(i.e. God is Love)**
31 And the second [is] like, [namely] this, Thou shalt love thy neighbor as thyself. There is no other commandment greater than these.	(30) Set your goodness before people, Then you are greeted by all; One welcomes the what is good, Spits upon what is bad. (31) Guard your tongue from harmful speech, Then others will love you. You will find your place in the Sanctuary, the house of God, Be kind to the poor. Get thee a seat in the sanctuary. Be strong to do the commandment of God. You will share in the offerings of your lord. ‡
Jesus on prayer Matthew 6:6 But thou, when thou prayest, enter into thy closet, and when thou hast shut thy door, pray to thy Father who is in secret; and thy Father who seeth in secret shall reward thee openly.	**Teachings of Sage Ani on prayer** Do not raise your voice in the house of god, He abhors shouting; (too much talking) Pray by yourself with a loving heart, Whose every word is in secret. He will grant your needs, He will hear your words, He will accept your offerings.

THE TRANSITORY AND ILLUSORY NATURE OF THE WORLD

Man fears time, and time fears the pyramids!
(Ancient Proverb)

In order to practice Yoga effectively, there must be a firm grasp of the philosophy concerning the true nature of the world, and indeed the universe. In the *Gospel of Thomas* and the *Gospel of Philip,* there are several teachings, which seek to convey the need to give up one's desires for worldly things due to their innate illusoriness and transitory nature. Further, this psychological dependency is the main cause of the mind's bondage to the world of time and space. This process of bondage is known as egoistic attachment. Everything in nature changes and eventually fades away, yet most people go through a great deal of mental strain and stress seeking to possess objects. Even when objects are acquired, the passion, which impelled one to strive for them, is often unfulfilled within a short time. Sometimes there seems to be an immediate feeling of satisfaction right after you get something you longed for, and at other times, you realize that the object is not what you expected and is, therefore, disappointing. Modern physicists are now saying that matter is not as solid and static as it appears. It is in constant change and decay. Even the pyramids and the Great Sphinx, the oldest known massive monuments in the world, are gradually decaying and will one day cease to be. So what does this mean in reference to people's desires and expectations from the world?

In Ancient Egyptian and Indian philosophy, the illusoriness of the world process was understood well by the Sages. Both solid (gross) objects (matter) as well as the mental process (subtle-matter) are understood to be manifestations of the Spirit. They are like the matter, which manifests in a dream—matter that seems so solid and real, but of course, is not. According to which reality should we live? Should we live according to what the senses are saying or according to what science is saying? This is where Yoga philosophy can be a great help. Many times people know a truth but cannot live in accordance with that truth. Instead, they live according to an illusion. For example, a person may have learned to smoke when he was an ignorant youth, but when he grew up he learned that smoking leads to an early grave. However, he could not or did not want to stop smoking. He was unable to stop because he was caught up in the illusion of pleasure, which he was deriving from smoking. In reality smoking was detrimental from the very first cigarette, and damaged the body more every time it was done. The smoker thinks he cannot calm down without it or he thinks he is addicted and has to have it. All of these are illusions because many people have been able to calm themselves in any situation by just quieting the body and practicing deep breathing exercises. Others have quit as soon as they learned that smoking was harmful. Still others have quit on the day they were told they have cancer. So from beginning to end there is merely an illusion of pleasure and happiness in his mind. It is illogical to seek to become attached to objects or to engage in activities, which are illusory and transitory, but people do exactly this every day, from the time of their birth to the time of their death. Further, since Jesus tells us that *"we and the Father are One"* and that *"the Kingdom of Heaven is all around us,"* then it is clear that physical objects are in reality manifestations of God-consciousness, which is essentially our own consciousness as well. Since the world of objects is in reality our own creation, as in a dream, then we need not grasp at them since we are already one with them. This grand truth is difficult for people to understand because they do not practice living in a detached manner and calming the mind from the distracting thoughts of ignorance in order to glimpse the higher reality.

In the following passage from the *Gospel of Thomas,* the illusoriness of the human personality is explained. Jesus speaks of images, which came before one's present existence, the existence that does not die.

88. Jesus says: "Now, when you see your appearance, you rejoice. But when you see your images which came into being before you, which do not die and do not show themselves, how will you be able to bear the greatness?"

From the *Gospel of Philip* on the illusoriness of language and of worldly objects:

Names given to worldly things are very deceptive, since they turn the heart aside from the real to the unreal. And whoever hears the word "God" thinks not of the reality, but has been thinking of what is not real: so also, with the words: "Father," "Son," "Holy Spirit," "life," "light," "resurrection," "church," etc., it is not the real that one thinks of but the unreal, although the words have referred to the real. The names that one has heard exist in the world and one is through them deceived. If the names were situated in the eternal realm, they would not be uttered on any occasion in the world, nor would they have been assigned to worldly things: their reference would be in the eternal realm.[101]

"Learn to distinguish the real from the unreal."
(Injunction to the Ancient Egyptian Initiates)

Perhaps the most important teaching of Gnosticism or any other high mystical philosophy is the illusoriness of the world. In the Biblical quote above, Jesus alludes to this very point. Applying the psycho-mythical understanding to the text, in the state of Christhood, all of our mental concepts of heaven and earth will indeed pass away. When they are transcended, they come to an end, as it were. Since the world is a projection of our own minds, the "Kingdom" cannot be found in one particular place or another, just as a dream experience cannot be found anywhere except in the mind, which itself does not exist in ordinary time and space. It must be discovered through a change in mental perception.

The world is an illusory modification of "Absolute Existence." The Kingdom is already "among us" therefore, it can only be discerned by the pure of heart. The heart must be purified by losing the desire for worldly involvements that distract the mind from eternal thoughts and aspirations (the Kingdom). The illusoriness of the world was such an important subject that the *Gospel of Thomas* devoted several verses to emphasize it. The traditional New Testament, Matthew 10:26, suggests that there is a mysterious piece of information that will be revealed to those who are faithful.

10:26 Fear them not therefore: for there is nothing covered, that shall not be revealed, and hid, that shall not be known.

In the verse below from the *Gospel of Thomas*, the intimation is that the mystery is already present and that if the disciple learns to "know" what is in front of her/him, then the revelation will inevitably be evident.

5. Jesus said: "Know what is before your face, and what is hidden from you will be revealed to you. For nothing hidden will fail to be revealed."

In verse 87, the teaching becomes more detailed as the illusoriness of worldly images is explained. It is remarkably similar to the following statement from *Mundaka Upanishad*, wherein Brahman (God) is described. It is similar even with respect to the description of the inner "light" which supports all objects but is hidden to ordinary human consciousness. However, once this light (God) is discovered, the existence of the object (image), as a separate and independent reality, is overshadowed by the knowledge of the true nature of the object (image), the light of God.

87. Jesus says: "Images are visible to man, but the light which is in them is hidden. In the image of the light of the Father, it {this light} will be revealed, and his image will be veiled by his light."

Mundaka Upanishad

"Self-luminous is that Being (God), and formless. He dwells within all and without all. He is unborn, pure, greater than the greatest, without breath, without mind."

From Hermetic Philosophy

"Knowledge derived from the senses is illusionary; true knowledge can only come from the understanding of the union of opposites."

The illusion of separation from the Self is the source of all other illusions. It gives rise to feelings such as fear, greed, hatred and anger, because the individual believes he/she must fight for his/her survival. Since the individual does not remember that he/she is immortal and a part of all other beings, he/she develops the idea of looking out for self only and of having a good time, since "you only live once." This psychic imbalance develops due to ignorance about one's spiritual nature; therefore, ignorance is seen as the root of all evils in the form of criminality, selfishness, greed, violence and malice.

Gospel of Thomas

11. Jesus says: This heaven will pass away, and the heaven, which is above it, will pass: but those who are dead will not live, and those who live will not die!

ATTACHMENT: THE SOURCE OF HUMAN PAIN AND SUFFERING

Matthew 6

19. Lay not up for yourselves treasures upon earth, where moth and rust doth corrupt, and where thieves break through and steal:

20 But lay up for yourselves treasures in heaven, where neither moth nor rust doth corrupt, and where thieves do not break through nor steal:

21 For where your treasure is, there will your heart be also.

The passages above point to some important principles of spiritual practice. Many times people become so involved with the world that they make themselves believe they cannot take time for serious spiritual practices. They may want to wait until retirement or until they get set in their job or hit the lottery, etc. These are all excuses and by the time they get old it is too late.

Attachment is a direct result of ignorance and egoism. People become attached to objects and other people because they do not realize that they already encompass them, just like the ocean encompasses all the waves. For this reason, Jesus emphasizes the idea of detachment from the world and from family relationships in order to free the mind (purify the heart) from the illusions of worldly attachments. This theme exists in the orthodox versions of the Bible, however, the church does not emphasize it. One of the reasons is that it is not well understood by the church. Also, the idea of developing detachment towards family members is often erroneously interpreted as not having love for others. This is evidence of the deep misunderstanding of the philosophy since physical or psychological attachment is not a measure of how much a person cares about another person. On the other hand, there is ample evidence that attachment is a cause of countless problems in society. So the philosophy of detachment must be profoundly understood in its yogic form and not with ignorant imaginations.

Gospel of Thomas

47. Jesus says: "You must be as passers by."

54. Jesus says: "Blessed are the solitary and the elect, for you will find the Kingdom! Because you have issued from it, and you will return to it again."

65. ...When {a person} finds him/herself solitary, they will be full of light; but when they find themselves divided, they will be full of darkness.

Attachment is any feeling which emotionally ties one to or causes desire for an object, including persons, places and things. The erroneous premise in modern society, which manifests as attachment is the idea that happiness comes from something outside of oneself, which can be acquired or experienced by the senses. As a result of this erroneous way of thinking, people try to hold objects close to themselves, hoping to secure happiness. However, in this world of constant gain and loss, people cannot really own or hold anything. In the morning a person may be informed that they have just been selected for a great job they always wanted, and then in the afternoon they may die of a heart attack. Nothing in life is certain except that some day everything will be given up—at the time of death, if not before. It is only due to ignorance and delusion that people do not reflect and live according to this truth and realize that they themselves are supremely full, and that nothing can really be gained or lost by anyone.

People project their happiness on objects. In effect, they surrender their power to objects and other people. How do they do this? Every time a person says: "I will not be happy until I get that car" or " I will not rest until I achieve that level of income" or " I can't relax because that person has a larger house than mine," etc., they are surrendering their power. There is no person in this world who is free from the ups and downs of life, no matter how wealthy they are or how many family members they may have around. Even if you enjoyed a relationship which was the best in the world, with no fighting, rivalries or animosities, in the back of your mind there would always be a fear lurking that you might lose that person or that the person would say or do something that would hurt you. Ultimately there is always a haunting thought in the back of the mind that someday it will all come to an end.

All of this reasoning is not intended to bring a feeling of morbidity to the mind. It is a reflective exercise on the truth in which most people refuse to engage. Its purpose is to allow a spiritual aspirant to let go of the world of illusions and, thereby, to cease wasting energy and time on things that are not real or worth pursuing. Then that energy and attention can be directed towards discovering that which is real and true. This is the true meaning of detachment is when the seemingly different objects of the world no longer delude one and therefore hold the illusion of being happy once they are acquired. The truth is that a person need not attach to anything or anyone because the Soul is already one with all. Therefore, all that is necessary is to discover and experience life at the level of the Soul, and then the feeling of oneness with all humanity will emerge.

Modern society considers that the more attachments a person has, the more prosperous a person is. In reality egoistic or sentimental attachments weaken people and render them incapable of resisting temptations from evil doing. Every object that you desire has a piece of your willpower locked up in it. So if that object comes into your view it will compel you to do something you do not really want to do. If you have a desire for sex, you will not be able to resist a certain temptation though you know it is wrong and will lead you to disaster. If you walk down the street and see a stereo you can't afford, you will feel compelled to get it, and when the bill comes you will suffer from the stress of not being able to pay it. If you are attached to a son or daughter you will feel compelled to give them whatever they want even if it is not right for them. You will not be able to think clearly and make the right decision, and this will lead you to future disaster.

Actions, which are characterized by a feeling of attachment (described above), are detrimental to spiritual attainment and to the enjoyment of life, because such actions invariably lead to disappointment, disillusionment and mental agitation. If one does something to please another person or even oneself with the idea of deriving some benefit from the person or situation, be it material or psychological, one is left open to the whims of others or to chance. One is attached to outside factors as determiners of one's mental state.

In this world of relativity, it is certain that not every situation will be pleasing or in keeping with our every expectation. Therefore, if one's intent is to achieve a state of equanimity, one must strive to find that balance within one's own heart (mind). One's own perceptions and reactions are the only thing that one can truly control. One must understand that, ultimately, one is the ruler of one's own self. That self is identical with all existence, and is supremely full. It has no need for outside approval or validation. Our ignorance of this fact leads us to make our happiness dependent on factors outside of ourselves.

Through the incorporation of these teachings in our daily activities and by practicing reflection and meditation, it is possible to intuitively discover real inner fulfillment, contentment and abiding happiness, which is not affected by the outer conditions of the world. One who understands this teaching would act because he or she wants to, out of the "goodness" of their heart, not because they are looking for happiness by making others happy or by expecting something in return from them. Outside factors are always variable and therefore illusory. Since all is the Self, when one acts in the interest of others or the world, one is acting for the Higher Self.

When a person has inner contentment, follows a virtuous course of action, and has relinquished their concern over the fruits of their actions, they will no longer suffer from mental agitation, anguish or frustration. Full enjoyment of the world and happiness are best achieved with a mental attitude of detachment, living in a way, which promotes purity of heart and increasing peace.

THE ILLUSORINESS OF FAMILY AND RELATIONSHIPS

Look at your own experience in relationships but look at the whole picture. Most people like to remember the fun and happy moments of relationships and prefer to forget the pain and sorrow. Is this an honest way to be? There is no relationship, which does not have some degree of pain, attached to it. If you overlook the pain, you are missing out on the spiritual wisdom that the relationship holds for you. Most people have experienced a relationship where everything is going perfectly. There is harmony, laughter and synchronicity with the other person. Things are clicking. Then all of a sudden one person says something, which the other person does not like, and that person becomes indignant, angry, or sullen, or disappointed with the other. What happened with that harmony and happiness? Ordinary human relationships are like a time bomb or a minefield. You never know when a disaster will be coming. However, most people overlook this, and when the blowup comes, they are surprised or shocked and they fall into the pits of animosity and despair. Worldly relations are imperfect by their very nature, and human emotions are unpredictable. Therefore, any relationship that is based upon them is also imperfect and unpredictable. Should we throw out relationships altogether? Is there a better way to live? The wisdom of Yoga and mystical religion provide some answers.

Matthew 12
46 while he was yet speaking to the people, behold, [his] mother and his brethren stood outside, desiring to speak with him.
47 then one said to him, Behold, thy mother and thy brethren stand outside, desiring to speak with thee.
48 But he answered and said to him that told him, Who is my mother and who are my brethren?
49 And he stretched forth his hand toward his disciples, and said, behold my mother and my brethren!
50 For whoever shall do the will of my Father whom is in heaven, the same is my brother, and sister, and mother.

A similar episode to Matthew 12:46-50 appears in the story of Buddha. After attaining Enlightenment, Buddha returned to the city where he grew up as a prince. Prior to becoming a Yogi, Buddha was a prince who would inherit a vast kingdom. However, in his youth he ventured out into the kingdom and saw how some people lived in luxury while others lived in misery, illness and pain, and how all living beings ultimately die, regardless of the glory or the riches attained. He developed dispassion and went into the forest to study the teachings of the Brahmins and Yogis. After enlightenment, Buddha continued the practice of wandering the countryside as a begging monk seeking for alms as a mode of survival. When his father, the King, heard of this he immediately went out with his entourage to find his son. Upon finding him, the King asked Buddha to return with him to the palace where they could live in a way befitting their royal family tradition. Buddha replied that in his family, meaning those who are Enlightened, there have always been beggars wandering freely.

Luke 14
    26 If any [man] cometh to me, and hateth not his father, and mother, and wife, and children, and brethren, and sisters, yea, and his own life also, he cannot be my disciple.

The passage from Luke 14:26 is almost exactly the same as the one in the *Gospel of Thomas* Verse 60, denoting its Gnostic concurrence. However there is one important additional statement in the Gnostic version of the parable.

    60. Whoever does not hate his father and his mother, as I do cannot become a disciple to me. And whoever loves his father and mother as much as he loves me cannot be a disciple to me. For my mother gave me falsehood, but my true mother gave me life.[14]

    How could Jesus ask us to hate our family? Statements such as this one have baffled Christian followers to such a degree that many have overlooked them completely. How many Sunday services are given with the subject of hating one's family? If Jesus is the embodiment of love and compassion, how can he speak of hating those who are closest to you?

From a Gnostic point of view, loving one's family is like loving a small piece of God. Since all things are within the Kingdom of Heaven, it is not possible to love one thing over another. Mental peace and spiritual realization cannot occur if one thing is preferred over another, for there arises in the mind thought vibrations of dislike for other things. The duality, which is set up in the mind, gives rise to feelings of separation, closeness, possession, loss, etc. These in turn, keep the mind clouded with thoughts related to its illusions, egoism, attachment, desire, imaginations and misconceptions, thus preventing it from perceiving the truth of existence. In reality there is no difference between any objects in creation except that which is created in the egoistic mind beset by ignorance of the truth. All objects have the same source and are composed of the same substance. Therefore, the wise do not crave any object over another and therefore they abide in perpetual peace of mind. No matter who is present or who is absent, the mind of an enlightened human being is always serene and fulfilled. A different translation of the same text from the *Gospel of Thomas* brings up deeper issues:

    ...And whoever does not love his father and his mother as I do cannot become a disciple to me.

In this translation the idea emerges that all things must be loved equally. Jesus seems to say that he loves his mother and father, but not in the egoistic, possessive sense which is the usual understanding of love. Jesus loves impersonally and without distinction. How can an ocean love one wave over another when it is all the waves?

The *Brihadaranyaka Upanishad* contains a similar statement, which lends deeper insight into the meaning of this teaching:

    As a man in the embrace of his loving wife knows nothing that is without, nothing that is within, so man in union with the Self knows nothing that is without, nothing that is within, for in that state all desires are satisfied. The Self is the only desire; he is free from craving, he goes beyond sorrow.

    Then father is no father, mother is no mother; worlds disappear, gods disappear, scriptures disappear; the thief is no more, the murderer is no more, castes are no more; no more is there monk or hermit. The Self is then untouched by good or evil, and the sorrows of the heart are turned into joy.

From the Upanishad we are to understand that in the state of intuitional realization (Enlightenment) one beholds one's essential nature from the Soul's perspective. From here the entire world, including one's family relations, dissolves into the totality of one's consciousness, which is one with the Universal Self. In Christian terminology, upon beholding the Kingdom of Heaven one's individual family relationships dissolve into the totality of the Kingdom, which includes all humanity and all creation. In order to achieve this state, it is necessary to live one's life according to this truth. In doing so, the bonds of attachment to the illusory worldly relationships are then loosened, and the realization of the higher truth becomes fact. Further, relationships are enjoyed in a more profound way because the mind is no longer burdened by the expectations which cause one to have "conditions" for loving others. An example of this is "I will love you if you love me or do this for me," etc.

Luke 18
> 28 Then Peter said, Lo, we have left all, and followed thee.
> 29 And he said to them, Verily I say to you, There is no man that hath left house, or parents, or brethren, or wife, or children, for the sake of the Kingdom of God,
> 30 who shall not receive much more in this present time, and in the world to come life everlasting.

Speaking on the family at the time of the coming of the Kingdom:

Matthew 24
> 19 And woe to them that are with child, and to them that nurse infants in those days!

Speaking on those who have risen from the dead (in consciousness):

Mark 12
> 25 For when they shall rise from the dead, they neither marry, nor are given in marriage; but are as the angels who are in heaven.

From the Dhahamapada of Buddha:

"These sons belong to me, and this wealth belongs to me;" with such thoughts a fool is tormented. He himself does not belong to himself, how much less sons and wealth?

The Bhagavad Gita contains the same teaching concerning detachment from worldliness and from family relationships.

Gita: Chapter 13 Kshetra-Kshetrajna Vibhag Yogah—The Division of Field and the Knower of the Field.

> 9. Detachment, absence of the feeling of mine-ness towards son, wife, house and the like and constant equanimity of mind in all happenings whether desirable or undesirable.
> 10. Unflinching devotion to Me through the Yoga of inseparability, abiding in solitary places, not delighting in the company of the worldly-minded.

It should be clear by now to you, the reader, that you are not the body, the mind, the senses, nor the ego-personality. Further, it must be clear that the world, as your senses perceive it, is not what it appears to be. At least intellectually, you must by now understand that your true identity is the Spirit which is neither male nor female, and that your transient physical body cannot own or be attached to anything since it is only a brief resident on earth. Therefore, what is the nature of relationships in the physical form and what is their purpose? You must understand that your Soul (your Higher Self) places you in situations and relationships based on your own karmic basis (thoughts and actions). Thus, it is your very own consciousness that draws your relationships to you. As that consciousness changes and evolves, so too will your relationships. Thus, your destiny is not pre-determined; rather, you create it at every moment. Free will and self-effort are the keys to attaining spiritual realization, because these are the keys to transforming yourself from one condition to another, regardless of what you may have done in the past.

In coming into the physical realm and vivifying matter (the physical body), the spirit gains experience through various situations in the process called human life. The spirit is continuously striving (evolving) to return to its original state of "Supreme Peace," which it lost when it became attached to a physical form and the constant movement of the ego. The problem arises when the mind "believes" itself to be a separate entity from the Self and develops an individual ego identity. In forgetting itself, the spirit searches for unity or oneness, but in believing what the mind tells it through the senses, the spirit (individual soul) "identifies" with that information. Thereby, it begins to search for unity and oneness in the way the limited senses and mind have convinced it to search. So people then look to human relationships and to the possession of wealth and physical objects in order to fill the void of the Soul, but of course this is not possible because nothing that is imperfect and limited (worldly relationships and objects) can satisfy that which is eternal and infinite (the Soul). Childhood is an important period in developing one's sense of identity and correct understanding about the nature of reality. The ego-personality develops desires and conjures up ideas as to how to achieve the fulfillment of those desires. Desire fulfillment is of two types, ignorant and wise.

The ignorant form of desire fulfillment is based on an erroneous understanding of the nature of one's desires and the way to resolve them. All desires arise from the need to regain the feeling of infinite bliss, which comes from achieving unity and supreme peace. Thus, the wise form of desire is the desire to attain Enlightenment. Due to identification with the mind and body, people search for fulfillment (bliss) by trying to satisfy the desires, which arise in the mind and body. When the spirit-based desire for unity becomes confused with the physical body-sense desires, the soul searches for unity by establishing intimate relationships with other individuals or by striving for worldly conditions which the ego considers to be good, while, at the same time, trying to avoid what it considers to be bad.

People become happy because the performance of sense-based activities temporarily allows them to release tension in the mind. This temporary release of mental tension (agitation) is a movement towards an illusion of peace, because once the tension has built back up, they must again seek situations, which will provide the same release over and over again. Sometimes this is attained through watching television, overeating, smoking, shopping, sexual activity, drugs or other activities.

Sometimes this ignorant form of life carries over into spirituality as well. People begin to feel satisfied when they have gone to church because they get a chance to sing, clap, dance or otherwise act in ways that they normally do not. Most often this is only an illusory release of tension and not a movement closer to the Spirit, as they would like to believe. Actually, this form of spiritual practice is agitating to the mind because it does not lead to real resolutions of the problems of life, but only a prolongation of them.

For some, when the frustration level builds beyond their ability to cope, they attempt suicide. Sometimes if a person perceives someone else is a threat to their happiness or if they harbor deep uncontrollable resentment towards someone, they may become violent with that person, even to the point of murder. Since this type of lifestyle is based on an erroneous understanding, the desires were never truly met and thereby resurfaced again and again, causing an endless cycle based on ignorance. The peace (release of tension) that people can experience through the mind and senses is only a glimpse of what is waiting in the Enlightened State. At some point all of the mental agitation must cease in order to allow the mind to experience the incomparable joy of the mind in which there are no thoughts. This is the only way to discover the deeper essence of the Self.

For these reasons, correct understanding of reality and of one's true identity is essential in conquering one's physical-sense desires in order to determine the true needs of the soul. The soul needs to expand beyond the confines of the physical body, family relationships and the physical world. From this position of freedom it experiences true peace and fulfillment which enables it to operate most effectively and peacefully in all realms (physical, mental, spiritual). Therefore, all relationships, including marriage and family, are good to the extent that they assist one in achieving the lofty goal of self-discovery through desire fulfillment based on wisdom rather than ignorance.

Every situation (good or bad) is a potential source of fulfillment. Dispassion, detachment, study, reflection and meditation, along with participation in the practical world when guided by the wisdom teachings, are the ways to achieve supreme fulfillment. One must cultivate dispassionate love, giving without expecting something in return. This provides the joy and peace that cannot come from possessive (ego-based) loving, which leaves one open for the inevitable pain of disappointment. One's own maturity and spiritual insight as well as spiritual guidance by the wise must assist one in deciding which relationships to engage in and to maintain. The wisdom teachings and guidance of a qualified spiritual preceptor are the best aids in making these choices.

Although seemingly a selfish venture, the pursuit of Enlightenment is the most selfless process in which one can engage, because if a person develops the qualities (virtues) necessary to achieve the coveted goal, all who come in contact with that person will benefit, just like in a dark room, everyone is able to see if only one person has light. Since all human beings are in reality expressions of the one Supreme Being, the best thing an individual can do is to free him/herself from the clutches of egoism and selfishness. These include feelings of machismo, feminism, immorality, hate, sadness, sexism, racism, etc., which are all ego-based mental conditions arising from ignorance. As each individual is saved, the world is thus one step closer to salvation. Therefore, doing one's best and then relinquishing the rest to the Self is the preferred course of spiritual life.

In relationships, as in any other area of life, the keys are honesty, patience and dispassionate love. One who aspires to achieve the greatest goal must realize that the road is full of obstacles and challenges. Relationships need to be prioritized according to the wisdom of Yoga philosophy. The relationship with the Self comes first. One cannot have a higher level of interactions if one is spiritually unfulfilled. When one discovers one's connection to the Kingdom, one's purpose in life will become clear. From this point, all other relationships will occur in harmony with this paramount priority. Otherwise, life situations will always seem to be in contradiction with one's deeper feelings and lead to constant mental unrest and anguish.

If a relationship is based on solid spiritual principles it will prosper, meaning that those in the relationship will grow spiritually and the happiness as well as the pain will lead them to greater heights of spiritual experience. A married person should live no differently than a single person who is practicing the teachings. They should also practice the spiritual disciplines to the extent that they can, including dispassion, celibacy, chanting, forgiveness, meditation, etc. When a relationship is spiritualized by the practice of the teachings it takes on a different path, a path that will lead to the resurrection (Enlightenment) of both partners in the relationship.[1]

HEALTH OF THE MIND AND BODY: VEGETARIANISM AND CHRISTIANITY, THE DIET OF CHRISTIAN INITIATES

As with the healing systems of Egypt and India, which encompassed Naturopathic approaches to health maintenance, and natural treatment of disease, the *Therapeuts*, another Egypto-Jewish sect in Ancient Egypt, were renowned for their mastery of the healing arts. For thousands of years the temples of Egypt had been centers for healing where the public could go for help in spiritual as well as physical health matters. For this reason they were called *Per Ankh,* "House of Life." Like Hippocrates, the famous Greek physician who studied with the Egyptian doctors, the Therapeuts assimilated the healing wisdom of Egypt, which included dietetics, fasting and surgery. Another important significance of the word "Therapeut" is its meaning: "servants of God" or priests of the mysteries.

The mind-body connection and its relation to physical and mental health, which was established in the health systems of Egypt for thousands of years before, was well understood by the Therapeutæ and the Essenes. The modern day medical establishment had until recently, rejected the idea of the mind-body connection. The ancient science of *Ayur-Veda* from India is similar in many respects to the therapeutic methods of preventative health care and holistic disease treatments described in the *Essene Gospel of Peace*. In much the same way as many Hindu sects promote vegetarianism, the *Gospel of Peace* emphasizes vegetarianism as a way to health. While there are a few passages in the Bible which declare that humans should eat fruits and vegetables, the *Gospel of Peace* devotes a great deal of attention to the subject and, in addition, considers food as a medicine.

Genesis 1
29. And God said, Behold, I have given you every herb bearing seed, which [is] upon the face of all the earth, and every tree, in which [is] the fruit of a tree yielding seed; to you it shall be for food.

Today, there are few, if any, Christian denominations which openly and actively promote vegetarianism, since it, like celibacy and detaching from family, friends and possessions, is not seen as a pleasant, attractive or pleasurable practice. It seems to cut into a person's enjoyment of life and is considered a "hard teaching" to follow by many. There is no doubt that many people who will read this book and explore the teachings of the Bible, in the context that they have been discussed, will find the teachings distasteful or even incongruous (not consistent with what is logical, customary, or expected; inappropriate). When people begin to realize that the goal of the teachings is to lead them to liberation or resurrection from the world of human experience, many become internally shaken with fear and immediately change the subject of conversation or leave the room. Talking about God and going to live with God in some kind of afterlife state is comfortable for many people, but the thought of actually giving up all and surrendering your very personality to God can cause a deep fear to enter the mind. This happens because the teachings are not correctly understood. Further, people are attached to their egoistic desires and to the illusory pleasures of the senses due to ignorance of the nature of the world. It should be understood that vegetarianism, prayer, rituals, etc., in and of themselves, do not make a person automatically "spiritual." However, they do aid in purifying the mind and body so that spiritual disciplines may be carried out more effectively.

The *Gospel of Peace* describes disease as the work of demons and indicates that it is caused by sinful behavior. The sinful behavior is usually related to lifestyles, which produce negative physical or mental conditions in the body. These may be too much worry, poor eating habits or poor hygiene. The prescribed treatment given by Jesus is to balance the spiritual through prayer and meditation, and the physical through vegetarianism (proper diet), regular fasting and internal cleansing (enema) according to the needs of the individual and then to: *"go in peace and sin no more."* Below Jesus emphasizes physical purification by keeping the laws of hygiene and diet (laws of the Earth

---

[1] For more on the Yogic teachings related to relationships, marriage, sublimation of sex desire, etc. see the book *Egyptian Tantra Yoga by* Dr. Muata Ashby.

Mother), and the spiritual, by keeping the practice of prayer and devotion to the Heavenly Father (the laws of the Father).

From the *Gospel of Peace*:

"Follow, therefore, first, the laws of your Earthly Mother, of which I have told you. And when her angels shall have cleansed and renewed your bodies and strengthened your eyes, you will be able to bear the light of our Heavenly Father."

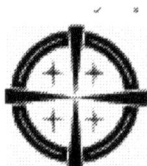

In the following passages from the *Gospel of Peace*, Jesus expands on the parable of Genesis 1:29.

For I tell you truly, he who kills, kills himself, and whosoever eats the flesh of slain beasts, eats of the body of death. For in his body every drop of their blood turns to poison; in his bones their bones to chalk; in his bowels their bowels to decay... And their death will become his death.

Behold, I have given you every herb bearing seed which is upon the face of all the earth, and every tree in which is the fruit of a tree yielding seed; to you it shall be for meat. And to every beast of the earth, and to every fowl of the air, and to everything that creepeth upon the earth, wherein there is breath of life, I give every green herb for meat...

But flesh, and the blood, which quickens it, shall ye not eat.

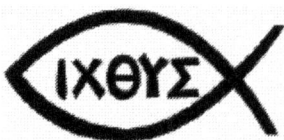

One more important aspect of the Christian doctrines related to vegetarianism is to be found in the ritual observance of *Lent*. Lent is a period of fasting, abstaining from eating meat and penitence which is traditionally observed by Christians in preparation for Easter. In the fourth century A.C.E., a tradition was established of eating only what was necessary to survive. The length of time was established as 40 days, beginning on Ash Wednesday and then extending (omitting Sundays) to the day before Easter. The observance varies within Anglican and Protestant churches. Also, the time of the observances has been questioned. According to an apostolic constitution in February 1966, issued by Pope Paul VI, fasting and abstinence during the Lent period are mandatory only on Ash Wednesday and Good Friday. However, in many other mystical traditions these observances were espoused as integral parts of the spiritual discipline to be followed all year around. Further, there is evidence to suggest that the Gnostic Christian sects also observed these vows perennially.

Above: The fish with the name of Jesus in Greek.

While it is true that Jesus fed the multitudes with fish, this episode should be understood for its deeper symbolism. The fish in Ancient Egyptian mythology was the symbol of guidance and chastity. Also, Jesus realized that he needed to reach the people at their current stage of culture. Therefore, he used what they would accept. However, it is to be understood that ordinary people who do not know any better may eat whatever they like. This is a factor of their ignorance. Thus, the Bible accepts them. However, the other teachings of the Bible clearly direct serious Christians toward the path of vegetarianism as a means to promote physical and mental purity and thereby spiritual evolution as well.

Many times people use the excuse that many cultures eat meat and have done so for generations, and so this means that anyone can. This is an expression of a person's egoistic desire to continue eating meat out of ignorance. Most people do not know that the human body is not designed to eat meat. Thus, it is no wonder that chronic degenerative illnesses are highest in countries with the highest meat consumption. Just because people live in areas with harsh climate where there is no other food available, it does not excuse others from following the better path for the reasons outlined here. If you have to eat meat in order to survive then of course you should eat meat. However, as soon as you are able to develop better conditions you should leave meat behind.

The Islamic faith has a similar tradition called *Ramadan.* The observance of Lent and Ramadan implies an understanding that fasting, vegetarianism and abstinence are means to bringing a person closer to their divine essence. So why wouldn't the church institute this policy every day of the year instead of just on Ash Wednesday and Good Friday?

One factor which shaped Western Christianity is the fact that the peoples of the European and Middle Eastern culture have lived for thousands of years on a diet which includes meat. Very possibly the practice of vegetarianism was difficult to institute since eating meat is somewhat addictive, like a drug. However, all vices need to be corrected if a human being expects to attain higher spiritual realization. How can a person profess to love humanity and nature if they promote killing and eating animals? Animals have minds, which are developed to a lesser degree than those of human beings are, but they feel pain and anguish nevertheless, and they express this in two ways when they are killed. First, the negative mental vibrations of anger, hatred and anguish go into the environment and degrade the planet. A sensitive person can feel these vibrations just as one feels vibrations of good will or ill will when entering a room filled with other people. Secondly, at the time of death the animals secrete toxins into their tissues, which act as poisons in the human body. Is it any wonder that Western countries have a higher incidence of gastrointestinal (colon) cancers? Meat also is very grounding to the soul. This means that it helps to intensify body-consciousness and dulls spiritual sensitivity.

Further, the meat industry is constantly experiencing scandals about antibiotics and hormones fed or implanted in cattle to make them grow faster, chemicals added to preserve the meat in stores, and deaths occurring from meat contaminated with deadly bacteria. Yet meat is advocated by the industry under the guise of serving the public health needs. Is it good service to humanity to promote something, which leads to death?

Greed plays an important part in deluding a person into selling poison to another. Delusion, ignorance and weak will play important roles in compelling a person to do things even when they know those things are not good for them. If you want to reach for spiritual heights you must strive to purify your physical body as well as your mind. If it means going against the norm of society, then Amen (so be it). Vegetarianism and the control of the sex-urge are two important ways of channeling the energies of the mind, enabling you to direct it towards spiritual realization. There is a vegetarian saying that goes "One should make one's stomach a garden and not a graveyard." When you eat meat, it rots (putrefies) in your guts because there is no proper digestion there to deal with it. When you see a dead animal on the side of the road reflect on what is happening to it and realize that you are poisoning yourself as if you were eating from that same carcass!

SIN, EVIL, THE DEVIL

Christian theology holds the belief of Original sin. It is said to be the condition of every human being which resulted from the original fall of Eve and Adam who were the first human beings created by God. However, the term 'original sin' is not found in the Bible. It is a concept which early Christian theologians developed to explain the need for redemption and salvation by Christ. They cite specific texts as implying original sin. These include Romans 7, 1 John 5:19, and Luke 11:13. Because of this first sin by Adam and Eve, all humanity is said to have lost the grace of God. Under this view it has been understood that the sin of Adam and Eve is endlessly transmitted to all human beings. In a sense this notion of original sin is correct, but not in the sense that the masses of Christian followers have come to understand. People have been guilty of committing the sin of eating from the tree of knowledge of good and evil from the beginning of time, that is, losing their sense of oneness with all Creation, but they have done so on their own and not as a form of evil inheritance from Adam and Eve. Human beings have tasted of the knowledge of duality and egoism, and these keep people separated from their knowledge of the Higher Self. In this respect people are committing the sin of ignorance and egoism. The soul came to believe that it was separate and individual, that it is not connected to God, and therefore, sin and its ramifications arise. Sin is the feeling of separation from God as well as the acts that arise out of this state of ignorance: egoism, selfishness, greed, anger, etc. In a broad context sin is anything that takes a person away from discovering their true Self or the knowledge of the truth.

The Judeo-Christian tradition has conceptualized the devil as a personality rather than as a concept to explain the negative or egoistic aspects of the human personality.

The devil in later Christian and Hebrew belief is equated with "the supreme spirit of evil," who for all time has been ruling over a kingdom of all evil spirits, and is in constant opposition to God. The word "Devil" is derived from the Latin *diabolus*, and from the Greek *diabolos,* which is an adjective that means *slanderous.* It is also used in ancient Greek as a noun to identify a specific person as being a slanderer. The term "diabolos" was used for the *Septuagint* or Greek translation of the Jewish Bible, not referring to human beings, but in order to translate the Hebrew word *ha-satan* (the satan), an expression which was originally used as the title of one of the members of the divine court whose function was to act as a roving spy for God. Satan gathered intelligence about human beings during his travels on earth just like the Hindu character Narada, a Sage who would relate information about the happenings on earth to Lord Vishnu.

Thus, originally, Satan meant "an opponent and not a particular being with actual existence. At around the 6th century B.C.E., Satan appears in the Old Testament as an individual angel who is subordinate to God. Gradually, as Jewish and Christian tradition developed around this idea, Satan became known as a personality who was the source of all evil, and was responsible for leading human beings into sin. This character was most likely influenced by the Ancient Egyptian God, Set (Seth), who killed his own brother. However, even Set was never seen as the "source of evil itself" until the late dynastic period, which was when the Jewish people were living in Egypt. This notion of a personality who causes evil in human beings is extremely dangerous because it allows people with poor moral development to shirk responsibility for their actions.

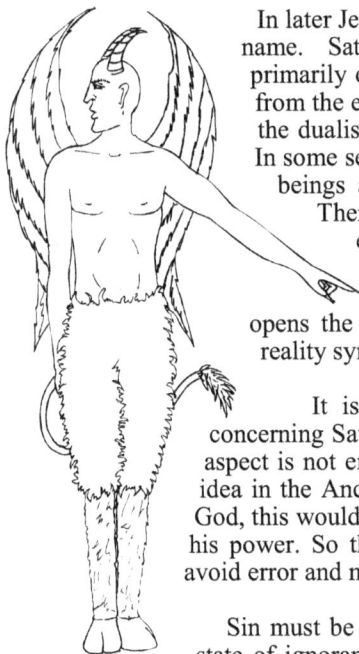

In later Jewish tradition, and therefore also in early Christian thought, this title became a proper name. Satan was then seen as a personified adversary not only of human beings, but also primarily of God. The development of the devil as a personified evil adversary probably arose from the early Jewish and Christian association with the dualistic theologies of Persia as well as the dualistic philosophy of Zoroaster and the misunderstanding of the Egyptian character *Set*. In some segments of Jewish theology, the idea of Satan developed as an "evil impulse." Human beings are seen as susceptible to a force, which is outside of, and separate from them. Therefore, with this view it is possible for a human being to become "possessed" by the evil force and coerced into wrongdoing. Jesus was seen as the savior who broke the power of the devil over human beings. This view is dangerous because it negates the power of the human mind to control itself, the power of free will. It also opens the door to superstition and imagination about evil supernatural beings, which are in reality symbols mistaken as real beings that exist in fact.

It is important to note that in both the Christian and Jewish systems, the dualism concerning Satan is always temporary since the devil is ultimately subject to God, even though this aspect is not emphasized in popular discourses. This view is more closely in tune with the original idea in the Ancient Egyptian teaching. Otherwise, if Satan were the true adversary of God, this would mean that God is not omnipotent because there is a being who can limit his power. So the teaching related to Satan must be correctly understood in order to avoid error and misunderstanding in one's spiritual movement.

Above: The classic depiction of the devil in Judeo-Christian iconography.

Sin must be understood, as the idea of separation between one's self and God, the state of ignorance about one's own spiritual essence. Evil must be understood as the actions of people who are ignorant of the higher spiritual reality within themselves. Such actions are based on anger, hatred, greed, lust, jealousy, etc. Each person must take responsibility for their actions while striving to engender a sense of Divine Presence within themselves. When this occurs, the very basis of sin and ignorance is dispelled from the mind. At this stage of spiritual development there is transcendence of the notion of good and evil. Understanding all to be part of oneself, there is no need to debate about one's treatment of others. One's treatment of others becomes a spontaneous act based on love, compassion, forgiveness and magnanimity, much like there is instant forgiveness of one's teeth when they bite one's tongue. This is the true goal of religion—to rise above ignorance (evil, egoism).

In Matthew Chapter 6, verses 9-13, Jesus instructs his followers as to how they should pray to God. The end of the prayer (verse 13) contains a peculiar statement, which seems, on the surface, to be very contradictory.

9. After this manner therefore pray ye: Our Father who art in heaven, Hallowed be thy name.
10 Thy kingdom come. Thy will be done on earth, as [it is] in heaven.
11 Give us this day our daily bread.
12 And forgive us our debts, as we forgive our debtors.
13 And lead us not into temptation, but deliver us from evil: For thine is the kingdom, and the power, and the glory, forever. Amen.

The ordinary Christian doctrine almost always presupposes the existence of an evil entity ordinarily referred to as the devil. However, verse 13 seems to refer to God as the source of temptation (evil). Why should the prayer asking not to be led into temptation be directed towards God and not the devil? The only answer, which is possible from a mystical point of view, is that God is the source of both evil and good. More accurately, God sustains Creation and Creation is the venue where good and evil can exist. However, human beings always have a choice to follow the path of good or of evil. Then this understanding also leads to the conclusion that there is no devil as such, only evil thoughts and actions. This teaching reflects the understanding and subtle exposition by the Christian Sages, of the highly advanced teaching known as non-duality. This is an understanding that in reality God has no rivals or contenders. God is Absolute and Supreme because God is the only reality behind good as well as evil. In reality God transcends these two concepts which the mind has created for the purpose of understanding and explaining human activities. In the final analysis, an advanced spiritual aspirant must understand that there is no outside force, which pushes an individual to evil actions. Evil is an expression of the level of the lack of understanding of one's true nature (God), just as darkness is an manifestation of the degree to which the sun is absent.

A serious follower of the teachings must develop a keen understanding of the true meaning of sin and its implications. Sinful acts are those acts *you* perform which carry you away from the discovery of your true being. They are characterized by pettiness, greed, anger, hard-heartedness, hatred, egoism, infatuation, etc. Virtuous acts are those acts which *you* perform which move you forward towards integration of your personality and eventual merging of your individual ego with the Cosmic Self, God. Virtue implies developing peace, contentment, selflessness, and finally, self-discovery. Virtuous acts are characterized by peacefulness, kindness, selflessness, sharing, giving, universal love, forgiveness, serenity and other lofty qualities.

In this perspective, that which takes you away from Divine-realization is demoniac (satanic), while that which brings you closer to God-realization is divine. Hence, just as there is no Jesus-like "savior" outside of yourself, likewise, there is no personality called "the devil" that exists in fact as a distinct personality outside of yourself. The thoughts and actions you choose are what you classify as either divine or demoniac. Therefore, your fate lies with the thoughts and actions by which you choose to live. Your present ego-personality is the creation of your past actions, feelings, thoughts and experiences.

WHAT IS THE EGO AND EGOISM?

The Indian Vedantic text Yoga Vasistha Vol. II describes the ego as follows.

When the Self (transcendental-Absolute consciousness) develops identification with the limited body, it assumes the form of *ahamkara* (egoism), which expresses in this manner: "I am this body. I am this mortal individual." This egoism is the true root of all evil. 86-p 63

Pride, vanity, conceit, narcissism, vainglory, superiority, insolence, presumption, arrogance, disdain, haughtiness, hauteur, loftiness, selfishness, lordliness, superciliousness, etc., represent various forms of intensification of the ego. Through the intensification of body-consciousness and through the pursuit of selfish acts in the hopes of fulfilling personal desires, the ego idea of self becomes inflated. The mind is more and more intensely turned towards the individual self, the body and the world for fulfillment rather than towards the transcendental Self, the spirit within.

The characteristics mentioned above are considered to be demoniac or satanic forms of behavior. On the other hand, selfless service, charity, inward renunciation of possessions, etc., represent saintly or virtuous qualities, which lead to the Divine because they cause effacement of the ego. This effacement leaves the soul free of the troubles, needs, concerns and sufferings of the ego-self and gives rise to the Christ-Self. It is this ego-body consciousness idea of self which produces the major obstacle to spiritual evolution. It is this very problem that mystical Christian wisdom and the ceremony of the Christian Eucharist is directed to solving.

Ego-effacement is the central point of attention in all rituals and mystical philosophies. At many times through the history of Christianity, this issue was dealt with directly by certain Christian Mystics who often found themselves ostracized by the mainstream members of the church. In some instances, the problem is described as the need to free the soul from the body, although the message of the church to the masses does not refer to it specifically in those terms nor does it describe a course of action to effect such a release. The following statement from *Gregory I* or *Gregory the Great* (c. 540-604 A.C.E.) illustrates the struggle of the mystic. Gregory was a writer and monk who became pope in 590 A.C.E.

"My sad mind, laboring under the sourness of its engagements, remembers how it went with me formerly in the monastery, how all perishable things were beneath it, how it rose above all that was transitory, and, though still in the body, went out in contemplation beyond the bars of the flesh" *(Dial. I Perf.)*.

Gregory's description of his contemplative (meditative) experiences show his understanding of a perception which lies beyond the ordinary bounds of the human sense organs and thinking mind. He understood the concept of the witnessing Self because he wrote about the mind as being separate from himself, as a possession rather than as himself. This is a very important distinction. If it were possible for you, the reader, to transcend your sense perceptions and identification with the body, it would be possible to perceive a vast expansive reality, which illumines all things and reveals them to be transitory and perishable.

There is a strong current of mystical thought within the Catholic church, although its practice has remained confined to the monastic orders, the unrecognized mystical Christian traditions and in the writings of certain Christian mystics such as Gregory, rather than in the main dogma and teaching to the masses. Some Christians such as St. Francis of Asisi were considered to be "fools." Many times, those such as St. Francis, who had known mystical experience, were the targets of strong rebuke and disbelief. They were ridiculed for their ascetic lifestyle and self-discipline, the very practices, which the mystics recognized as the mechanism for achieving purity of heart, which ultimately frees the soul from bondage to the body.

This situation has led to a practice of religion which tends to remain at the level of ritual and myth, centering around the Christian Mass, the Eucharist, and holidays celebrating the story of Jesus, rather than focusing on the meaning of the mass ritual and the mystical symbolism of the story. This meaning is supposed to be revealed to the individual through the metaphysical and mystical aspects of religious practice. The mystical mechanism for leading the individual to have the kind of realizations that Gregory had is now less defined and consequently less available to those who seek to deepen their spirituality through the Christian faith. Great Christian mystics who were in their time reviled, but who are now accepted as pre-eminent Christian theologians, sought to directly confront the question of the ego. This was accomplished primarily through devotion to and identification with Christ. This devotion is first directed to the personality of Jesus, and then goes beyond that identification, entering into the transcendental reality which is, as Gregory puts it, *beyond the bars of the flesh.* This is the Christ. In the following text from the Bible, Jesus' opinion about the "personality" of people is given.

Matthew 22

16 And they sent out to him their disciples with the Herodians, saying, Master, we know that thou art true, and teachest the way of God in truth, neither carest thou for any [man]: for thou regardest not the person of men.

Jesus does not regard the personality or the ego as real *(neither carest thou for any [man]: for thou regardest not the person of me*n). He ascribes truth and reality to the Self (God) who is eternal. To Jesus it is the feeling of identification with the transcendental Self which breaks the bonds of mental attachment to that which is transitory and facilitates the perception of that which is absolute. This is the true meaning of the practice of the communion.

Matthew 24

35 Heaven and earth shall pass away, but my words shall not pass away.

THE GREATEST SECRET: GOD IS THE MYSTERY, THE LIGHT WITHIN

Gospel of Thomas:
2. Jesus says: "If those who seek to attract you say to you: "See, the Kingdom is in Heaven!" then the birds of heaven will get there before you. If they say to you: "It is in the sea!" then the fish will get there before you. But you need to understand, the Kingdom is both within you and it is outside of you as well."
3. When you know yourselves, then you will be known, and you will know {realize} that it is you who are the sons of the living Father. But if you do not know yourselves, then you will be in a state of poverty, and it is you who are the poverty.

The Gospel of Thomas continuously points the aspirant to her/himself as the knower and enlightener of Self. Here Jesus emphasizes that knowing oneself is the key to the Kingdom of the Living Father in much the same way as Buddhist Sages refer to the Living Buddha. The discovery of that Self is the result of realizing the wisdom {Gnosis} within oneself.

New Testament John 11

25 Jesus said to her, I am the resurrection, and the life: he that believes in me, though he were dead, yet shall he live.

When Jesus states that he is the resurrection and the life he is in reality stating that anyone who realizes the wisdom within themselves, which he represents, will attain Enlightenment {*though dead, shall he live*}. This point is confirmed in the following verse from the Gospel of Thomas, where Jesus acknowledges Thomas as his equal since he has realized that Jesus is beyond any description or categorization. In this realization, Thomas himself has recognized the transcendental aspect of Jesus, the Christ, which is also within him and beyond any categorization. Similarly, the Taoist and Upanishadic texts say that those who experience the Self cannot define it.

14. Jesus says to his disciples: "Compare me and tell me whom I am like." Simon Peter says to him: "You are like a just angel!" Matthew says to him: "You are like a wise man and a philosopher!" Thomas says to him: "Master, my tongue cannot find words to say whom you are like!" Jesus says: "I am no longer thy master; for you have drunk, and you are inebriated from the bubbling spring which I have measured out."

The *Bhagavad Gita* contains similar passages to the *Gospel of Thomas.* In the *Gita*, Arjuna, the disciple of Krishna, is told of the secret wisdom.

Gita: Chapter 11 Vishwarup Darshan Yogah—the Yoga of the Vision of the Cosmic Form

1. Arjuna said, "O Krishna, the Supreme Secret concerning the Self which you have graciously presented before me, has dispelled my delusion.

In the same chapter of the *Gita* Arjuna is given a vision of the cosmic form of Krishna. It encompasses all things, like the Kingdom of Heaven that is spoken of by Jesus. As we will see, this vision is similar to those reported in the Bible and in the Gnostic Gospels in very important ways.

Gita: Chapter 11

3. O Supreme Being, whatever You say about Yourself is indeed so. But still, O best of the souls, I would like to behold Your Divine Form.

4. If You consider that it is possible for me to behold your Divine Form, then, O Lord of Yoga, please reveal to me Your imperishable Form.

5. Lord Krishna said, Behold, O Arjuna, My hundreds and thousands of divine forms, of different colors and shapes.

6. Behold the sun gods, the Vasus, the Rudras, the Ashwini-kumaras, and the wind-gods. Behold many more wonders that you have never seen before.

7. O conqueror of sleep, today, even in my body beholds the entire universe consisting of movables and immovables centered in Me, and also behold what you would wish to see.

8. But, you cannot behold My Divine Form with your physical eyes, therefore, I am bestowing upon you the intuitional vision by which you will be able to behold my Divine Glory and Cosmic Powers.

9. Sanjaya said, O King, then Sri Hari, the Great Lord of Yoga, thus saying revealed His Divine Form to Arjuna.

10. With numerous faces and eyes, with numerous wondrous scenes, dazzling with divine ornaments, with uplifted divine weapons (such is the form he revealed).

16. O Lord of the universe, the Deity of Cosmic Form, I behold you everywhere having countless forms, countless arms, stomachs, faces and eyes. I do not see the beginning, middle or end of Your Being.

19. I behold You as one devoid of beginning, middle and end; endowed with limitless valor, with innumerable arms, having sun and moon as Your eyes, with faces blazing with fire, scorching this world with your radiance.

20. All the directions as well as that which is in the middle of the earth and sky are filled with You alone. O Great Soul, beholding this terrible and strange form of Yours, the three worlds are being agitated.

23. Seeing Your great form with many faces, many eyes, many arms, many thighs and feet, and many terrible tusks and stomachs, O Mighty Armed, the worlds are terrified and so am I.

The preceding text from the Gita parallels the vision of Peter, James, and John as they explain how *"he was transfigured before them."* This moment of *"transfiguration"* is the moment wherein Christ reveals itself to the seeker. Compare statements 20 and 23 from the Gita where Arjuna, the seeker (aspirant, initiate, disciple) beholds the multiform vision of God and describes it as a *"terrible and strange form"*(20) and *"great form"*(23), to the following segment from the *Apocalypse of Peter* which describes how Peter, in trance, experiences Christ with *"fear and joy"*:

{the Savior} said to me... "...put your hands upon {your} eyes ... and say what you see!" But when I had done it, I did not see anything. I said, "No one sees {this way}." Again he told me, "Do it again." And there came into me fear and joy, for I saw a new light, greater than the light of day.

In the *Gospel of Thomas*, Jesus gives further insight into the meaning of the light:

29. There is light within a man of light, and he lights up the whole world. If he does not shine, then he is in darkness.

The following statement from the *Gita* elucidates further on the meaning of light and the sun:

Gita—Chapter 3; Karma Yogah—the Yoga of Action:
The intellect lit up with...the light of wisdom is superior to the path of selfless action...

Gita Chapter 5
16. For those whose ignorance has been destroyed by the knowledge of the Self, wisdom shines forth like the sun, revealing the Reality of the Transcendental Self.

Such Gnostic statements as those proceeding were available to the writers of the traditional New Testament as evidenced by John 11:9-10:

If someone walks in the day he does not stumble, because he sees the light of this world. But if someone walks in the night, he stumbles because the light is not with him.

There is an important difference between the Gnostic and Biblical statements presented above. The Bible points the reader in the direction of a physical light and, therefore, to exoteric or worldly conceptions about the wisdom being imparted. For instance, from this statement we might conclude that we simply need to understand the stories about Jesus' life and the other church doctrines in order to be resurrected. On the other hand, the statement from the *Gospel of Thomas* leads us to a broader and more explicit understanding of the light. It implies that if there is light within *"a man,"* he may illuminate the entire planet. This statement does not suggest that an illuminated person actually becomes a huge lamp, which can light up the entire world. Rather, it is a figurative way of describing the magnanimity and divinity within *"the man"* who has the light of wisdom and intuitive knowledge *"within."* It refers to a complete transformation in consciousness. Further, there is a clear implication that Jesus himself acknowledges the existence of others beside himself who also carry the *"light within."* This understanding that divinity does not belong exclusively to Jesus is an important feature of Gnostic teachings. It is also an inherent factor of Indian as well as Ancient Egyptian mystical philosophy.

In the following segments from the Gita, the same explicit feeling about the light "within" is also found.

Gita: Chapter 5 Karma Sanyas Yoga—The Yoga of Renunciation of Action

24. One who finds bliss within, rejoices within, and finds the light of wisdom within himself — such a Yogi becomes Brahman, and attains absolute freedom (Nirvana).

Gita: Chapter 8 Akshara Brahma Yogah—the Yoga of Imperishable Brahman

26. These two paths—the path of Light and that of Darkness are considered beginningless. Following the path of Light one does not return, while following the path of darkness one returns.

In the following statements we are to understand that God, as represented by the deity Krishna, is himself the light. Further, a new parallel to the character of Jesus emerges with the *"I Am"* formula in which Jesus declares that he is, or from a Gnostic perspective, what he represents, is Christhood, the teaching, the light of wisdom itself.

Gita: Chapter 7 Jnana Vijnana Yogah—the Yoga of Wisdom and Realization

8. O Son of Kunti! I am the taste in the waters, I am the light in the sun and the moon; I am Pranava (Om) in the Vedas, the sound in the Ether element, and manliness in men.

9. I am the pure fragrance in earth, I am the effulgence in fire,[I] I am the life in all living beings, and I am the austerity in the ascetics.

10. O Partha, know Me to be the eternal seed of all beings. I am the intellect in the wise, the valor of those who are valiant.

11. O Best of the Bharatas! Among the strong, I am their strength that is devoid of lust and passion. Among all beings I am the desire that is not opposed to Dharma (the ethical law).

[I] Fire of worldly desire.

Compare the statements in the Gita to the following "I am" statements from the traditional New Testament. Using the Yogic principles inherent in mystical Christianity it is clear to see that these statements are referring to the same mystical ideal.

Revelations 1
   8 I am Alpha and Omega, the beginning and the ending, saith the Lord, who is, and who was, and who is to come, the Almighty.

John 1:23
   23 He said, I [am] the voice of one crying in the wilderness, Make straight the way of the Lord, as said the prophet Isaiah.

John 6:35
   35 And Jesus said to them, I am the bread of life: he that cometh to me shall never hunger; and he that believes on me shall never thirst.

John 6:41
   41 The Jews then murmured at him, because he said, I am the bread which came down from heaven.

John 6:51
   51 I am the living bread, which came down from heaven: if any man shall eat of this bread, he shall live forever: and the bread that I will give is my flesh, which I will give for the life of the world.

John 8:12

   12. Then Jesus spoke again to them, saying I am the light of the world: he that followeth me shall not walk in darkness, but shall have the light of life.

John 9:5
   5 As long as I am in the world, I am the light of the world.

John 10:7
   7 Then said Jesus to them again, Verily, verily, I say to you, I am the door of the sheep.

John 10:9
   9 I am the door: by me if any man shall enter, he shall be saved, and shall go in and out, and find pasture.

John 10:11
   11 I am the good shepherd: the good shepherd[1] giveth his life for the sheep.

John 10:14
   14 I am the good shepherd, and know my [sheep], and am known by mine.

John 11:25
   25 Jesus said to her, I am the resurrection, and the life: he that believes in me, though he were dead, yet shall he live...

John 14:6
   6 Jesus saith to him, I am the way, and the truth, and the life: no man cometh to the Father, but by me.

John 15:1
   1. I am the true vine, and my Father is the vinedresser.

John 15:5
   5 I am the vine, ye [are] the branches: He that abideth in me, and I in him, the same bringeth forth much fruit: for without me ye can do nothing. {without me: or, severed from me}
Compare the previous statements to the following Egyptian Hermetic teaching. The *I am* statement in all of them is pointing to the same mystical truth.

---

[1] Death of the physical body. State of ignorance about God, The Kingdom of Heaven (God).

"I am the Mind - the Eternal Teacher. I am the begetter of the Word - the Redeemer of all humankind - and in the nature of the wise, the Word takes flesh. By means of the Word, the world is saved. I, Thought - the begetter of the Word, the Mind - come only unto they that are holy, good, pure and merciful, and that live piously and religiously, and my presence is an inspiration and a help to them, for when I come, they immediately know all things and adore the Universal Spirit. Before such wise and philosophic ones die, they learn to renounce their senses, knowing that these are the enemies of their immortal Souls.[16]

The idea of the *Word* or *Logos* being the savior of the world existed before Christianity. The main difference in Orthodox Roman Christianity was that the *"word"* or saving wisdom became flesh in the personality of Jesus, the man. This was an idea that Gnostic Christianity and other mystery religions rejected. The more ancient idea holds that the *word* itself is not only the Divine Presence, but its power of manifestation as well. With this understanding, the entire universe, including the human personality, body and mind are all manifestations of the *"Living Word"* itself—not just Jesus. The new Christian idea that emerged sees the *word* as being embodied in the person of Jesus himself and nowhere else. This is a more egoistic view. Jesus is a symbol of the potential realization of the divine word or essence in every human being.

In relation to the term *"word,"* another Biblical term, *"Dabhar,"* is of interest. This word implies creation, deeds, actions, and accomplishments as opposed to talk. It relates to the creative power of the Divine, of which human beings partake. Biblical scholars have often confused the meanings of these terms. However, a thorough understanding of the writings of the Hellenistic period known as *"Hermetic"* and the more ancient writings of Egypt reveal the correct interpretation. The following verses come from various chapters throughout the Egyptian *Book of Coming Forth By Day*, which show the initiate's gradual realization that the gods are in reality aspects of him/herself. This is the earliest known form of the *"I am"* formula used in philosophy. Thus, the I am (God) is the source of all action and all existence. Further, the initiate understands his/her true nature and its power:

"I am the Great God, the self created one, Nun...I am Ra...I am Geb...I am Atum...I am Asar...I am Min...I am Shu...I am Anubis...I am Aset...I am Hathor...I am Sekhmet...I am Orion...I am Saa...I am the Lion... I am the young Bull...I am Hapi who comes forth as the river Nile..."

In the following segments from Chapter 23 of the Ancient Egyptian *Book of Coming Forth By Day*, the initiate, having understood his oneness, and having identified with God in the form of Asar, exclaims the following:

"I am yesterday, today and tomorrow. I have the power to be born a second time. I am the source from which the gods arise."

This is the moment of great realization to which the entire religious system of the Ausarian Resurrection was directed. The aspirant or initiate was to understand his identity with the transcendental reality properly before death, but if not, then on the way through the Duat (after-death state or astral plane of mind). As with the Gnostics, the Ancient Egyptians considered those who had not had this mystical experience as *"Mortals"* while those who had it were called *"Sons of Light."*[44]

The following verse from the traditional New Testament reveals a close similarity in the idea of being an offspring or follower of the light.

John 12:36
36 While ye have light, believe in the light, that ye may be the children of light. These things spoke Jesus, and departed, and was hidden from them.

PURIFICATION BY THE FIRE OF WISDOM

The metaphor of fire is used extensively in Christian, Hebrew and other mythologies. The following quotes from India further clarify the meaning of fire as a symbol of the knowledge, which burns away karmas or mental obstructions in the path of the spiritual seeker:

Bhagavad Gita Chapter 4

37. Oh Arjuna, just as blazing fire turns fuel into ashes, so the fire of wisdom turns all actions into ashes.

Teachings of Hermes

"The Mind being builder doth use the fire as tool for the construction of all things, but that of man only for things on earth. Stripped of its fire the mind on earth cannot make things divine, for it is human in its dispensation. And such a Soul, when from the body freed, if it have fought the fight of piety-to Know God and to do wrong to no one-such a Soul becomes entirely mind. Whereas the impious Soul remains in its own essence, chastised by its own self."

In Chapter 9, Krishna (God) states that he himself is the fire as well as the one who makes sacrifices (referring to the aspirant on the spiritual path) as well as the object which is thrown into the fire. Krishna is everything.

16. I am Kratu, I am Yajna, I am Swadha, I am the medicinal herb, I am the sacred Mantra, the clarified butter that is poured in fire; as well as I am the fire, and the very act of offering oblation.

Similarly, as Buddha is *"The awakened one,"* Jesus claims to be not only *"The way"* and *"The light,"* but he also claims to be the fire itself and proclaims that anyone who is near him is also near the fire:

86. Jesus says: "He who is near me is near the fire, and he who is far from me is far from the Kingdom.[51]

The philosophy of the "field" is also very important in both Christian and Hindu mythology. It is an expression referring to the field of consciousness within which the soul plays out various roles and carries out various actions as well as interacts with others and with objects in time and space. This teaching emphasizes learning the rules by which this field operates and then changing one's attitude and behavior in such a way as to not be trapped by or caught up in the enslaving factors within it through ignorance. In the Hermetic Texts and Chapter 13 of the *Bhagavad Gita*, a more detailed explanation of Jesus' statement in Matthew 13:38 and 13:44 may be found in reference to the *field*:

"I am the lotus pure coming forth from the god of light, the guardian of the nostril of Ra, the guardian of the nose of Hathor; I make my journey; I run after him who is Horus. I am the pure one coming forth from the fields."

Gita: Chapter 13, Kshetra-Kshetrajna Vibhag Yogah—the Division of Field and the Knower of the Field

1. The Blessed Lord said, O Arjuna, this body is known as the Field, and the One who knows this body is the Knower of the Field. Thus do the Sages say who have discerned into the nature of both.

2. Know Me as the Knower of the Field in all beings. It is My view that true knowledge consists in knowing the distinction between the Field and the Knower of the Field.

6. Desire, aversion, pleasure, pain, the aggregate (of body and senses), consciousness, firmness—this in brief is the Field along with its effects.

7. Absence of pride, absence of hypocrisy, non-violence, forbearance, uprightness, service of preceptor, purity, steadiness, control over the body and senses.

8. Dispassion towards the objects of the senses, absence of egoism, and reflection upon the evils associated with birth, death, old age, disease and pain.

9. Detachment, absence of the feeling of mine-ness towards son, wife, house and the like and constant equanimity of mind in all happenings whether desirable or undesirable.

10. Unflinching devotion to Me through the Yoga of inseparability, abiding in solitary places, not delighting in the company of the worldly-minded.

12. I will relate to you that which is to be known,[I] knowing which one attains immortality. It is the Supreme Brahman, who is without beginning, who is said to be neither existent nor non-existent.

13. With His hands and feet everywhere, head and eyes and faces everywhere, ears everywhere thus permeating all that Brahman dwells in this world.

[I] Compare with Matthew 16:19

From the Bible:

Leviticus 19:19

19. Ye shall keep my statutes. Thou shalt not let thy cattle mate with another kind: thou shalt not sow thy field with mixed seed: neither shall a garment mingled of linen and woolen come upon thee.

Matthew 13:24

24. Another parable he told to them, saying, The Kingdom of Heaven is likened to a man who sowed good seed in his field...

Matthew 13:31

31 Another parable he put forth to them, saying, The Kingdom of Heaven is like a grain of mustard seed, which a man took, and sowed in his field.

Matthew 13:38

38 The field is the world; the good seed are the children of the Kingdom; but the tares are the children of the wicked [one];

1 Corinthians 3:9

9 For we are laborers together with God: ye are God's field, [ye are] God's building. {husbandry: or, tillage}

Matthew 16:19

And I will give to thee the keys of the Kingdom of Heaven: and whatever thou shalt bind on earth shall be bound in heaven: and whatever thou shalt loose on earth shall be loosed in heaven.

In Leviticus 19:19 we are told that sowing mixed seed or allowing the cattle to mate with another kind is prohibited because it will bear mixed crops. This parable relates to sowing good and evil thoughts in the mind and it goes along with Matthew 6:24 - *No man can serve two masters: for either he will hate the one, and love the other; or else he will hold to the one, and despise the other. Ye cannot serve God and money.*

The other parables and injunctions clarify this teaching, explaining that life itself (including the personality and the world of time and space) is the field, and that there is a necessity to sow good seed in the form of righteous actions and positive thinking. In Mark 10:25, presented in an earlier chapter, Jesus talks about the difficulty of discovering the Kingdom of Heaven when there is an abundance of prosperity. In the following quotations from the Gita, the need to control one's desire for wealth is further elucidated:

Gita: Chapter 1

33. People, for whom I would have desired to gain kingdom, enjoyments and prosperity, are here assembled having given up their concern for their life and wealth.

Gita: Chapter 7

16. O Best of the Bharatas! There are four types of virtuous men who worship Me—Arta (distressed), Jinjasu (inquirer), Artharthi (desirer of wealth), and Jnani (the man of wisdom).

17. Of these four the Jnani who is ever united with God, and has one-pointed devotion to God is the best. Because, I am supremely dear to the man of wisdom, and he is dear to Me.

18. All these (four types) are indeed the best; however, I consider the man of wisdom as My very Self. For with his mind fully established in My Self, he considers Me as his highest goal.

CHAPTER XII: INTRODUCTION TO CHRISTIAN YOGA MEDITATION

THE NEXT STEP IN THE JOURNEY FROM JESUS TO CHRIST

We have seen how the teachings of the Bible and the Nag Hammadi Library contain almost direct correlations to the mystical teachings of Ancient Egypt and India. We have also seen that the main objective of Christianity is far more profound, personal and sublime than the ordinary message usually given by the church. Indeed, we are not just to practice being good for the sake of waiting for some savior at the end of time, but we are to realize our divinity, our oneness and unity in, and as, Christ, even before death, and in so doing, discover the Kingdom of Heaven here and now.

This volume in the Christian Yoga series represents the Jesus aspect of the "Journey from Jesus to Christ." It has presented the origins and history of Christianity from Ancient Egypt up to the present day, and has introduced the mystical aspects of Christianity as it was originally intended to be understood. This first volume in the study of the history and wisdom teachings of Christian Yoga (Gnostic Christian mysticism) has prepared you for the second part of the journey, the movement towards Christ. The second volume in this series will expand into the deeper aspects of the teachings presented here. This volume is the foundation for understanding the higher teachings of mysticism and it is a tribute to the glorious efforts of the early Egyptian Gnostic Christian Sages who brought forth the eternal mystical principles of life in the form of Christianity.

You must now continue the journey of spiritualizing your life by practicing the affirmations of Christian wisdom, applying Christian teachings to your day to day activities and meditating on the Christian teachings daily. The following section is an introduction to meditation.

HOW TO BEGIN THE JOURNEY FROM JESUS TO CHRIST

The following is an introduction to meditation using the wisdom teachings presented in this volume. A more advanced instruction on the art of meditation will be presented in Christian Yoga Volume II. The presentation below will serve to get the serious aspirant started on the path of meditation. Audio tapes will be available through the Sema Institute for those desiring a guided Gnostic Christian meditation experience.

Meditation may be thought of or defined as the practice of mental exercises and disciplines to enable the meditator to achieve control over the mind, specifically, to stop the vibrations of the mind due to unwanted thoughts, imaginations, etc.

The theory of meditation is that when the mind and senses are controlled and transcended, the awareness of the transcendental state of consciousness becomes evident. From here, consciousness-awareness expands, allowing the meditator to discover the latent abilities of the unconscious mind. When this occurs, an immense feeling of joy emerges from within, the desire for happiness and fulfillment through external objects and situations dwindles and a peaceful, transcendental state of mind develops. Also, the inner resources are discovered which will allow the practitioner to meet the challenges of life (disappointments, disease, death, etc.) while maintaining a poised state of mind.

Meditation and Yoga Philosophy are disciplines which are directed toward increasing awareness. Awareness or consciousness can only be increased when the mind is in a state of peace and harmony. Thus, the disciplines of Meditation (which are part of the Yoga) are the primary means of controlling the mind and allowing the individual to mature psychologically and spiritually.

Modern scientific research has proven that one of the most effective things anyone can do to promote mental and physical health is to sit quietly for 20 minutes twice each day. This is more effective than a change in diet, vitamins, food supplements, medicines, etc. It is not necessary to possess any special skill or training. All that is required is that one achieves a relaxed state of mind, unburdened by the duties of the day. You may sit from a few minutes up to an hour in the morning and in the late afternoon. Begin by sitting quietly for five minutes each day and building up your meditation time every week.

This simple practice, if followed each day, will promote above average physical health and spiritual evolution. One's mental and emotional health will be maintained in a healthy state as well. The most important thing to remember during this meditation time is to just relax and not try to stop the mind from pursuing a particular idea but also not trying to actively make the mind pursue a particular thought or idea. If a Hekau or Mantra (Chanting-Prayer) is recited, or if a special icon is meditated upon, the mind should not be forced to hold it. Rather, one should direct the mind and when one realizes that one has been carried away with a particular thought, bring the mind gently back to the original object of meditation, in this way, it will eventually settle where it feels most comfortable and at peace.

During the practice, sometimes one will know that one has been carried away into thoughts about what one needs to do, or who needs to be called, or is something burning in the kitchen?, etc. These thoughts are worldly thoughts. Simply bring the mind back to the original object of meditation or the hekau. With more practice, the awareness of the hekau or object of meditation (candle, mandala, etc.) will dissipate as you go deeper. This is the positive, meditative movement that is desired. The goal is to relax to such a degree that the mind drifts to deeper and deeper levels of consciousness, finally reaching the source of consciousness, the source of all thought; then the mind transcends even this level of consciousness and there, communes with the Absolute Reality, God. This is the state of "Cosmic Consciousness", the state of enlightenment. After a while, the mental process will remain at the Soul level all the time. This is the Enlightened Sage Level.

The following are Christian words of power and affirmations. You will notice that they all correspond to the ancient Egyptian and Indian teachings. It should be noted here that Christian monasticism first began in Egypt and Asia minor around the years 200-350 ACE. Hesychasm, from the Greek word *hesychia* or "quietness", is a term designating a contemplative tradition which dates from the 4th century ACE in Eastern Christian monasticism. The Hesychast monks, in particular, the ones from the monasteries of Mount Athos, engaged in a practice of devoting themselves to continuous mental prayer as a means to achieve union with God. The most popular form of prayer in this system was the Jesus Prayer, which was also known as "prayer of the heart." It generally consists of the words: "Lord, Jesus Christ, Son of God, have mercy on me, a sinner."

The following lines of scripture come from the traditional Christian Bible and the Gnostic Christian gospels from Ancient Egypt. The following affirmations may be used as uplifting utterances and as words of power in the same manner as the Egyptian hekau or the Indian mantras. It is up to you to choose an appropriate form of the teaching which best suits your personality. When you begin to understand that the destination of the spiritual journey may be reached through various paths, you will be able to incorporate various elements from different traditions without guilt, shame or hesitation. The most important point to keep in mind is the goal itself that is to be reached. Use the symbols and practices which you feel most comfortable with but always remember that the goal of all spiritual paths is to achieve realization of the transcendental Self which lies beyond all symbols and concepts, even of the highest philosophies.

Materials needed for Christian Yoga Meditation.

To assist your meditation efforts you may use icons and symbols which will serve to draw your mind towards the Divine. You may use a picture of Jesus, a cross (Ankh cross preferably), a candle, a comfortable pillow or chair and some incense. Also, you should create an altar in a special corner of your room where you will practice your meditations. This area is to be used for no other purpose.

Take a comfortable seated posture. After uttering some inspiring prayers from the Bible or the Gnostic texts begin by chanting. The word "Amen" may be chanted repeatedly. Then choose one of the following special affirmations for your concentration-meditation practice.

Jesus said:

"Thou shalt love thy neighbor as thyself."

"Is it not written in your law, I said, Ye are gods?"

"The Kingdom of God is within of you."

"I and [my] Father are one."

"The Kingdom of the Father is spread upon the earth and men do not see it!"

Since all of the teachings of Jesus are directed to you personally, you should recite these special teachings in the first person affirmative.

Thus meditate and assert:

I love my neighbor as myself.

"I am the embodiment of service; I care for all human beings and all living beings in the universe as I care for my very self; I care for all of nature, as I care for my very own body."

Assert within yourself:

I am Divine.

"I am not this mind and body with their negative thoughts and desires"; "I am the Self, who is like a bird that is free to roam the vast expanse of the sky"; "I am not this perishable body that is a conglomeration of earthly elements that will some day return to the earth; I am the spirit which is subtle and free of all associations of the body"; "I am free from all associations of the body, be they of family, country, etc.; these associations of the body may have a practical value in the world of time and space but they do not in any way affect or hamper the real me."

Thus assert:

The Kingdom of God is within me.

"I have nowhere to go, nowhere to seek, nowhere to search for the greatest treasure of all existence because it is within me already and it always was"; "Within my heart lies the source of all happiness. I am the abode of all fulfillment!"; "All I need to do in order to discover this treasure is to open my heart by discarding the illusions and ignorance which cloud my mind"; "I look not to the world of time and space but to the eternity and infinity which is within me"; "I look not to the vanity of my body but to the peace of my innermost self: I am That I am!"

I and the Father are one.

This statement has a most ancient origin and it is one of the highest spiritual teachings. It exists in the Egyptian Mysteries and in the Indian Vedantic teachings and is used as a *hekau* or *mantra* to be repeated with deep understanding and feeling by those aspirants who want to direct their minds toward their essential nature.

You must, by now, realize that you are the focus of the Christian movement. Not you, your ego-personality, body, name, family, etc., but the innermost Self within you. When Jesus stated that he and the Father are one, he was not referring to his personality. He was referring to his innermost Self. He was also not referring to God as the "Creator-Father", sitting on the throne in heaven somewhere, because these are mental concepts that human beings have created. The terms "The Father" and "God" are metaphors to explain that which transcends all human conceptions. When we think of God using this new understanding, we should begin to think about that which is

261

without name or form, that which is all pervasive and eternal and that, which is not personal. Look within yourself; your soul is all of these things also. When you sleep your ego is not there. You do not have a name or form and yet you continue to exist, therefore, you are not the ego. Reflect constantly on this relationship between your innermost Self and the innermost Self of all creation (God) because they are one and the same. Teresa de Jesus also popularly known as Teresa of Avila beautifully described this ecstatic union with the divine:

> "The soul neither sees, hears, nor understands while she is united to God - God establishes himself in the interior of this soul in such a way that when she comes to herself, it is impossible for her to doubt that she has been in God and God in her. So does that Beauty and Majesty stamped on the soul that nothing can drive it from her memory. The soul is no longer the same, always enraptured."

Thus assert: "I, the innermost Self, not the ego, am one with the innermost reality of all that exists which transcends all outer manifestations, all names and all forms!" This is the internal realization of Divinity within you.

Assert boldly:

"The Kingdom of the Father is spread upon the earth, and I see it!"

"This world, this universe, my body, my loved ones, all human beings are manifestations of Divine consciousness!"; "All this is a reflection of the innermost Self who is eternal and infinite!"; "I (the innermost Self) am the sustainer of this reality as I sustain my dreams in the vastness of the mind"; "All that I see is a reflection of the innermost self."; "All this is the Kingdom/Queendom of Heaven!"; "Therefore, both internally and externally I have discovered the transcendental reality!"; "I am all this!" This is the external realization of Divinity in all creation.

Amen

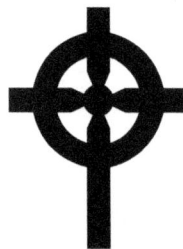

TIME-LINE OF MAJOR WORLD RELIGIONS AND MYSTICAL PHILOSOPHIES AND SELECTED WORLD EVENTS

c. >36,766 B.C.E-10,858 B.C.E	Egyptian Pre-dynastic history
c. 10,000 B.C.E.	The Sphinx: Horus in the Horizon.
c. 10,500 - 5,700 B.C.E.	Egyptian Pre-dynastic history
c. 5,700 - 342 B.C.E.	Egyptian Dynastic History
c. 5,500 B.C.E.	Egyptian Philosophy (Yoga), Pyramid Texts, Egypt.
c. 2,500 B.C.E	Pre-Aryan Dravidian Religion -Yoga, India.
c. 1,700 B.C.E.	Invasion of Egypt, Europe, Persia and India by the Indo-Europeans (Aryans).
c. 1,400-900 B.C.E	Aryan Vedas, India.
c. 1,350 B.C.E.	Canaanite Religion.
c. 1,200-500 B.C.E.	Old Testament- Moses, Egypt.
c. 1,200 B.C.E.	Olmecs. Central America.
c. 1,200 B.C.E.	Jainism, India.
c. 1,030 B.C.E.	Druids.
c. 800 B.C.E.	Upanishads-Classical Indian Vedanta-, India.
c. 800 - 500 B.C.E.	Vasudeva - Krishna, India
c. 700 B.C.E.	Samkhya-Yoga philosophy, India.
c. 700 BCE-500 ACE	Greek mythology and Mystery religions, Greece-Egypt.[I]
c. 600 B.C.E.	Zoroaster, Persia.
c. 600 B.C.E.	Buddhism (Theravada), India.
c. 550 B.C.E.	Confucianism, China.
c. 500 B.C.E.	Taoism- Lao Tsu, China.
c. 500-51 B.C.E.	Celtic Religion.
c. 500-100 B.C.E.	Hinduism- Mahabharata, Bhagavad Gita, Patanjali- India.
c. 324 B.C.E.	Invasion of Egypt, Persia and India by Alexander the Great.
c. 300 B.C.E.-300 C. E	Gnosticism, Jewish Essene and Therapeut cults throughout: Egypt, Palestine, Greece and Rome. Buddhists send missionaries to Egypt, Persia, China Greece and Rome.
c. 200 B.C.E.	Roman composite and Mystery religions, Greece-Egypt-India.[II]
c. 100 B.C.E -100 A.C.E.	Hermeticism
c. 100 B.C.E -100 A.C.E. to Present	Mahayana Buddhism develops becomes dominant religion in India. Missionaries sent to Egypt, Persia, China Greece and Rome.
c. 200 A.C.E.	Shaivism (Saivism)- Puranas and Agamas, Hindu scriptures in India.
c. 300 A.C.E.	Mayas (central America-decedents of the Olmecs).
c. 325 A.C.E.	Christianity accepted in Rome.
c. 400 A.C.E.	Theodosius of Rome decrees that Orthodox Christianity is the only form of Christianity allowed in the Roman Empire. All other forms of Christianity and all other religions and cults are outlawed. Dark ages of Europe begin. An exodus of religious leaders, artists, scientists out of increased contact with the Orient and the European renaissance.
c. 476 A.C.E.	Roman Empire overrun by barbarians from northern and northeastern Europe. Christianity almost dies out.
c. 1,000-1,500 A.C.E.	Invasion of India by Muslims.
c. 1,200 A.C.E.	Cabalism, Jewish.
c. 1,300 A.C.E.	European Renaissance.
c. 1,450 A.C.E.	Sikhism (combination of Islam and Hinduism), India.
c. 1,517 A.C.E.	Protestant Christian Movement.
c. 1,611 A.C.E.	King James Version of Old and New Testament.
c. 1,800 A.C.E. - Present	Modern Vedanta Attempts to integrate dual and non-dual philosophy, Buddhist psychology and yoga.
	The preceding dates are approximations. They represent the approximate date in which the religious precepts were first codified. Archeological and sociological history suggest that all of these systems undoubtedly existed for a long time before actually being "written down."

[I] Mystery religions based on the Egyptian mysteries of Isis and Osiris and those of Buddha and Krishna (India).
[II] Mystery religions based on the Egyptian mysteries of Isis and Osiris and those of Buddha and Krishna (India).

INDEX

1,000 year intervals, 125

12 tribes, 19

Ab, 121, 122, 133, 226

Abhyasa, 192

Above and Below, 229

Abraham, 16, 19, 20, 24, 25, 27, 51, 65, 68, 75, 78, 83, 84, 86, 87, 88, 94, 103, 126, 127, 130, 136, 151, 210

Absolute, 13, 36, 37, 48, 49, 110, 122, 133, 134, 168, 169, 170, 179, 181, 184, 196, 199, 200, 202, 203, 204, 221, 233, 239, 241, 250, 260

Absolute Existence, 241

Absolute reality, 13, 48

Absolute Reality, 134, 233

Absolute Self, 170

Absolute Truth, 133

Abstinence, 131

Abyssinia, 76

Acquiescence to the will of God, 131

Acts, 15, 27, 43, 54, 66, 67, 70, 97, 104, 117, 164, 193, 200

Acts of Judas Thomas, 104

Acts of Paul, 193

acupuncture, 166

Adam and Eve, 197, 229, 249

adhimatra, 177

adhimatratama, 177

Adolf Bastian, 48

Adonai, 74

Adonis, 221

Adultery, 118

Advaya-Taraka- Upanishad, 178

Aegean Sea, 140

Africa, 10, 11, 12, 25, 27, 29, 39, 40, 44, 48, 50, 51, 52, 56, 57, 76, 77, 81, 82, 83, 85, 86, 87, 92, 104, 128, 136, 138, 141, 142, 146, 149, 150, 151, 154, 161, 162, 163, 174, 185, 186, 188, 198, 199, 218, 219, 225, 280

African Americans, 130, 151

African Methodist Episcopal Church, 153

African Methodist Episcopal Zion Church, 153

Against the Heresies, 116

Agastya, 191

Agitated personality, 99

Agni, 125

Agnostic, 18, 63

Ahura Mazda, 124

Air, 73

Akhenaton, 72, 74, 198, 199, 200, 201

Akhenaton, Pharaoh, 74

Aksum, 76

Albert Einstein, 48, 195

Alchemy, 166

Alexander, 139

Alexander the Great, 24, 138, 141, 142, 263

Alexandria, 24, 79, 92, 115, 132, 139, 142, 280

Allah, 13, 19, 20, 24, 49, 89, 106, 111, 127, 128, 129, 130, 134, 135, 202, 204, 205, 216, 240, 244

all-encompassing God, 58

almond, 1

Alpha and Omega, 136, 166, 205, 229, 255

Ambrose, 46

Amen, 57, 62, 94, 140, 198, 199, 204, 249, 250, 260, 262

Amenta, 284

Amentet, 285

Americas, 11, 25, 150, 161, 163

Amma, 49

Ammit, 122

Amun, 43, 44, 57, 59, 62, 76, 78, 79, 81, 94, 96, 139, 140, 169, 170, 176, 189, 198, 199, 203, 204, 210, 239, 280

Amun-Ra-Ptah, 62, 188, 203, 205

Anabaptists, 149

Ancient Egypt, 1, 2, 10, 11, 12, 13, 16, 18, 19, 23, 24, 28, 29, 30, 31, 33, 36, 37, 39, 40, 41, 42, 43, 44, 47, 48, 49, 50, 51, 52, 53, 54, 55, 56, 57, 58, 59, 60, 61, 62, 63, 64, 65, 67, 68, 69, 70, 71, 72, 73, 74, 75, 76, 78, 79, 80, 81, 82, 83, 84, 86, 87, 88, 89, 92, 93, 94, 95, 96, 98, 100, 103, 105, 106, 107, 108, 111, 115, 116, 117, 118, 119, 120, 121, 122, 123, 125, 126, 127, 129, 131, 133, 134, 135, 139, 140, 141, 142, 143, 144, 149, 153, 161, 163, 164, 166, 167, 169, 170, 173, 176, 177, 180, 181, 183, 184, 186, 187, 188, 189, 191, 192, 195, 198,

199, 200, 201, 202, 203, 204, 208, 209, 210, 215, 217, 219, 222, 224, 225, 226, 228, 229, 230, 231, 233, 234, 236, 237, 238, 239, 240, 247, 248, 249, 250, 254, 256, 259, 260, 279, 280, 281, 282, 283, 284, 285, 286, 289, 290, 291

Ancient Egyptian Mystery Religion, 31

Ancient Egyptian mystical philosophy, 129, 164

Ancient Egyptian Mystical Philosophy, 11

Ancient Egyptian Pyramid Texts, 31, 60, 61

Ancient Egyptian Wisdom Texts, 13, 234

Ancient mystical philosophy, 11, 63, 164, 205, 209

Ancient Mystical Philosophy, 46, 47, 48

Androgyny, 56

Angels, 130, 191, 215

anger, 35, 58, 59, 60, 123, 124, 177, 178, 184, 185, 196, 197, 209, 223, 226, 227, 229, 241, 248, 249, 250

Anger, 45, 136, 192

Anglican, 148, 149, 150, 153, 162, 180, 248

Anglican Church, 148, 149, 150

Angra Mainyu, 124

Ani, 119, 222, 239, 279

Ankh, 1, 2, 96, 97, 100, 101, 107, 189, 233, 247, 260, 279

Annunciation, 95, 96, 189

anointed one, 94

Anointed One, 221

Anointing of Asar Ani, 222

anthropomorphic forms, 188

Anu, 284

Anu (Greek Heliopolis), 54, 73, 79, 284

Anubis, 59, 81, 122, 210, 256

Apocalypse of Peter, 253

Apocrypha, 19, 78, 115, 148, 157, 193, 279

Apocryphon, 28, 116

Apophis, 229

apostle, 127

Apostle, 116, 191

Apostles, 116

Apostles Creed, 90

Apostolic Letters, 194
Apostolic Tradition, 194
Appolonius of Tyana, 103
Apuat, 80
Aquarian Gospel, 78, 80, 83, 85, 103, 128
Arabia, 166
Arabs, 19, 26, 51, 79, 86, 129
Aramaic, 20, 65, 148
Arati, 187
Ardhanari, 107
Arianism, 64, 92
Aristotelian, 141, 187
Aristotle, 32, 33, 48, 138, 142
Arius, 64, 92, 139, 204
Arjuna, 12, 30, 110, 117, 133, 193, 227, 252, 253, 256, 257
Ark of the Covenant, 80
Armageddon, 60, 217
Arthur, 144
Arthurian Legend, 144
Aryan, 282
Aryans, 69, 86, 124, 125, 192, 263
asana, 171
Asar, 9, 24, 40, 54, 57, 58, 59, 60, 61, 62, 72, 76, 78, 79, 80, 81, 83, 88, 89, 92, 94, 95, 100, 104, 105, 114, 121, 122, 132, 135, 139, 142, 165, 176, 183, 184, 190, 194, 199, 203, 204, 205, 210, 216, 220, 221, 229, 230, 256, 284, 285, 290, 291
Asarian Resurrection, 284, 285, 286
Aset, 24, 54, 55, 58, 59, 60, 61, 78, 79, 92, 95, 96, 141, 144, 164, 176, 181, 182, 183, 184, 185, 186, 187, 188, 189, 190, 194, 204, 210, 230, 256, 284, 285, 290
Aset (Isis), 284, 285
Ash Wednesday, 248
Asha, 125
Ashoka, 142
Asia Minor, 55, 83, 86, 116, 138, 142, 224
Asians, 86
Asiatic, 80, 83
Aspirant, 175
Assyrians, 61, 67
Astral, 170, 210, 230, 284
Astral Body, 170
Astral Plane, 284
astral travel, 166

astrology, 166
Atheist, 10, 18
Atheists, 18, 38
Athens, 141
Atlantis, 55
Atom, 40
Aton or Aten, 198
Attachment, 242
Attis, 59, 61, 62, 221
Augustus, 51, 52
Ausarian mystery, 57, 60
Ausarian Mystery, 61
Ausarian religion, 131
Ausarian salvation story, 78
Austerity, 34, 105, 113, 123, 254
Avatars, 203
Avidya, 108
AVIDYA, 172
awakened one, 257
Awareness, 34, 47, 62, 106, 110, 113, 166, 176, 180, 203, 216, 225, 229, 232, 259
Ayur-Veda, 247
Ba (also see Soul), 133, 226
Baal Shem Tov, 165
Balance, 108, 123
Balance of Mind, 123
Bandlet of Righteousness, 111
Beautiful West, 169
Being, 11, 13, 30, 33, 40, 48, 53, 54, 56, 57, 58, 63, 68, 74, 93, 105, 106, 119, 122, 129, 135, 140, 143, 156, 163, 169, 176, 182, 188, 198, 201, 202, 204, 205, 206, 209, 241, 246, 253, 285
Benares, 218
Benu, 80
Bhagavad Gita, 12, 30, 33, 42, 89, 105, 113, 117, 133, 152, 183, 192, 195, 206, 225, 227, 245, 252, 256, 257, 263, 279
Bhagavata Purana, 183
Bhagavata-Purana, 177
Bhakti or Devotional Surrender To God, 89
Bhakti Yoga, 30, 131
Bhakti Yoga See also Yoga of Divine Love, 30, 131
bhav, 217
bhavana, 177
Bhoga, 191, 224, 225
Bhoga Tyaga, 191, 225
Bible, 1, 12, 15, 16, 18, 19, 20, 21, 22, 23, 24, 25, 27, 28, 31,

40, 41, 42, 43, 44, 45, 48, 50, 51, 55, 56, 58, 60, 61, 62, 63, 65, 66, 67, 68, 70, 71, 73, 75, 76, 77, 78, 79, 80, 81, 83, 84, 85, 86, 87, 88, 92, 94, 113, 115, 116, 117, 118, 122, 125, 126, 128, 132, 138, 147, 148, 149, 150, 152, 153, 154, 155, 156, 157, 159, 160, 162, 165, 169, 171, 182, 183, 186, 188, 193, 194, 197, 200, 201, 205, 209, 210, 215, 217, 220, 226, 228, 229, 234, 237, 238, 239, 241, 242, 247, 248, 249, 252, 253, 254, 258, 259, 260, 279, 280, 285
BIBLE, 280
Big Bang, 53
Billy Graham, 154
biofeedback, 166
Bishops, 22, 28, 50, 97, 138, 174
Black, 105
Black land, 140
Black Madonna, 162, 185, 189, 190, 280
Black Muslims, 130
Black One, 88
Black Virgin, 190
Bliss, 179, 202
Bodhisatva, 109
bodily resurrection, 90
Book of Coming forth by day, 279
Book of Coming forth by Day, 64, 198
Book of Coming Forth by Day, 31, 226
Book of Coming Forth By Day, 12, 30, 104, 111, 121, 122, 123, 133, 169, 188, 198, 217, 222, 256, 284
Book of Coming Forth by Day and Night, 31
Book of the Dead, see also Rau Nu Prt M Hru, 284
Book of Thomas, 168, 230
Brahma, 41, 56, 57, 125, 184, 203, 254
Brahman, 13, 14, 49, 59, 104, 105, 107, 108, 112, 117, 119, 134, 152, 167, 168, 169, 170, 171, 179, 181, 184, 192, 202, 203, 204, 206, 216, 225, 227, 241, 254, 257
BRAHMAN, 171
Brahmin, 104, 113, 184

Brahmins, 107
Breath control, 33, 171
bridegroom, 185
brides, 185
Brihadaranyaka Upanishad, 192
Britain, 143
Britanni, 143
British Commonwealth of
  Nations, 144
British Isles, 143
Britons, 144
Buber, Martin, 165
Buddha, 12, 14, 29, 32, 35, 41,
  69, 99, 104, 105, 106, 107,
  108, 109, 110, 112, 113, 123,
  135, 165, 192, 194, 198, 203,
  205, 207, 221, 222, 229, 244,
  245, 252, 257, 263, 279
BUDDHA, 207
Buddhi, 104
Buddhism, 104, 141, 142, 192,
  202
Buddhist, 24, 31, 37, 50, 63, 69,
  104, 107, 108, 109, 110, 111,
  113, 123, 125, 132, 142, 167,
  168, 197, 203, 226, 230, 252,
  263
Budge, Wallis, 189, 279, 280
Buto, 188
Byzantine Empire, 138
Byzantines, 146
Byzantium, 164
Cabalism, 41
Cabalists, 165
Caduceus, 230
Campbell, Joseph, 165
Canaan, 81
Canaanites, 85
Cannan, 126
Canonized, 28, 146, 147, 148,
  164, 191
Capra, Frijot, 195
Capstone, 229
Caribbean, 76
Carl Jung, 12, 50, 165, 189, 207,
  219
Catholic, 10, 11, 18, 19, 21, 22,
  23, 28, 29, 31, 48, 50, 54, 61,
  65, 90, 97, 104, 111, 113,
  116, 131, 138, 144, 147, 148,
  150, 157, 163, 164, 165, 174,
  180, 182, 186, 187, 191, 194,
  203, 224, 251, 285
Catholic schools, 10
Catholic-Celtic, 144
Causal Body, 170

Celsus, 103
Celtic, 86, 100, 143, 144, 146,
  148, 163, 180, 263
Celtic Christianity, 144
Celtic cross, 100
Celtic Kingdom, 144
Celtic tribes of Ireland, 180
Celts, 143
Chakra, 111, 112
chakras, 58
Chakras (see energy centers of the
  body), 111, 112, 113, 132, 223,
  230
Chakras of Kundalini, 230
Chaldeans, 68, 83
Channel Islands, 144
Chanting, 33, 139, 166, 174, 247
chaotic, 56
Charismatic, 155
Charlemagne, 146
Chi, 134, 135
Chi Kung, 135
children of Israel, 126
China, 10, 29, 41, 69, 125, 135,
  150, 169, 263
Chitta, 172
Chou Dynasty, 135
Christ, 1, 2, 9, 10, 12, 14, 15, 17,
  22, 23, 28, 35, 41, 44, 46, 50,
  58, 60, 62, 64, 81, 87, 88, 89,
  90, 91, 92, 93, 94, 99, 100,
  101, 104, 105, 106, 107, 112,
  113, 116, 123, 125, 127, 128,
  139, 145, 149, 151, 152, 155,
  156, 160, 161, 169, 174, 180,
  182, 183, 186, 191, 192, 193,
  194, 207, 209, 210, 220, 221,
  222, 223, 228, 233, 249, 252,
  253, 259, 284
Christ as the Son of God, 89
Christ consciousness, 223
Christ Consciousness, 35, 41, 93,
  104, 112, 149, 156, 160, 174,
  223
Christhood, 12, 28, 41, 92, 99,
  100, 104, 107, 146, 159, 209,
  221, 222, 223, 241, 254
Christian church, 11, 23, 55, 65,
  90, 92, 96, 97, 100, 104, 115,
  116, 128, 138, 146, 147, 148,
  164, 180, 188, 223
Christian Church, 11, 23, 55, 61,
  68, 90, 92, 96, 97, 101, 104,
  115, 116, 128, 147, 148, 150,
  153, 155, 156, 157, 164, 180,
  188, 208, 223

Christian church denominations,
  147
Christian cross, 100
Christian Cross, 97, 100, 166,
  229
Christian Fathers, 46, 62, 174
Christian Mystical Philosophy,
  11, 158
Christian philosophy, 65
Christian Theology, 78
Christian Yoga, 2, 10, 14, 16, 18,
  21, 22, 37, 40, 41, 44, 49, 74,
  82, 93, 161, 163, 167, 173,
  174, 195, 217, 234, 259, 260
Christian Zealots, 177
Christianity, 1, 2, 10, 11, 12, 13,
  15, 16, 18, 19, 22, 23, 24, 25,
  27, 28, 29, 30, 31, 32, 33, 35,
  36, 44, 45, 46, 48, 49, 50, 54,
  55, 56, 57, 59, 60, 62, 64, 67,
  68, 75, 76, 77, 78, 79, 80, 81,
  82, 90, 91, 92, 93, 94, 96,
  100, 101, 103, 104, 109, 110,
  111, 113, 115, 116, 119, 122,
  123, 125, 126, 127, 128, 131,
  132, 137, 138, 139, 140, 141,
  143, 144, 145, 146, 149, 150,
  153, 154, 155, 156, 157, 158,
  160, 161, 162, 163, 164, 165,
  166, 167, 168, 172, 173, 175,
  179, 182, 183, 184, 185, 186,
  187, 188, 189, 191, 194, 195,
  198, 199, 202, 203, 204, 205,
  207, 208, 209, 210, 215, 219,
  220, 224, 225, 229, 230, 234,
  247, 248, 251, 255, 256, 259,
  263, 280, 281, 285
Christology, 16, 62, 91, 139, 223
CHRISTOLOGY, 62, 223
Christos, 222
Church, 11, 19, 21, 22, 23, 28,
  31, 46, 65, 68, 78, 90, 92,
  100, 113, 115, 116, 138, 139,
  146, 147, 148, 149, 150, 152,
  153, 154, 155, 160, 162, 163,
  165, 191, 285
church fathers, 63
Church Fathers, 113
church leadership, 92
Church of England, 22, 148, 150,
  152, 153, 155
Clement of Alexandria, 139
Cloud of Unknowing, 165
Cobra Goddess, 188
Coffined One, 81

Company of gods and goddesses, 53, 54

Concentration, 171

Conception, 96, 186, 189

Conflict, 279

Confucianism, 202

Confucius, 29

Congregationalists, 149

Consciousness, 12, 13, 14, 23, 32, 33, 34, 35, 37, 40, 41, 47, 48, 49, 58, 59, 60, 61, 62, 63, 64, 93, 99, 101, 103, 104, 106, 109, 110, 111, 112, 113, 121, 122, 132, 133, 134, 135, 137, 160, 167, 168, 169, 171, 186, 191, 192, 193, 195, 196, 202, 204, 205, 216, 219, 220, 222, 223, 228, 229, 230, 260, 284

Constantine, 23, 100, 116, 138

Constantinople, 138, 147

Contentment (see also Hetep), 108, 123

Coptic, 28, 76, 78, 80, 96, 123, 136, 138, 139, 147, 204, 284

Coptic church, 78, 139

Coptic Church, 78, 138, 139, 147

Copts, 96

Corinthians, 23, 27, 43, 80, 116, 210, 258

Corinthians, Romans, Philippians, Hebrews, 116

Cornwall, 144

Corpus Hermeticum, 164

Cosmic consciousness, 48, 49, 122, 171, 172, 219, 222, 223

Cosmic Consciousness, 23, 122, 205

Cosmic Illusion, 104, 195

cosmic order, 125

cosmic Self, 251

Cosmic Self, 251

Cosmology, 33

Council at Nicea, 92

Council of Chalcedon, 101, 139

Counseling, 279, 280

Course in Miracles, 166

Creation, 1, 18, 33, 36, 40, 41, 44, 46, 48, 49, 55, 56, 57, 62, 63, 65, 67, 73, 80, 93, 96, 105, 107, 119, 125, 129, 134, 135, 149, 172, 196, 200, 201, 202, 204, 210, 217, 219, 228, 229, 230, 249, 250, 284

creative visualization, 166

Cross, 97, 100, 101, 165, 229, 233

crucifixion, 145

Crusades, 23, 25, 147, 153, 161, 163, 164

Culture, 283

Cushite, 81

Cybele, 61, 132

Cymbals, 290, 291

Dabhar, 256

Daisetz Suzuki, 165

Dark Ages, 146, 193

Day of Judgment, 130

De Anima, 142

De Trinitate, 62

de, Cosimo Medici, 164

Dead Sea Scrolls, 21, 24, 28, 90, 157, 279

Death, 226, 238, 255

December, 61, 95, 104, 285

December 25, 95

December 25th, 61

Deism, 34, 163

Delphi, 55

Delusion, 249

Demotic, 55

Denderah, 284

Desire, 42, 170, 197, 246, 257

detachment, 246

Detachment, 34, 174, 245, 257

Devi Sukta, 187

Devil, 101, 249

Devotional Love, 132

Dhahamapada, 245

dharana, 171

Dharma, 110, 113, 123, 192, 254

Dharmakaya, 49, 203

dhyana, 171

Di, Huang, 135

Diabolos, 111

diabolus, 249

Dialogue of the Savior, 194

Diet, 282

Diodorus, 51, 52, 53, 71, 72, 86

Diodorus Siculus, 52

Dionysius, 24, 164, 207

Dionysius the Areopagite, 24

Dionysius the Areopagite, 24, 164, 207

Dionysius, Pseudo, 164

Dionysus, 103

Discipline, 37, 167

dispassion, 113, 171, 172, 173, 175, 223, 226, 230, 231, 244, 247

Dispassion, 174, 246, 257

Divali, 191

divination, 166

Divine Cow, 188

Divine Sport, 171

Djed Pillar of Asar, 230

Djehuti, 56, 59, 74, 94, 107, 122, 125, 134, 138, 164, 189, 210

Djehuti-Hermes, 184, 230

DNA, 45

Docetism, 101

Dodonian, 100

dogma, 13, 64, 65, 127, 186, 251

Dogon, 49, 141

Dove, 1

Dravidian, 125, 263

dream, 216

Dream, 137

Druid, 100, 143, 144

Druid crosses, 100

Druidism, 143

Druids, 29, 143, 263

Dualism, 34, 93, 139, 206, 250

dualism and egoism, 34

Duality, 35, 41, 93, 106, 124, 133, 135, 171, 196, 204, 206, 220, 221, 228, 229, 244, 249

duat, 230

Duat, 73, 94, 230, 256, 284

Dull personality, 98

Durga, 182

dux bellorum, 145

Dynastic period, 51

Early Christianity, 11, 100

Earth, 47, 73, 188, 247

Easter, 11, 248

Eastern Orthodox Church, 19, 147, 150

Eastern religions, 29

Eckhart, Meister, 165

Ecumenical, 65

Edfu, 284

Edmond Bordeaux Szekeley, 23

Egoism, 34, 35, 44, 59, 60, 64, 79, 93, 112, 113, 121, 176, 180, 188, 197, 204, 209, 223, 229, 242, 244, 246, 249, 250, 251, 257

Egyptian Book of Coming Forth By Day, 12, 67, 111, 122, 133, 169, 188, 198, 217, 256, 284

Egyptian Christians, 139

Egyptian civilization, 55, 68, 78, 83, 86, 141, 143, 144, 199

Egyptian Civilization, 86

Egyptian dynasties, 31

Egyptian High Priests, 53

Egyptian Mysteries, 16, 50, 133, 142, 261, 282, 286
Egyptian Physics, 285
Egyptian proverbs, 283
Egyptian religion, 10, 11, 29, 36, 54, 55, 67, 71, 72, 79, 80, 111, 119, 126, 127, 129, 142, 187, 198, 204
Egyptian Yoga, 3, 36, 37, 62, 141, 176, 192, 199, 279, 280, 281, 282, 284, 289, 290, 291
Egyptian Yoga see also Kamitan Yoga, 281, 282, 284
Egyptians, 85
Einstein, Albert, 48, 195
Elamites, 87
Elementary Ideas, 48
Elijah, 67, 92, 130, 131, 220
Elijah Muhammad, 130, 131
Elohim, 56, 74, 188, 189
energy center, 132
Enlightened Sages, 49, 116, 149, 160
Enlightenment, 12, 35, 41, 62, 81, 92, 99, 100, 107, 108, 109, 111, 112, 113, 117, 122, 138, 141, 142, 172, 174, 176, 178, 180, 191, 196, 206, 209, 221, 222, 224, 229, 230, 244, 246, 247, 252, 280, 282, 283, 284, 285, 286
Ennead, 53, 54
epistles, 116
Equanimity, 109
esoteric, 137
Essene Gospel of Peace, 23, 24, 28, 247, 279, 280
Essenes, 28, 90, 132, 137, 141, 222, 247
Eternal Teacher, 225
eternal witness, 203, 204
Ethiopia, 16, 27, 52, 53, 70, 72, 75, 76, 77, 81, 83, 84, 85, 86, 88, 93, 111, 128, 129, 140, 154, 161, 162, 177, 188, 199
Ethiopian priests, 52
Ethiops, 140
Eucharist, 60, 61, 89, 94, 204, 251, 284
Eudoxus, 140
Euphrates River, 65, 67, 126, 218
Eusebius, 53, 68
Evil, 101, 197, 229, 249, 250
Exercise, 33, 284
Existence - Knowledge - Bliss, 202

exoteric, 137
extrasensory perception, 166
extraterrestrial life, 166
Eye of Heru, 59, 176, 188
Eye of Horus, 61
Eye of intuitional vision, 60
Faith, 10, 11, 18, 20, 24, 59, 63, 92, 96, 103, 104, 116, 125, 128, 143, 144, 174, 177, 185, 204, 224, 226, 232, 233, 252
Falashas, 27, 75, 76
Fard, W. D., 130
Fasting, 33, 111, 112, 247, 248
Father-Son-Holy Ghost, 57
Fear, 241
Female, 182, 191, 203
Festival of Lights, 191
Fetters, 192
Fetters of the soul, 192
Ficino, Marsilio, 164
Fiction, 35
Fields of Reeds, 188
filed, the, 257
First Intermediate Period, 51
Fish, 1
Flood, 55
Folk Ideas, 48
forgiveness, 251
Forgiveness, 123
formlessness, 42
Fornication, 136
Four Christian Fathers, 46
fourteen pieces, 59
France, 143, 144
Francis of Assisi, 165, 182
Francis, Saint of Assisi, 165
French Arthurian romances, 145
Freud, Sigmund, 219
G., C. Jung, 207
Galileans, 91
Galilee, 91
Galli, 143
Garden of Eden, 197, 229
Gaul, 143, 146, 180, 189
Gauls, 143
Gautama, 107
Gautama, Siddhartha, 113
Geb, 54, 56, 73, 256, 284
General, Roman Titus, 89
Germany, 143, 144
Gita Govinda, 184
Giza, 40, 51, 65
Giza Plateau, 51
Gnosis, 28, 124, 132, 133, 134, 137, 219, 221, 252

Gnostic, 13, 18, 21, 23, 24, 27, 28, 29, 30, 31, 36, 38, 41, 48, 55, 60, 61, 64, 65, 79, 89, 90, 91, 92, 96, 100, 101, 103, 104, 105, 107, 116, 117, 122, 123, 124, 125, 129, 131, 132, 134, 135, 137, 138, 142, 152, 153, 156, 157, 163, 164, 166, 168, 169, 170, 174, 175, 184, 185, 187, 191, 193, 194, 195, 196, 201, 202, 203, 205, 219, 220, 223, 224, 225, 226, 230, 233, 244, 248, 253, 254, 256, 259, 260, 279, 280
Gnostic Book of Thomas, 168, 230
Gnostic Christianity, 28, 48, 64, 90, 96, 100, 101, 104, 131, 134, 137, 157, 164, 175, 184, 185, 195, 219, 220, 224, 256
Gnostic gospels, 90, 96, 193
Gnostic Gospels, 18, 90, 96, 122, 193, 202, 203, 253, 279
Gnostics, 18, 63, 64, 65, 116, 124, 153, 186, 256, 279
God, 1, 10, 12, 13, 14, 15, 16, 18, 19, 21, 23, 24, 25, 26, 27, 28, 29, 30, 32, 33, 34, 36, 37, 38, 41, 43, 44, 48, 49, 50, 53, 54, 55, 56, 57, 58, 59, 60, 61, 62, 63, 64, 65, 66, 67, 69, 70, 73, 74, 76, 77, 78, 79, 80, 81, 84, 85, 86, 88, 89, 90, 91, 92, 93, 94, 96, 97, 98, 99, 100, 103, 104, 105, 106, 108, 111, 112, 118, 119, 120, 121, 122, 123, 124, 125, 126, 127, 128, 129, 130, 131, 132, 133, 134, 138, 140, 142, 145, 146, 147, 149, 151, 152, 153, 155, 156, 157, 158, 159, 160, 162, 163, 164, 165, 166, 167, 168, 169, 170, 173, 174, 176, 177, 178, 179, 181, 182, 183, 184, 185, 186, 187, 188, 189, 190, 191, 192, 193, 194, 195, 196, 197, 198, 199, 200, 201, 202, 203, 204, 205, 206, 207, 208, 209, 210, 215, 217, 218, 219, 220, 221, 222, 223, 224, 225, 226, 227, 228, 229, 230, 231, 232, 233, 235, 236, 238, 239, 240, 241, 244, 245, 247, 249, 250, 251, 252, 253, 254, 255, 256, 257, 258, 260, 261, 262, 280, 283, 284, 285, 291
God of Light, 56, 200

Goddess, 1, 13, 54, 61, 95, 103, 119, 134, 176, 179, 182, 187, 188, 189, 221, 229, 285, 289, 291, 292

Goddesses, 54, 284

Godhead, 62, 188

Gods, 40, 52, 53, 54, 64, 67, 69, 118, 119, 120, 129, 133, 188, 191, 198, 199, 205, 236, 279, 280, 284

Golden Age, 146

Good, 22, 94, 124, 161, 174, 197, 229, 233, 248

Good and evil, 29, 105, 124, 196, 226, 229, 249, 250

Good and Evil, 197, 229

Good Association, 174

Good Friday, 248

Good God, 124

Good religion, 124

good shepherd, 184

Good Shepherd, 94

goodness of man, 124

Gopi, 184, 279

Gopis, 183, 185

Gospel Music, 154

Gospel of John, 164

Gospel of Luke, 193

Gospel of Mary, 28, 185, 193, 279

Gospel of Peace:, 248

Gospel of Philip, 135, 185, 191, 240

Gospel of Thomas, 240, 241, 242, 244, 252

Gospel of Truth, 224

Gospel to the Egyptians, 28

Gospels, 18, 21, 22, 23, 28, 61, 63, 79, 81, 91, 92, 115, 122, 123, 145, 156, 157, 159, 192, 198, 202, 203, 253, 279, 285

Govinda, 94, 184

Great Mother, 188

Great Mystery, 165

Great Pyramid, 40, 55, 80

Great Pyramids, 40, 55

Great Spirit, 13, 49

Greece, 48, 53, 55, 72, 80, 103, 138, 139, 140, 141, 142, 161, 163, 176, 180, 189, 219, 263, 280, 282

greed, 35, 46, 58, 60, 88, 89, 171, 178, 185, 196, 197, 223, 229, 241, 249, 250

Greed, 153, 192, 249

Greek Empire, 138, 141, 147

Greek philosophers, 12, 29, 33, 51, 138, 139, 140, 141, 142

Greek philosophy, 31, 132, 139, 141, 281

Greek Philosophy, 139

GREEK PHILOSOPHY, 139

Greeks, 100

Green, 201

Greenfield papyrus, 279

Gregory, 46, 190, 193, 251, 252

Gregory the Great, 190, 251

Grimaldi, 52

guru, 191

Guru, 12, 144, 168, 175, 178, 179, 180

Guru - Disciple Relationship, 168

Guru-yoga, 179

Haile Selassie, 76, 77

Ham, 81

Hammurabi, 69, 84

Harmony, 35, 47

Hasidim, 165

Hatha Yoga, 135

hatha-yoga, 177

Hathor, 59, 96, 144, 183, 188, 189, 191, 256, 257, 284, 285, 286

hatred, 35, 58, 59, 123, 178, 209, 217, 227, 241, 248, 250

Hawk, 79, 207

Health, 174, 247, 281

Heart, 10, 13, 31, 34, 40, 49, 61, 63, 74, 91, 93, 105, 110, 111, 117, 118, 119, 121, 122, 123, 125, 133, 136, 145, 168, 172, 173, 178, 182, 184, 192, 193, 197, 202, 204, 206, 223, 225, 226, 232, 233, 240, 241, 242, 243, 244, 251, 279, 285

Heart (also see Ab, mind, conscience), 122, 133, 168, 226, 279, 285

Heaven, 12, 27, 41, 63, 73, 80, 99, 109, 129, 155, 169, 174, 185, 188, 196, 197, 203, 204, 206, 216, 225, 230, 231, 240, 244, 252, 253, 255, 258, 262, 285

Hebrew religion, 204

Hebrews, 24, 65, 66, 67, 68, 70, 74, 75, 78, 81, 83, 86, 90, 116, 119

Heinrich Zimmer, 14

Hekau, 40, 122, 177, 260, 291

Helena, Saint, 100

Heliopolis, 79

Hell, 129, 155, 188

Hellenism, 141

Heraclian emperors, 146

heresies, 142

Heresies, 116

Heretical, 11, 12, 48, 64, 101, 128, 142

Hermes, 12, 30, 31, 94, 107, 134, 164, 227, 256, 279

Hermes (see also Tehuti, Thoth), 12, 30, 31, 94, 107, 134, 164, 227, 256, 279

Hermes Trismegistos, 134

Hermetic, 31, 32, 107, 138, 164, 169, 205, 241, 255, 256, 257

Hermetic Books, 164

Hermetic philosophy, 31

Hermetic Philosophy, 241

Hermeticism, 24, 164, 166, 205, 224, 263

Herodotus, 27, 51, 53, 68, 71, 72, 82, 83, 86, 87, 141, 143, 279, 280

Heru, 24, 40, 43, 54, 56, 57, 59, 60, 61, 79, 89, 94, 95, 96, 103, 104, 105, 106, 125, 135, 169, 183, 185, 186, 188, 189, 191, 203, 205, 207, 210, 221, 222, 229, 230, 284, 285, 290, 291

Heru - Set, 135

Heru (see Horus), 24, 40, 43, 54, 56, 57, 59, 60, 61, 79, 89, 94, 95, 96, 103, 104, 105, 106, 125, 135, 169, 183, 185, 186, 188, 189, 191, 203, 205, 207, 210, 221, 222, 229, 230, 284, 285, 290, 291

Hetheru, 59, 286, 290

HetHeru (Hathor), 59

HetHeru (Hetheru , Hathor), 290

Hetheru (Hetheru, Hathor), 286

Hieroglyphic Writing, language, 283

Hieroglyphs, 13

Hierophant, 79

High God, 62, 94, 140, 163, 182, 188, 203

Higher Self, 172

Hinayana, 110

Hinayana,, 36, 107, 110

Hindu, 12, 30, 31, 36, 40, 41, 55, 56, 57, 59, 66, 94, 105, 106, 110, 123, 125, 137, 145, 167, 168, 184, 188, 191, 195, 199, 203, 204, 223, 247, 249, 257, 263, 279, 280

Hindu mythology, 55, 59, 94, 167, 195, 204, 257

Hinduism, 36, 37, 49, 69, 108, 123, 125, 134, 141, 142, 165, 168, 180, 202, 204, 215, 223, 231, 263, 280

Hindus, 100, 119, 125, 132, 191

Holy Communion, 89

Holy Grail, 145

Holy Land, 25, 87, 163

Holy of Holies, 81, 96, 189

Holy of Holies or Mesken, 189

holy spirit, 240

Holy spirit, 204

Holy Spirit, 1, 15, 54, 62, 63, 93, 96, 155, 156, 189, 201, 202, 203, 204, 232, 240

Horus, 24, 43, 56, 57, 59, 60, 61, 62, 79, 94, 95, 103, 104, 105, 106, 125, 135, 169, 176, 183, 186, 188, 189, 191, 203, 207, 210, 221, 222, 229, 230, 257, 263, 290

HORUS, 205, 207

Horus in the Horizon, 263

Horushood, 35, 41

Houses of Life, 247

HOW THIS BOOK WAS WRITTEN, 15

Humility, 15, 235

Hymns of Amun, 43, 79, 170, 199, 239, 280

I and the Father are One, 62, 204

Iam formula, 256

Iamblichus, 71, 140, 279

ice age, 39

Ice Age, 52

Identification, 168, 228

Ignorance, 44, 108, 168, 172, 174

Illusion, 35, 104, 107, 108, 112, 121, 122, 133, 134, 171, 172, 181, 195, 197, 207, 219, 221, 223, 224, 225, 228, 231, 240, 241, 246

immaculate conception, 186

Inculturation, 190

India, 10, 12, 24, 29, 30, 32, 33, 41, 42, 48, 51, 53, 54, 64, 69, 72, 82, 83, 86, 89, 93, 103, 104, 105, 107, 109, 113, 116, 117, 120, 122, 123, 124, 125, 128, 131, 132, 134, 135, 141, 142, 150, 154, 161, 166, 167, 168, 169, 171, 173, 181, 182, 183, 191, 192, 195, 199, 202, 203, 209, 217, 218, 219, 224,

229, 247, 256, 259, 263, 282, 283, 291

Indian Mystical Philosophy, 11

Indian Yoga, 12, 16, 37, 108, 122, 142, 192, 230, 281, 282, 291

Individual consciousness, 33, 196, 219

Indo Europeans, 125

Indus, 282

Indus Valley, 282

Initiate, 282

Intellect, 104, 123

Intellectual, 46, 47, 57, 61, 65, 91, 108, 113, 132, 175, 176, 183, 195, 219, 221

Intelligence, 49

Intuition, 132

intuitional, 47, 49, 59, 60, 79, 132, 133, 137, 195, 196, 230, 244, 253

Intuitional, 219

Iraq, 68, 72, 78, 83, 84, 86, 126

Ireland, 143, 144, 150, 151, 180

Ireland, Northern, 144

Irenaeus, 116

Isha Upanishad, 108

Ishmael, 19

Isis, 24, 32, 54, 55, 57, 58, 59, 60, 61, 79, 92, 95, 141, 144, 164, 176, 177, 181, 182, 183, 184, 186, 187, 188, 189, 190, 210, 230, 256, 263, 279, 284, 285, 290

ISIS, 176, 186

Isis, See also Aset, 284, 285

Islam, 13, 19, 24, 29, 36, 38, 63, 65, 67, 76, 127, 128, 129, 130, 131, 153, 158, 165, 176, 198, 199, 202, 204, 215, 263, 279, 281

Isle of Man, 144

Israel, 19, 24, 25, 26, 66, 67, 68, 71, 75, 76, 78, 80, 81, 83, 86, 89, 91, 113, 119, 126, 127, 130, 154, 210, 237, 238, 239

Israelites, 188

Italy, 144

Jah, 77

Jain, 107, 203

Jain philosophy, 107

Jainism, 107, 141, 142

Jamaica, 76

Japa, 177

Japheth, 81

jealousy, 58, 178, 250

Jealousy, 192

Jeanne Marie Bouvier de la Motte Guyon, 165

Jehovah, 13, 73, 74, 119, 151

Jerome, 46

Jerusalem, 91, 218

Jerusalemites, 91

Jesus, 1, 2, 10, 11, 13, 14, 15, 16, 17, 19, 22, 23, 24, 27, 28, 29, 31, 41, 44, 48, 54, 57, 59, 60, 61, 62, 63, 64, 65, 66, 67, 68, 78, 79, 80, 81, 86, 87, 88, 89, 90, 91, 92, 93, 94, 95, 96, 97, 98, 99, 101, 102, 103, 104, 105, 106, 107, 109, 110, 111, 112, 113, 114, 115, 116, 117, 118, 122, 123, 125, 126, 127, 128, 130, 132, 133, 134, 135, 137, 138, 139, 142, 145, 146, 147, 148, 149, 150, 152, 156, 157, 158, 159, 160, 161, 162, 163, 165, 166, 168, 169, 170, 173, 174, 175, 179, 180, 182, 183, 184, 185, 186, 188, 189, 191, 192, 193, 194, 198, 201, 203, 204, 205, 208, 209, 210, 217, 219, 220, 221, 223, 224, 229, 230, 231, 233, 234, 235, 239, 240, 241, 242, 244, 247, 248, 250, 251, 252, 253, 254, 255, 256, 257, 258, 259, 260, 261, 284, 285

Jesus ben Pandera, 103

Jesus Christ, 10, 28, 41, 66, 81, 89, 90, 91, 93, 94, 105, 125, 137, 145, 160, 186, 191, 208, 209, 223, 260, 284

Jesus of Nazareth, 81, 91, 101, 103

Jesus, baptized, 88

Jewish, 1, 15, 19, 22, 23, 24, 25, 27, 28, 40, 55, 56, 59, 65, 66, 67, 68, 69, 70, 73, 74, 75, 78, 79, 80, 81, 83, 87, 88, 89, 90, 91, 94, 96, 100, 103, 115, 118, 119, 125, 126, 127, 128, 129, 131, 132, 141, 147, 148, 157, 159, 162, 165, 184, 188, 192, 199, 203, 208, 217, 247, 249, 250, 263

Jewish Bible, 55, 56, 80, 115, 147, 148, 249

Jewish Mysticism, 40

Jewish religion, 15, 65, 67, 68, 83, 89, 90, 119, 199

JHVH, 74

JHWH, 74

JHWH or JHVH, 74
Jivan mukti, 171
Jnana Yoga, 181, 195, 279
John of the Cross, 165
John the Baptist, 81, 88, 92, 111, 186, 220
Jordan River, 88
Joseph Campbell, 165, 279
Joseph of Arimathea, 145
Josephus, 1, 88
Joshua, 67, 81
Joy, 109
Judaism, 15, 19, 24, 26, 27, 28, 29, 36, 38, 51, 65, 67, 68, 70, 71, 72, 74, 75, 76, 77, 80, 82, 86, 90, 115, 125, 126, 127, 128, 131, 148, 159, 165, 182, 184, 189, 198, 204, 208, 215, 234, 281
JUDAISM, 65
Judeo-Christian-Islamic, 29
Julius Caesar, 143
Jung, Carl, 165
Justinian, Emperor I, 146
Ka, 103, 128, 133, 226
Kaba, 19
Kabah, 103, 128
Kabbalah, 41, 49, 101, 281
Kali, 182, 203, 204
Kalki Avatara, 125
Kamit, 51, 58, 140, 218
Kamit (Egypt), 51, 58, 140, 218
Kamitan, 282
Kamsa, King, 106
Kant, 33
Karma, 104, 107, 172, 225, 254, 283
KARMA, 171, 172
Karma Yoga, 225
karmic entanglements, 113
Kemetic, 106, 288, 290, 291
Kether, 49
Khepera, 40
Khepra, 40
Khepri, 129, 197, 226
Ki (see also Life ForceRaButoKundalini), 73
King Amasis, 55
King David, 67
King James Bible, 22, 148
Kingdom, 1, 12, 27, 28, 35, 41, 49, 51, 63, 65, 76, 79, 80, 83, 93, 99, 100, 107, 109, 122, 134, 137, 144, 147, 152, 156, 158, 160, 164, 168, 169, 173, 174, 185, 196, 197, 201, 203,

204, 206, 215, 216, 217, 223, 224, 225, 226, 230, 231, 232, 233, 240, 241, 242, 244, 245, 247, 252, 253, 255, 257, 258, 259, 261, 262, 285
Kingdom of God, 203
Kingdom of heaven, 27, 113, 185, 258
Kingdom of Heaven, 12, 27, 35, 41, 49, 63, 65, 80, 99, 100, 109, 122, 158, 168, 169, 174, 185, 196, 197, 203, 204, 206, 216, 225, 230, 240, 244, 253, 255, 258, 259, 285
Kingdom of Heaven of Christianity, 49
Kingdom of the Father, 1, 93, 134, 137, 224, 261, 262
Kings Chamber, 80
Kmt, 58
KMT (Ancient Egypt), 52
KMT (Ancient Egypt). See also Kamit, 52
Know thyself, 134, 225
Know Thyself, 35
KNOW THYSELF, 168
Knowledge, 28, 117, 123, 131, 135, 195, 197, 202, 206, 227, 229, 241
Knum, 73, 94, 96, 189
Koran, 19, 20, 66, 111, 127, 128, 129, 130
Krishna, 12, 30, 32, 42, 69, 94, 104, 105, 106, 110, 117, 125, 165, 169, 183, 184, 185, 191, 194, 195, 198, 203, 204, 205, 206, 216, 221, 223, 229, 252, 253, 254, 257, 263, 279, 285
Kula-Arnava-Tantra, 179
Kundalini, 111, 122, 132, 135, 230, 279
Kundalini Yoga, 132, 135
Kung Fu, 135
Kush, 111, 201
Kybalion, 41, 42, 107, 279
Lake Victoria, 52, 85
Lamb, 94
Land of Ham, 85
Lao Tzu, 198
Lao-Tsu, 29
Lao-Tzu, 41
Last Supper, 145
Latin Cross, 100
Laws of Manu, 41
Laya, 177
laya-yoga, 177
Laziness, 136

Learning, 11
left brained thinking, 187
Lent, 248
Liberation, 12, 35, 171, 181
Libya, 55, 81, 85, 87, 92, 93
Libyans, 51
Life Force, 45, 56, 96, 134, 135, 136, 171, 189, 200, 201, 204, 279, 283
light, The, 257
Lila, 171
Listening, 168, 181
Logos, 256
Lord of Darkness, 124
Lord, The of the Perfect Black, 88
Lotus, 3
Love, 3, 30, 33, 132, 154, 172, 173, 239, 280, 283
Lucid personality, 99
Lucifer, 101, 125
Lust, Thirst, and Delight, 112
Luther, Martin, 165
Lycurgus, 140
Maat, 47, 56, 60, 73, 108, 118, 119, 120, 121, 122, 123, 129, 135, 149, 192, 236, 283, 285
MAAT, 236, 283
Maati, 108, 121, 215, 280
MAATI, 3, 283
Maccabees, 67, 148, 165
Macedonian epoch, 146
madhya, 177
Madonna, 1, 186, 189
Magdalene, Mary, 183, 191, 192, 193, 221
Magic, 280
Mahabharata, 30, 69, 125, 263
Mahanirvanatantra, 184
Mahavakyas, 169
Mahavakyas or Great Utterances, 169
Mahavira, 29, 41
Mahayana, 110
Mahayana, 107
Mala, 192
Mala or gross impurity, 192
Malcolm X, 130
Male, 203
Maltese Cross, 100
Manana: Reflection, 181
Mandorla, 1
Manetho, 51, 53, 54, 79
mantra, 177
mantra-yoga, 177
Manu, 41, 56, 123, 169

Mara, 112

Marcus Garvey, 76, 130

Mars, 164

martial arts, 166

Martin Buber, 165

Martin Luther, 131, 147, 165

Martin Luther King, 131

Mary Magdalene, 17, 29, 114, 183, 184, 191, 192, 193, 221, 279

Masoretic Hebrew text, 74

massage, 166

Masters, 49

Matter, 3, 228, 280, 285

Matthew, 15, 16, 27, 61, 62, 63, 64, 78, 81, 87, 88, 90, 91, 92, 93, 94, 96, 99, 110, 113, 117, 138, 147, 150, 152, 158, 159, 161, 170, 185, 186, 189, 194, 202, 215, 226, 227, 231, 232, 234, 235, 239, 241, 242, 243, 244, 245, 250, 252, 257, 258

Maya, 104, 134, 195, 196

MAYA, 170

Mecca, 19, 103, 128, 131, 218

Medieval Greek Empire, 138

Meditating, 181

Meditation, 10, 11, 33, 34, 41, 56, 60, 80, 81, 107, 108, 109, 111, 133, 135, 159, 168, 171, 172, 173, 174, 176, 178, 181, 184, 193, 218, 219, 227, 230, 243, 246, 247, 259, 260, 280, 282, 283, 291

Mediterranean, 142

Meister Eckhart, 165, 182

Memphis, 140

Memphite Theology, 57, 59, 142

Mental agitation, 34, 113, 170, 197, 243, 246

Merlin, 144

Mesken, 96, 189

Mesolithic, 39

Mesolithic Age, 39

Mesopotamia, 40, 65, 67, 69, 72, 84, 86, 87, 125, 126, 141, 208

Mesopotamian, 125

messiah, 81, 89, 90

Messiah, 115

messiahs, 89

Metamorphosis, 35

Metaphysical Neters, 203

Metaphysics, 10, 32, 33, 139, 142, 285

Metempsychosis, 141

Methodist, 153, 154

Metu Neter, 13, 122, 169

Middle Ages, 144, 146, 165

Middle East, 10, 25, 27, 29, 39, 65, 67, 68, 82, 84, 128, 131, 135, 139, 163, 210, 221, 248, 281

Middle Kingdom, 51, 83

middle path, 108

middle way, 113

Min, 256, 284

Mind, 1, 42, 48, 106, 108, 123, 169, 185, 187, 196, 204, 205, 210, 225, 247, 256, 257, 279

mindfulness, 203

Mindfulness, 109, 203

missionaries, 111

Mithra, 125

Modern physics, 61

Modern scholarship, 115

Modern science, 11, 33, 34, 137

Moksha, 35

monism, 198

Monism, 29, 36, 37, 38, 199

Monistic, 29

Monophysitism, 139

Monotheism, 36, 198

Moon, 52, 106, 210

Mortals, 256

Moses, 15, 16, 19, 24, 51, 66, 67, 68, 69, 70, 71, 73, 74, 75, 79, 80, 83, 86, 88, 103, 115, 118, 125, 126, 127, 151, 198, 199, 234, 263

Mother Mary, 188

Mount Sinai, 80

Muhammad, 19, 113, 128, 129, 130, 131, 147, 165

Muhammad, Prophet, 128

Mundaka Upanishad, 69, 167, 241

Music, 35, 47, 139, 149, 154, 290, 291

Muslim, 129

Mysteries, 40, 60, 132, 164, 204, 207, 279, 282, 286

Mysterium Magnum, 165

Mystery religions, 11, 12, 32, 61, 89, 92, 100, 219, 256, 263

Mystery Religions, 279

Mystic Knowledge of GOD, 131

Mystical Christianity, 56, 194

mystical experience, 17, 34, 61, 64, 65, 133, 169, 197, 251

Mystical experience, 61, 169

Mystical religion, 55, 65, 81, 168, 243

Mysticism, 12, 13, 20, 29, 34, 37, 40, 60, 65, 80, 128, 131, 134, 144, 160, 163, 164, 165,

166, 167, 173, 174, 189, 194, 198, 203, 279, 282, 284, 285, 286

Myth - Ritual - Mystical, 180

Mythology, 12, 13, 14, 35, 54, 56, 57, 59, 79, 80, 94, 100, 101, 103, 104, 105, 106, 125, 129, 134, 140, 141, 143, 144, 166, 167, 176, 183, 186, 188, 191, 192, 193, 195, 198, 199, 203, 204, 205, 208, 210, 215, 217, 224, 225, 226, 228, 229

Mythology is a lie, 35

Nag Hammadi, 18, 21, 22, 24, 27, 28, 96, 157, 187, 259, 279, 280

Nagarjuna, 168

Narayana, 41, 59

Nation of Islam, 130, 131

Native American, 25, 43, 49, 68, 147, 150, 162, 163

Native Americans, 25

Nativity, 100

Nature, 66, 104, 110, 135, 156, 205, 220, 240

Neberdjer, 40, 44, 73, 78, 80, 118, 119, 188, 203

Nebertcher, 40, 188, 203, 204

Nebertcher means, 203

Nefer, 290, 291

negative confessions, 120

Negative Confessions, 120

Nehast, 230

Neolithic, 39

Neolithic Age, 39

Neo-Platonism, 141, 164

Neo-Pythagoreanism, 141

Nephthys, 59, 176, 188

Nesi-Khensu, 198

Neter, 13, 48, 71, 119, 169, 203, 284

neters, 203

Neteru, 3, 118, 119, 290, 291

Netherworld, 230

New Age, 12, 144, 166, 219, 225

New Age Movement, 166

New Kingdom, 51, 54

New Stone Age, 39

New testament, 89

New Testament, 10, 15, 19, 20, 21, 23, 27, 28, 44, 60, 63, 66, 81, 89, 92, 96, 115, 116, 125, 130, 135, 145, 147, 148, 152, 155, 156, 157, 164, 186, 189, 191, 192, 202, 203, 230, 233,

241, 252, 254, 255, 256, 263, 279
New World, 163
Nicean council, 23, 50
Nicean Council, 23
Nicomachean Ethics, 142
Niddidhyasana: Meditation, 181
Nirvana, 12, 35, 108, 110, 113, 152, 176, 184, 224, 254
NIRVANA, 108
niyama, 171
Noah, 81
Noah's Ark, 81
Noahs Ark, 55
Noble Eight-fold Path, 108
Noble Truth, 108
Noble Truth of Suffering, 108
Noble Truth of the Cause of Suffering, 108
Noble Truth of the End of Suffering, 108
non-dualist Divinity, 198
Non-dualistic, 34, 93, 139, 204, 205
Non-stealing, 123
non-violence, 257
Non-violence, 123
North Asia, 125
North East Africa, 39, 51, 135
North East Africa . See also Egypt Ethiopia
       Cush, 135
Nothingness, 109
Novena, 54
Nubia, 53, 83, 201
nun, 92
Nun (primeval waters-unformed matter), 40, 256
Nut, 54, 56, 73, 188, 190, 284
Odin, 100
of , Republic Ireland, 144
Ogdoad, 40
oikoumene, 65
Old Kingdom, 51, 65
Old Testament, 19, 20, 21, 25, 56, 63, 65, 67, 70, 75, 76, 77, 79, 80, 83, 86, 88, 89, 90, 115, 118, 125, 127, 128, 148, 157, 162, 188, 249, 263
Om, 9, 42, 254, 290, 291
On the Trinity, 62
One God, 127, 128, 198, 201
Oneness, 13, 30, 174
Ontology, 33
opposites (duality), 106
Opposites of creation, 174, 196

Origen, 139
original sin, 249
Orion Star Constellation, 285
Orpheus, 103
Orthodox church, 31, 65, 92, 117, 141, 182, 194
Orthodox Church, 19, 31, 64, 65, 92, 116, 117, 141, 147, 182, 194, 219
Osarisiph, 79
Osiris, 24, 32, 40, 52, 53, 54, 55, 57, 58, 59, 60, 61, 76, 79, 80, 81, 83, 88, 89, 92, 94, 95, 100, 104, 105, 121, 122, 132, 135, 139, 141, 142, 165, 176, 183, 184, 190, 199, 203, 205, 210, 216, 220, 221, 222, 229, 230, 256, 263, 284, 290, 291
Ottoman Turks, 138
Overdrinking, 136
ownership, 113
Pa Neter, 13, 48, 129, 203, 204
pagan, 141
pagan religions, 142
Pain, 170, 242
Paleolithic, 39, 40
Palermo Stone, 51
Palestine, 25, 28, 67, 68, 70, 72, 76, 79, 81, 82, 83, 85, 86, 90, 91, 113, 115, 126, 140, 161, 263
Palestinians, 25, 26
Pan, 103
Pandora, 103
panentheism, 198
Panentheism, 29, 36, 200
Panentheistic, 29, 94, 140
Pantheism, 36, 200
Papyrus of Nesi Amsu, 56
Papyrus of Nesi-Khensu, 64
Papyrus of Nes-Menu, 176
Papyrus of Turin, 51
Paraclete, 203
Passion, 220
Passion of Jesus, 220
Patanjali, 108, 109, 168, 171, 172, 263
Patañjali, 33
Patanjali, Sage, 167, 172
Patience, 131
Patrick, St., 144
Paul, 15, 23, 28, 115, 161, 164, 193, 210, 248
Paul, St., 164

Peace (see also Hetep), 20, 23, 24, 28, 227, 245, 247, 248, 279, 280
Pentateuch, 67, 80, 115, 199
Pentecost Sunday, 54
Per Ankh, 247
Percival, 145, 146
Persia, 29, 67, 84, 93, 100, 103, 124, 125, 126, 128, 142, 146, 218, 250, 263
Persia,, 29
Persian Gulf, 67, 85, 87, 126
personality integration, 180
PERT EM HERU, SEE ALSO BOOK OF THE DEAD, 284
phallus, 59
Pharisee, 115
Pharisees, 89
phenomenal world, 61
Philae, 55, 177, 284
Philippians, 23, 116
Philo of Alexandria, 79, 132
Philosophy, 9, 10, 11, 12, 13, 16, 29, 32, 35, 36, 37, 46, 47, 48, 49, 69, 107, 108, 109, 132, 135, 139, 141, 165, 168, 169, 170, 176, 195, 202, 219, 241, 259, 263, 280, 282, 283, 284, 285
Philosophy of, 109
Philosophy of Oneness, 13, 30
Phoenix, 54, 80, 210
Phrygians, 61
Phut, 81
Physical Body, 170
Pillar of Osiris, 132, 230
Pir Vilayat Inayat Khan, 209
Pistis Sophia, 185, 194, 279
Plato, 33, 53, 55, 71, 139, 140, 141, 142, 164
Platonic Academy, 164
Pleasure and pain, 49
Plotinus, 141, 164
Plutarch, 79, 140, 176
Point (see also Black Dot and Bindu), 196
Polytheism, 36
Pontius Pilate, 89, 90, 91, 145
Pope Gregory, 193
Porphyry, 141
Poverty, 131
Prakriti, 134
Prana, 135
Prana (also see Sekhem and Life Force), 134, 135
pranayama, 171

pratyahara, 171
pre-dynastic, 188
Pre-dynastic, 55
Presbyterians, 149
Priests and Priestesses, 282
Primeval Hill, 40
Primeval waters, 40, 41, 56, 57, 59, 226
Primeval Waters, 139, 228
promised land, 126, 218
Protestant, 19, 63, 65, 144, 147, 148, 150, 153, 155, 162, 165, 248, 263
Protestant mystics, 165
Protestantism, 65, 147, 148, 149, 153, 155
Protestants, 19, 144, 147, 148, 150, 153, 163
Psalms, 63, 85, 86, 125, 149
Psyche, 11, 12, 14, 32, 33, 219, 223
psychiatrists, 180
psychic healing, 166
psychic paranormal powers, 177
psychologists, 180
Psychology, 12, 32, 33, 219
Psycho-mystical, 31
Psycho-mythology, 229
Psycho-Mythology, 12
Psycho-spiritual transformation, 12
Ptah, 40, 44, 57, 59, 62, 76, 78, 134, 140, 188, 198, 203, 204, 205, 285
PTAH, 203
Ptolemy II, 53, 115, 142
Purana, 177, 183
Pure consciousness, 195, 196, 202, 204, 228
Pure Consciousness, 13, 48, 49, 196, 228
Purified mind, 48
Puritans, 148, 149
Purusha, 41, 56
Pyramid texts, 279
Pyramid Texts, 12, 31, 60, 176, 204, 263, 279
Pyramids, 199
Pythagoras, 29, 53, 71, 139, 140
Pythagorean, 141
queen of the Gods, 188
Quetzalcoatle, 49
Quietism, 165
Ra, 24, 44, 53, 54, 55, 56, 57, 58, 59, 62, 73, 79, 106, 122, 129, 140, 142, 188, 198, 199,

202, 203, 205, 210, 216, 226, 256, 257, 284, 290, 291
racism, 10, 25, 104, 110, 246
Racism, 45, 150, 151
Radha, 183, 184, 191
Rahab, 87
Raising the Tet, 230
Raja Yoga, 209
Ram, 94
Rama, 12, 69, 145, 176, 183, 204
Ramadan, 248
Ramakrishna, 49
Ramses, 71
Ramses II, 141
Rastafarianism, 76, 77
Rati, 184
Reality, 48, 134, 195, 202, 204, 233, 254, 260
Realization, 105, 168, 254
Realm of Light, 188
Red Sea, 74, 201
Reflecting, 181
Reflection, 11, 59, 88, 106, 109, 132, 137, 168, 172, 176, 181, 196, 231, 243, 246, 257
refuge doctrine, 110
reincarnation, 24, 49, 50, 62, 100, 104, 121, 141, 166, 171, 203, 205, 218, 220, 224, 226
Reincarnation, 49, 219
Relationships, 243, 246
Relegare, 34
Religion, 9, 16, 18, 24, 31, 33, 34, 35, 37, 39, 47, 49, 50, 65, 68, 69, 71, 73, 76, 94, 115, 116, 129, 131, 141, 153, 162, 202, 203, 209, 210, 215, 230, 231, 263, 284, 285, 290
Renaissance, 146, 164, 263
Renunciation, 34, 113, 128, 131, 191, 224, 225, 251, 254
Repentance, 131
rest, 134
resurrection, 34, 126
Resurrection, 3, 12, 35, 43, 54, 57, 58, 61, 80, 113, 162, 183, 210, 215, 256, 280, 284, 285, 286
resurrection from the grave, 91
Revival Movement, 153, 162
Rig (Rik) Veda, 42
Rig Veda, 42, 187, 191, 279
Right Action, 109
Right Effort, 109
Right Livelihood, 109
Right Meditation, 109

Right Mindfulness, 109
Right Speech, 109
Right thinking, 47
Right Thinking, 123
Right Thought, 109
Right Understanding, 109
Righteous action, 173, 184
Righteous Action, 172, 173, 174, 280
Righteousness, 28, 89, 111, 192, 232, 280
ritual identification, 58
Ritualism, 38
Rituals, 13, 19, 24, 33, 60, 61, 74, 103, 131, 137, 139, 165, 184, 206, 217, 218, 224, 225, 226, 247, 251, 285
Roman, 10, 11, 19, 22, 23, 24, 28, 48, 50, 51, 54, 55, 60, 62, 64, 65, 67, 68, 76, 86, 89, 90, 91, 92, 97, 100, 103, 104, 111, 113, 115, 116, 132, 137, 138, 139, 140, 142, 143, 144, 145, 146, 147, 148, 149, 150, 157, 160, 161, 162, 164, 165, 174, 180, 182, 186, 187, 220, 229, 256, 263
Roman Catholic, 10, 19, 22, 28, 48, 54, 55, 67, 104, 111, 113, 138, 144, 147, 148, 150, 160, 162, 164, 165, 174, 180, 182, 186, 187, 220
Roman empire, 55, 65, 92, 116, 142, 143, 146, 147
Roman Empire, 23, 24, 50, 51, 55, 62, 65, 67, 86, 90, 111, 116, 138, 142, 144, 145, 146, 161, 229, 263
Romans, 23, 43, 44, 45, 47, 51, 54, 86, 89, 90, 97, 116, 132, 140, 143, 144, 145, 146, 164, 193, 228, 232, 249
Rome, 21, 27, 29, 40, 51, 55, 61, 67, 92, 100, 103, 116, 132, 138, 139, 140, 146, 147, 148, 149, 150, 161, 176, 180, 184, 189, 203, 263
Saa (spiritual understanding faculty), 176, 256
Sabbath, 88, 226
Sage, 191, 221
Sages, 10, 13, 16, 20, 34, 37, 44, 46, 47, 48, 49, 61, 67, 103, 106, 107, 108, 113, 116, 125, 132, 139, 157, 158, 160, 165, 167, 168, 169, 176, 180, 183,

187, 204, 205, 207, 223, 228,
231, 240, 250, 252, 257, 259,
279, 284, 286
Saint, 221
Sainthood, 218
Saints, 10, 13, 16, 30, 34, 47, 65,
66, 107, 108, 132, 168, 169,
176, 179, 187, 191, 215, 231,
284
Saints and Sages, 10, 30, 65, 66,
168, 187, 231
Sakshin, 203
salvation, 34
Salvation, 23, 34, 35, 38, 154,
168
Salvation . See also resurrection, 23,
35, 38, 154, 168
samadhi, 171, 172
Samadhi (see also
KiaSatori), 172
Samkhya, 37, 106, 134
Samkhya philosophy, 106, 134
Samnyasa, 107
SAMNYASA, 171
Samothracians, 61
Samsara, 224
Sanga, 110
Sanskrit, 33, 179, 181, 184
Santeria, 154
Saraswati, 203
Saraswati - Kali - Lakshmi, 203
Sargon I, 66
Sat samkalpa, 171
Satan, 112, 249
Sat-Chit-Ananda, 202
Satsanga, 168, 173, 192
saviors, 191
Schopenhauer, 179
Scotland, 144
Scotus, John Erigena, 164
Sebek, 80
Second Council of
Constantinople, 164
Second Intermediate Period, 51
Secret Book of James, 116
Secret Book of John, 169
Secret of the Golden Flower, 279
See also Ra-Hrakti, 284
Seer, seen and sight, 205
Seers, 34, 49
seer-seen-sight, 203
Sefirotic Tree of Life, 230
Sehu, 180
Sekhem, 132, 134, 135
Sekhmet, 134, 188, 203, 256
Seleucia, 193

Self (see Ba, soul, Spirit,
Universal, Ba, Neter, Heru).,
282, 283, 284
Self (seeBasoulSpiritUniversal
BaNeterHorus)., 12, 13, 15, 32,
33, 34, 35, 37, 38, 41, 44, 47,
48, 49, 50, 54, 56, 60, 61, 63,
64, 70, 79, 95, 106, 108, 110,
112, 113, 122, 123, 124, 132,
133, 134, 135, 137, 168, 169,
170, 171, 172, 174, 176, 178,
179, 180, 181, 183, 185, 191,
195, 196, 197, 198, 203, 204,
205, 216, 219, 221, 225, 226,
227, 228, 229, 230, 231, 232,
241, 243, 244, 245, 246, 249,
251, 252, 253, 254, 258, 260,
261, 262
Self control, 135, 171
Self Control, 123, 174
Self Existent Spirit, 41, 56
self knowledge, 223
selfless service, 178
Self-realization, 35, 177
Self-realized, 179
Sema, 35, 259, 281
Semite, 52
Semitic, 69
Senses, 123
Separatists, 149, 150
Sepher (Sefir) Yezirah, 41
Septuagint, 115, 249
Serapion, the bishop of Antioch,
101
Serapis, 100
Serpent, 111, 112, 113, 132
Serpent of Ignorance, 229
Serpent Power, 111, 112, 113,
132
Serpent Power (see also Kundalini and
Buto), 111, 112, 113, 132
Set, 54, 58, 59, 60, 61, 79, 105,
135, 176, 210, 229, 230, 239,
249, 250
Seti I, 283
seven deadly sins, 192
seven demons, 192
Sex, 43, 183, 225, 280, 284
sexism, 10, 110, 192, 246
Sex-Sublimation, 123
sexual energy, 59, 185
Sexuality, 24, 280
Shabaka Inscription, 40, 41
Shakti (see also Kundalini), 134
Shaktis, 184
SHAMA, 171

shamanism, 166
Shang Dynasty, 135
Shankaracarya, 279
Shaolin Temple, 135
Sheba, 75, 77
Shem, 81
Shem, Baal Tov, 165
Shen, 101, 135
Shepherd, 94, 184
Shetaut Neter, 16, 36, 54, 284
Shetaut Neter See also Egyptian
Religion, 16, 35, 36, 37, 38,
54, 68, 71, 131, 135, 215, 284
Sheti, 173
Shinto, 180
Shintoism, 180, 202
Shiva, 57, 59, 142, 175, 177,
184, 203, 204
Shiva-Samhita, 175, 177
Shravana: Listening, 181
Shrimad-Bhagavata, 183
Shu (air and space), 40, 54, 56, 73,
80, 256
Shunya, 109
siddhis, 177
Sikhism, 141, 202, 263
Sin, 27, 222, 249, 250
Sirius, 95, 285
Skeptics, 33
skin, 88
Sky, 73
Slave Trade, 11, 162
Slavery, 151
Smrti, 30
Society, 22, 106, 151
Socrates, 141, 179
Solomon, 80
Solon, 53, 55, 139
son of God, 89
Song of Govinda, 184
Sons of Light, 256
Sophia, 185
soteriology (saving work), 91
Soul, 45, 47, 64, 100, 199, 226,
242, 244, 245, 253, 257, 260,
279
South West Asia, 39, 81, 83
Southeast Asia, 39, 85
Sphinx, 39, 40, 51, 55, 70, 240,
263, 279
Spirit, 1, 15, 16, 32, 41, 45, 49,
54, 55, 56, 57, 58, 59, 62, 63,
79, 93, 96, 100, 127, 134,
135, 169, 189, 202, 203, 204,
205, 210, 226, 227, 228, 232,
240, 245, 246, 256

Spiritual discipline, 282
Spiritual preceptor, 144
Spiritual transformation, 10, 12, 91, 115, 135, 176
Spiritual Transformation, 35
Sri Yantra, 54
Sruti, 30
St. Augustine, 46, 62, 148, 165
St. Catherine of Siena, 165
St. Clementin, 80
St. Hildegard, 165
St. Polycarp, 116
St. Teresa of Ávila, 165
State of Israel, 25
Stoic, 141
Stone Age, 39
Study, 123
study of scriptures, 178
Sublimation, 284
Suffering, 108, 170, 242
Sufi, 13, 131, 132, 176, 209
Sufism, 38, 131, 132, 153, 165
Sun, 56, 106, 201, 210
Sun and the Moon, 106
Supreme being, 24, 57
Supreme Being, 1, 11, 13, 29, 30, 33, 40, 48, 50, 53, 54, 56, 57, 58, 63, 73, 74, 78, 79, 93, 105, 106, 119, 122, 125, 127, 129, 135, 140, 143, 163, 169, 176, 182, 188, 198, 201, 202, 204, 205, 215, 236, 246, 253, 285
surrender, 129
Suzuki, Daisetz, 165
Svetasvatara Upanishad, 183, 206
Swami, 9, 12, 165, 179, 279, 280
Swami Jyotirmayananda, 9, 12, 165, 179, 279, 280
Swami Vivekananda, 165
Swastika, 100
Switzerland, 144
synchretic view, 142
Synoptic Gospels, 23
Syria, 58, 68, 72, 78, 83, 86, 93, 138, 164, 201, 230
Talking, 247
Talmud, 75, 103, 165, 215
Talmudic tradition, 103
Tammuz, 221
Tantra, 3, 59, 174, 179, 184, 247, 279, 284
Tantra Yoga, 3, 174, 247, 284
Tantric, 191
Tantric Yoga, 33

Tanzania, 52
Tao, 13, 14, 35, 49, 134, 135, 167, 169, 170, 202, 203, 204, 216, 279
TAO, 135
Tao Te Ching, 13, 134, 135, 167, 170, 279
Taoism, 35, 38, 41, 49, 134, 135, 166, 202, 231, 263, 281
Taoist, 203
tarot, 166
Tarsus, 115
Tau Cross, 100
Teacher of Righteousness, 89
Tefnut, 40, 54, 73, 80
Tefnut (moisture), 40, 54, 73, 80
Tehorn, 56
Tehuti, 134
Tehuti-Hermes, 184
Tem, 40, 54, 56, 59, 129
Temple of Aset, 284
Temple of Delphi, 55
Temple of Luxor, 189
Ten Commandments, 67, 69, 70, 80, 118, 234, 236
Ten Lost Tribes, 67
ten thousand things, 135
Tenseness, 136
Teresa, St. of Ávila, 165
Tertulian, 62
Testimony of Truth, 223, 224, 280
TET pillar, 58
Thales, 29, 53, 139, 140
Thamte, 56
the , Dionysius Aropagite, 207
The Absolute, 202, 203, 205
The All, 194, 205
The Apocalypse of Paul, 28
The Apocalypse of Peter, 28
The awakened one, 257
The Bhagavad Gita, 12, 30, 113, 152, 245, 252, 279
The Black One, 105
The Demigods, 53
The Dhahamapada, 12
The Egyptian Book of Coming forth by Day, 198
The Egyptian Book of Coming Forth By Day, 12, 122, 133, 169, 188, 198, 217
The Egyptian Book of Coming Forth By Day and By Ni, 12
The Enlightened One, 107
The Existing One, 74

The God, 53, 54, 121, 129, 203, 236, 279, 284
The Gods, 53, 279, 284
The Gospel of Philip, 28, 29, 185
the Gospel of Thomas, 23, 24, 31, 80, 92, 93, 104, 134, 137, 186, 205, 224, 227, 240, 241, 244, 252, 253, 254
The Gospel of Thomas, 13, 28, 30, 117, 142, 185, 226, 227, 252
The Gospel of Truth, 28, 224
The Hymns of Amun, 43, 280
The Letter of Peter to Philip, 28
the occult, 166
The Philosophy of Oneness, 13
The Pyramid Texts, 12
The Secret Book of James, 24, 28
The Self, 32, 41, 48, 54, 56, 169, 171, 178, 205, 228, 244
The Spirits of the Dead, 53
The Unmoved Mover, 142
The Varieties of Religious Experience, 165
the way, 205
The way, 99, 104, 108, 134, 257
The Word, 157
The WORD, 94
The Yoga Vasistha, 12, 113, 181, 218
the, John Baptist, 175, 186, 220
Theban Theology, 62
Thebes, 28, 62, 140, 204, 283
Thecla, 193
Theists, 18
Themis, 53, 56
Theodosius, 55, 142, 263
Theory of the Forms, 142
Theosophy, 166
Therapeuts, 28, 29, 247
Thoughts (see also Mind), 60, 112
three Kings, 95
Thrice Greatest Hermes, 12, 30, 31, 279
Thucydides, 141
Thunder, Perfect Mind, 169, 185, 187
Tiamat, 56
Tibetan Buddhism, 107
Time, 279, 280
time-space-causation, 61
Tomb, 283
Tomb of Seti I, 283, 291

Torah, 67, 74, 80, 115, 125, 128, 215
Transcendental Self, 93, 195, 254
transfiguration, 253
transformation, 132
transpersonal psychology, 166
Transpersonal Psychology, 12, 219
Tree of Knowledge of Good and Evil, 229
Tree of Life, 189, 206, 229, 230
Triad, 57, 62, 195, 202, 203, 205, 216, 228
Trinity, 44, 57, 58, 62, 63, 67, 77, 92, 93, 102, 111, 127, 128, 140, 155, 188, 202, 203, 204, 215, 284, 291
Trust in God, 131
Truth, 28, 48, 108, 123, 124, 125, 127, 133, 223, 224
Turkey, 68, 103, 115, 128, 139, 140
Uddhism, Kingdom of Heaven of Christianity, Kether, 49
Uganda, 85
Unas, 61
Understanding, 109, 250
Underworld or Astral Plane, 230
undifferentiated, 42
undifferentiated consciousness, 205, 229
Unformed Matter, 228
Unified Field Theory, 48
union with GOD, 131
Union with the Divine, 16, 37
United Kingdom, 143, 144
Universal consciousness, 33, 35, 122
Universal Consciousness, 33, 284
universal love, 251
Unmoved Mover, 142
Upanishad, Brihadaranyaka, 244
Upanishad, Kena, 170
Upanishad, Mundaka, 241
Upanishad, Prasna, 218
Upanishad, Svetasvatara, 206
Upanishads, 30, 33, 42, 48, 69, 107, 122, 166, 167, 168, 169, 170, 178, 179, 192, 195, 199, 218, 279, 284
Uraeus, 132
VAIRAGIA, 171
Vaishnavism, 192
Vandals, 128, 146
Varuna, 125

Vatican, 11, 23, 193
Veda, 178
Vedanta, 9, 12, 32, 35, 36, 37, 38, 49, 50, 69, 131, 142, 152, 167, 168, 169, 170, 181, 199, 202, 224, 226, 263
Vedanta, Advaita, 224
Vedantic, 12, 169
Vedantic. See also Vedanta, 12, 35, 59, 104, 137, 169, 176, 192, 203, 230, 251, 261
Vedas, 30, 42, 69, 167, 168, 169, 191, 254, 263
Vedic, 282
Vedic Aryan, 125
Vegetarianism, 249
Vesica Piscis, 1
Vessel of the Fish, 1
Vesta, 53, 184
Vestal Virgins, 184
Viking, 144
Vikings, 128, 146
vikshepa, 177
Vikshepa, 170
VIKSHEPA, 170
Vilayat, Pir Inayat Khan, 209
Virgin birth, 29
Virgin Birth, 59, 186
Virgin Mary, 54, 78, 79, 90, 130, 186, 210
Virgin's Well, 79
Vishnu, 69, 125, 145, 178, 183, 184, 192, 203, 204, 249
Visigoths, 128
VIVEKA, 171
waking, dream and dreamless states, 216
Wales, 144
Waset, 204
Washing the heart, 226
Washing the heart . See also Purity of Heart, 226
Water, 47, 218
Way of Nature, 135
Welsh, 144
West Indies, 150
Western civilization, 27, 29, 51, 139
Western Europe, 164
Western religions, 24, 36, 174, 198, 208, 219
Wheel of Life, 168
Wheel of the Law, 108
Whirling Dervishes, 131
Whirling Dervishes (see also !Kung of Afrika), 131

Whitehead, 33
Will, 20, 64, 119, 128, 202
Wisdom, 283
Wisdom (also see Djehuti), 13, 16, 33, 62, 67, 106, 108, 119, 135, 148, 167, 168, 174, 185, 219, 234, 236, 256, 280
Wisdom (also see Djehuti, Aset), 283
Wisdom teachings, 28, 30, 33, 67, 113, 137, 168, 171, 178, 181, 195, 234, 246
Word, Living, 256
Word, the, 256
Worry, 110, 136
Y, 39
Yahweh, 24, 67, 73, 74, 119, 125, 127, 142, 182, 189, 199, 200, 204
Yajnas, 217
Yajnas or ritual, 217
yama, 171
Yamas and Nyamas (See Yoga of Righteous Action and Maat Philosophy, 123
Ying and Yang, 41, 135
Yoga, 2, 9, 10, 11, 12, 14, 16, 18, 22, 30, 32, 33, 34, 35, 37, 40, 41, 46, 47, 48, 49, 50, 54, 61, 64, 69, 71, 74, 75, 77, 93, 105, 108, 109, 111, 113, 116, 117, 132, 133, 135, 142, 151, 157, 158, 159, 166, 167, 168, 169, 171, 172, 173, 174, 175, 176, 177, 178, 179, 180, 181, 195, 196, 197, 202, 203, 205, 206, 209, 217, 219, 220, 221, 223, 224, 225, 230, 231, 232, 233, 240, 243, 245, 246, 247, 251, 253, 254, 257, 259, 263, 279, 280, 281, 282, 283, 284, 285, 289, 290, 291
YOGA, 219
Yoga counselor, 175
yoga instructors, 180
Yoga of Action, 167, 219, 254
Yoga of Devotion, 219
Yoga of Devotion (see Yoga of Divine Love), 33, 167, 172, 173, 219
Yoga of Devotional Love, 173
Yoga of Divine Love, 30, 174
Yoga of Divine Love (see Yoga of Devotion), 30, 174
Yoga of Meditation, 33, 167, 172, 173, 174, 219
Yoga of Righteous, 172, 173, 174

Yoga of Righteous . See also Karma
    Yoga, 172, 173, 174
Yoga of Selfless Action, 33
Yoga of Selfless Action. See also Yoga
    of Righteous, 33
Yoga of wisdom, 33
Yoga of Wisdom, 33, 105, 117,
    133, 172, 173, 174, 181, 195,
    219, 254
Yoga of Wisdom (see also Jnana Yoga),
    33, 105, 117, 133, 167, 172,
    173, 174, 181, 195, 219, 254
Yoga Philosophy, 35

Yoga Sutra, 172, 177
Yoga Sutras, 172
Yoga Vasistha, 12, 113, 176, 196,
    217, 218, 224, 225, 251, 280
Yoga, Raja, 209
Yogi, 225
Yogic, 10, 16, 18, 31, 44, 56, 77,
    97, 104, 108, 166, 171, 175,
    178, 179, 247, 255
Yogic spiritual discipline, 16
Yogic Spiritual Preceptor, 175
Yoruba, 141, 154
Yorubas, 49

Zen, 166
Zen Buddhism, 107, 165
Zeus, 100, 140
Zion, 25, 182
Zionism, 25
Zohar, 41
Zoomorphic, 210
Zoroaster, 24, 29, 124, 250, 263
Zoroastrian, 128, 187, 199
Zoroastrianism, 29, 38, 93, 124,
    125, 126
Zoroastrians, 124

BIBLIOGRAPHY

1- Egyptian Pyramid Texts
2- Egyptian Coffin texts
3- Egyptian Book of Coming forth by day of Anhai
4- Egyptian Book of Coming forth by day of Ani
5- Egyptian Book of Coming forth by day of Kenna
6- Egyptian Book of Coming forth by day of Ankhwahibre
7- Stele of Djehuti-nefer
8- Stele of abu
9- The Greenfield papyrus
10- The Ebers papyrus
11- The Turin Papyrus
12- Herodotus: The Histories
13- "The Meaning of the Dead Sea Scrolls" by A. Powell Davies
14- "The Other Bible" translated by Wilhelm Schneemelcher, New Testament Apocrypha
15- "Rig Veda" by Aryan and Indian Sages
16- "TemTTchaas: Egyptian Proverbs" by Muata Ashby
17- "Woman's Dictionary of Sacred Symbols" by Barbara Walker
18- "Gnostic Gospels" by Elaine Pagels
19- "The Mystery of the Sphinx" on video by John Anthony West
20- "The Ancient Egyptians" by Sir J. Gardner Wilkinson
21- "Woman's Encyclopedia of Myths and Secrets" by Barbara Walker
22- "Ancient Egypt the Light of the World " by Gerald Massey
23- "The Gods of the Egyptians Vol. I,II" by E. Wallis Budge
24- "Hindu Myths" by Wendy O'Flaherty
25- "The Great Book of Tantra" by Indra Sinha
26- "SADHANA" by Swami Sivananda
27- "The Kybalion" by Hermes Trismegistos
28- "Vivekacudamani" by Shankaracarya
29- "African Presence in Early Asia" edited by Ivan Van Sertima and Runoko Rashidi
30- "Jnana Yoga" by Swami Jyotirmayananda
31- "Four Gnostic Gospels" Translated by Marvin Meyer
32- "Pistis Sophia"
33- "Civilization or Barbarism" by Cheikh Anta Diop
34- "Smithsonian Magazine" June 1993
35- "Echoes of the Old Darkland" by Dr. Charles Finch
36- "The Bhagavad Gita" translated by Antonio DE Nicolas
37- "The Opening of the Way" by Isha Schwaller DE Lubicz
38- "Gospel of Mary" by Mary Magdalene, Nag Hammadi Library 473
39- "Hippolytus," ref 1.24
40- "Life Force" by Leo Ludzia
41- "Recovering the Soul" by Dr. Larry Dossey
42- "Egyptian Book of the Dead" by Gerald Massey
43- "Mind- It's Mysteries and Control" BY Swami Sivananda
44- "Stolen Legacy" by George G.M. James
45- "Egyptian Book of the Dead" by E. Wallis Budge
46- "Egyptian Book of the Dead" by R.O. Faulkner
47- "The Upanishads" by Swami Prabhavananda
48- "African Presence in Early Asia" by Dr. Ivan Van Sertima
49- "Hero of a Thousand Faces" by Dr. Joseph Campbell
50- "Encyclopedic Dictionary of Yoga" by Georg Feurstein
51- "The Bhagavad Gita" translated by Swami Jyotirmayananda
52- "The Tantric Way" by Ajit Mookerjee and Madhu Khanna
53- "Kundalini" by Gopi Krishna
54- "Myths and Symbol in Ancient Egypt" by R.T. Rundle Clark
55- "The Secret of the Golden Flower: A Chinese Book of Life" Translation by Richard Wilhelm
56- "Theory and Practice of Counseling and Psychotherapy" by Gerald Corey
57- "The Tao of Physics" by Frijot Capra
58- "Transformations of Myth Through Time" by Joseph Campbell
59- "Integral Yoga" by Swami Jyotirmayananda
60- "Time Magazine" March 14, 1994
61- "Ancient Egyptian Literature" Volume I and II, by Miriam Lichtheim
62- "Ruins of Empires" by C.F. Volney
63- "Thrice Greatest Hermes" by G.R.S. Mead
64- "Egyptian Yoga" by Reginald Muata Ashby
65- "The Origin of Western Barbarism" by Michael Wood
66- "Encyclopedia of Mysticism and Mystery Religions" by John Ferguson
67- "Dancing With Siva" by S. S. Subramuniyaswami
68- "Merriam-Webster Dictionary"
69- "Tao Te Ching" by Lao Tsu
70- "The Isis Papers" by Dr. Frances Cress-Welsing
71- "Tibetan Book of the Dead" by Francesca Fremantle and Chögyam Trungpa
72- "Essene Gospel of Peace" translated by Edward Bordeau Szakeley
73- "Islam and the Sciences"
74- "On the Mysteries" by Iamblichus
75- "Funk and Wagnals New Encyclopedia"
76- "Christian and Islamic Spirituality" by Maria Jaoudi
77- "The Story of Islam"
78- "Conflict of the Gods" by Carlos Fuentes
79- "Middle Passage" BET Television
80- "Egyptian Book of the Dead" by Gerald Massey
81- "Testament" by John Romer
82- "Secret Book of Egyptian Gnostics" by Jean Doresse
83- "Buddha: the Intelligent Heart" by Alistair Shearer
84- "Ferdmand's Handbook to the World's Religions"

85- "Yoga Vasistha Vol. I" by Sage Valmiki - Translation by Swami Jyotirmayananda

86- "Yoga Vasistha Vol. II" by Sage Valmiki - Translation by Swami Jyotirmayananda

87- "Yoga Vasistha Vol. III" by Sage Valmiki - Translation by Swami Jyotirmayananda

88- HOLY BIBLE- New Revised Standard Version

89- HOLY BIBLE- King James Version

90- Essene *Gospel of Peace* by Edmund Bordeaux Szekely

91- Gospel of Thomas

92- "Am I a Hindu?: the Hinduism Primer" by Ed. Viswanathan

93- Nag Hammadi Library, edited by James Robinson

94- Irenaeus, AH

95- Tertulian, De Pudicitia

96- Testimony of Truth, Nag Hammadi Library

97- Clement of Alexandria, Stromata 4.71ff

98- "Love and Sexuality Vol. I-II" by O.M. Aivanov

99- "How did sex begin?" by R. Brasch

100-"The Subordinate Sex" by Vern L. Bullough

101- "The Gnostic Scriptures" by Bentley Leyghton

102- "Pastoral Counseling" edited by Barry K Estadt, Melvin C. Blanchette, John R. Compton

103- "Refutation of all heresies" V

104- On the Cessation of the Oracles 14

105- Exhortation II

106- Fo-Sho-Hing 1299

107- Blackwell's book of Philosophy; Zeller's History of Philosophy; Diogenes Laertius; Kendrick's Ancient Egypt.

108- Herodotus Book III 124; Diogenes VIII 3; Pliny N. H., 36, 9; Antipho recorded by Porphyry.

109- "Legends of the Egyptian Gods" by E. Wallis Budge

110- "From Fetish to God" by E. Wallis Budge

111- "Ancient, Medieval and Modern Christianity" by Charles Guignebert

112- "The Priests of Ancient Egypt" by Serge Sauneron, Grove p114

113- "Egyptian Magic" by E.W. Budge

114- "The Hymns of Amun" by Dr. Muata Ashby

115- American Heritage Dictionary.

116- "The Cycles of Time" by Dr. Muata Ashby

117- Random House Encyclopedia.

118- "The Bandlet of Righteousness: An Ethiopian Book of the Dead" translated by E.A. Wallis Budge

119- "The Ausarian Resurrection: The Ancient Egyptian Bible" by Dr. Muata Ashby

120- "Meditation: The Ancient Egyptian Path to Enlightenment" by Dr. Muata Ashby

121- "The Wisdom of Maati: Spiritual Enlightenment Through the Path of Righteous Action" by Dr. Muata Ashby

122- "The Hidden Properties of Matter" by Dr. Muata Ashby

123- Copton's Encyclopedia

124- Strong's Exhaustive Concordance of the Bible.

125- Sex and Race by J.A. Rogers

126- Websters Encyclopedia

127- "From Egypt to Greece" by Dr. Muata Ashby

128- "Christians of the Copperbelt (SCM, London 1961) p 287. By J. V. Taylor and D. Lehmann

129- New Blackfriars, "Comment", Jan., 1984, p. 3, by J. O. Mills

130- "The Cult of The Black Madonna" by Ean Begg

131- "A History of Christianity in Africa" by Elizabeth Isichei

132- "Egyptian Yoga: Volume II" by Reginald Muata Ashby

COPYRIGHTS

OTHER BOOKS FROM C M BOOKS

P.O.Box 570459
Miami, Florida, 33257
(305) 378-6253 Fax: (305) 378-6253

This book is part of a series on the study and practice of Ancient Egyptian Yoga and Mystical Spirituality based on the writings of Dr. Muata Abhaya Ashby. They are also part of the Egyptian Yoga Course provided by the Sema Institute of Yoga. Below you will find a listing of the other books in this series. For more information send for the Egyptian Yoga Book-Audio-Video Catalog or the Egyptian Yoga Course Catalog.

Now you can study the teachings of Egyptian and Indian Yoga wisdom and Spirituality with the Egyptian Yoga Mystical Spirituality Series. The Egyptian Yoga Series takes you through the Initiation process and lead you to understand the mysteries of the soul and the Divine and to attain the highest goal of life: ENLIGHTENMENT. The *Egyptian Yoga Series*, takes you on an in depth study of Ancient Egyptian mythology and their inner mystical meaning. Each Book is prepared for the serious student of the mystical sciences and provides a study of the teachings along with exercises, assignments and projects to make the teachings understood and effective in real life. The Series is part of the Egyptian Yoga course but may be purchased even if you are not taking the course. The series is ideal for study groups.

Prices subject to change.

1.   EGYPTIAN YOGA: THE PHILOSOPHY OF ENLIGHTENMENT An original, fully illustrated work, including hieroglyphs, detailing the meaning of the Egyptian mysteries, tantric yoga, psycho-spiritual and physical exercises. Egyptian Yoga is a guide to the practice of the highest spiritual philosophy which leads to absolute freedom from human misery and to immortality. It is well known by scholars that Egyptian philosophy is the basis of Western and Middle Eastern religious philosophies such as *Christianity, Islam, Judaism,* the *Kabala,* and Greek philosophy, but what about Indian philosophy, Yoga and Taoism? What were the original teachings? How can they be practiced today? What is the source of pain and suffering in the world and what is the solution? Discover the deepest mysteries of the mind and universe within and outside of your self. 8.5" X 11" ISBN: 1-884564-01-1 Soft $19.95

2.   EGYPTIAN YOGA II: The Supreme Wisdom of Enlightenment by Dr. Muata Ashby ISBN 1-884564-39-9 $23.95 U.S. In this long awaited sequel to *Egyptian Yoga: The Philosophy of Enlightenment* you will take a fascinating and enlightening journey back in time and discover the teachings which constituted the epitome of Ancient Egyptian spiritual wisdom. What are the disciplines which lead to the fulfillment of all desires? Delve into the three states of consciousness (waking, dream and deep sleep) and the fourth state which transcends them all, Neberdjer, "The Absolute." These teachings of the city of Waset (Thebes) were the crowning achievement of the Sages of Ancient Egypt. They establish the standard mystical keys for understanding the profound mystical symbolism of the Triad of human consciousness.

3.   THE KEMETIC DIET: GUIDE TO HEALTH, DIET AND FASTING Health issues have always been important to human beings since the beginning of time. The earliest records of history show that the art of healing was held in high esteem since the time of Ancient Egypt. In the early 20th century, medical doctors had almost attained the status of sainthood by the promotion of the idea that they alone were "scientists" while other healing modalities and traditional healers who did not follow the "scientific method' were nothing but superstitious, ignorant charlatans who at best would take the money of their clients and at worst kill them with the unscientific "snake oils" and "irrational theories". In the late 20th century, the failure of the modern medical establishment's ability to lead the general public to good health, promoted the move by many in society towards "alternative medicine". Alternative medicine disciplines are those healing modalities which do not adhere to the philosophy of allopathic medicine. Allopathic medicine is what medical doctors practice by an large. It is the theory that disease is caused by agencies outside the body such as bacteria, viruses or physical means which affect the body. These can therefore be treated by

medicines and therapies The natural healing method began in the absence of extensive technologies with the idea that all the answers for health may be found in nature or rather, the deviation from nature. Therefore, the health of the body can be restored by correcting the aberration and thereby restoring balance. This is the area that will be covered in this volume. Allopathic techniques have their place in the art of healing. However, we should not forget that the body is a grand achievement of the spirit and built into it is the capacity to maintain itself and heal itself. Ashby, Muata ISBN: 1-884564-49-6 $28.95

4. INITIATION INTO EGYPTIAN YOGA Shedy: Spiritual discipline or program, to go deeply into the mysteries, to study the mystery teachings and literature profoundly, to penetrate the mysteries. You will learn about the mysteries of initiation into the teachings and practice of Yoga and how to become an Initiate of the mystical sciences. This insightful manual is the first in a series which introduces you to the goals of daily spiritual and yoga practices: Meditation, Diet, Words of Power and the ancient wisdom teachings. 8.5" X 11" ISBN 1-884564-02-X Soft Cover $24.95 U.S.

5. *THE AFRICAN ORIGINS OF CIVILIZATION, MYSTICAL RELIGION AND YOGA PHILOSOPHY* HARD COVER EDITION ISBN: 1-884564-50-X $80.00 U.S.   81/2" X 11" Part 1, Part 2, Part 3 in one volume 683 Pages Hard Cover First Edition Three volumes in one. Over the past several years I have been asked to put together in one volume the most important evidences showing the correlations and common teachings between Kamitan (Ancient Egyptian) culture and religion and that of India. The questions of the history of Ancient Egypt, and the latest archeological evidences showing civilization and culture in Ancient Egypt and its spread to other countries, has intrigued many scholars as well as mystics over the years. Also, the possibility that Ancient Egyptian Priests and Priestesses migrated to Greece, India and other countries to carry on the traditions of the Ancient Egyptian Mysteries, has been speculated over the years as well. In chapter 1 of the book *Egyptian Yoga The Philosophy of Enlightenment,* 1995, I first introduced the deepest comparison between Ancient Egypt and India that had been brought forth up to that time. Now, in the year 2001 this new book, *THE AFRICAN ORIGINS OF CIVILIZATION, MYSTICAL RELIGION AND YOGA PHILOSOPHY,* more fully explores the motifs, symbols and philosophical correlations between Ancient Egyptian and Indian mysticism and clearly shows not only that Ancient Egypt and India were connected culturally but also spiritually. How does this knowledge help the spiritual aspirant? This discovery has great importance for the Yogis and mystics who follow the philosophy of Ancient Egypt and the mysticism of India. It means that India has a longer history and heritage than was previously understood. It shows that the mysteries of Ancient Egypt were essentially a yoga tradition which did not die but rather developed into the modern day systems of Yoga technology of India. It further shows that African culture developed Yoga Mysticism earlier than any other civilization in history. All of this expands our understanding of the unity of culture and the deep legacy of Yoga, which stretches into the distant past, beyond the Indus Valley civilization, the earliest known high culture in India as well as the Vedic tradition of Aryan culture. Therefore, Yoga culture and mysticism is the oldest known tradition of spiritual development and Indian mysticism is an extension of the Ancient Egyptian mysticism. By understanding the legacy which Ancient Egypt gave to India the mysticism of India is better understood and by comprehending the heritage of Indian Yoga, which is rooted in Ancient Egypt the Mysticism of Ancient Egypt is also better understood. This expanded understanding allows us to prove the underlying kinship of humanity, through the common symbols, motifs and philosophies which are not disparate and confusing teachings but in reality expressions of the same study of truth through metaphysics and mystical realization of Self. (HARD COVER)

6. AFRICAN ORIGINS BOOK 1 PART 1 African Origins of African Civilization, Religion, Yoga Mysticism and Ethics Philosophy-Soft Cover $24.95 ISBN: 1-884564-55-0

7. AFRICAN ORIGINS BOOK 2 PART 2 African Origins of Western Civilization, Religion and Philosophy(Soft) -Soft Cover $24.95 ISBN: 1-884564-56-9

8. EGYPT AND INDIA (AFRICAN ORIGINS BOOK 3 PART 3) African Origins of Eastern Civilization, Religion, Yoga Mysticism and Philosophy-Soft Cover $29.95 (Soft) ISBN: 1-884564-57-7

9. THE MYSTERIES OF ISIS: **The Ancient Egyptian Philosophy of Self-Realization** - There are several paths to discover the Divine and the mysteries of the higher Self. This volume details the mystery

teachings of the goddess Aset (Isis) from Ancient Egypt- the path of wisdom. It includes the teachings of her temple and the disciplines that are enjoined for the initiates of the temple of Aset as they were given in ancient times. Also, this book includes the teachings of the main myths of Aset that lead a human being to spiritual enlightenment and immortality.   Through the study of ancient myth and the illumination of initiatic understanding the idea of God is expanded from the mythological comprehension to the metaphysical. Then this metaphysical understanding is related to you, the student, so as to begin understanding your true divine nature. ISBN 1-884564-24-0 $22.99

10. EGYPTIAN PROVERBS: TEMT TCHAAS *Temt Tchaas* means: collection of——Ancient Egyptian Proverbs How to live according to MAAT Philosophy. Beginning Meditation. All proverbs are indexed for easy searches. For the first time in one volume, ——Ancient Egyptian Proverbs, wisdom teachings and meditations, fully illustrated with hieroglyphic text and symbols. EGYPTIAN PROVERBS is a unique collection of knowledge and wisdom which you can put into practice today and transform your life. 5.5"x 8.5" $14.95 U.S   ISBN: 1-884564-00-3

11. THE PATH OF DIVINE LOVE The Process of Mystical Transformation and The Path of Divine Love This Volume focuses on the ancient wisdom teachings of "Neter Merri" –the Ancient Egyptian philosophy of Divine Love and how to use them in a scientific process for self-transformation. Love is one of the most powerful human emotions. It is also the source of Divine feeling that unifies God and the individual human being. When love is fragmented and diminished by egoism the Divine connection is lost. The Ancient tradition of Neter Merri leads human beings back to their Divine connection, allowing them to discover their innate glorious self that is actually Divine and immortal. This volume will detail the process of transformation from ordinary consciousness to cosmic consciousness through the integrated practice of the teachings and the path of Devotional Love toward the Divine. 5.5"x 8.5" ISBN 1-884564-11-9 $22.99

12. INTRODUCTION TO MAAT PHILOSOPHY: Spiritual Enlightenment Through the Path of Virtue Known as Karma Yoga in India, the teachings of MAAT for living virtuously and with orderly wisdom are explained and the student is to begin practicing the precepts of Maat in daily life so as to promote the process of purification of the heart in preparation for the judgment of the soul. This judgment will be understood not as an event that will occur at the time of death but as an event that occurs continuously, at every moment in the life of the individual. The student will learn how to become allied with the forces of the Higher Self and to thereby begin cleansing the mind (heart) of impurities so as to attain a higher vision of reality. ISBN 1-884564-20-8 $22.99

13. MEDITATION The Ancient Egyptian Path to Enlightenment   Many people do not know about the rich history of meditation practice in Ancient Egypt. This volume outlines the theory of meditation and presents the Ancient Egyptian Hieroglyphic text which give instruction as to the nature of the mind and its three modes of expression. It also presents the texts which give instruction on the practice of meditation for spiritual Enlightenment and unity with the Divine. This volume allows the reader to begin practicing meditation by explaining, in easy to understand terms, the simplest form of meditation and working up to the most advanced form which was practiced in ancient times and which is still practiced by yogis around the world in modern times. ISBN 1-884564-27-7 $24.99

14. THE GLORIOUS LIGHT MEDITATION Technique of Ancient Egypt ISBN: 1-884564-15-1$14.95 (PB) New for the year 2000. This volume is based on the earliest known instruction in history given for the practice of formal meditation. Discovered by Dr. Muata Ashby, it is inscribed on the walls of the Tomb of Seti I in Thebes Egypt. This volume details the philosophy and practice of this unique system of meditation originated in Ancient Egypt and the earliest practice of meditation known in the world which occurred in the most advanced African Culture.

15. THE SERPENT POWER: The Ancient Egyptian Mystical Wisdom of the Inner Life Force.   This Volume specifically deals with the latent life Force energy of the universe and in the human body, its control and sublimation. How to develop the Life Force energy of the subtle body. This Volume will introduce the esoteric wisdom of the science of how virtuous living acts in a subtle and mysterious way to cleanse the latent psychic energy conduits and vortices of the spiritual body. ISBN 1-884564-19-4 $22.95

16. EGYPTIAN YOGA *The Postures of The Gods and Goddesses* Discover the physical postures and exercises practiced thousands of years ago in Ancient Egypt which are today known as Yoga exercises. This work is based on the pictures and teachings from the Creation story of Ra, The Asarian Resurrection Myth and the carvings and reliefs from various Temples in Ancient Egypt 8.5" X 11" ISBN 1-884564-10-0 Soft Cover $21.95   Exercise video $20

17. EGYPTIAN TANTRA YOGA: The Art of Sex Sublimation and Universal Consciousness This Volume will expand on the male and female principles within the human body and in the universe and further detail the sublimation of sexual energy into spiritual energy. The student will study the deities Min and Hathor, Asar and Aset, Geb and Nut and discover the mystical implications for a practical spiritual discipline. This Volume will also focus on the Tantric aspects of Ancient Egyptian and Indian mysticism, the purpose of sex and the mystical teachings of sexual sublimation which lead to self-knowledge and Enlightenment. 5.5"x 8.5" ISBN 1-884564-03-8 $24.95

18. ASARIAN RELIGION: RESURRECTING OSIRIS The path of Mystical Awakening and the Keys to Immortality NEW REVISED AND EXPANDED EDITION! The Ancient Sages created stories based on human and superhuman beings whose struggles, aspirations, needs and desires ultimately lead them to discover their true Self. The myth of Aset, Asar and Heru is no exception in this area. While there is no one source where the entire story may be found, pieces of it are inscribed in various ancient Temples walls, tombs, steles and papyri. For the first time available, the complete myth of Asar, Aset and Heru has been compiled from original Ancient Egyptian, Greek and Coptic Texts. This epic myth has been richly illustrated with reliefs from the Temple of Heru at Edfu, the Temple of Aset at Philae, the Temple of Asar at Abydos, the Temple of Hathor at Denderah and various papyri, inscriptions and reliefs. Discover the myth which inspired the teachings of the *Shetaut Neter* (Egyptian Mystery System - Egyptian Yoga) and the Egyptian Book of Coming Forth By Day. Also, discover the three levels of Ancient Egyptian Religion, how to understand the mysteries of the Duat or Astral World and how to discover the abode of the Supreme in the Amenta, *The Other World*   The ancient religion of Asar, Aset and Heru, if properly understood, contains all of the elements necessary to lead the sincere aspirant to attain immortality through inner self-discovery. This volume presents the entire myth and explores the main mystical themes and rituals associated with the myth for understating human existence, creation and the way to achieve spiritual emancipation - *Resurrection.* The Asarian myth is so powerful that it influenced and is still having an effect on the major world religions. Discover the origins and mystical meaning of the Christian Trinity, the Eucharist ritual and the ancient origin of the birthday of Jesus Christ. Soft Cover ISBN: 1-884564-27-5 $24.95

19. THE EGYPTIAN BOOK OF THE DEAD MYSTICISM OF THE PERT EM HERU $26.95   ISBN# 1-884564-28-3 Size: 8½" X 11" I Know myself, I know myself, I am One With God!–From the Pert Em Heru "The Ru Pert em Heru" or "Ancient Egyptian Book of The Dead," or "Book of Coming Forth By Day" as it is more popularly known, has fascinated the world since the successful translation of Ancient Egyptian hieroglyphic scripture over 150 years ago. The astonishing writings in it reveal that the Ancient Egyptians believed in life after death and in an ultimate destiny to discover the Divine. The elegance and aesthetic beauty of the hieroglyphic text itself has inspired many see it as an art form in and of itself. But is there more to it than that? Did the Ancient Egyptian wisdom contain more than just aphorisms and hopes of eternal life beyond death? In this volume Dr. Muata Ashby, the author of over 25 books on Ancient Egyptian Yoga Philosophy has produced a new translation of the original texts which uncovers a mystical teaching underlying the sayings and rituals instituted by the Ancient Egyptian Sages and Saints. "Once the philosophy of Ancient Egypt is understood as a mystical tradition instead of as a religion or primitive mythology, it reveals its secrets which if practiced today will lead anyone to discover the glory of spiritual self-discovery. The Pert em Heru is in every way comparable to the Indian Upanishads or the Tibetan Book of the Dead." Muata Abhaya Ashby

20. ANUNIAN THEOLOGY THE MYSTERIES OF RA The Philosophy of Anu and The Mystical Teachings of The Ancient Egyptian Creation Myth Discover the mystical teachings contained in the Creation Myth and the gods and goddesses who brought creation and human beings into existence. The Creation Myth

holds the key to understanding the universe and for attaining spiritual Enlightenment. ISBN: 1-884564-38-0 40 pages $14.95

21. MYSTERIES OF MIND AND MEMPHITE THEOLOGY Mysticism of Ptah, Egyptian Physics and Yoga Metaphysics and the Hidden properties of Matter   This Volume will go deeper into the philosophy of God as creation and will explore the concepts of modern science and how they correlate with ancient teachings. This Volume will lay the ground work for the understanding of the philosophy of universal consciousness and the initiatic/yogic insight into who or what is God? ISBN 1-884564-07-0 $21.95

22. THE GODDESS AND THE EGYPTIAN MYSTERIESTHE PATH OF THE GODDESS THE GODDESS PATH The Secret Forms of the Goddess and the Rituals of Resurrection The Supreme Being may be worshipped as father or as mother. *Ushet Rekhat* or *Mother Worship*, is the spiritual process of worshipping the Divine in the form of the Divine Goddess. It celebrates the most important forms of the Goddess including *Nathor, Maat, Aset, Arat, Amentet and Hathor* and explores their mystical meaning as well as the rising of *Sirius,* the star of Aset (Aset) and the new birth of Hor (Heru). The end of the year is a time of reckoning, reflection and engendering a new or renewed positive movement toward attaining spiritual Enlightenment. The Mother Worship devotional meditation ritual, performed on five days during the month of December and on New Year's Eve, is based on the Ushet Rekhit. During the ceremony, the cosmic forces, symbolized by Sirius - and the constellation of Orion ---, are harnessed through the understanding and devotional attitude of the participant. This propitiation draws the light of wisdom and health to all those who share in the ritual, leading to prosperity and wisdom. $14.95 ISBN 1-884564-18-6

23. *THE MYSTICAL JOURNEY FROM JESUS TO CHRIST* $24.95   ISBN# 1-884564-05-4 size: 8½" X 11" Discover the ancient Egyptian origins of Christianity before the Catholic Church and learn the mystical teachings given by Jesus to assist all humanity in becoming Christlike. Discover the secret meaning of the Gospels that were discovered in Egypt. Also discover how and why so many Christian churches came into being. Discover that the Bible still holds the keys to mystical realization even though its original writings were changed by the church. Discover how to practice the original teachings of Christianity which leads to the Kingdom of Heaven.

24. THE STORY OF ASAR, ASET AND HERU: An Ancient Egyptian Legend (For Children)   Now for the first time, the most ancient myth of Ancient Egypt comes alive for children. Inspired by the books *The Asarian Resurrection: The Ancient Egyptian Bible* and *The Mystical Teachings of The Asarian Resurrection, The Story of Asar, Aset and Heru* is an easy to understand and thrilling tale which inspired the children of Ancient Egypt to aspire to greatness and righteousness. If you and your child have enjoyed stories like *The Lion King* and *Star Wars you will love The Story of Asar, Aset and Heru.* Also, if you know the story of Jesus and Krishna you will discover than Ancient Egypt had a similar myth and that this myth carries important spiritual teachings for living a fruitful and fulfilling life. This book may be used along with *The Parents Guide To The Asarian Resurrection Myth: How to Teach Yourself and Your Child the Principles of Universal Mystical Religion.* The guide provides some background to the Asarian Resurrection myth and it also gives insight into the mystical teachings contained in it which you may introduce to your child. It is designed for parents who wish to grow spiritually with their children and it serves as an introduction for those who would like to study the Asarian Resurrection Myth in depth and to practice its teachings. 41 pages 8.5" X 11"   ISBN: 1-884564-31-3 $12.95

25. THE PARENTS GUIDE TO THE AUSARIAN RESURRECTION MYTH: How to Teach Yourself and Your Child the Principles of Universal Mystical Religion.   This insightful manual brings for the timeless wisdom of the ancient through the Ancient Egyptian myth of Asar, Aset and Heru and the mystical teachings contained in it for parents who want to guide their children to understand and practice the teachings of mystical spirituality. This manual may be used with the children's storybook *The Story of Asar, Aset and Heru* by Dr. Muata Abhaya Ashby. 5.5"x 8.5"   ISBN: 1-884564-30-5 $14.95

26. HEALING THE CRIMINAL HEART BOOK 1 Introduction to Maat Philosophy, Yoga and Spiritual Redemption Through the Path of Virtue   Who is a criminal? Is there such a thing as a criminal heart? What is the source of evil and sinfulness and is there any way to rise above it? Is there redemption for those who have committed sins, even the worst crimes?   Ancient Egyptian mystical psychology holds

important answers to these questions. Over ten thousand years ago mystical psychologists, the Sages of Ancient Egypt, studied and charted the human mind and spirit and laid out a path which will lead to spiritual redemption, prosperity and Enlightenment.   This introductory volume brings forth the teachings of the Asarian Resurrection, the most important myth of Ancient Egypt, with relation to the faults of human existence: anger, hatred, greed, lust, animosity, discontent, ignorance, egoism jealousy, bitterness, and a myriad of psycho-spiritual ailments which keep a human being in a state of negativity and adversity. 5.5"x 8.5"   ISBN: 1-884564-17-8 $15.95

27.   THEATER & DRAMA OF THE ANCIENT EGYPTIAN MYSTERIES: Featuring the Ancient Egyptian stage play-"The Enlightenment of Hathor' Based on an Ancient Egyptian Drama, The original Theater - Mysticism of the Temple of Hetheru $14.95 By Dr. Muata Ashby

28.   GUIDE TO PRINT ON DEMAND: SELF-PUBLISH FOR PROFIT, SPIRITUAL FULFILLMENT AND SERVICE TO HUMANITY Everyone asks us how we produced so many books in such a short time. Here are the secrets to writing and producing books that uplift humanity and how to get them printed for a fraction of the regular cost. Anyone can become an author even if they have limited funds. All that is necessary is the willingness to learn how the printing and book business work and the desire to follow the special instructions given here for preparing your manuscript format. Then you take your work directly to the non-traditional companies who can produce your books for less than the traditional book printer can. ISBN: 1-884564-40-2 $16.95 U. S.

29.   Egyptian Mysteries: Vol. 1, Shetaut Neter ISBN: 1-884564-41-0 $19.99 What are the Mysteries? For thousands of years the spiritual tradition of Ancient Egypt, *Shetaut Neter,* "The Egyptian Mysteries," "The Secret Teachings," have fascinated, tantalized and amazed the world. At one time exalted and recognized as the highest culture of the world, by Africans, Europeans, Asiatics, Hindus, Buddhists and other cultures of the ancient world, in time it was shunned by the emerging orthodox world religions. Its temples desecrated, its philosophy maligned, its tradition spurned, its philosophy dormant in the mystical *Medu Neter,* the mysterious hieroglyphic texts which hold the secret symbolic meaning that has scarcely been discerned up to now. What are the secrets of *Nehast* {spiritual awakening and emancipation, resurrection}. More than just a literal translation, this volume is for awakening to the secret code *Shetitu* of the teaching which was not deciphered by Egyptologists, nor could be understood by ordinary spiritualists. This book is a reinstatement of the original science made available for our times, to the reincarnated followers of Ancient Egyptian culture and the prospect of spiritual freedom to break the bonds of *Khemn,* "ignorance," and slavery to evil forces: *Såaa* .

30.   EGYPTIAN MYSTERIES VOL 2: Dictionary of Gods and Goddesses ISBN: 1-884564-23-2 $21.95 This book is about the mystery of neteru, the gods and goddesses of Ancient Egypt (Kamit, Kemet). Neteru means "Gods and Goddesses." But the Neterian teaching of Neteru represents more than the usual limited modern day concept of "divinities" or "spirits." The Neteru of Kamit are also metaphors, cosmic principles and vehicles for the enlightening teachings of Shetaut Neter (Ancient Egyptian-African Religion). Actually they are the elements for one of the most advanced systems of spirituality ever conceived in human history. Understanding the concept of neteru provides a firm basis for spiritual evolution and the pathway for viable culture, peace on earth and a healthy human society.   Why is it important to have gods and goddesses in our lives? In order for spiritual evolution to be possible, once a human being has accepted that there is existence after death and there is a transcendental being who exists beyond time and space knowledge, human beings need a connection to that which transcends the ordinary experience of human life in time and space and a means to understand the transcendental reality beyond the mundane reality.

31.   EGYPTIAN MYSTERIES VOL. 3 The Priests and Priestesses of Ancient Egypt ISBN: 1-884564-53-4 $22.95 This volume details the path of Neterian priesthood, the joys, challenges and rewards of advanced Neterian life, the teachings that allowed the priests and priestesses to manage the most long lived civilization in human history and how that path can be adopted today; for those who want to tread the path of the Clergy of Shetaut Neter.

32. THE KING OF EGYPT: The Struggle of Good and Evil for Control of the World and The Human Soul ISBN 1-8840564-44-5 $18.95 This volume contains a novelized version of the Asarian Resurrection myth that is based on the actual scriptures presented in the Book Asarian Religion (old name –Resurrecting Osiris). This volume is prepared in the form of a screenplay and can be easily adapted to be used as a stage play. Spiritual seeking is a mythic journey that has many emotional highs and lows, ecstasies and depressions, victories and frustrations. This is the War of Life that is played out in the myth as the struggle of Heru and Set and those are mythic characters that represent the human Higher and Lower self. How to understand the war and emerge victorious in the journey o life? The ultimate victory and fulfillment can be experienced, which is not changeable or lost in time. The purpose of myth is to convey the wisdom of life through the story of divinities who show the way to overcome the challenges and foibles of life. In this volume the feelings and emotions of the characters of the myth have been highlighted to show the deeply rich texture of the Ancient Egyptian myth. This myth contains deep spiritual teachings and insights into the nature of self, of God and the mysteries of life and the means to discover the true meaning of life and thereby achieve the true purpose of life. To become victorious in the battle of life means to become the King (or Queen) of Egypt.Have you seen movies like The Lion King, Hamlet, The Odyssey, or The Little Buddha? These have been some of the most popular movies in modern times. The Sema Institute of Yoga is dedicated to researching and presenting the wisdom and culture of ancient Africa. The Script is designed to be produced as a motion picture but may be addapted for the theater as well. $19.95 copyright 1998 By Dr. Muata Ashby

33. FROM EGYPT TO GREECE: The Kamitan Origins of Greek Culture and Religion ISBN: 1-884564-47-X $22.95 U.S. FROM EGYPT TO GREECE This insightful manual is a quick reference to Ancient Egyptian mythology and philosophy and its correlation to what later became known as Greek and Rome mythology and philosophy. It outlines the basic tenets of the mythologies and shoes the ancient origins of Greek culture in Ancient Egypt. This volume also acts as a resource for Colleges students who would like to set up fraternities and sororities based on the original Ancient Egyptian principles of Sheti and Maat philosophy. ISBN: 1-884564-47-X $22.95 U.S.

34. THE FORTY TWO PRECEPTS OF MAAT, THE PHILOSOPHY OF RIGHTEOUS ACTION AND THE ANCIENT EGYPTIAN WISDOM TEXTS ADVANCED STUDIES This manual is designed for use with the 1998 Maat Philosophy Class conducted by Dr. Muata Ashby. This is a detailed study of Maat Philosophy. It contains a compilation of the 42 laws or precepts of Maat and the corresponding principles which they represent along with the teachings of the ancient Egyptian Sages relating to each. Maat philosophy was the basis of Ancient Egyptian society and government as well as the heart of Ancient Egyptian myth and spirituality. Maat is at once a goddess, a cosmic force and a living social doctrine, which promotes social harmony and thereby paves the way for spiritual evolution in all levels of society. ISBN: 1-884564-48-8 $16.95 U.S.

MUSIC BASED ON THE PRT M HRU AND OTHER KEMETIC TEXTS

Available on Compact Disc $14.99 and Audio Cassette $9.99

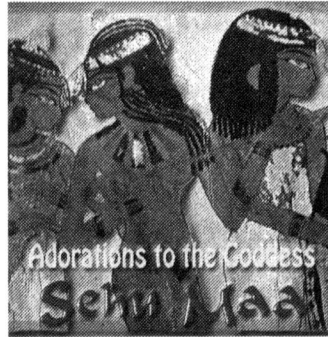

Adorations to the Goddess

Music for Worship of the Goddess

NEW Egyptian Yoga Music CD
by Sehu Maa
Ancient Egyptian Music CD
Instrumental Music played on reproductions of Ancient Egyptian Instruments– Ideal for <u>meditation</u> and reflection on the Divine and for the practice of spiritual programs and <u>Yoga exercise sessions.</u>

©1999 By Muata Ashby
CD $14.99 –

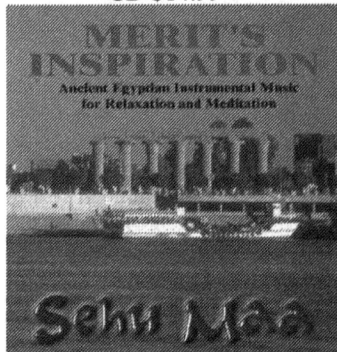

MERIT'S INSPIRATION
NEW Egyptian Yoga Music CD
by Sehu Maa
Ancient Egyptian Music CD
Instrumental Music played on
reproductions of Ancient Egyptian Instruments– Ideal for <u>meditation</u> and
reflection on the Divine and for the practice of spiritual programs and <u>Yoga exercise sessions.</u>
©1999 By
Muata Ashby
CD $14.99 –
UPC# 761527100429

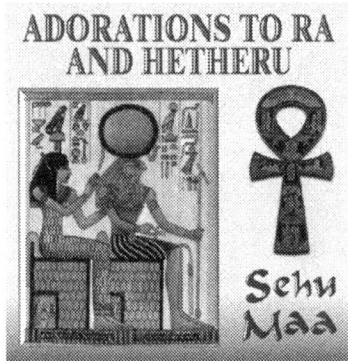

ANORATIONS TO RA AND HETHERU
NEW Egyptian Yoga Music CD
By Sehu Maa (Muata Ashby)
Based on the Words of Power of Ra and HetHeru
played on reproductions of Ancient Egyptian Instruments **Ancient Egyptian Instruments used: Voice, Clapping, Nefer Lute, Tar Drum, Sistrums, Cymbals** – The Chants, Devotions, Rhythms and Festive Songs Of the Neteru – Ideal for meditation, and devotional singing and dancing.

©1999 By Muata Ashby
CD $14.99 –
UPC# 761527100221

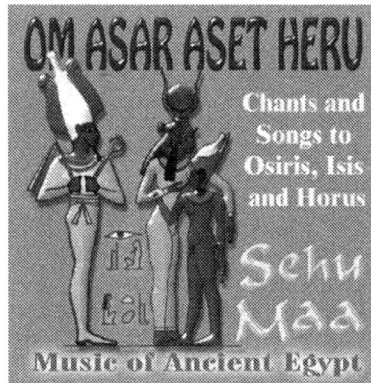

SONGS TO ASAR ASET AND HERU
NEW
Egyptian Yoga Music CD
By Sehu Maa
played on reproductions of Ancient Egyptian Instruments– The Chants, Devotions, Rhythms and Festive Songs Of the Neteru - Ideal for meditation, and devotional singing and dancing.
Based on the Words of Power of Asar (Asar), Aset (Aset) and Heru (Heru) Om Asar Aset Heru is the third in a series of musical explorations of the Kemetic (Ancient Egyptian) tradition of music. Its ideas are based on the Ancient Egyptian Religion of Asar, Aset and Heru and it is designed for listening, meditation and worship. ©1999 By Muata Ashby

CD $14.99 –
UPC# 761527100122

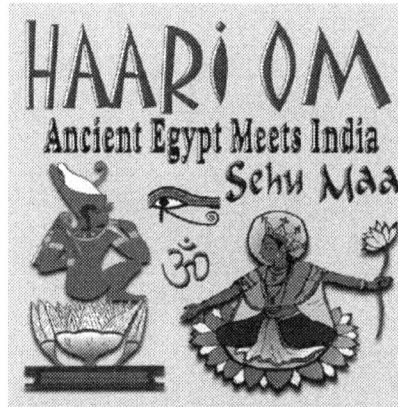

HAARI OM: ANCIENT EGYPT MEETS INDIA IN MUSIC
NEW Music CD
By Sehu Maa

The Chants, Devotions, Rhythms and
Festive Songs Of the Ancient Egypt and India, harmonized and played on reproductions of ancient instruments along with modern instruments and beats. Ideal for meditation, and devotional singing and dancing.
Haari Om is the fourth in a series of musical explorations of the Kemetic (Ancient Egyptian) and Indian traditions of music, chanting and devotional spiritual practice. Its ideas are based on the Ancient Egyptian Yoga spirituality and Indian Yoga spirituality.

©1999 By Muata Ashby
CD $14.99 –
UPC# 761527100528

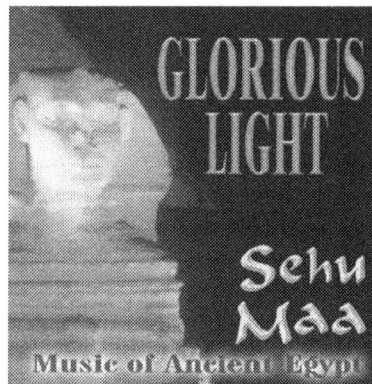

RA AKHU: THE GLORIOUS LIGHT
NEW
Egyptian Yoga Music CD
By Sehu Maa
The fifth collection of original music compositions based on the Teachings and Words of The Trinity, the God Asar and the Goddess Nebethet, the Divinity Aten, the God Heru, and the Special Meditation Hekau or Words of Power of Ra from the Ancient Egyptian Tomb of Seti I and more...
played on reproductions of Ancient Egyptian Instruments and modern instruments - **Ancient Egyptian Instruments used: Voice, Clapping, Nefer Lute, Tar Drum, Sistrums, Cymbals**
– The Chants, Devotions, Rhythms and Festive Songs Of the Neteru – Ideal for meditation, and devotional singing and dancing.
©1999 By Muata Ashby
CD $14.99 –
UPC# 761527100825

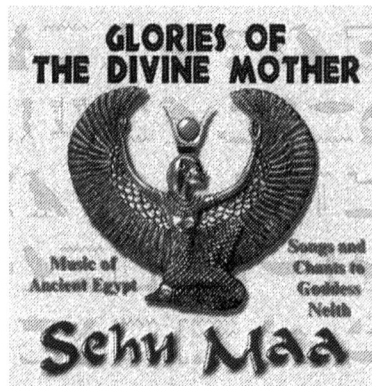

GLORIES OF THE DIVINE MOTHER
Based on the hieroglyphic text of the worship of Goddess Net.
The Glories of The Great Mother
©2000 Muata Ashby
CD $14.99 UPC# 761527101129`

Order Form

Telephone orders: Call Toll Free: 1(305) 378-6253. Have your AMEX, Optima, Visa or MasterCard ready.

    Fax orders: 1-(305) 378-6253   E-MAIL ADDRESS: Semayoga@aol.com

Postal Orders: Sema Institute of Yoga, P.O. Box 570459, Miami, Fl. 33257. USA.

               Please send the following books and / or tapes.

ITEM

_____Cost $_____

_____Cost $_____

_____Cost $_____

_____Cost $_____

_____Cost $_____

                    Total $_____

Name:_____

Physical Address:_____

City:_____ State:_____ Zip:_____

Sales tax: Please add 6.5% for books shipped to Florida addresses

_____Shipping: $6.50 for first book and .50¢ for each additional

_____Shipping: Outside US $5.00 for first book and $3.00 for each additional

_____Payment:_____

_____Check -Include Driver License #:

       _____

_____Credit card: _____ Visa, _____ MasterCard, _____ Optima,
      _____ AMEX.

Card number:_____

Name on card:_____ Exp. date:_____ / _____

Copyright 1995-2005 Dr. R. Muata Abhaya Ashby
Sema Institute of Yoga
P.O.Box 570459, Miami, Florida, 33257
(305) 378-6253 Fax: (305) 378-6253

www.ingramcontent.com/pod-product-compliance
Lightning Source LLC
Chambersburg PA
CBHW080245030426

42334CB00023BA/2707